Cooking with yogurt

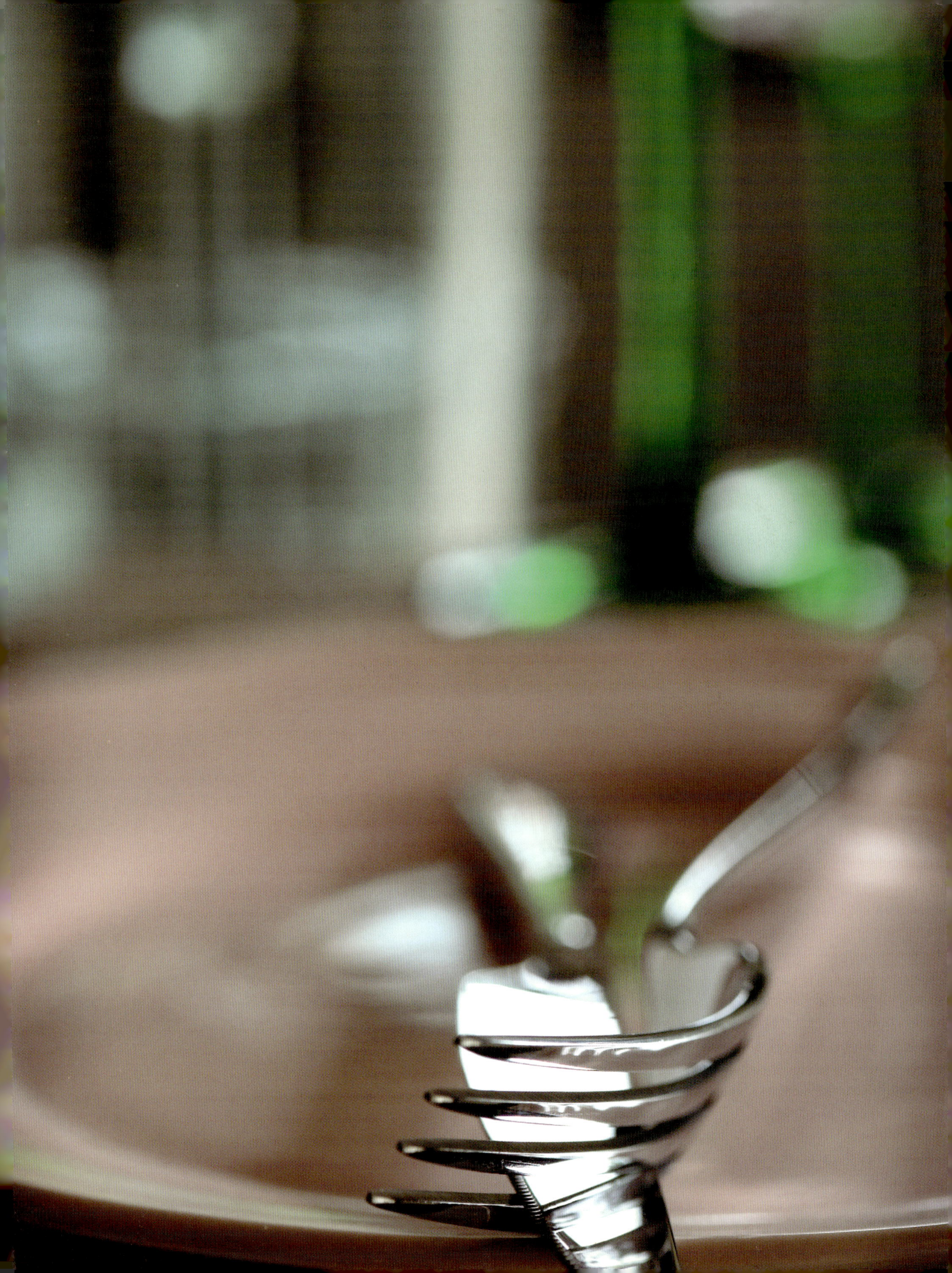

Cooking with yogurt

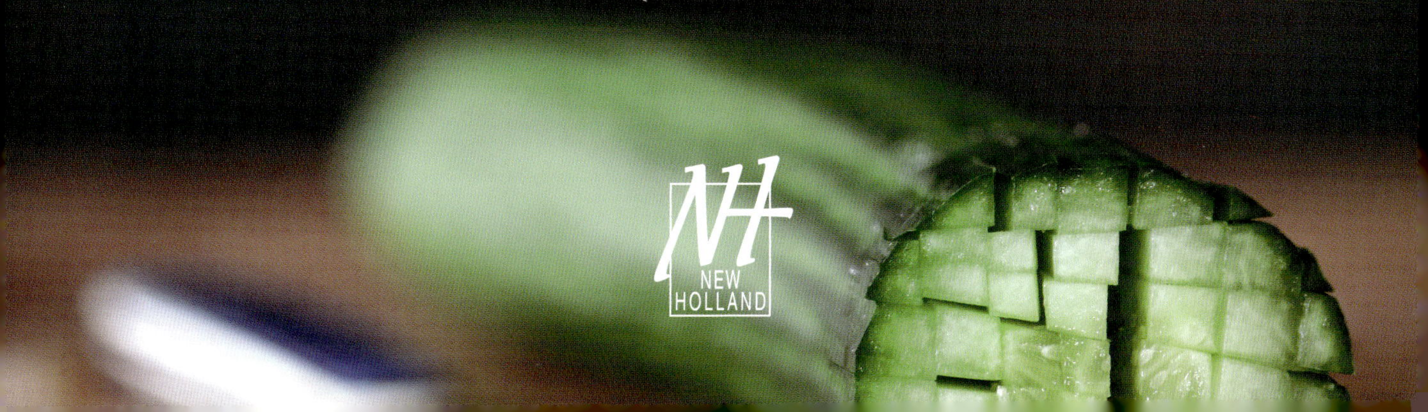

NEW HOLLAND

First published in 2015 by New Holland Publishers Pty Ltd
London • Sydney • Auckland

The Chandlery Unit 009 50 Westminster Bridge Road London SE1 7QY United Kingdom
1/66 Gibbes Street Chatswood NSW 2067 Australia
5/39 Woodside Ave Northcote, Auckland 0627 New Zealand

www.newhollandpublishers.com

A record of this book is held at the British Library and the National Library of Australia.

ISBN 9781742577401

Managing Director: Fiona Schultz
Publisher: Alan Whiticker
Project Editor: Holly Willsher
Cover Designer: Peter Guo
Production Director: Olga Dementiev
Printer: Toppan Leefung Printing Limited

10 9 8 7 6 5 4 3 2 1

Keep up with New Holland Publishers on Facebook
www.facebook.com/NewHollandPublishers

Acknowledgments

I feel like it was only yesterday when I cooked my first scrambled eggs and I had my first camera in my hands. Did I ever expect that I would be here now, finishing my first cookbook? I am grateful to all of the amazing people who have helped me over the years to perfect my cooking, create beautiful images and grow to become a good person. A big thank you to all of you, I will never forget all the support have given me.

I am extremely lucky to be surrounded by experienced and friendly professionals in my career and an incredibly supportive family. I will never forget my first steps into the kitchen with my grandfather Peter and my mother Dora. Also I will never forget the photographers Valia Chrankina, Jimmy Wormser and Alan King who opened the door of the professional photography for me.

Once again a big thank you to my friends Susanna Tee and Sian Riley for your enormous professional help and support during the creation of my book.

And last but not least I would like to say thank you to all the crew at New Holland Publishers who trust me to publish my first cookbook, especially to Fiona Schultz and Alan Whiticker.

This book is dedicated to my family, to my daughter Amelie and my wife Tsveta, to my sons Peter and Hristo.

Introduction

Yogurt for breakfast, yogurt for lunch, yogurt for dinner! I remember as a child at home, my parents bringing yogurt to the table with every meal. Even when I was ill and not feeling very well, my mother would say, "Don't eat anything, just have some yogurt." I remember those words so well and yogurt for me is not just a food, it is a guardian of good health. It helps when you need to recover your energy, something you can enjoy when you are hungry or thirsty. Yogurt is good for everybody young or old, busy exercising or relaxing and recovering.

What exactly is yogurt? A dairy, thick, creamy and sour product made mainly from cow milk using the good Lactobacillus bulgaricus and Streptococcus thermophilus bacteria. The process of preparation involves heating the milk first to kill the bad bacteria present in the milk and help the fermentation. The essential role of the lactic acid bacteria is to convert the lactose in the milk into lactic acid, which increases the acidity and helps to preserve the milk for longer. Although cow milk is most commonly used, there are also sheep, goat and buffalo yogurt and some more exotic like camel yogurt which I have never tried.

Yogurt – how to make it? I would say the best yogurt is a homemade yogurt. You will find a recipe in my book. The market is full of so many brands and styles of yogurt. Natural, low fat, sweetened, fruit flavored or even frozen yogurt. To choose the right product for your needs, my suggestion is to read the label and the nutrition info. All yogurts should contain live bacteria unless they are heat treated after fermentation (to prolong shelf life) and this should be clearly stated on the label. The important suggestion I can make is that the good natural yogurt has to be slightly sour and has short durability. Here, less is more: less durability of the product more quality natural yogurt.

There is not a lot of historical evidence about the origin of yogurt. It probably all happened unintentionally as most things do. What we know is that in 1905, in a microbiology laboratory in Geneva, Stamen Grigorov, a Bulgarian medical student, first examined the microflora of the yogurt and discovered a certain strain of lactic acid bacteria which was essential for the creation of yogurt and which he named Bacillus Bulgaricus. Later on, the Russian biologist Élie Metchnikoff, director of the institute Pasteur in Paris and a Nobel laureate, developed a theory that the toxic bacteria in the gut cause ageing and that lactic acid could prolong life. He believed that Lactobacillicus is essential for healthy living and thought that a regular consumption of yogurt was responsible for the long lifespans of peasants living in Balkan Peninsula, especially Bulgaria. Also according the Persian scripts 'Abraham owed his fertility and longevity to the regular ingestion of yogurt'.

Regarding the health benefit of eating yogurt, I'd rather leave that part to the professional dietitian Sian Riley who has written a chapter on it. She was also so kind to make the nutrition calculation for all the recipes in this book.

How did I combine the photography with the food? I was born in a small town close to river Danube and healthy good food was part of the local lifestyle. My grandfather and his brothers were in the restaurant business and as a child, I spent a lot of time around the professional kitchens which made me grow up with respect for quality cuisine. All this reflects in the way I relate to food, the way I choose and cook recipes, the way I style and shoot my food images.

For me, cooking is part of my culture. Having good food is a social tool that brings different people together around the table. I started my professional photography carrier more than thirty years ago, but I discovered my talent for cooking after I moved to the UK and specialized in still life and food photography. Being surrounded by food all day in my studio, creating my images step by step, I experimented and gradually discovered good quality ingredients.

I always add love to the plate I prepare. Regardless if I prepare food for an advertising picture or just a dinner for my kids, cooking is always a pleasure for me; an expression of happiness.

The idea for this book appeared spontaneously. I wanted to share my collection of recipes with healthy food lovers around the world. Simple combinations of the smartest food I know - the yogurt - and well-chosen ingredients, together with precisely chosen spices will satisfy the most fastidious taste. In this book I present to you ideas of how to add yogurt to your every day diet and make it even more exciting. I have replaced products like cream, mayonnaise, cream cheese and buttermilk with low fat yogurt. You can find 170 of my favorite recipes using yogurt in this book. The recipes are sourced from my family, friends and some are simply my creations. Most recipes contain yogurt as part of the ingredients and others use yogurt as a final touch to finish the symphony of flavor of well-prepared good food.

Along with the delicious taste, I hope you will enjoy the styling and photography I have done for all the food. Working in food photography I can tell you, the presentation of the food is most important. I am not a fan of the saying 'looks awful tastes great'. You have to enjoy the food on the plate. Sight is first and then is the scent and taste. I do work mostly with natural light in my kitchen studio and shooting yogurt that way gives me the chance to emphasize its natural creamy structure and the richness of colors and texture of the food. In my photography I always try to tell a story. I try to bring the food out of the picture. Some people think the food photographers never eat anything on set, but I will tell you one secret. All the recipes on this book are cooked, styled and photographed by myself and have passed home and friend critics. Most of these recipes are part of my every day family menu. I am really lucky to be surrounded by people who share and indeed support my passion for food.

The food has to deliver positive emotions. You have to enjoy your food, and nowadays people are so much more careful with what they eat. So many experts tell you not to eat this or drink that. My book is the opposite, it positively encourages eating good food by using yogurt, always more vegetables, less meat and just a pinch of salt!

I am sure you will love this book. The recipes are simple, the ingredients are easy to get, and everybody can cook them! Also, I hope this book will give to the pro healthy-food lovers an inspiration to experiment with different ingredients and create amazing tasty new recipes using yogurt.

Now, my suggestion is whatever you eat just have a spoonful of yogurt every day and that will give you healthier life and maybe longevity!

Food and art never end!
ilian

Contents

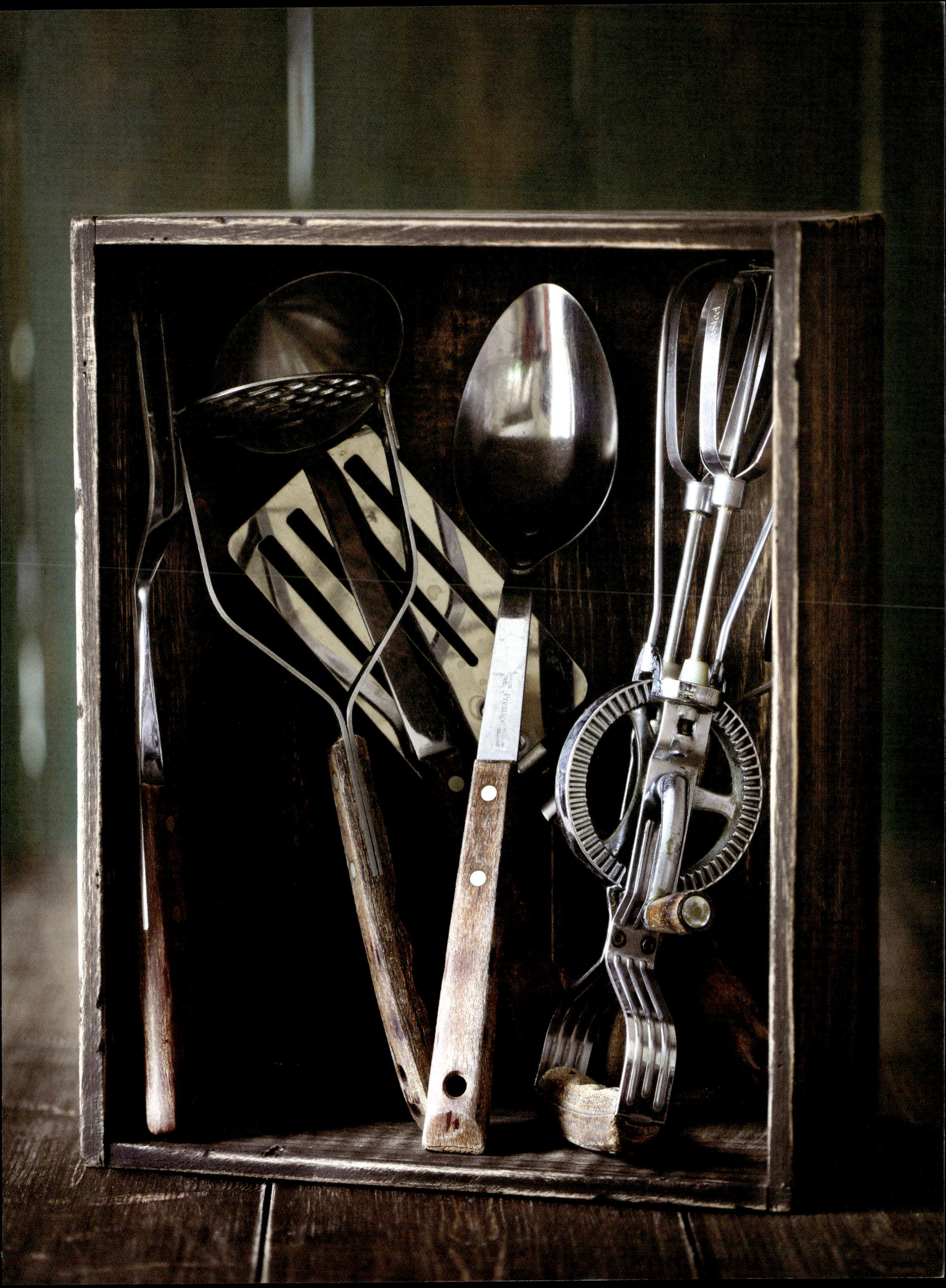

Ilian's recipes in this book are inspiring and creative, using a range of nutritional ingredients blended together to complement their flavors and textures. His Bulgarian roots and authentic culinary training ooze through his recipes, providing you with accessible dishes that bring mouth-watering results to adorn your dining table.

Nutritionally, Ilian's recipes include many wholesome and healthy ingredients such as eggs, nuts, garlic and oats. His use of a variety of fruits and vegetables creates a visually stunning masterpiece to our eyes, as well as their many nutritional qualities. As a dietitian, it has been a real pleasure digging deeper into the nutrition of Ilian's recipes, particularly due to his use of yogurt as a foundation for these creations, further enhancing the goodness of his dishes. Eaten for hundreds of years, yogurt has been a staple food for many of our European and worldwide neighbours, who have long recognised yogurt's culinary versatility as well as its health benefits. As part of a healthy balanced diet, yogurt can provide you with this nutritional goodness to benefit your health. Here is a taster of some of yogurt's nutritional qualities:

- Yogurt can be used to replace other high fat ingredients in recipes. Adding a creamy taste, without the extra calories and saturated fat. Great news for our waist line and our hearts.
- Yogurt contains high quality proteins that are used by our bodies to maintain muscle mass. This is important as we age, and a necessity in optimum sports performance. The protein in yogurt has also been shown to promote satiety, encourage weight maintenance and control our blood sugar levels. All good news for our general health.
- Yogurt provides our bodies with the full set of essential and non-essential amino acids and is rich in branched chained essential amino acids, such as Leucine, Isoleucine and Valine. These branched chained amino acids are vital for muscle growth and repair. Furthermore, the natural fermentation process of yogurt increases the concentration of the non-essential amino acids, Proline and Glycine, aiding immune function and nutrient absorption.
- Yogurt helps to balance out our good and bad bacteria. With over a hundred trillion bacteria in our gut, live bacteria in yogurt plays an important role in maintaining this balance and may also play a role in improving digestive function in people with gut problems such as Irritable Bowel Syndrome.
- Yogurt contains a number of nutrients required for the growth and maintenance of our bones – protein, phosphorus, magnesium and, of course, calcium. Yogurt, when included in a healthy balanced diet, helps to provide a good portion of our requirements for these nutrients.
- Yogurt is a good source of potassium, which is required by our bodies for normal muscle and nerve function, and essential for optimal blood pressure control.
- Yogurt provides our bodies with numerous vitamins and minerals, including: iodine, vitamin B1, vitamin B2, and vitamin B12, all important for bones, as well as our general health.

As Ilian shows, yogurt can be made at home by the fermentation of milk with harmless bacteria, or it can be purchased from the wide range of natural yogurts available on our supermarket shelves. The nutritional calculations in this book have been carried out using your 'average' yogurt, however, if purchasing yogurt, closer scrutiny of the labels will help you to adjust the nutritional content of your culinary masterpieces. For example, lower fat yogurt provides a greater reduced-calorie alternative. Or why not try strained yogurt? With a rich creamy taste and fabulous protein content, it will complement your hard work in the kitchen.

What is my favourite recipe from this book? As a mother and a dietitian, it has to be the Roasted Peppers Dip. Not only because of my love of the humble red pepper(!), but also because I appreciate Ilian's adventurous use of yogurt in this savoury dish, utilizing its natural fermented bacterial content. This recipe provides a tasty and nutritious snack or starter that the whole family can make and enjoy. Embrace the nutritional qualities of the recipes in this book and enjoy creating and eating your culinary masterpieces, whilst discovering a healthful and accessible method of cooking and dining.

Disclaimer

Food isn't simply a list of ingredients, but a unique combination of nutrients and flavors that vary and develop, depending on their growing, storage and cooking conditions. The nutritional calculations provided with these recipes are to be used as a guide to the nutrition within. These figures are not an exact science and will vary each and every time the meal is prepared and cooked. Paying close attention to, and comparing food labels, is a great way to optimise the nutrition of your own culinary creations. As a dietitian, I have to say, "Go easy on the salt - one man's pinch is another man's handful!" and always measure out high energy foods such as oil, butter, sugar and syrup. And after all that is done - please do ENJOY! It's what cooking and food is all about!

Sian Riley MSc Registered Dietitian

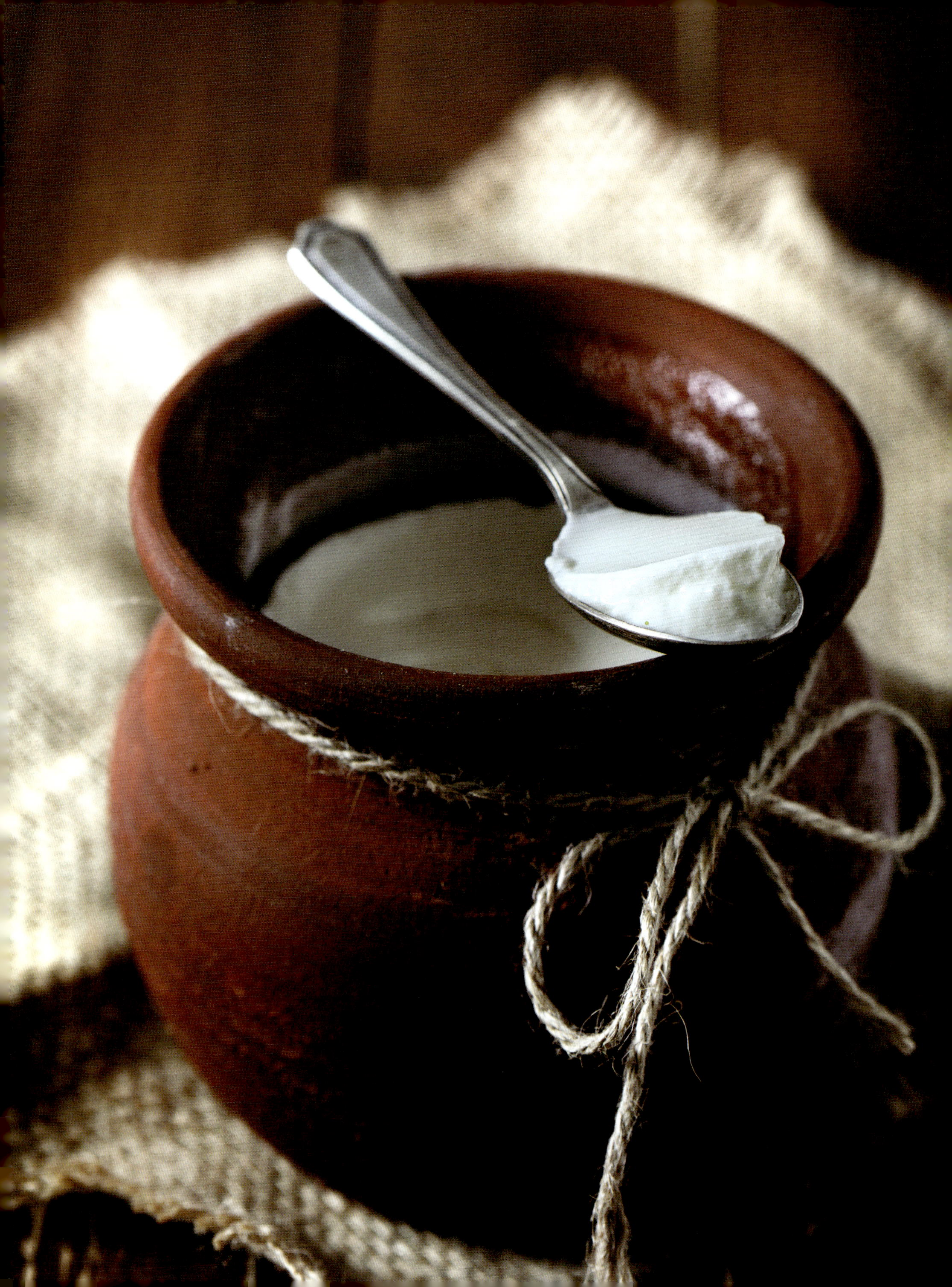

Homemade Yogurt

Homemade Yogurt

1 litre (1¾ pints) whole cow's milk
4 tablespoons plain whole milk yogurt with live and active culture

First sterilize a small, non-metallic, heatproof pot or two jars by pouring in boiling water and leaving for 2-3 minutes, then drain and set aside to dry.
Pour the milk into a medium saucepan and cook over the high heat, stirring well. Use a thermometer, if you have one. Heat the milk until it reaches 82°C (180°F) or just before it boils and then remove from the heat. Leave it to cool to about 45°C (115°F) or the temperature of the milk is okay to be touched with a finger for few seconds. Add the yogurt and stir well. Pour the mixture into the sterilized jars and cover it with a clean tea towel. Leave it to rest and ferment in a warm place for about 6 hours or overnight.
Then put it in the refrigerator and chill the yogurt thoroughly for about 3 hours or longer. That's it! Now you have your own home-made yogurt. If you use a clay pot to store the yogurt, on the second day in the refrigerator the yogurt will become really thick like a strained yogurt because the pot will have absorbed all the excess moisture.

Makes 800 g (28 oz)

632 kcal, 24 g fat (15.3g saturated), 45.6 g protein, 62.4 g carbs (62.4 g sugar), 0.0 g fibre, 1.6 g salt

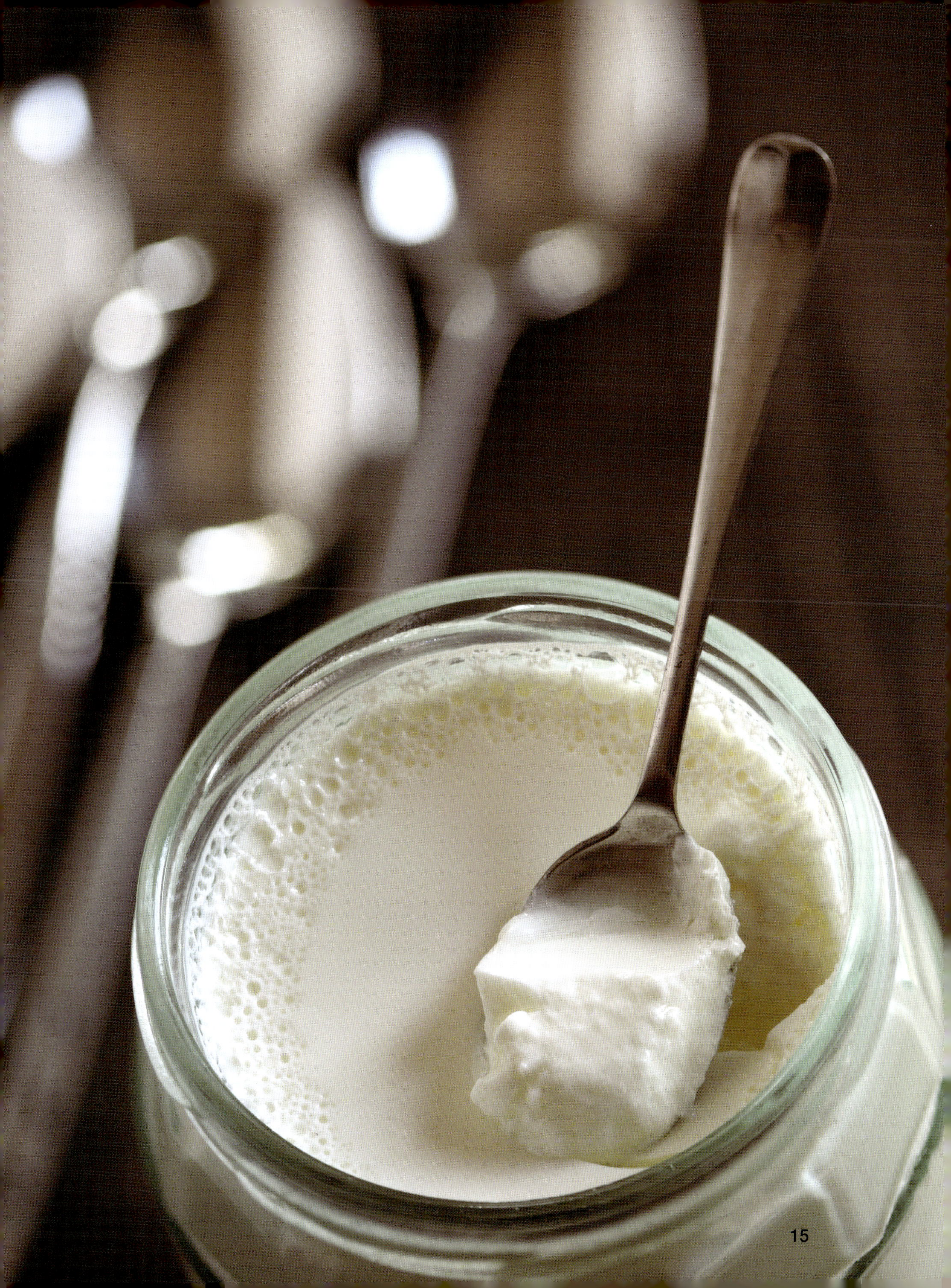

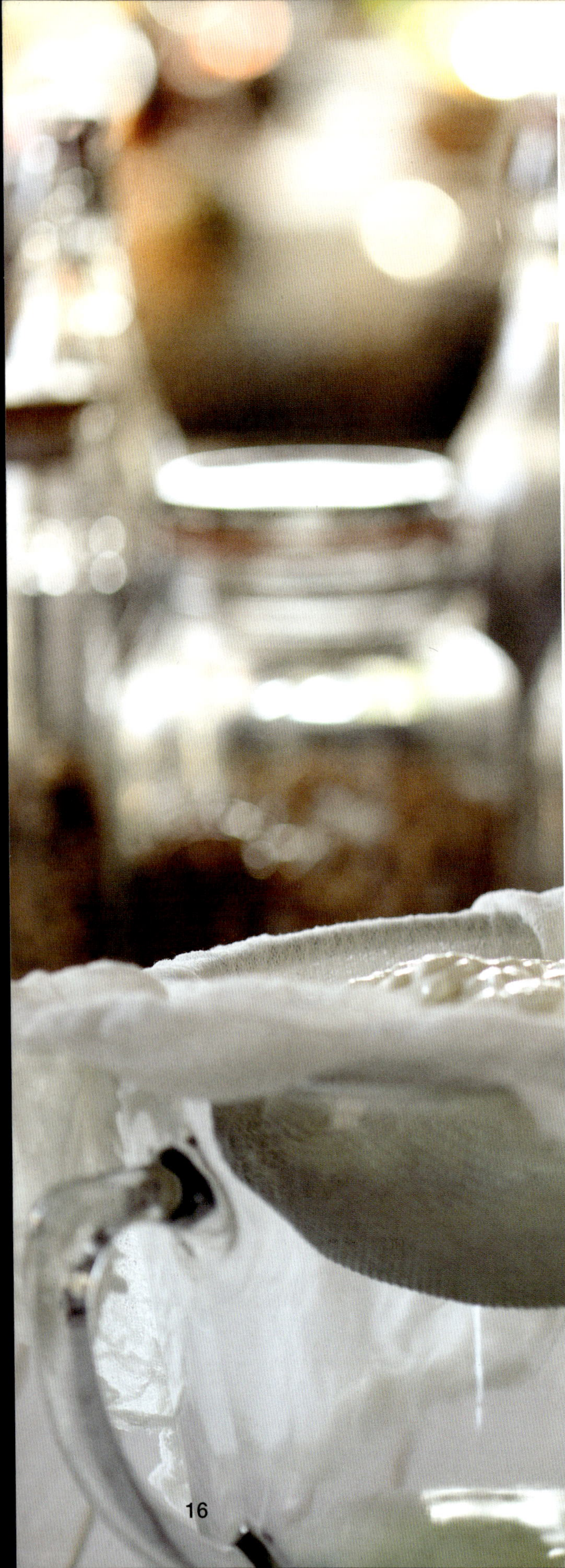

Strained Yogurt

1 kg (2.2 lb) plain whole yogurt

To make a strained yogurt you need some simple kitchen equipment.

Medium bowl big enough to put a colander or large cooking strainer inside.
80/80 cm (31/31 inches) Muslin or any knit fabric will work, even a coffee filter.

Put the large cooking strainer over the bowl and line the strainer with the muslin making four layers. Then pour the yogurt over the muslin. Do not squeeze or stir just let it rest inside the muslin. The bowl will collect the excess liquid. Cover the yogurt with the ends of the muslin and place the bowl in the refrigerator to rest. After about 30 minutes check it to make sure the liquid that is dripping is slightly milky but not too white. If the liquid is dripping white that means you are losing yogurt together with the liquid and need to add a few more layers. The yogurt is normally strained for about 6 hours but the longer you strain the thicker it gets.

700 g (24½ oz) strained yogurt

Per 100 g (3½ oz)
118k cal, 5 g fat (3 g saturated), 9 g protein, 10 g carbs (10 g sugar), 0.0 g fibre, 0.2 g salt

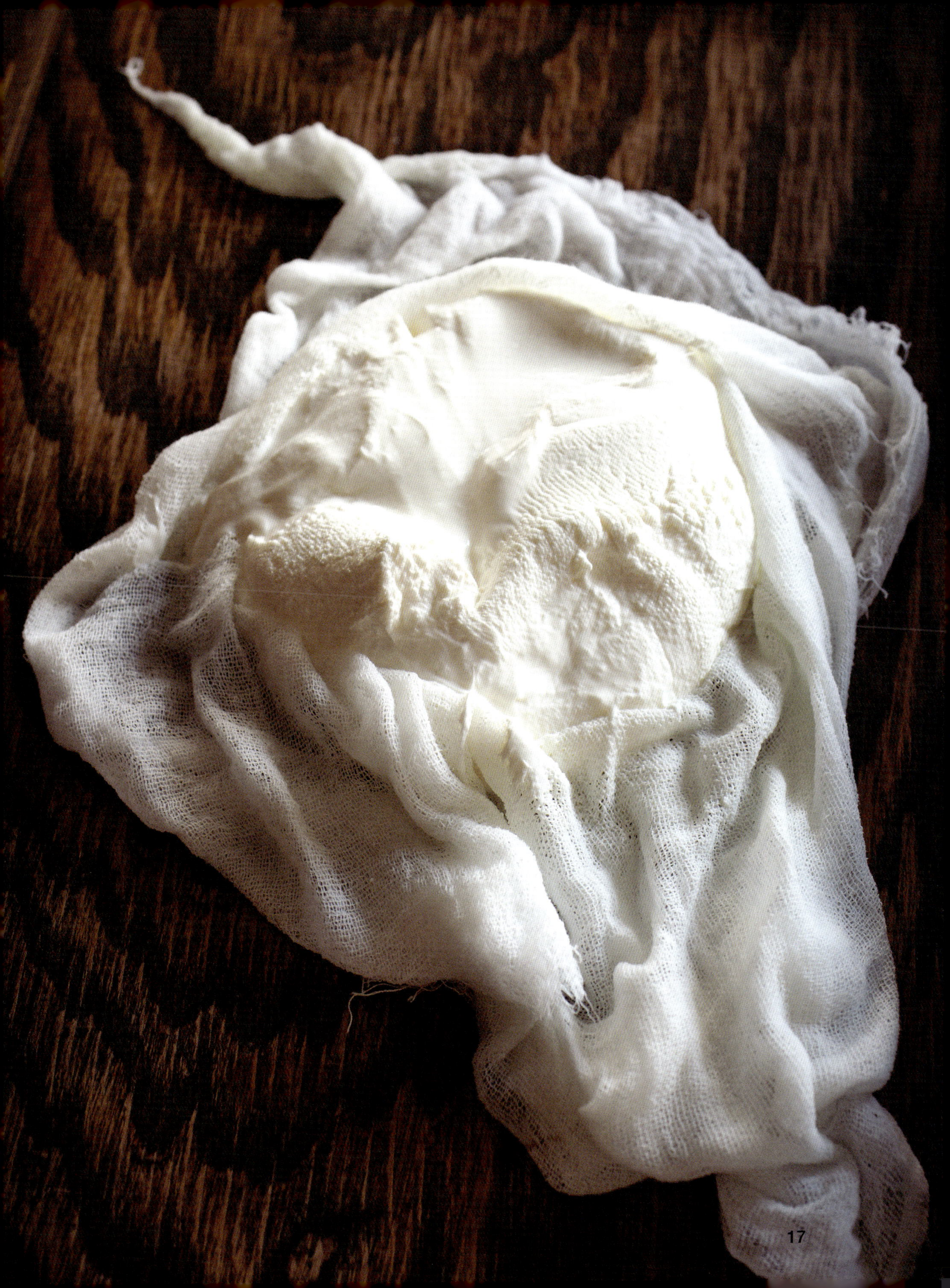

Snow White Yogurt

400 ml (13½ fl oz) buffalo whole milk
800 ml (27 fl oz) cow whole milk
4 tablespoons plain whole yogurt with live and active culture
3 tablespoons sugar

If you struggle to find buffalo whole milk, you can swap with goat whole milk, slightly different but still tastes great!

First sterilize small non-metal cups, heatproof glasses or small jars by pouring boiling water into them, leave for a couple of minutes, then drain, let them dry well and set aside.
Pour the buffalo whole milk and the cow whole milk into a medium saucepan and cook stirring well over high heat. Use a thermometer, if you have one. Heat the milk until it reaches 82°C (180°F) or just before boiling and remove from the heat. Leave it to cool to 45°C (115°F) or temperature is okay to touch with a finger for few seconds. Add the sugar and the plain whole yogurt with live and active culture and stir well. Then pour the mixture into the sterilized cups and cover with clean kitchen towel. Leave it to rest and ferment in a slightly warm place for about 6 hours or overnight. Then put it into the refrigerator to chill thoroughly for about 3 hours. Serve for breakfast or as a dessert together with some fresh berries.

Serves 6
Per serving
192 kcal, 8.6 g fat (5.5 g saturated), 8.1 g protein, 21.6 g carbs (21.6 g sugar), 0.0 g fibre, 0.3 g salt

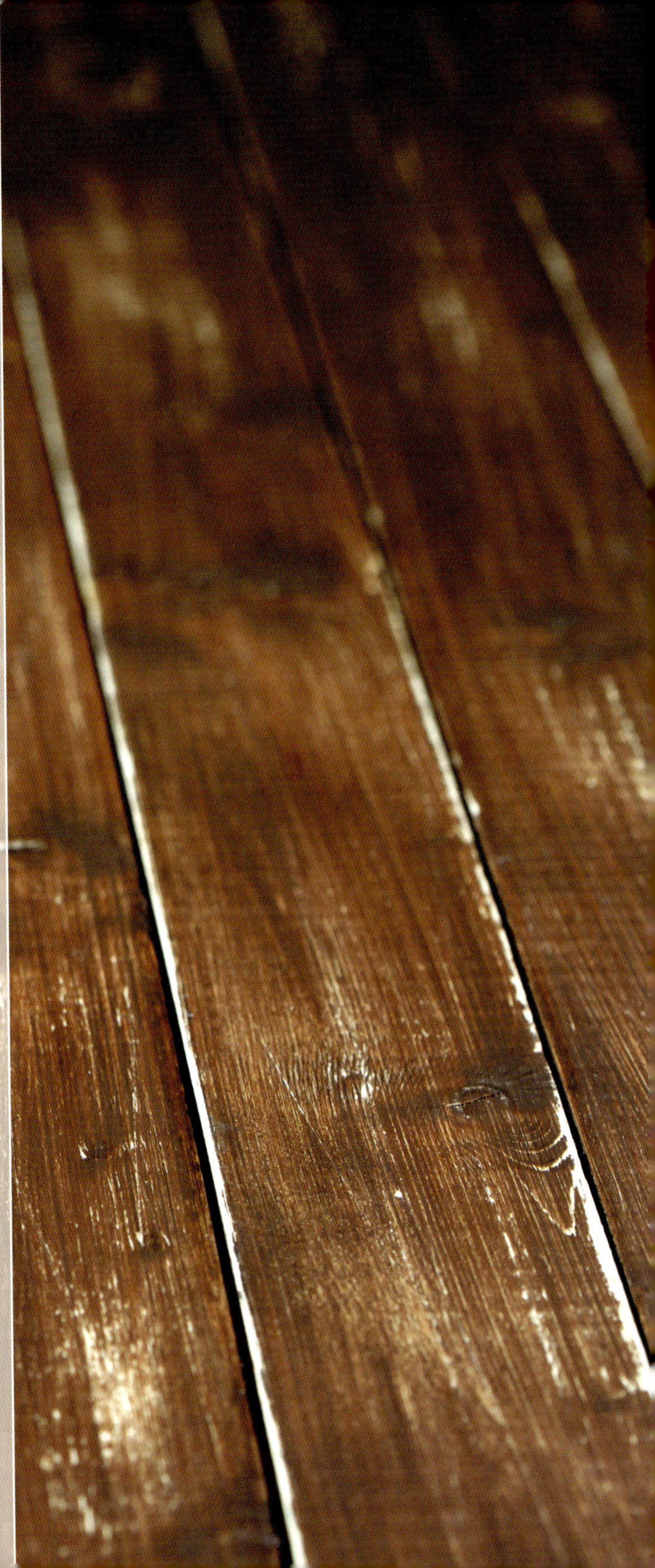

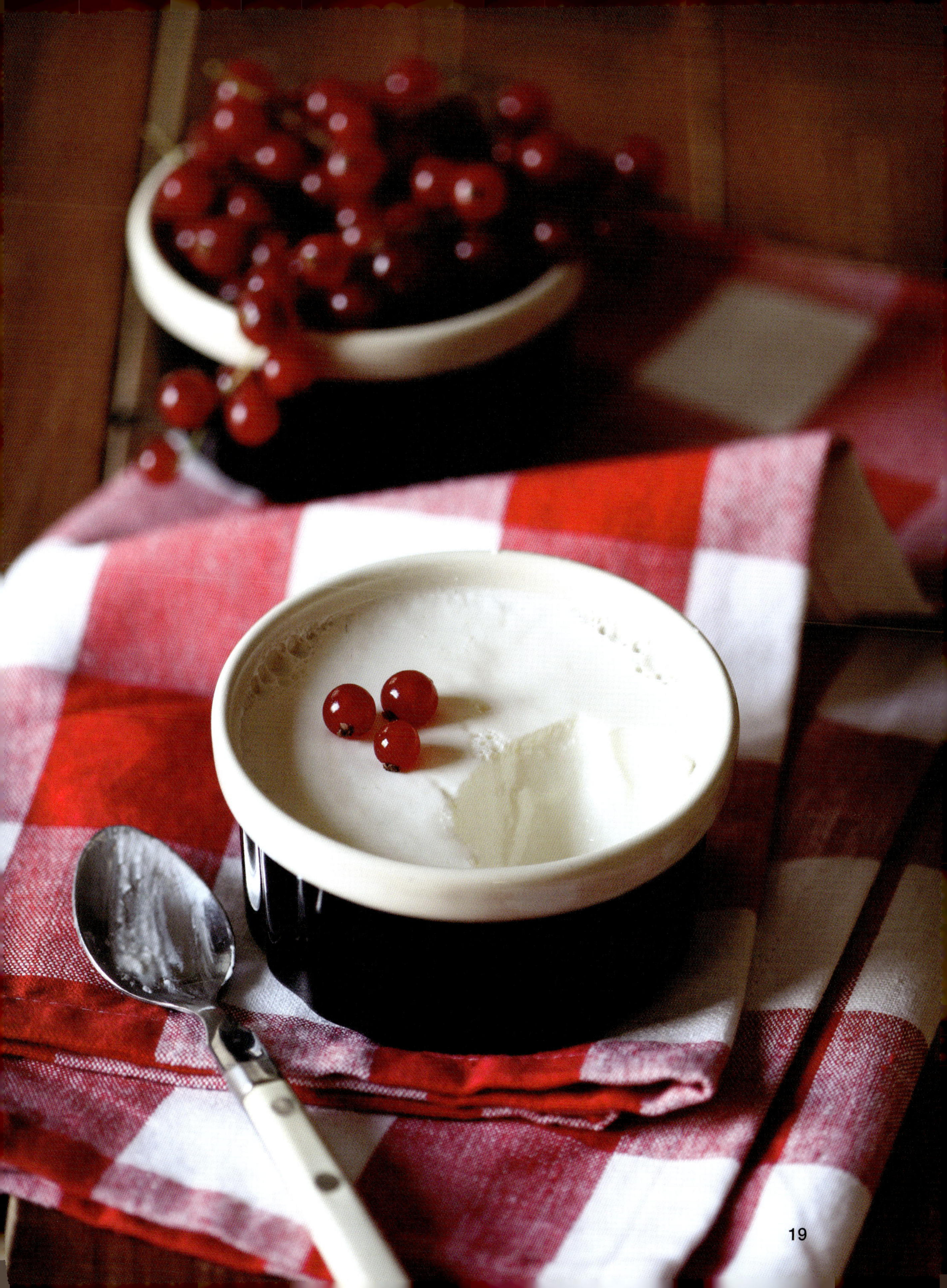

Coconut Goat Yogurt

1 litre (1¾ pints) goat whole milk
5 tablespoons plain whole yogurt with live and active culture
3 tablespoons coconut, desiccated

First sterilize small non-metal cups, heatproof glasses or small jars by pouring boiling water into them, leave for a couple of minutes, then drain, let them dry well and set aside.
Into a medium saucepan pour the goat whole milk and cook stirring well, over a high heat. It is useful to have a thermometer. Heat the milk until it reaches 82°C (180°F) or just before it boils then remove from the heat. Leave it to cool to 45°C (115°F) or temperature is okay to touch with a finger for few seconds. Add the desiccated coconut and the plain whole yogurt with live and active culture and stir well. Then pour the mixture into the sterilized cups and cover them with clean kitchen towel. Leave them to rest and ferment in a slightly warm place for about 6 hours or overnight. Then put in the refrigerator to chill the yogurt thoroughly for about 3 hours. Serve for breakfast or as a dessert together with some biscuits.

Serves 6

Per serving
160 kcal, 10.3 g fat (7.3 g saturated), 7.3 g protein, 10.3 g carbs (10.3 g sugar), 0.9 g fibre, 0.2 g salt

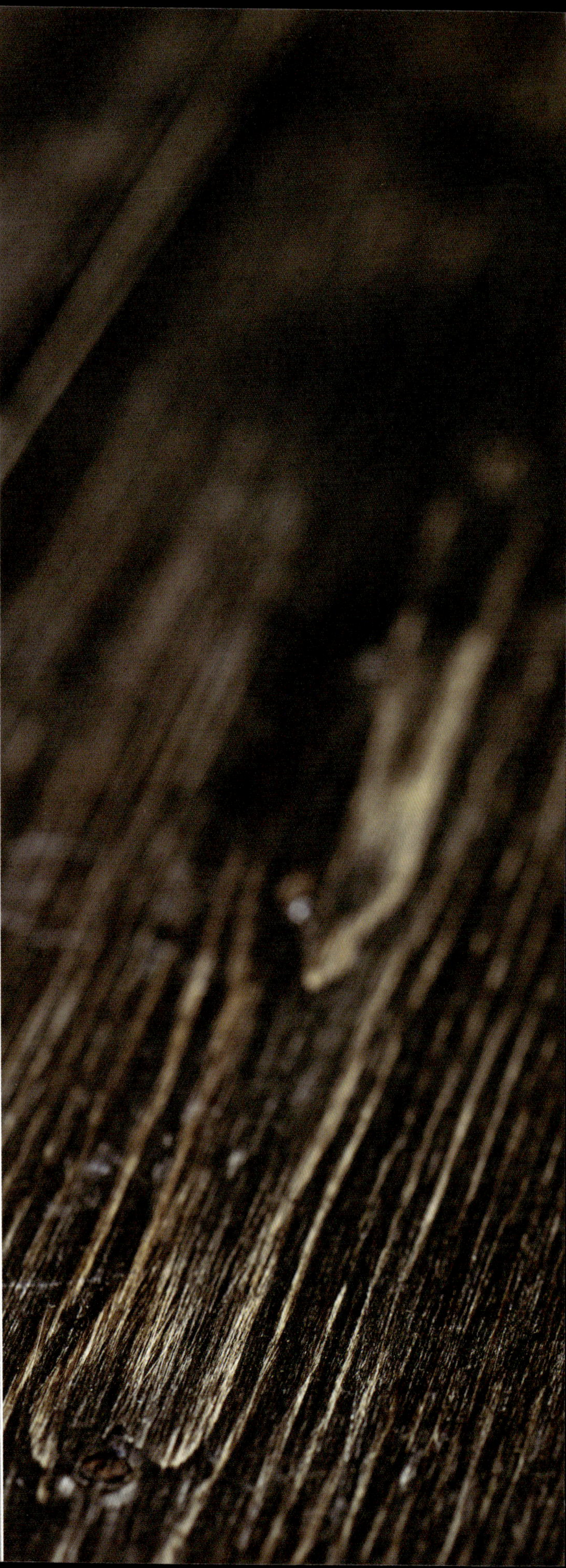

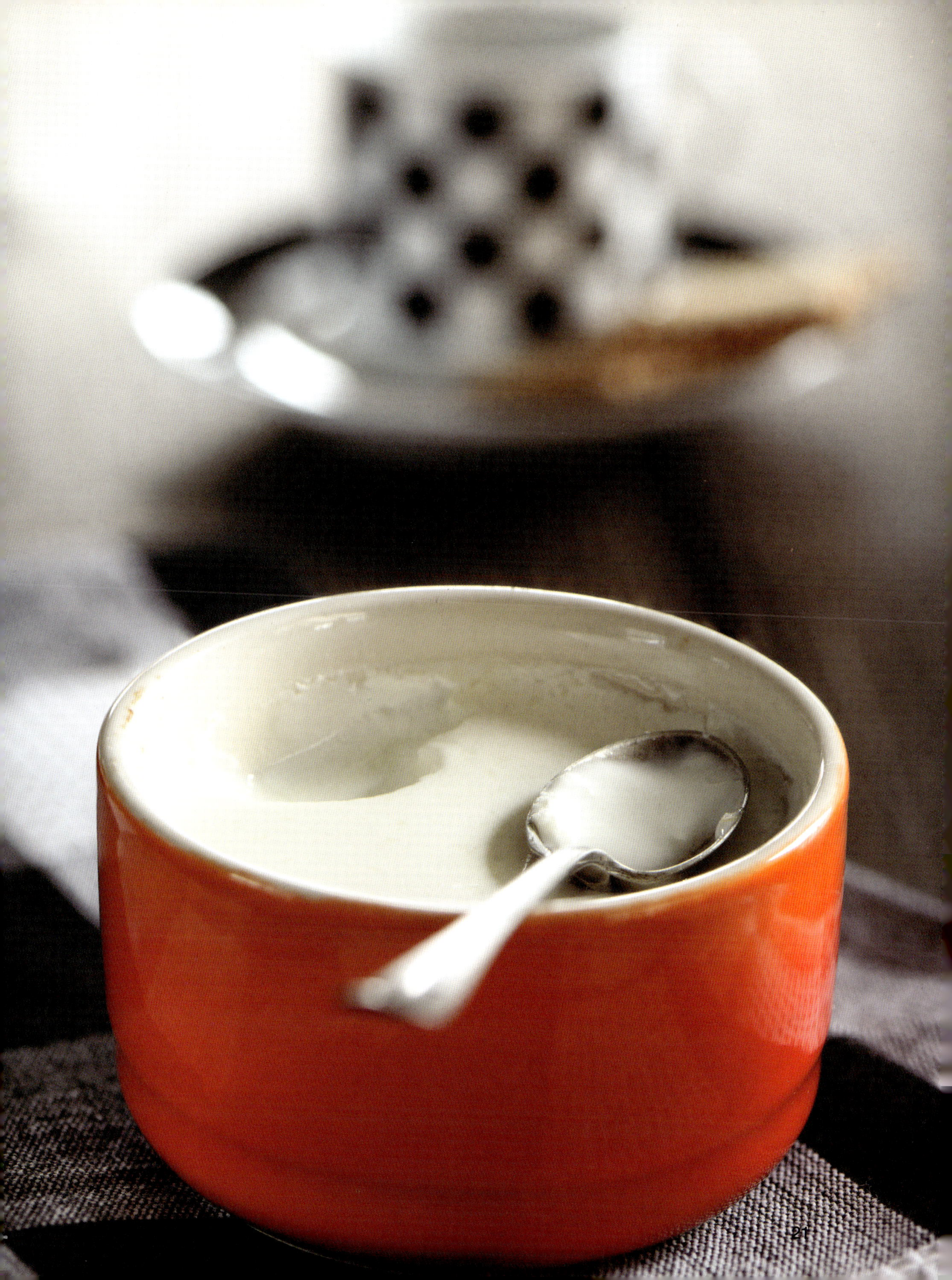

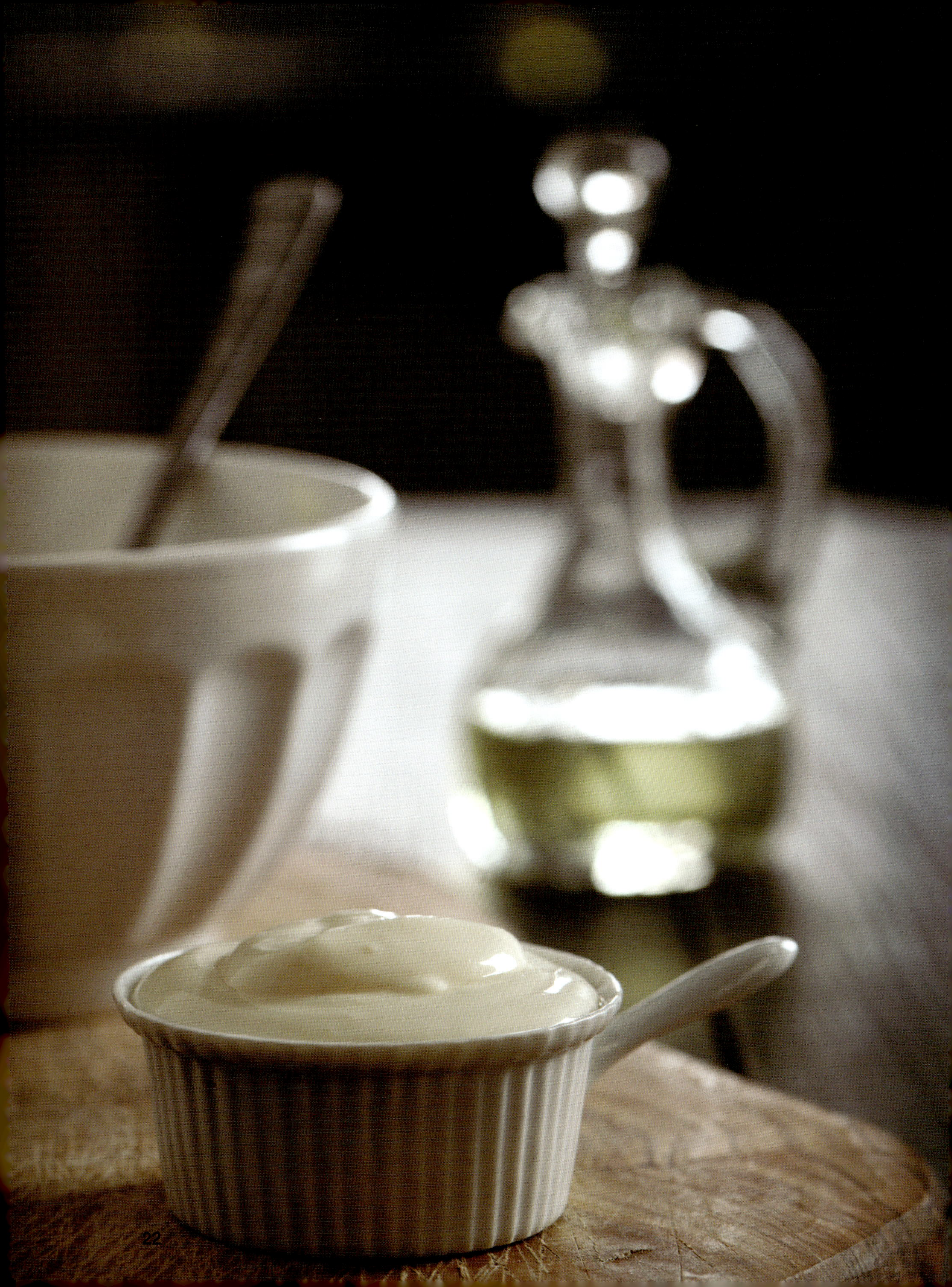

Yogurt and Horseradish Homemade Mayo

250 g (9 oz) low fat yogurt
2 egg yolks
200 ml (6¾ fl oz) extra virgin olive oil
pinch of salt
1 tablespoon horseradish

In a medium bowl combine the egg yolks, pinch of salt and whisk together. Then, very gently, gradually drizzle in the extra virgin olive oil and keep stirring with a whisk - slow in the beginning and faster once the first quarter of the oil is added. Then add to the mayonnaise, the horseradish, the yogurt and mix it well. The more yogurt you add, the lighter mayonnaise you will produce. Yogurt is naturally sour and the horseradish will give a really appetizing taste to the mayonnaise.

500 g (17½ oz)

Per 100 g (3½ oz)
414 kcal, 43 g fat (7g saturated), 4 g carbs (4 g sugar), 0.2 g fibre, 0.7 g salt

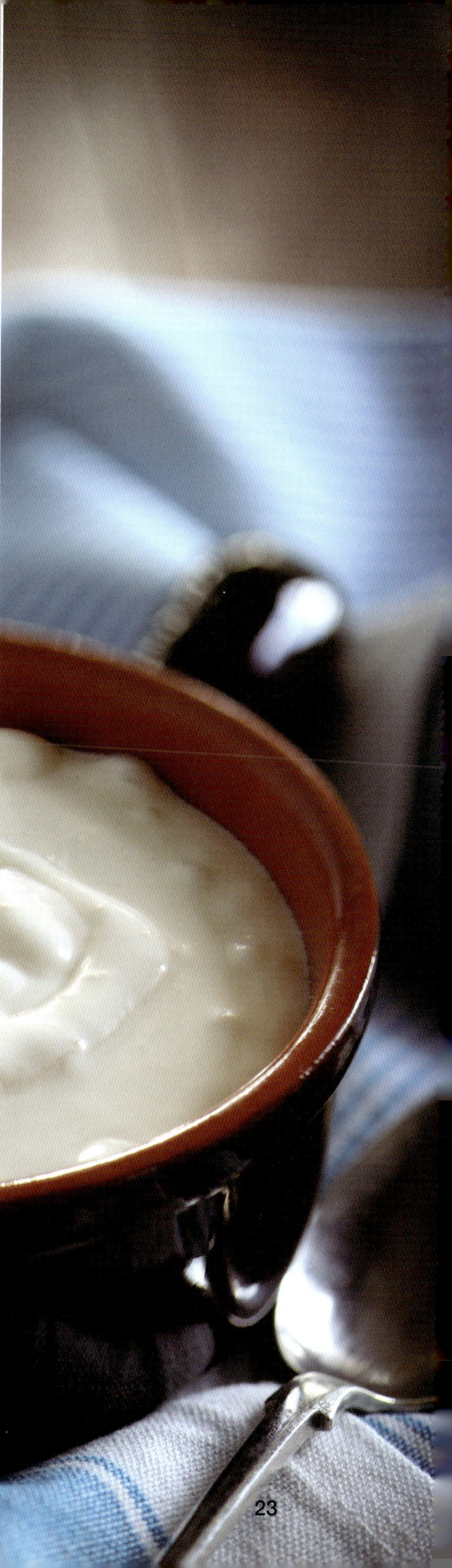

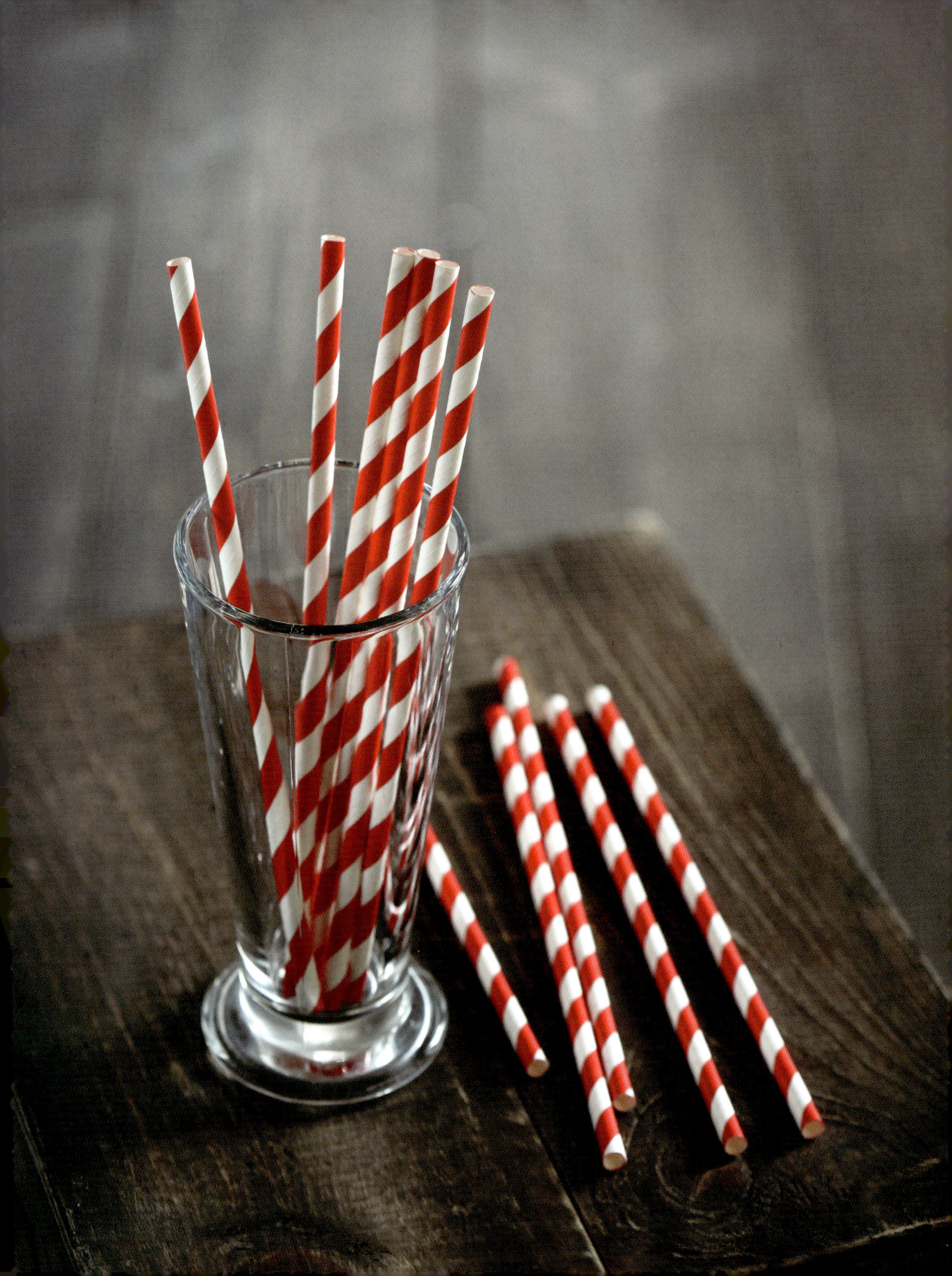

Drinks

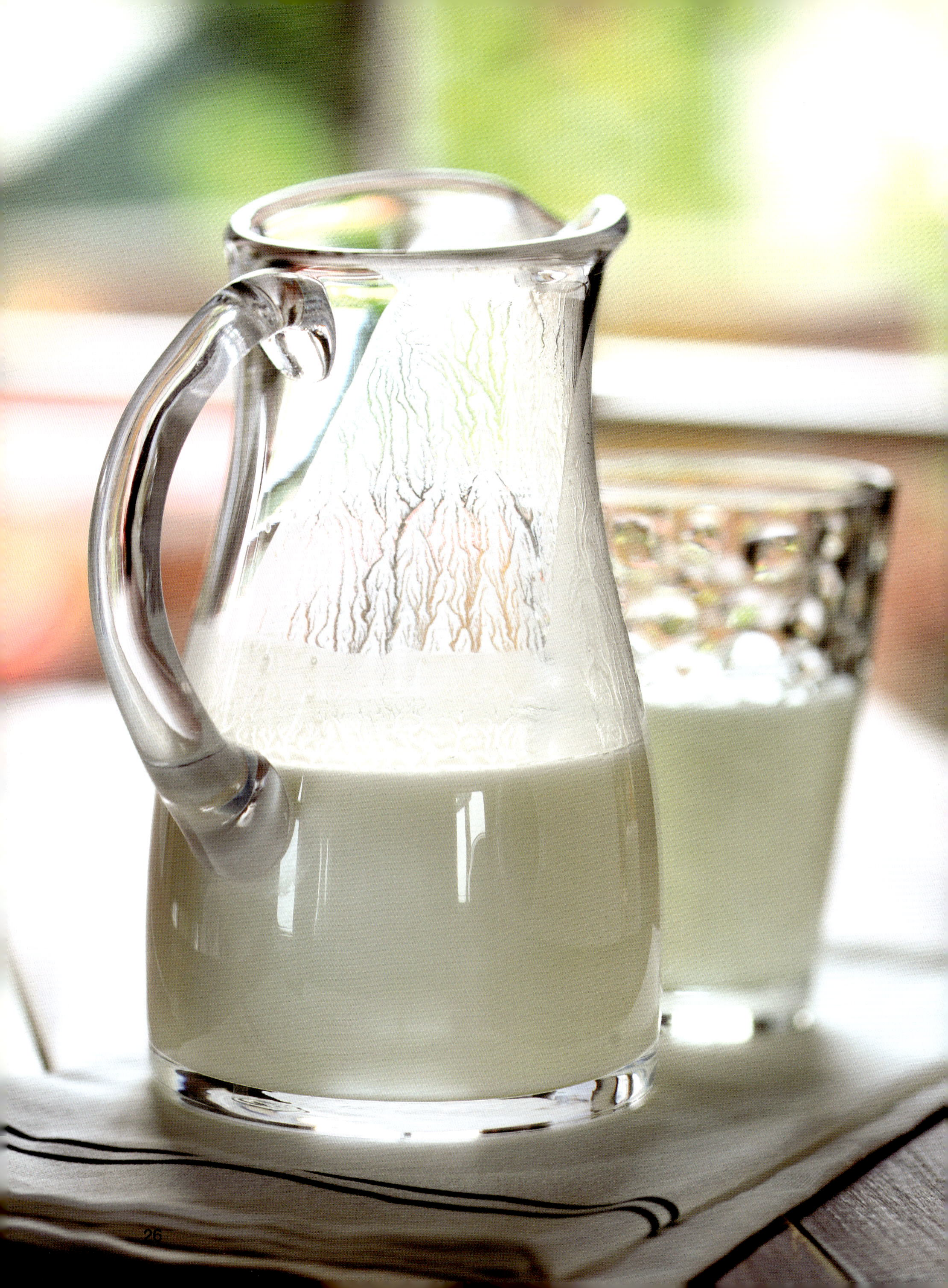

Airyan

500 g (17½ oz) low fat yogurt
500 ml (17 fl oz) mineral water
5 ice cubes
pinch of salt

Mix the yogurt, the mineral water and the salt in a jug. Stir well until there are no lumps. Add the ice cubes and serve.

This Balkan traditional summer drink is a brilliant idea for warm days! Some people make it with fizzy mineral water but I prefer still water.

Serves 5
Per serving
187 kcal, 1 g fat (0.7 g saturated), 4.8 g protein, 7.5 g carbs (7.5 g sugar), 0 g fibre, 0.7 g salt

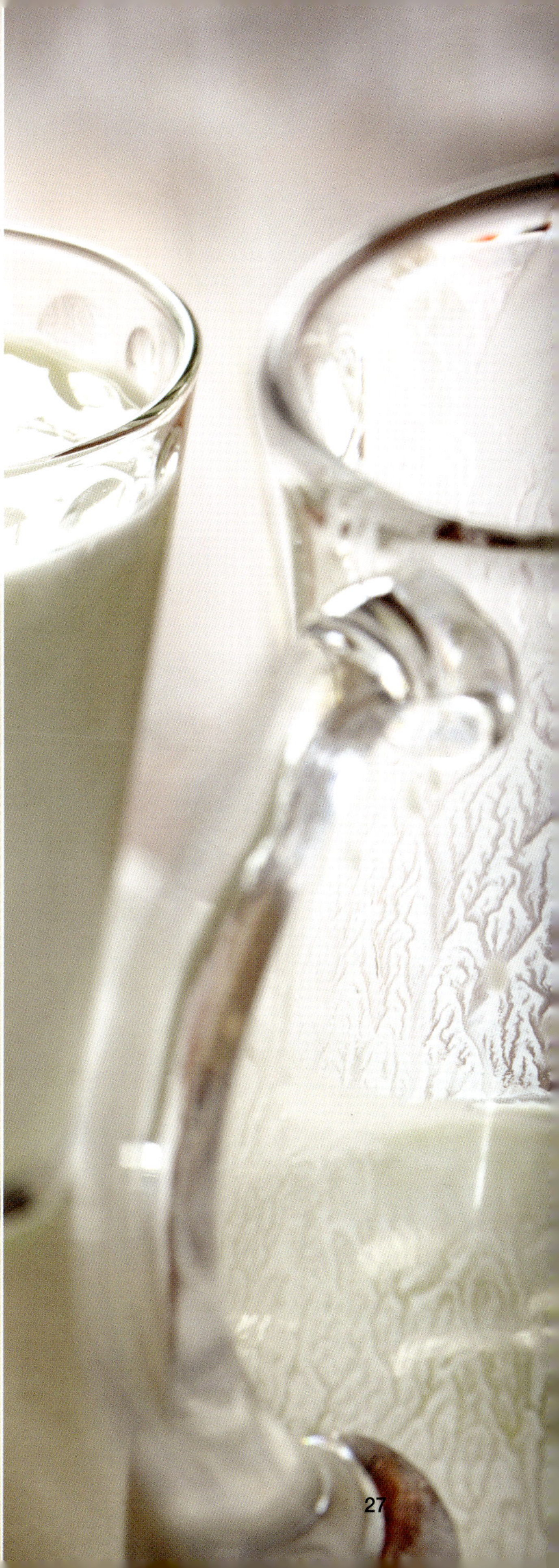

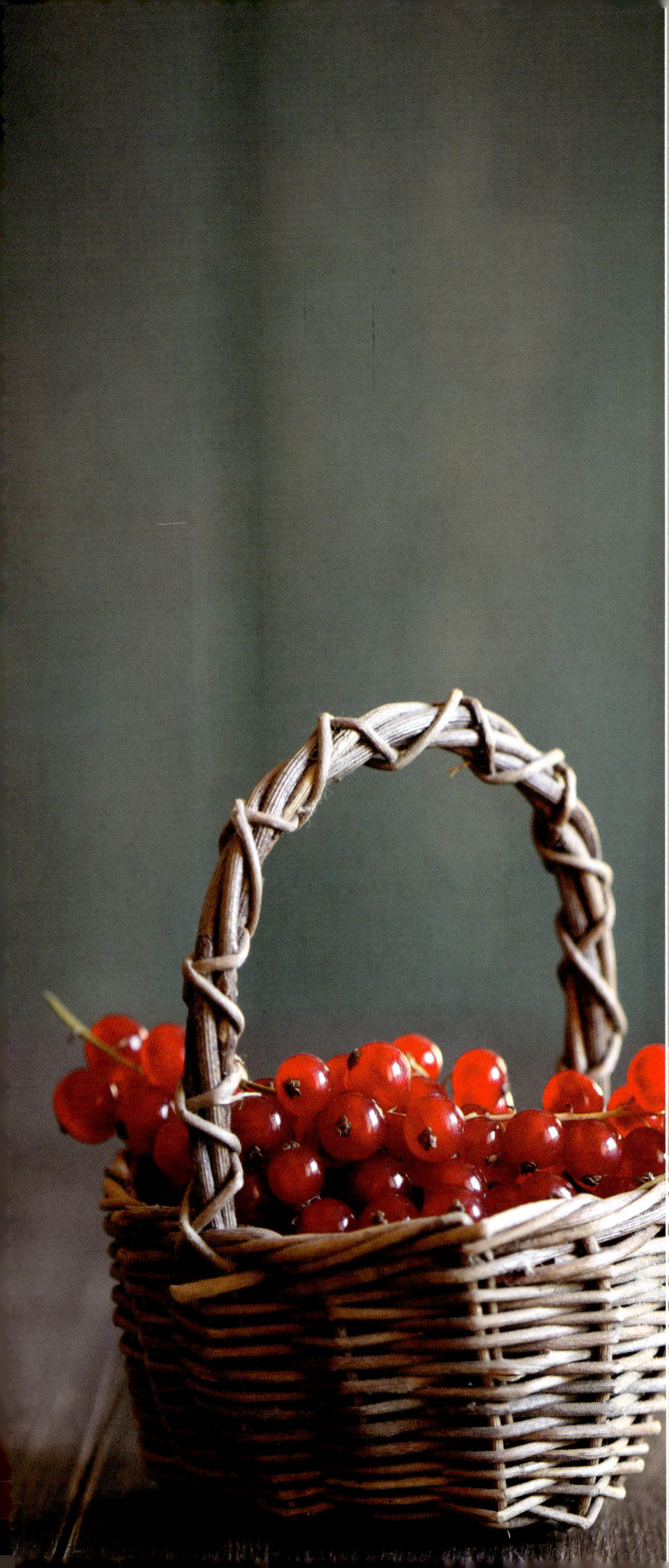

Redcurrant Rum Lassi

400 g (14 oz) low fat yogurt
50 g (2 oz) redcurrants
50 g (2 oz) golden syrup
25 ml (¾ fl oz) rum
pinch of salt
5 ice cubes
50 g (2 oz) pistachios nuts, finely chopped

Pour the yogurt into a blender and add the redcurrants, golden syrup, rum, salt and finally the ice cubes, blend until smooth. Serve quickly with the chopped pistachios on the top.

Lassi is a traditional, refreshing yogurt-based drink from the South Asian Panjab region. Redcurrant and Rum Lassi is my adaptation. I really like it, especially on hot days.

Serves 2
Per serving
431 kcal, 15.9 g fat (3.2 g saturated), 14.7 g protein, 53.8 g carbs (53.1 g sugar), 2.7 g fibre, 2.3 g salt

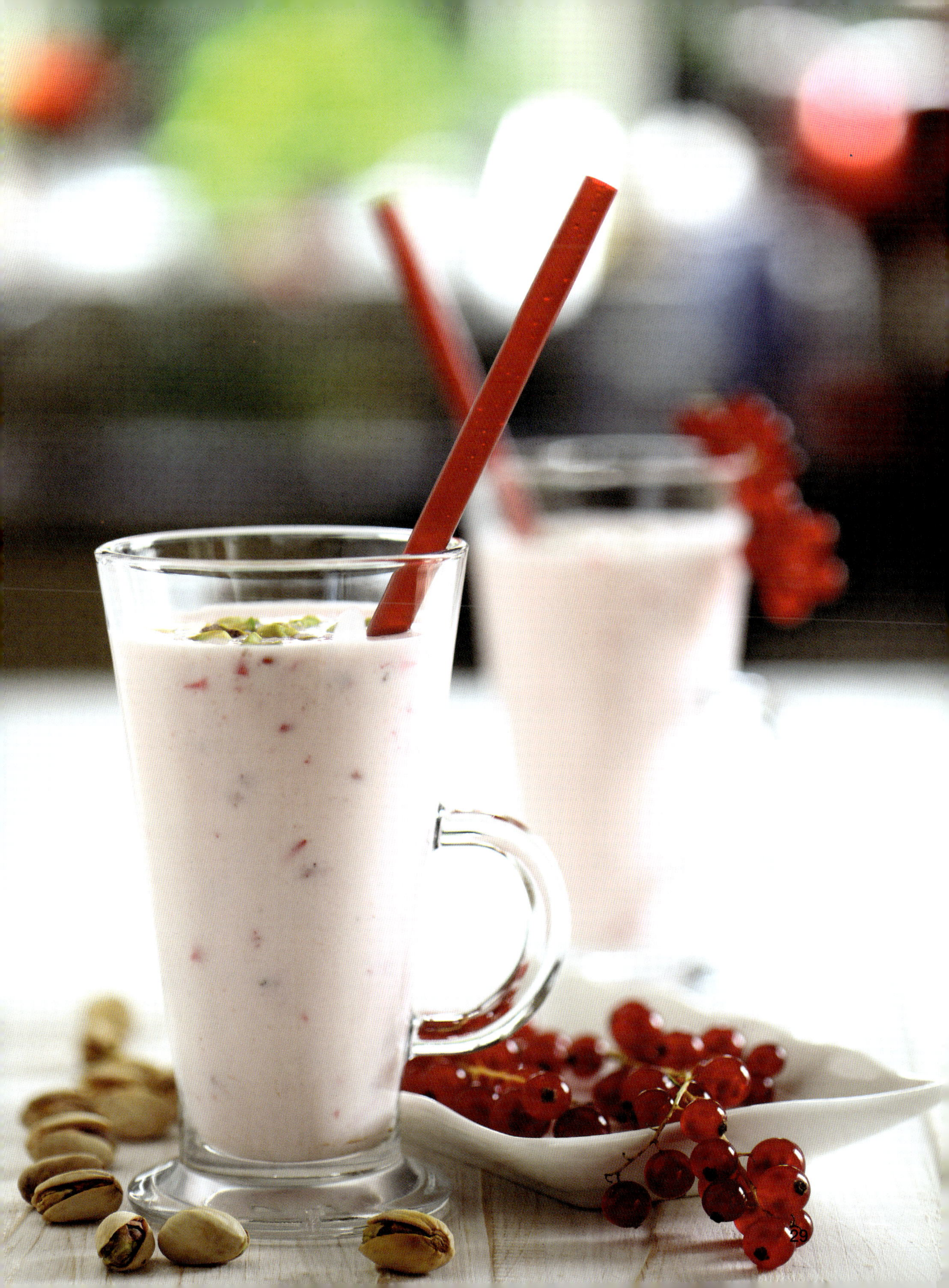

Very Berry Smoothie

100 g (3½ oz) strawberries
100 g (3½ oz) raspberries
50 g (2 oz) blueberries
2 small bananas
200 g (7 oz) low fat yogurt
200 ml (6¾ fl oz) semi-skimmed milk
1 tablespoon runny honey
½ teaspoon vanilla extract
5 ice cubes

In a blender throw in all the berries and peeled and chopped bananas. Pour in the yogurt and the milk, add the honey and vanilla flavoring and then the ice cubes. Blend the ingredients until smooth. Pour into glasses and serve immediately.

Serves 4

Per serving
122 kcal, 1.6 g fat (0.9 g saturated), 5.3 g protein, 23.2 g carbs (22.3 g sugar), 2.2 g fibre, 0.1 g salt

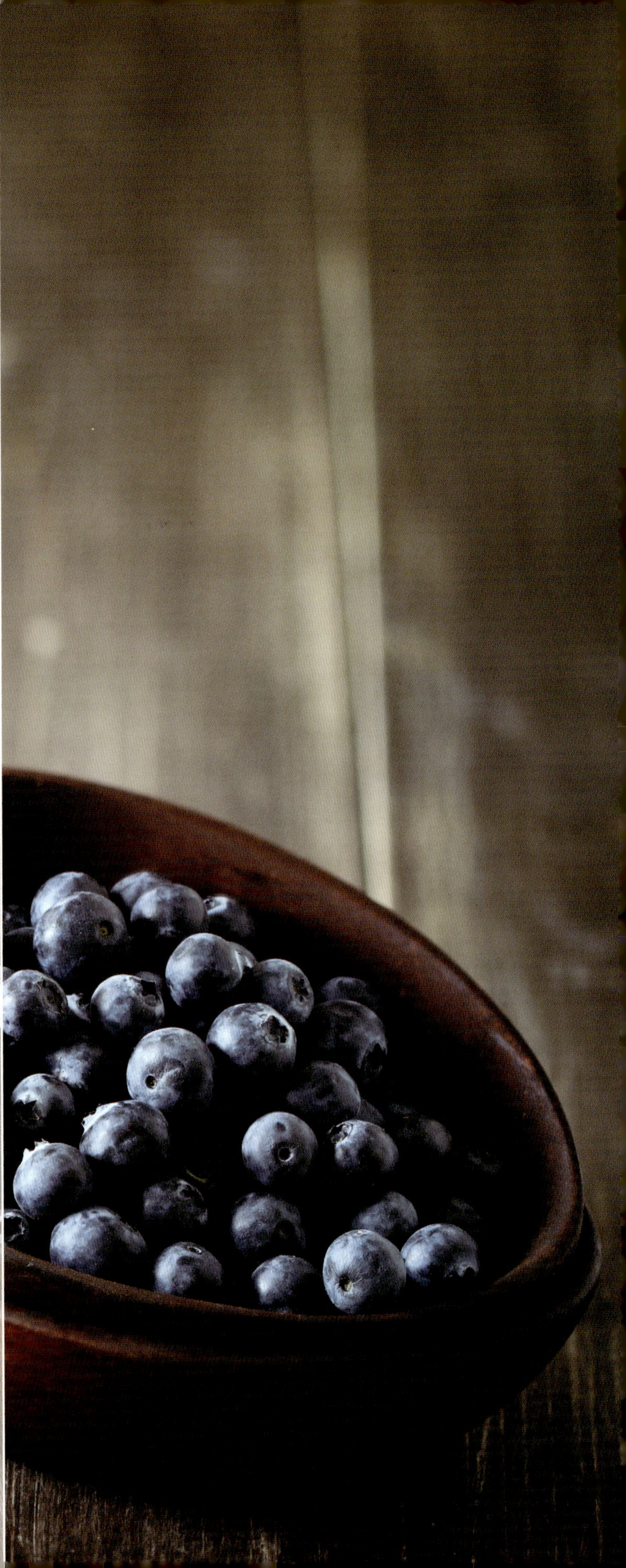

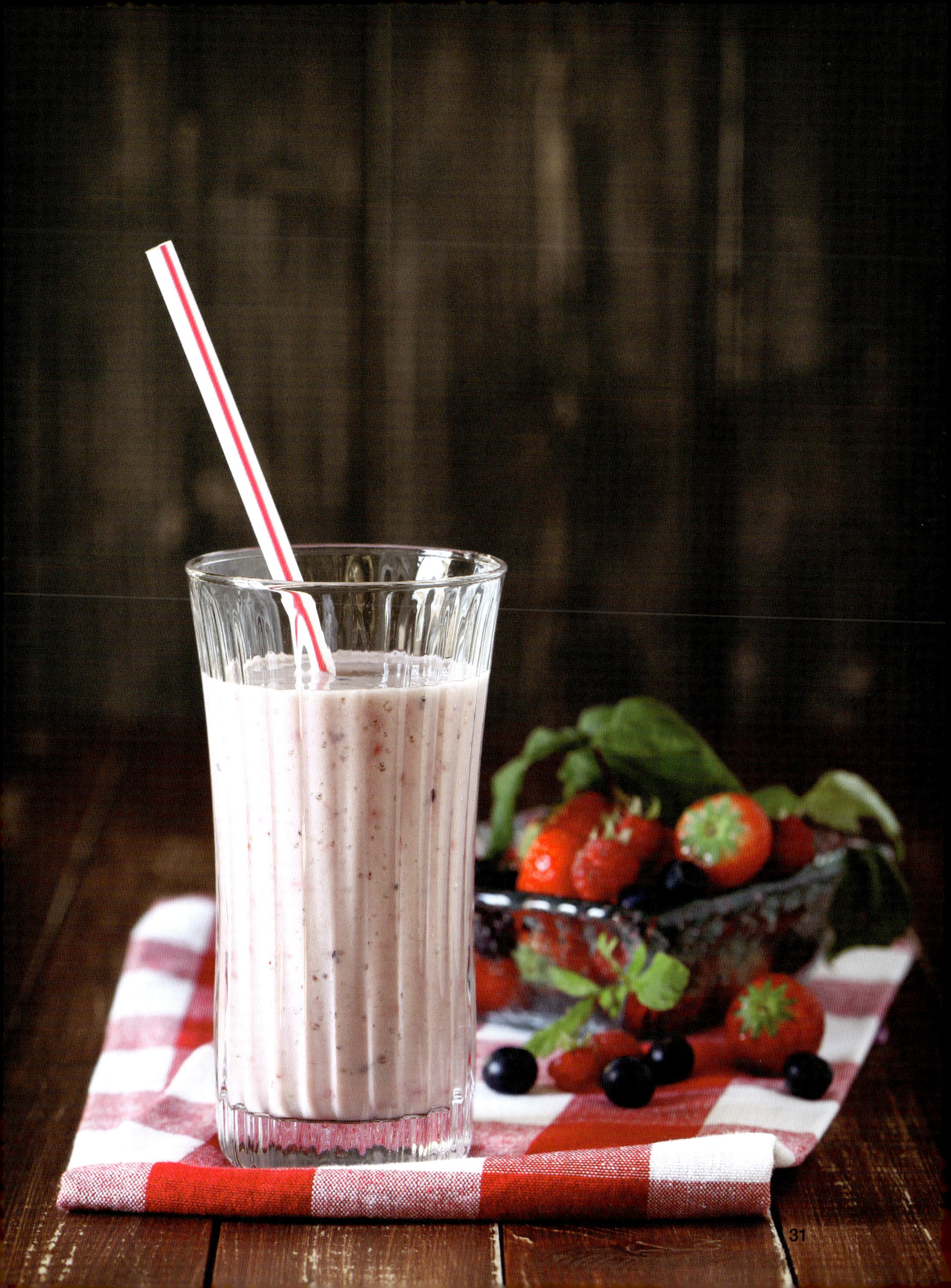

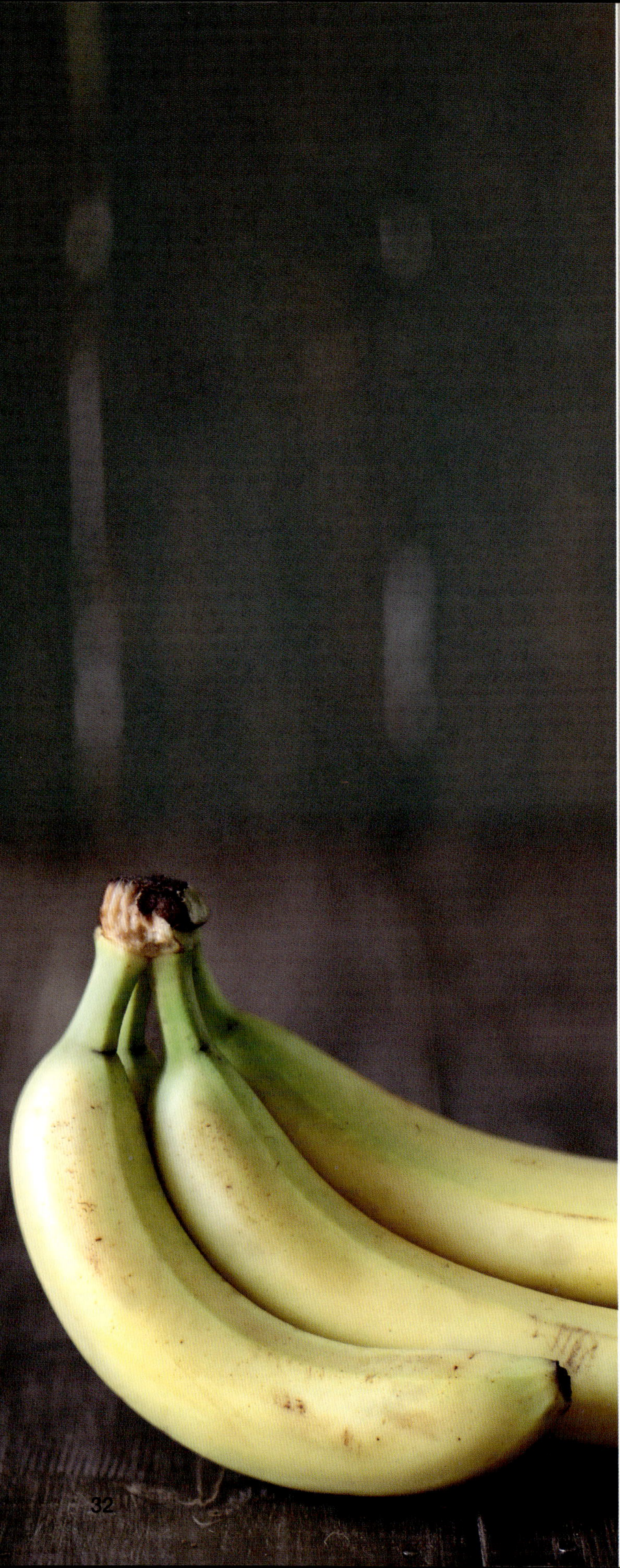

Avocado Smoothie

1 large avocado, peeled and diced
2 ripe bananas, peeled
200 g (7 oz) low fat yogurt
100 ml (3½ fl oz) skimmed milk
1 teaspoon honey
1 teaspoon ground cinnamon
4 ice cubes

Throw the avocado and bananas into the blender jar then pour in the yogurt and milk and add honey and cinnamon. Blend on high speed until smooth and frothy, serve cold.

Serves 4

Per serving
182 kcal, 10.2 g fat (2.4 g saturated), 4.8 g protein, 18.9 g carbs (17.4 g sugar), 0.1 g salt

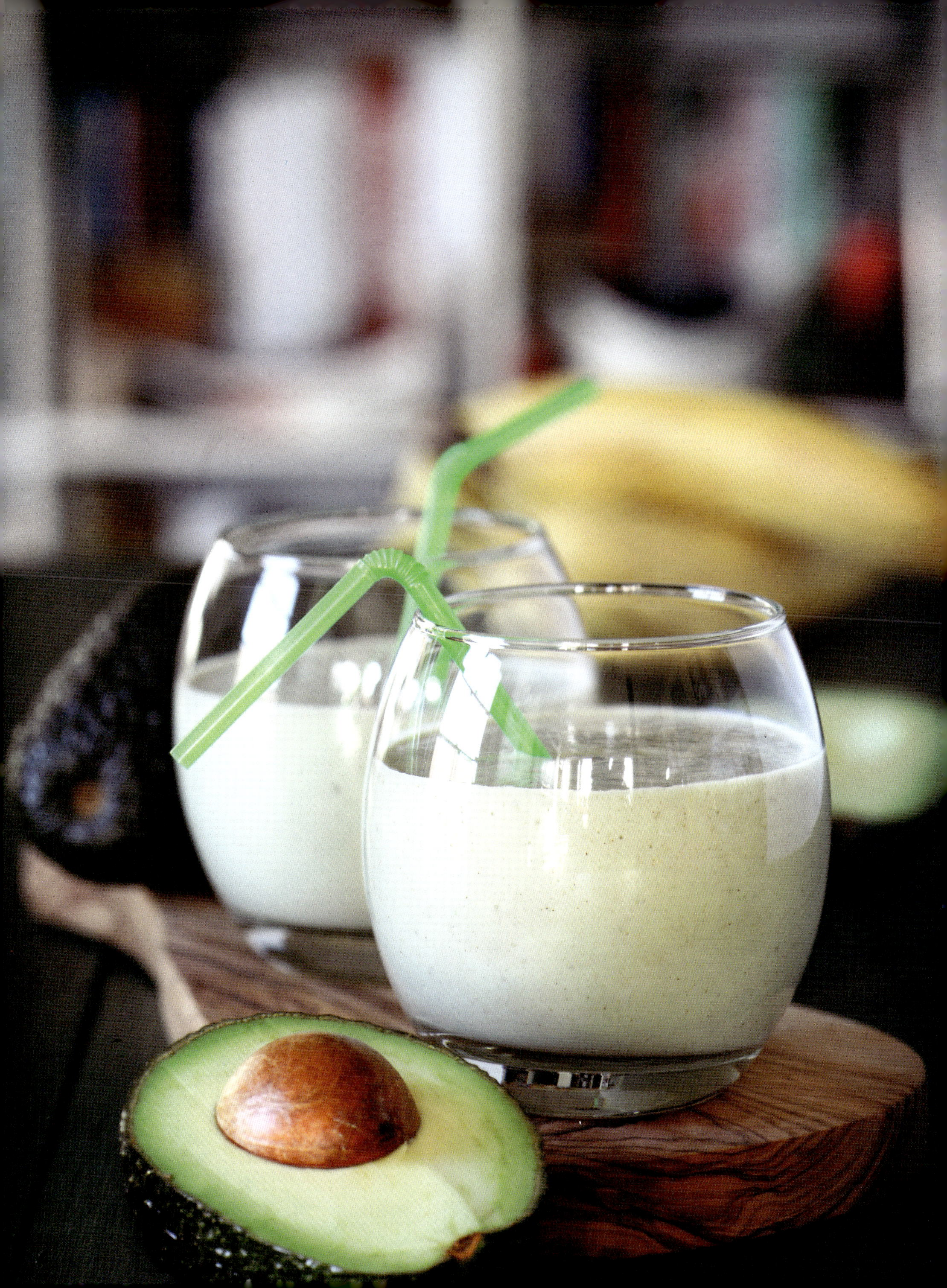

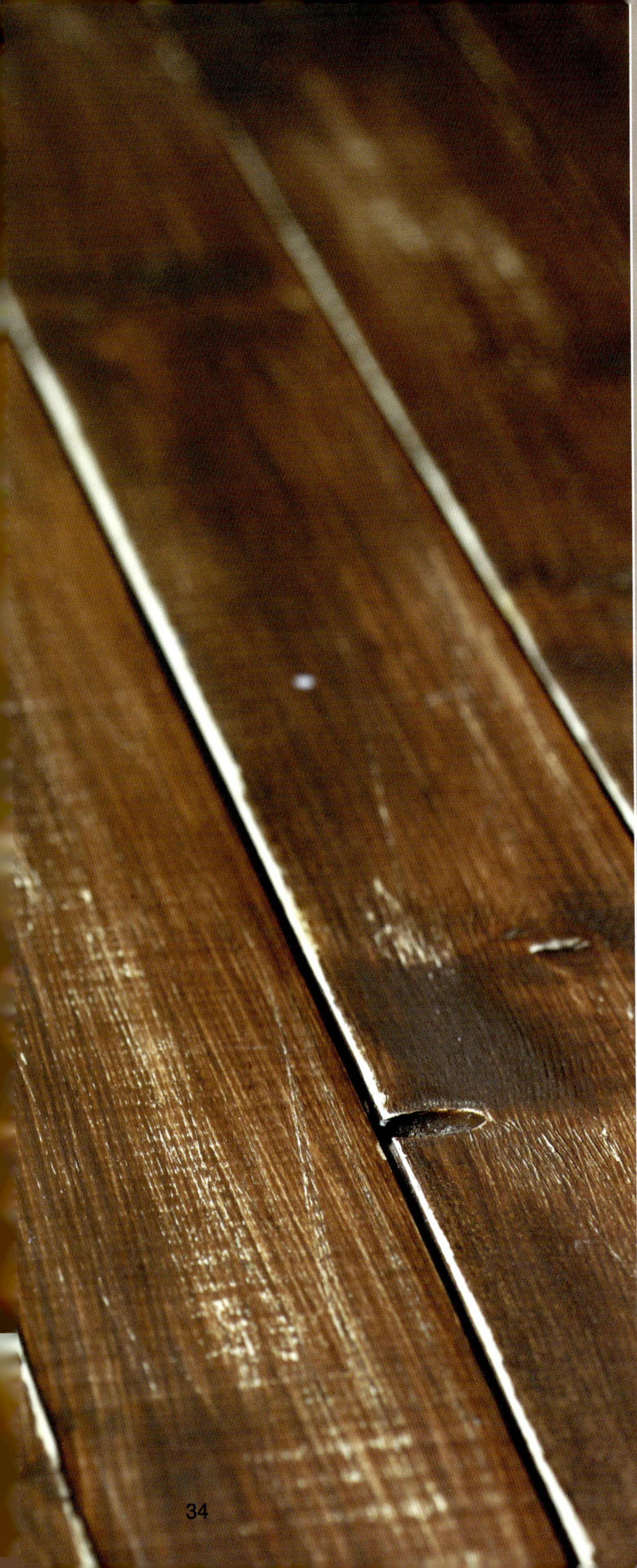

Cardamom Smoothie

1 banana
500 g (17½ oz) low fat yogurt
2 teaspoons brown sugar
1 tablespoon cardamom, grounded
4 tablespoons corn cereal
5 ice cubes

In a blender, combine the banana, yogurt, sugar, ground cardamom, corn cereal and ice cubes. Blend all ingredients together and serve in chilled glasses. Garnish with some cereal.

Serves 4

Per serving
125 kcal, 1.5 g fat (0.9 g saturated), 7.0 g protein, 23.1 g carbs (17.6 g sugar), 0.5 g fibre, 0.4 g salt

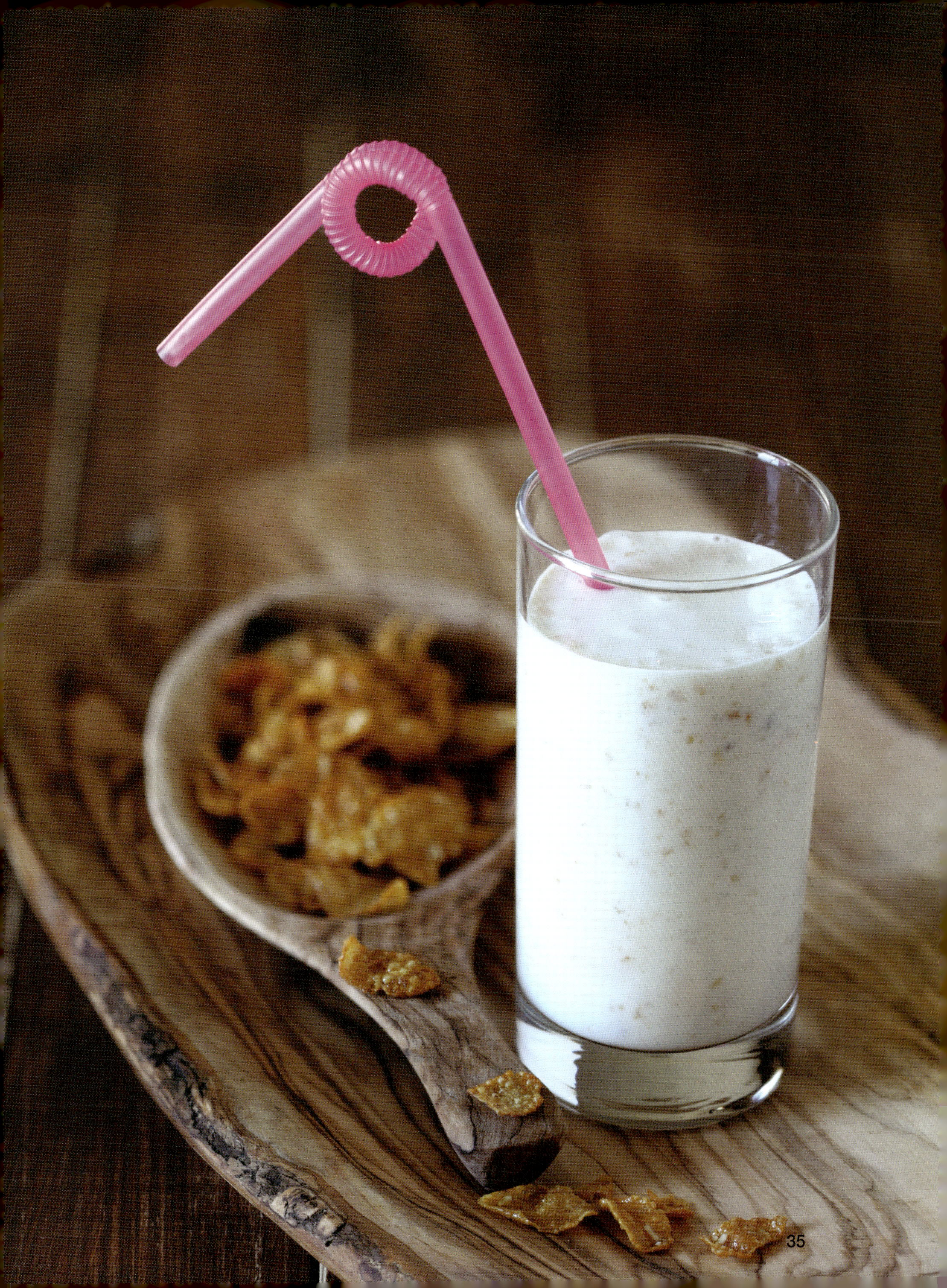

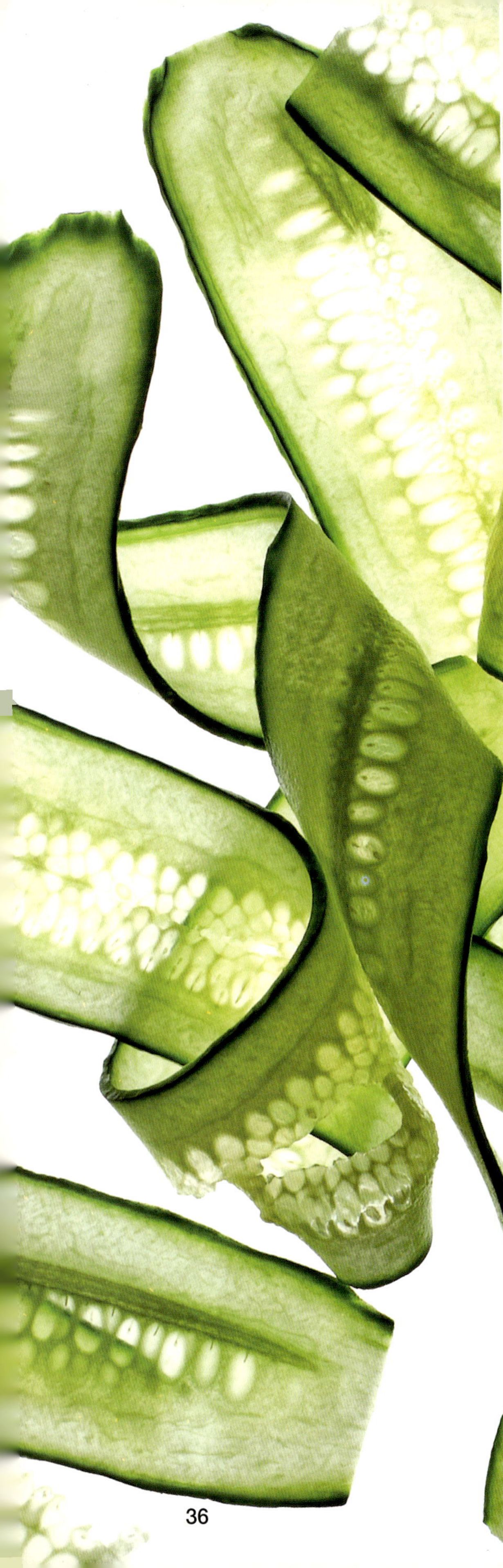

Cucumber and Pear Smoothie

1 medium cucumber
2 pears, peeled, chopped and seeded
1 pink lady apple, peeled, chopped and seeded
handful of chopped fresh coriander
100 ml (3½ fl oz) fizzy mineral water
300 ml (10 fl oz) low fat yogurt
juice of 1 small lime
pinch of salt, optional
5 ice cubes

Combine the chopped and seeded pears and apple into the blender and then add the chopped coriander, lime juice, fizzy water and yogurt. Blend all ingredients together until smooth and creamy.

Serves 4

Per serving
83 kcal, 0.9 g fat (0.5 g saturated), 4.1 g protein, 15.6 g carbs (15.5 g sugar), 2.8 g fibre, 0.9 g salt

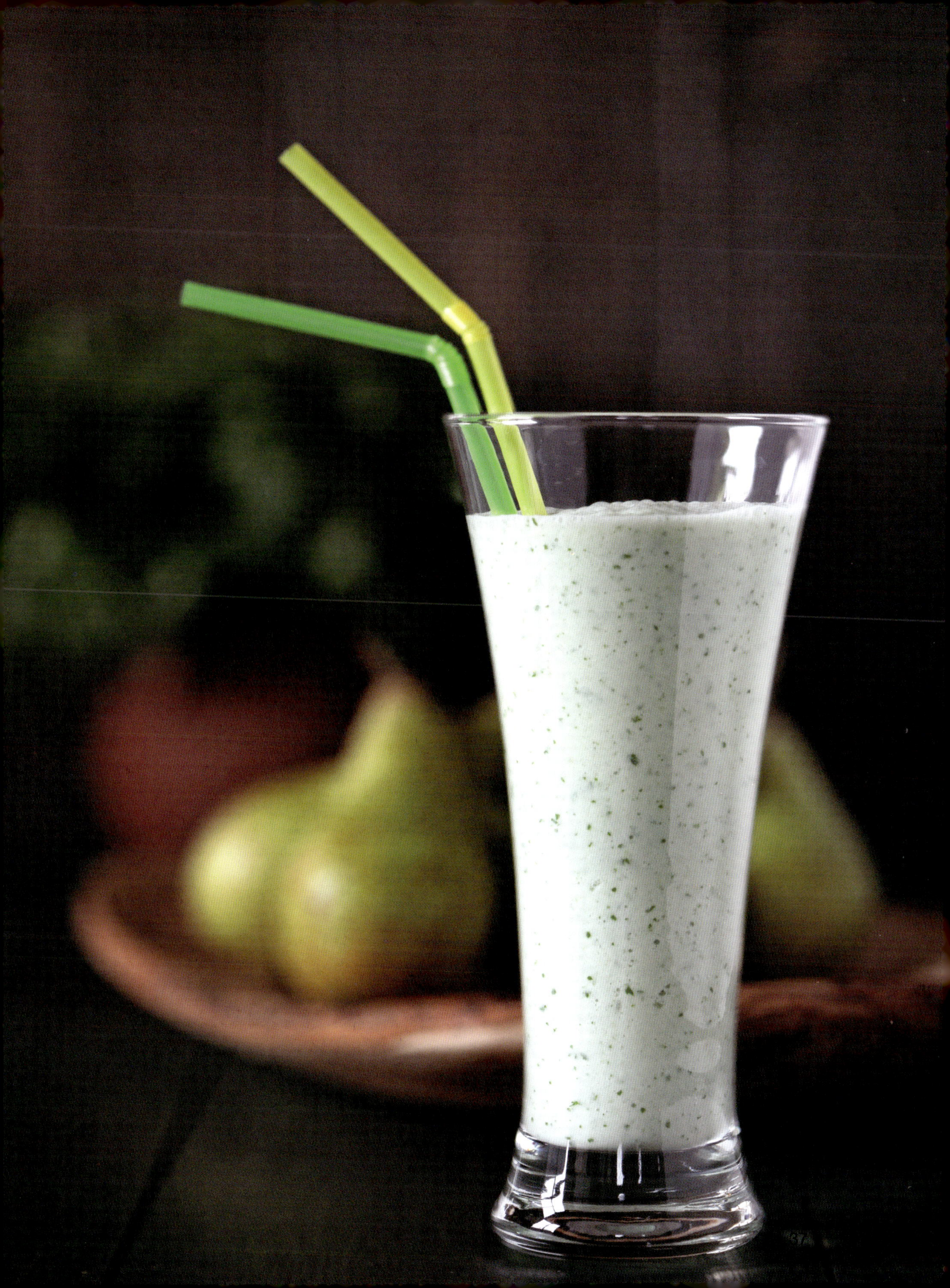

Dragon Fruit Smoothie

2 large dragon fruits, peeled and sliced
2 bananas, peeled
100 g (3½ oz) raspberries
400 g (14 oz) low fat yogurt
2 tablespoons honey
6 ice cubes

In a blender, combine the sliced dragon fruits, bananas, raspberries, yogurt, honey and ice cubes. Blend all ingredients together and serve into chilled glasses.

Serves 8

Per serving
107 kcal, 0.9 g fat (0.4 g saturated), 3.9 g protein, 22.2 g carbs (21.1 g sugar), 0.8 g fibre, 0.1 g salt

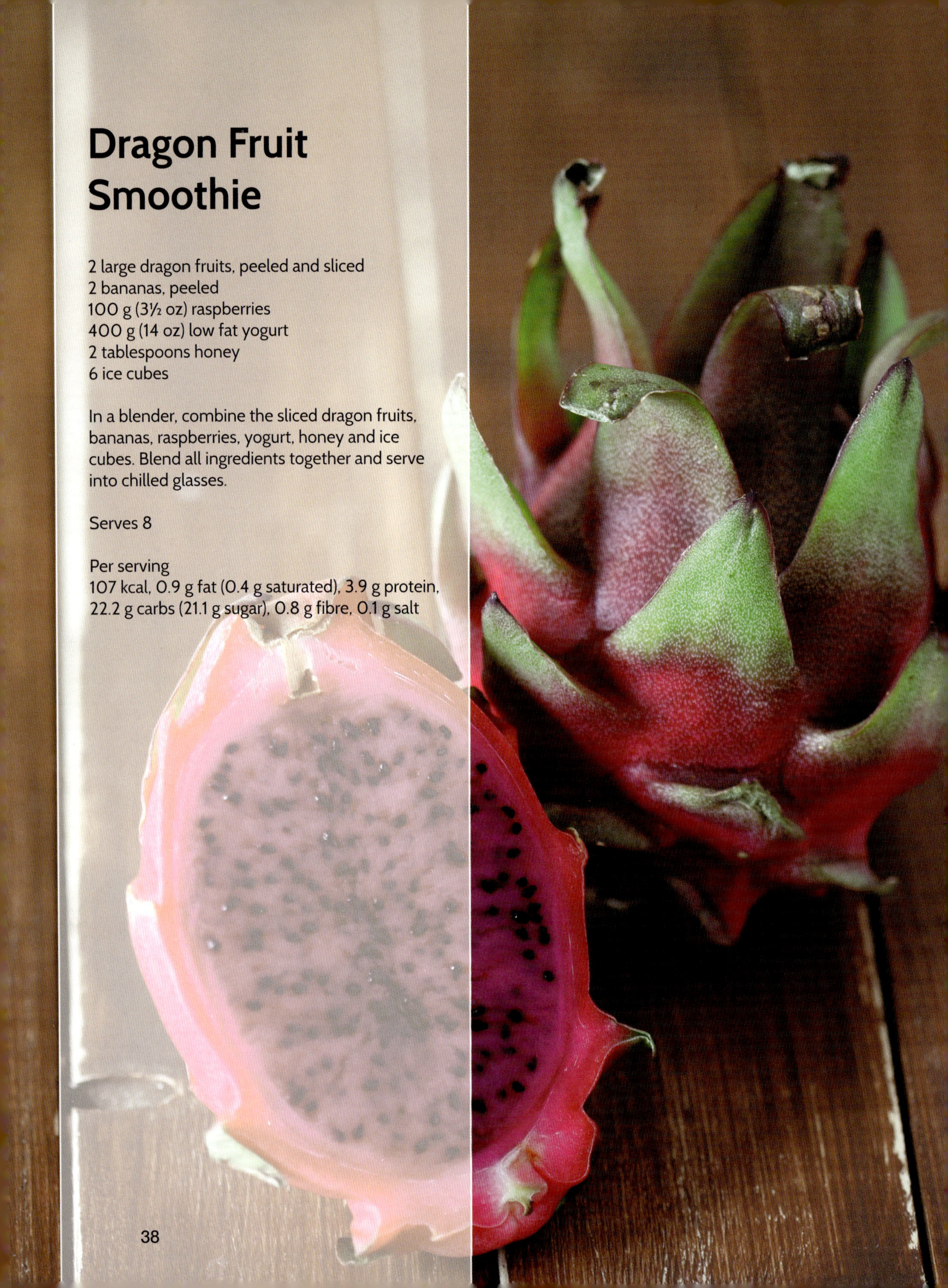

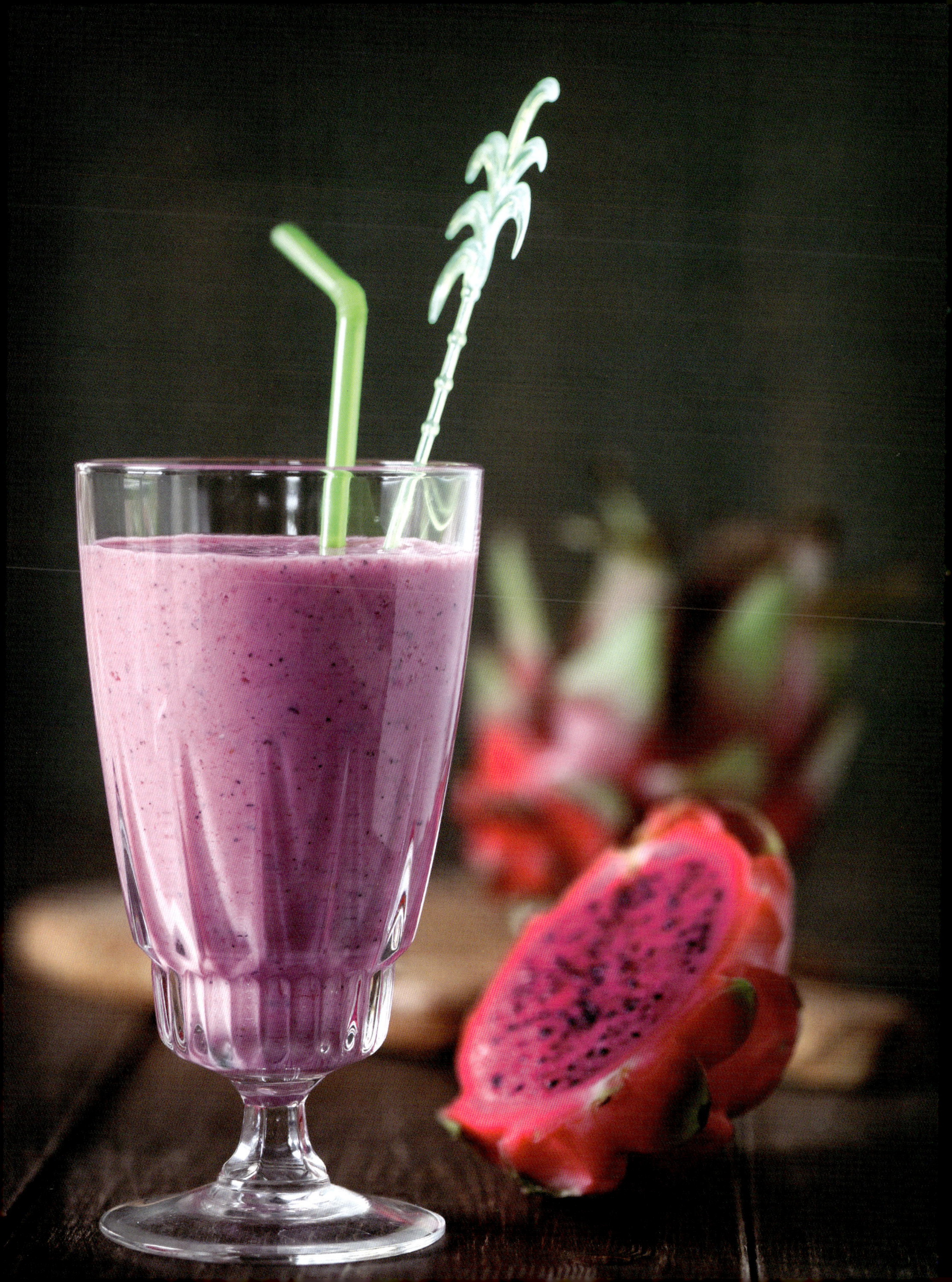

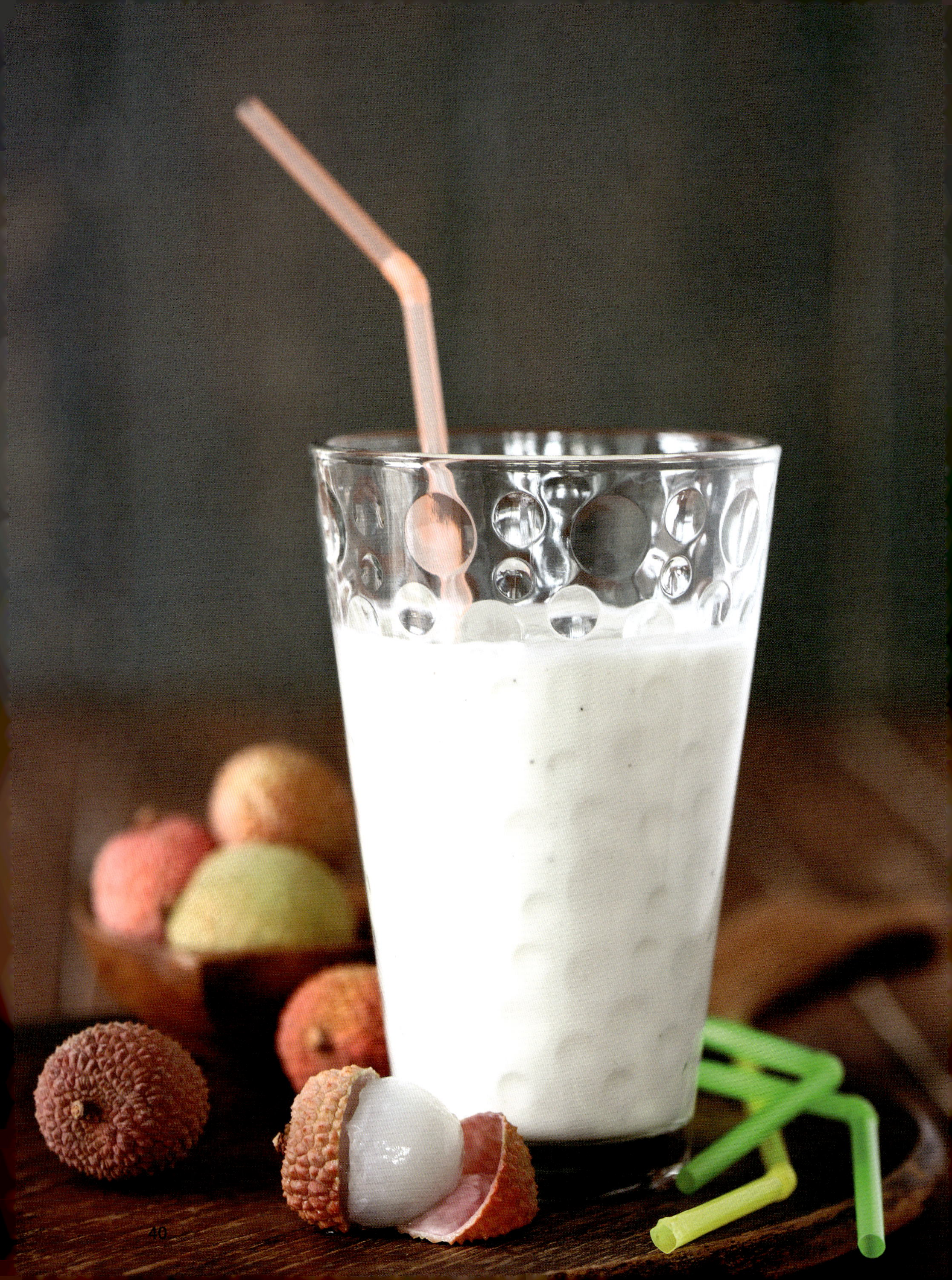

Lychee Yogurt Drink

8 lychees, peeled and seeded
400 g (14 oz) low fat yogurt
400 ml (13½ fl oz) mineral water
6 ice cubes
1 lemon, fresh juice
1 tablespoon honey
½ teaspoon cardamom, grounded

Combine the chopped lychees, yogurt, water, ice, lemon juice, honey and cardamom in the blender. Blend until smooth and frothy.

Perfect refreshing drink for warm days.

Serves 4

Per serving
91 kcal, 1.0 g fat (0.7 g saturated), 5.1 g protein, 16.5 g carbs (16.5 g sugar), 0.3 g fibre, 0.2g salt

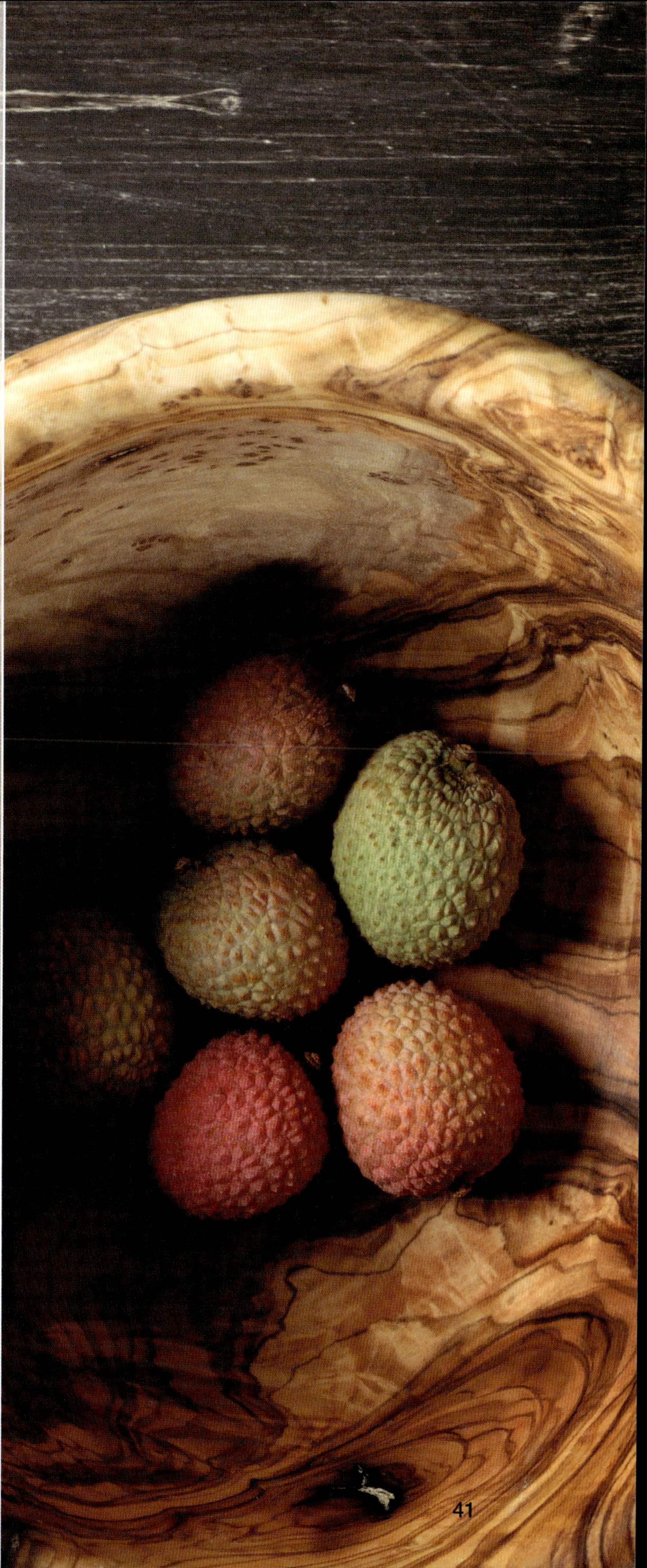

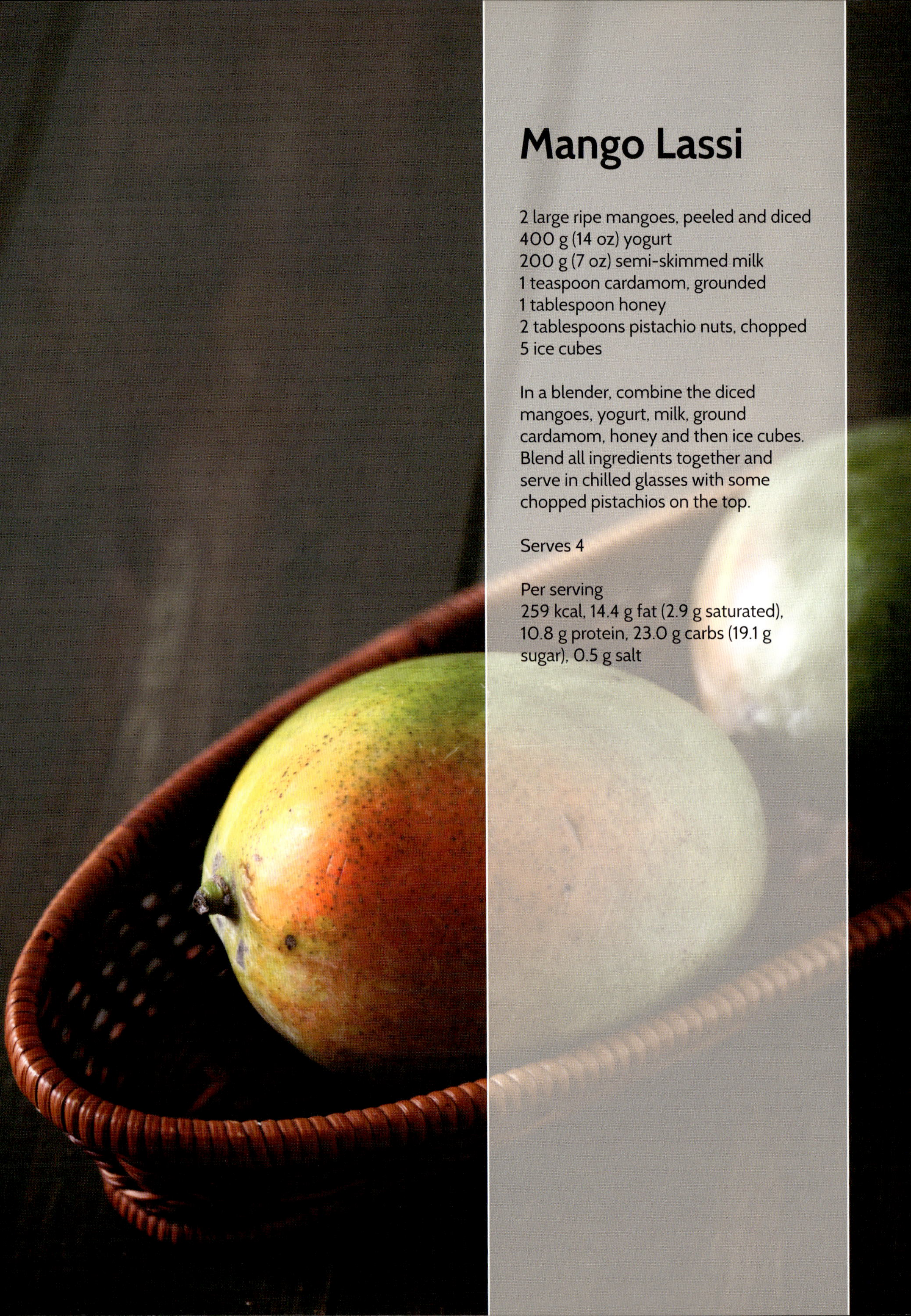

Mango Lassi

2 large ripe mangoes, peeled and diced
400 g (14 oz) yogurt
200 g (7 oz) semi-skimmed milk
1 teaspoon cardamom, grounded
1 tablespoon honey
2 tablespoons pistachio nuts, chopped
5 ice cubes

In a blender, combine the diced mangoes, yogurt, milk, ground cardamom, honey and then ice cubes. Blend all ingredients together and serve in chilled glasses with some chopped pistachios on the top.

Serves 4

Per serving
259 kcal, 14.4 g fat (2.9 g saturated), 10.8 g protein, 23.0 g carbs (19.1 g sugar), 0.5 g salt

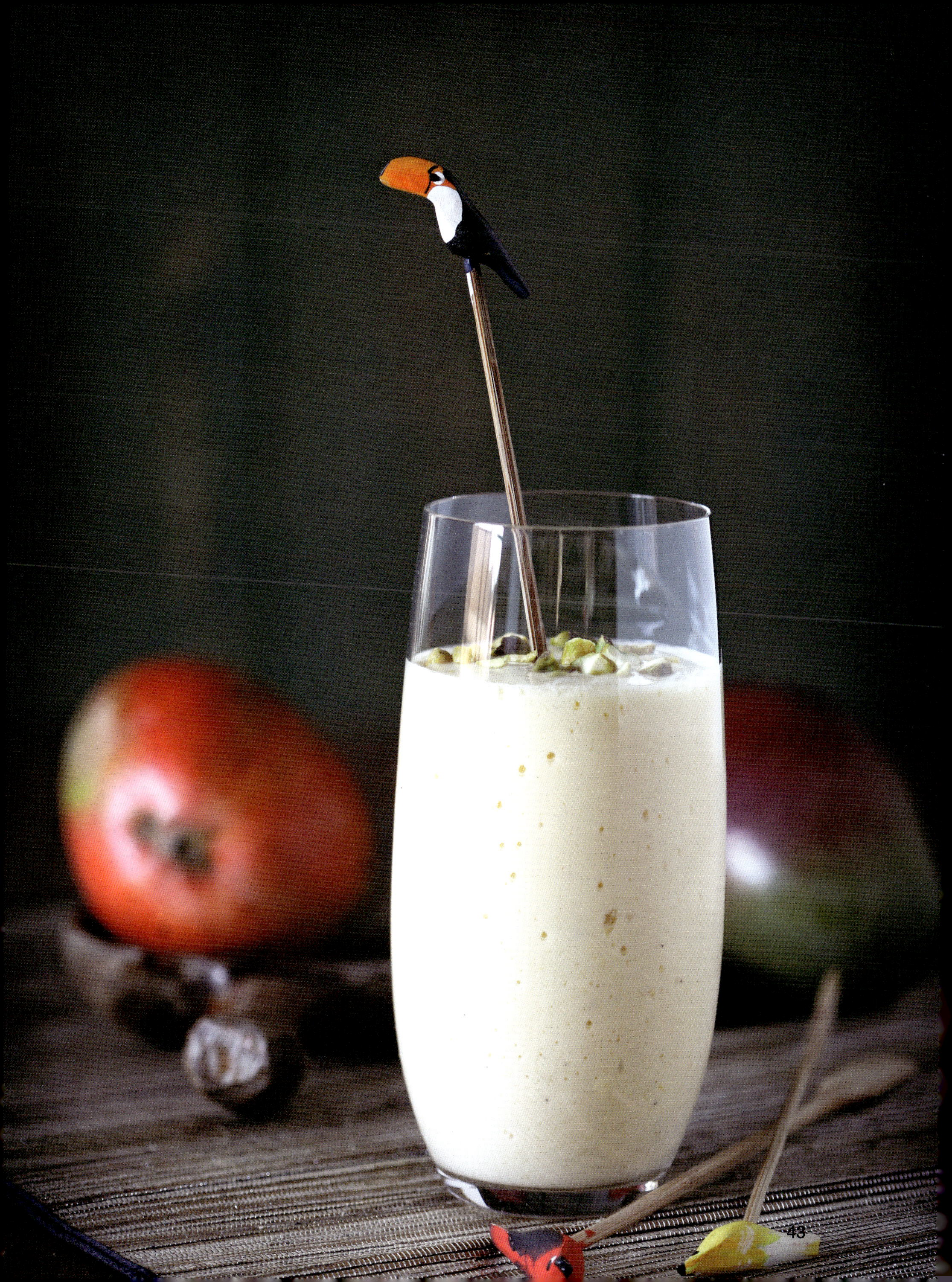

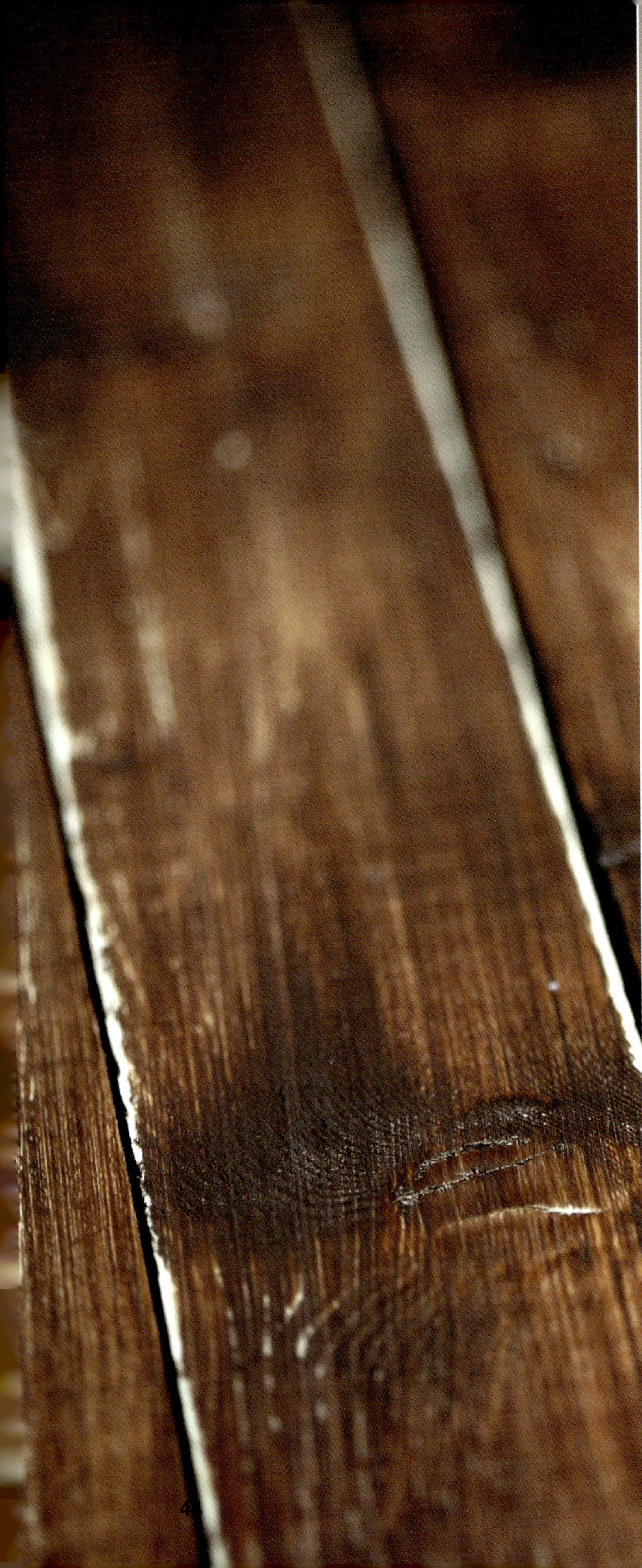

Persimmon Smoothie

2 medium persimmons, de-stemmed and peeled
200 ml (6¾ fl oz) semi-skimmed milk
½ teaspoon ground cinnamon
½ teaspoon pure vanilla extract
1 teaspoon lime juice
200 g (7 oz) plain yogurt
2 tablespoons brown sugar
5 ice cubes, crushed

In a blender, combine the persimmons, milk, cinnamon, vanilla extract, lime juice, yogurt, brown sugar and ice. Blend all ingredients together and serve in chilled glasses.

Serves 4

Per serving
122 kcal, 1.5 g fat (0.9 g saturated), 4.5 g protein, 23.6 g carbs (21.2 g sugar), 2.3 g fibre, 0.1 g salt

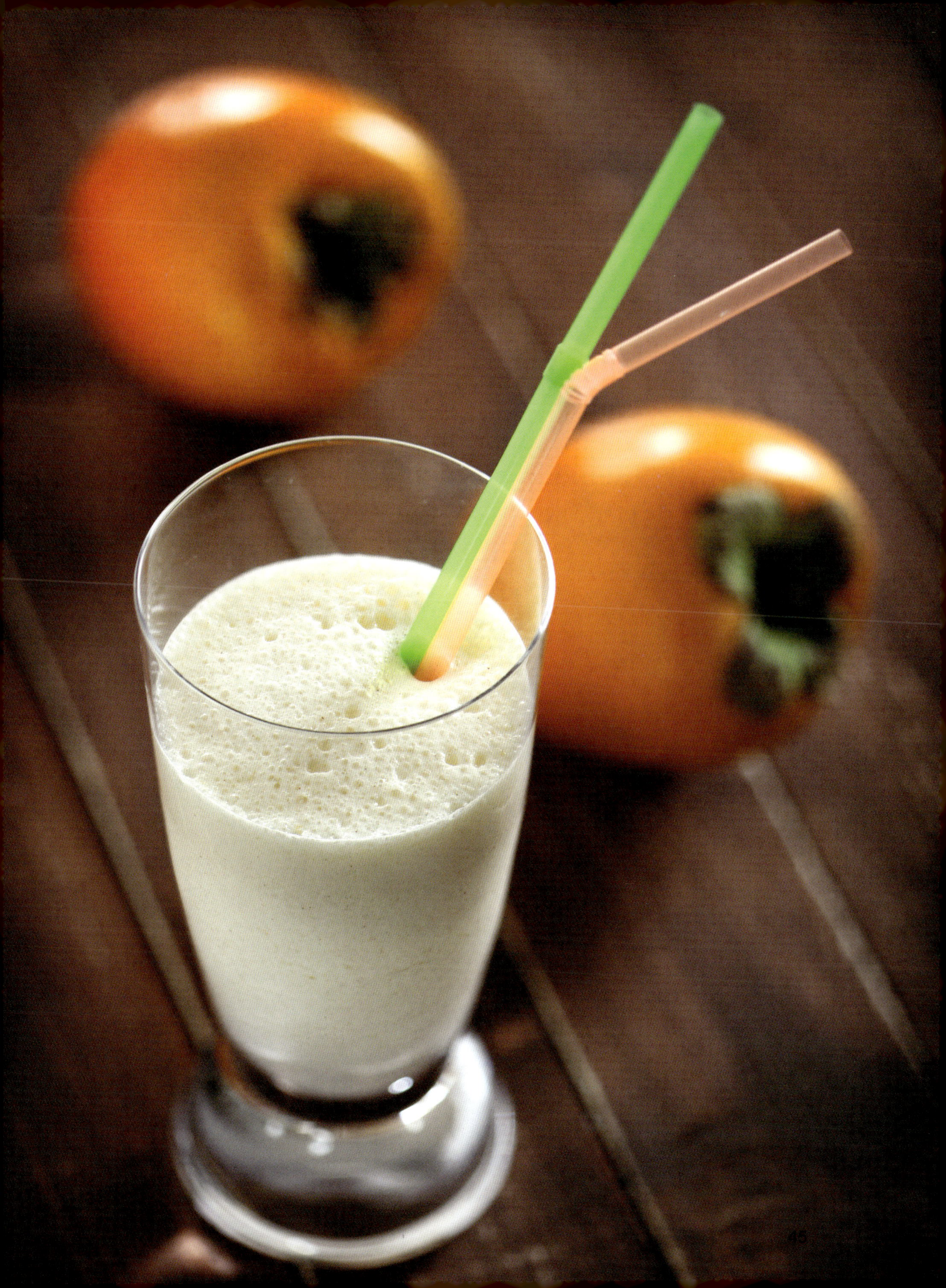

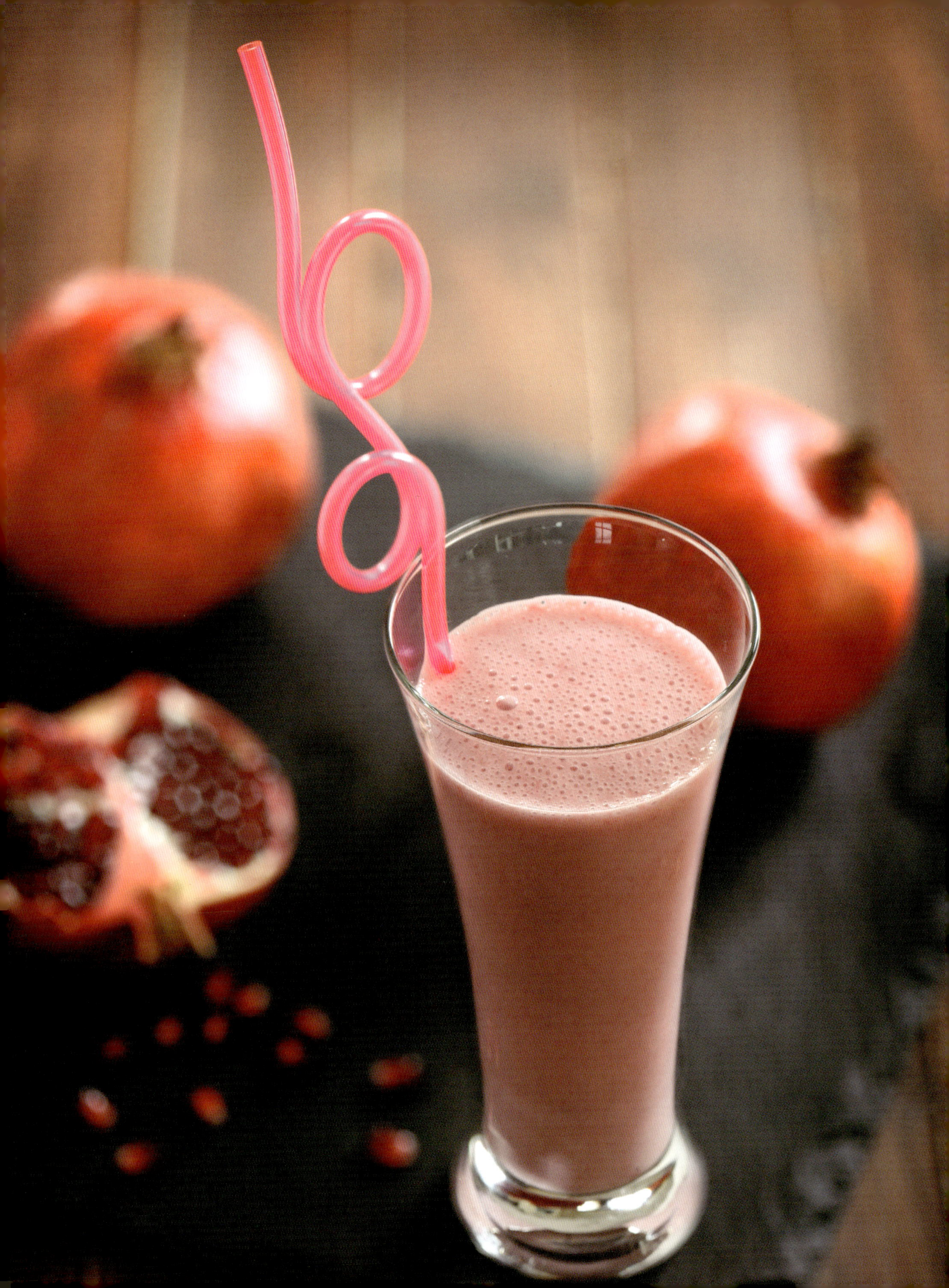

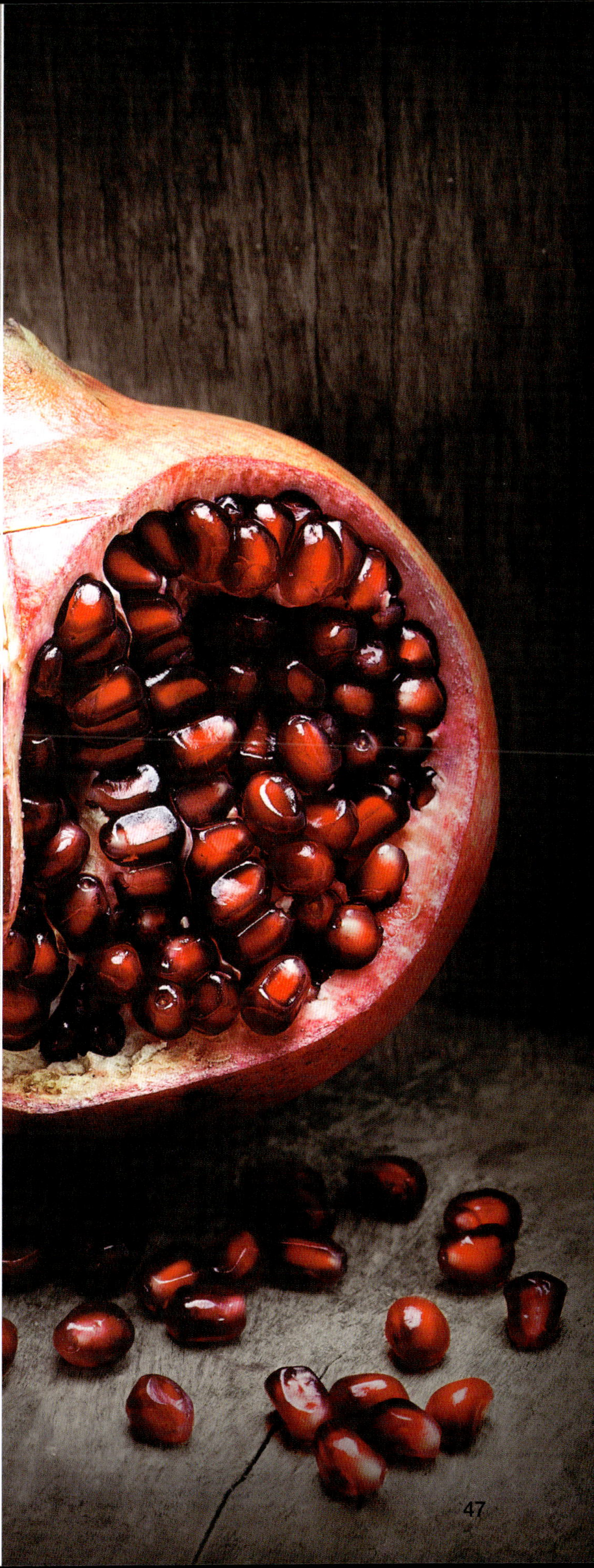

Pomegranate Smoothie

200 g (7 oz) plain yogurt
Squeezed juice from 2 pomegranates
2 large bananas
1 tablespoon brown sugar
6 ice cubes, crushed

In a blender, combine the yogurt with the pomegranate juice. Add the sliced bananas and blend together. Serve the smoothie in chilled tall glasses.

Serves 4

Per serving
115 kcal, 0.7 g fat (0.4 g saturated), 3.2 g protein, 25.8 g carbs (24.4 g sugar), 0.9 g fibre, 0.1 g salt

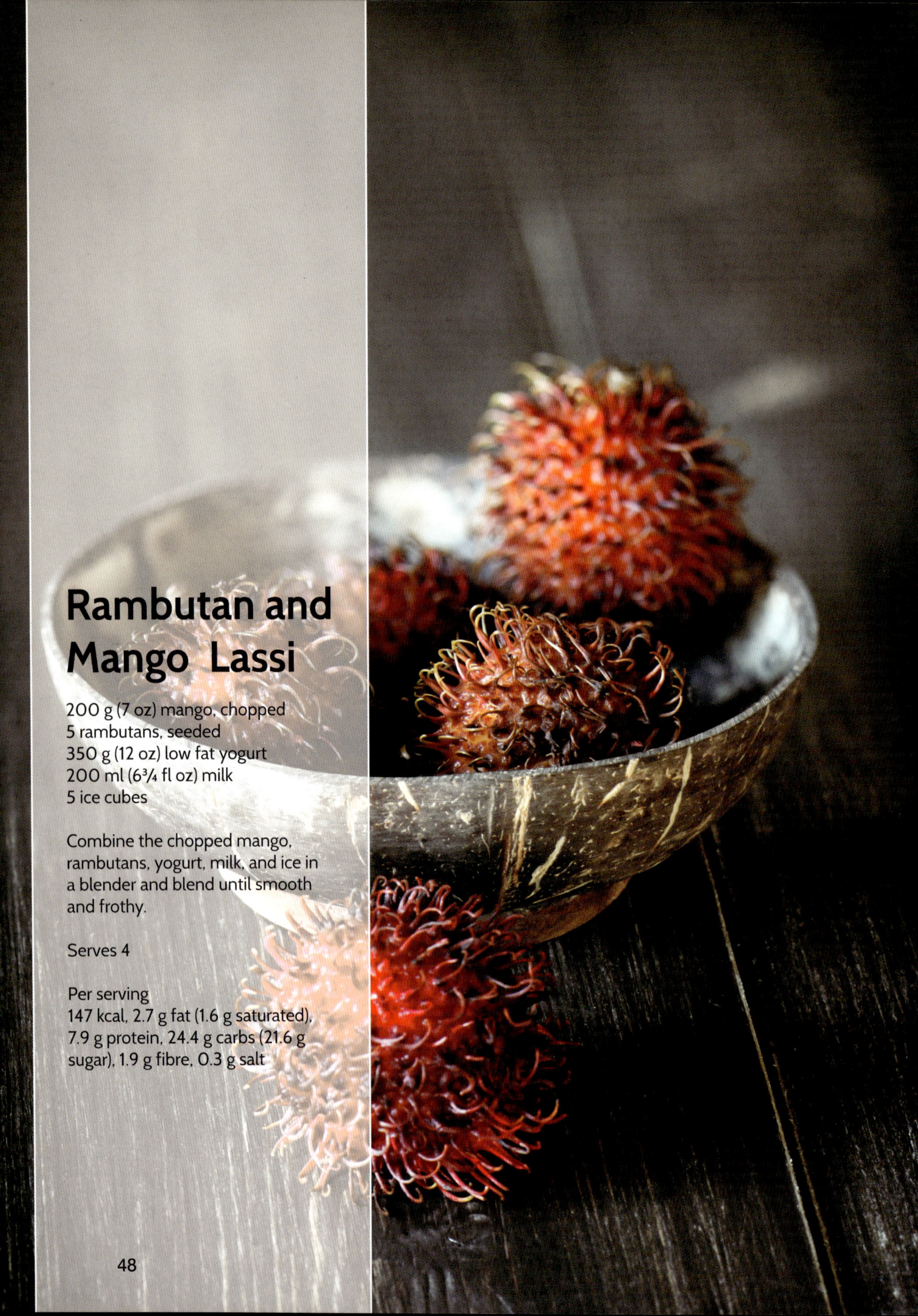

Rambutan and Mango Lassi

200 g (7 oz) mango, chopped
5 rambutans, seeded
350 g (12 oz) low fat yogurt
200 ml (6¾ fl oz) milk
5 ice cubes

Combine the chopped mango, rambutans, yogurt, milk, and ice in a blender and blend until smooth and frothy.

Serves 4

Per serving
147 kcal, 2.7 g fat (1.6 g saturated), 7.9 g protein, 24.4 g carbs (21.6 g sugar), 1.9 g fibre, 0.3 g salt

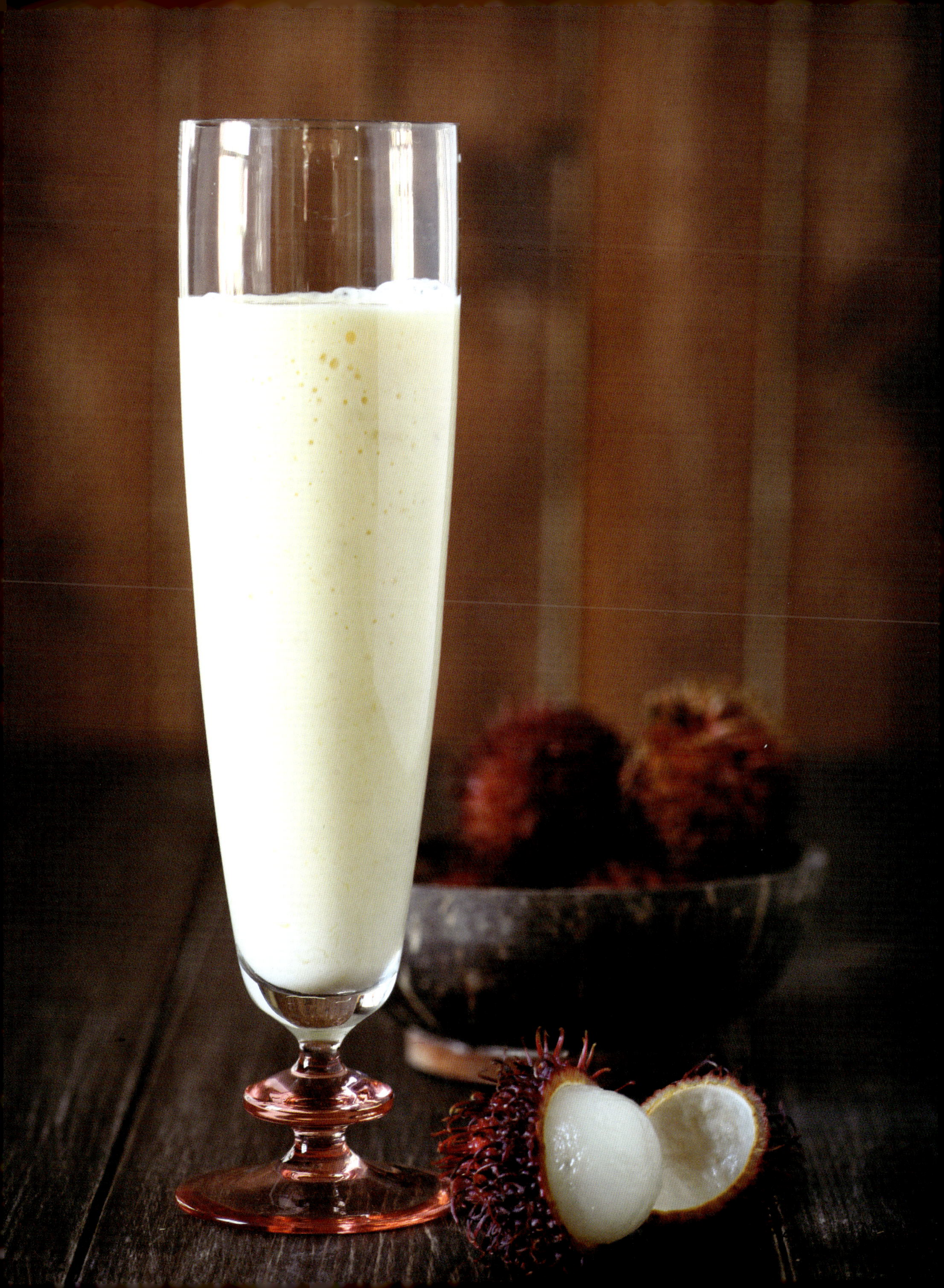

Rose Lassi

400 g (14 oz) low fat yogurt
300 ml (10 fl oz) sparkling water
2 tablespoons brown sugar
4 tablespoons rose water
½ teaspoon ground cardamom
½ teaspoon ground cinnamon
6 ice cubes

Pour the yogurt, sparkling water, sugar, rose water, ground cardamom, ground cinnamon and the ice cubes into the blender jar. Then blend until smooth and serve cold decorated with some rose petals.

Serves 4

Per serving
130 kcal, 1.0 g fat (0.7 g saturated), 4.8 g protein, 18.8 g carbs (18.8 g sugar), 0.0 g fibre, 0.2 g salt.

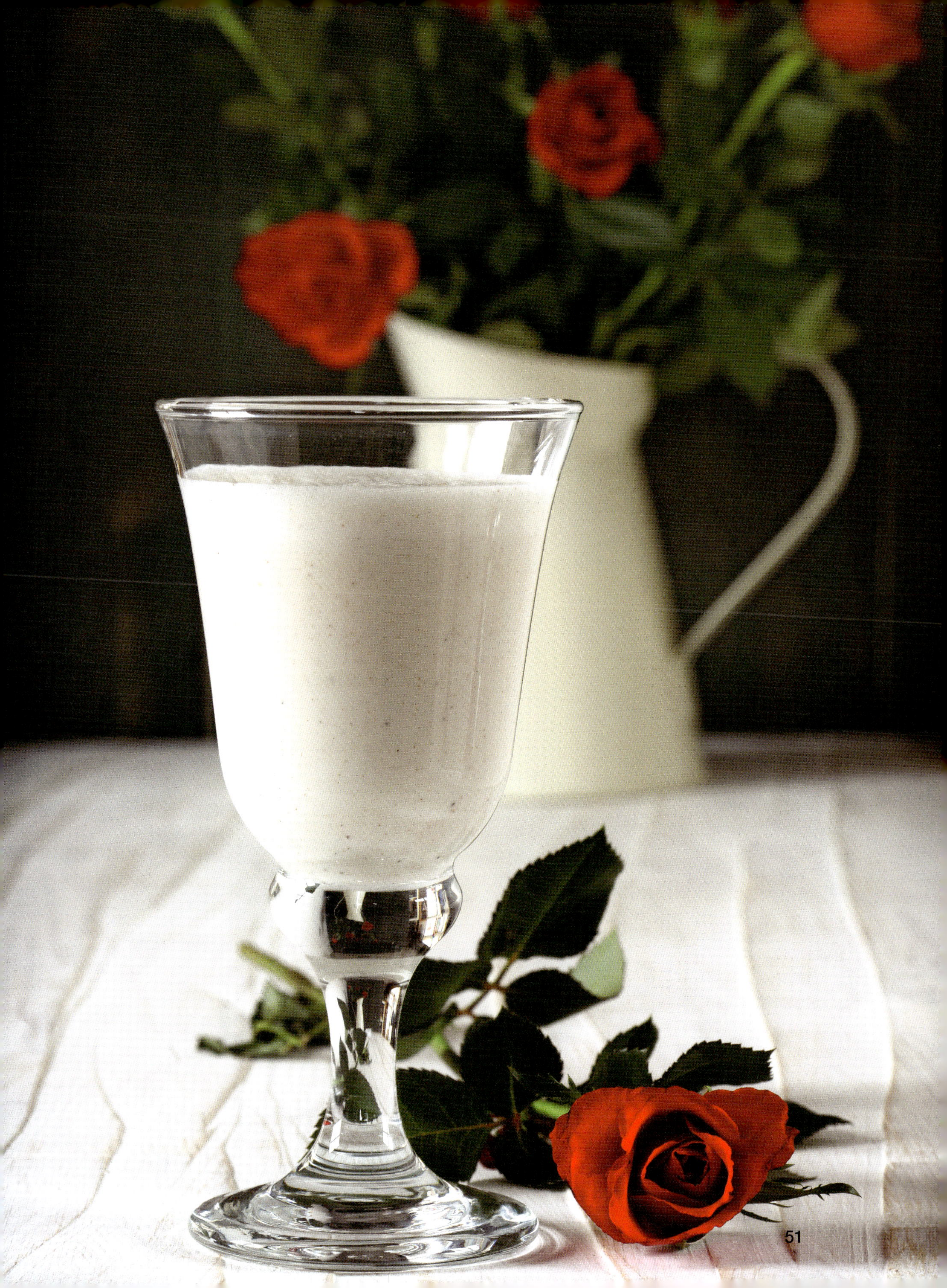

Spring Drink

150 g (5 oz) low fat yogurt
100 ml (3½ fl oz) milk
50 ml (1½ fl oz) coffee liqueur / Tia Maria (optional)
¼ teaspoon baking soda
1 teaspoon running honey
1 tablespoon lime fresh juice
1 teaspoon ground sumac
Fresh mint leaves
4 ice cubes, crushed

Pour the yogurt, milk, liqueur and honey into a medium bowl. Mix well then add the ice, lime zest and sumac and mix it again. Serve in a chilled glass decorated with fresh a fresh mint leaf.

You can swap the coffee liqueur with black coffee if is too early for alcohol!

Serves 2

Per serving
159 kcal, 1.6 g fat (1.0 g saturated), 5.6 g protein, 17.8 g carbs (17.3 g sugar), 0.1 g fibre, 0.3 g fat

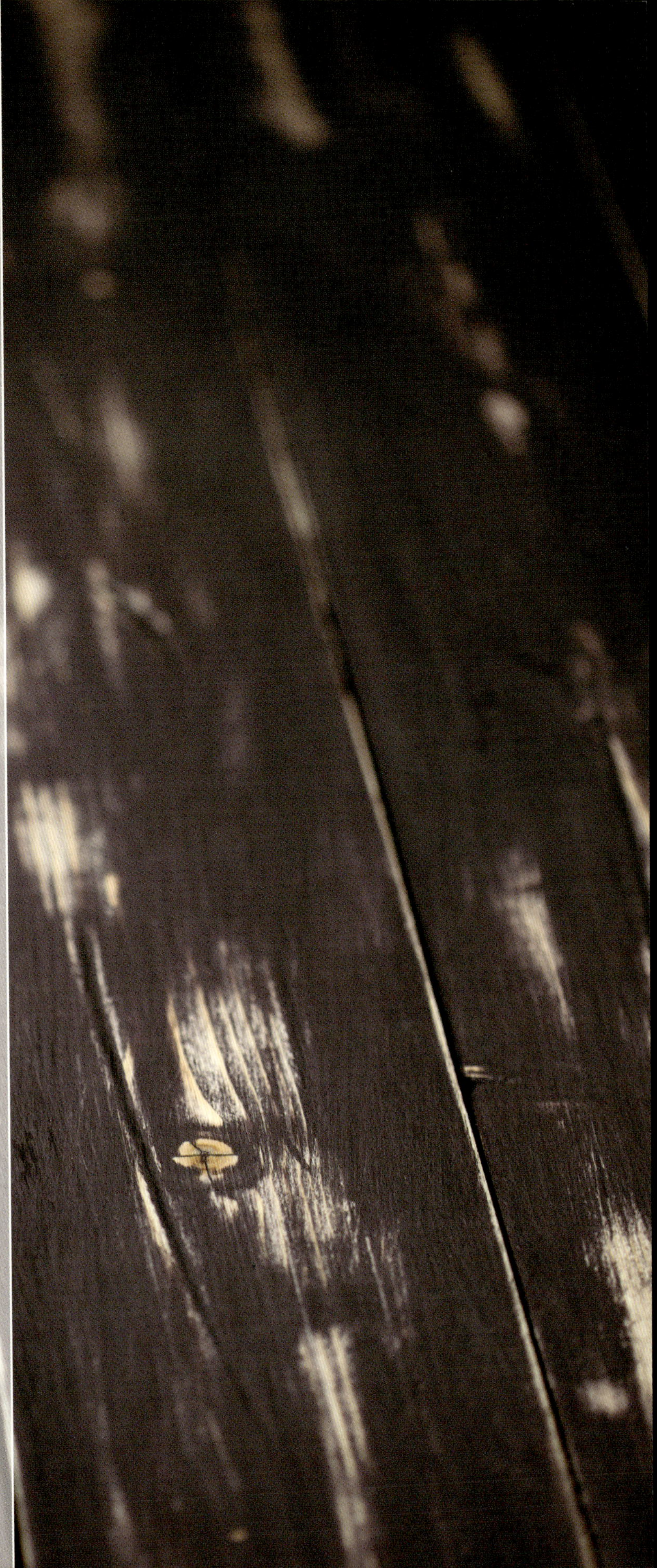

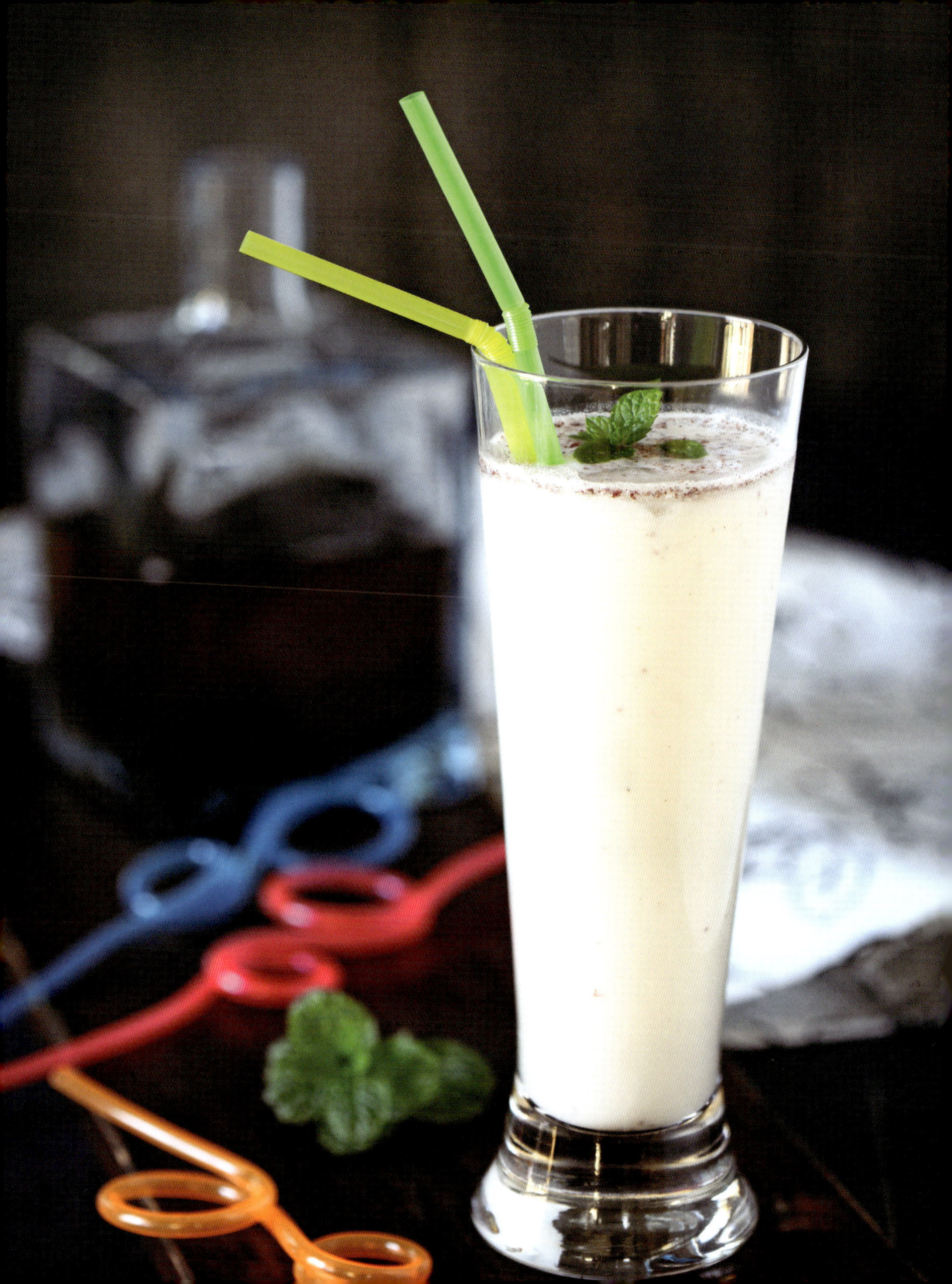

Yogurt Coffee

200 g (7 oz) low fat yogurt
100 ml (3½ fl oz) semi-skimmed milk
1 tablespoon honey
1 teaspoon cinnamon powder
1 teaspoon instant coffee powder
1 tablespoon ground almonds
½ teaspoon vanilla flavoring
2 ice cubes

Combine the yogurt, milk, honey, cinnamon, coffee, ground almonds, vanilla flavoring and ice cubes in the blender. Blend until smooth and frothy.

This is a very tasty and refreshing drink. For late afternoons, I sometimes swap the vanilla flavoring with 50 ml (1½ fl oz) cognac.

Serves 2

Per serving
175 kcal, 7.5 g fat (1.6 g saturated), 8.8 g protein, 19.7 g carbs (19.4 g sugar), 1.2 g fibre, 0.2 g salt

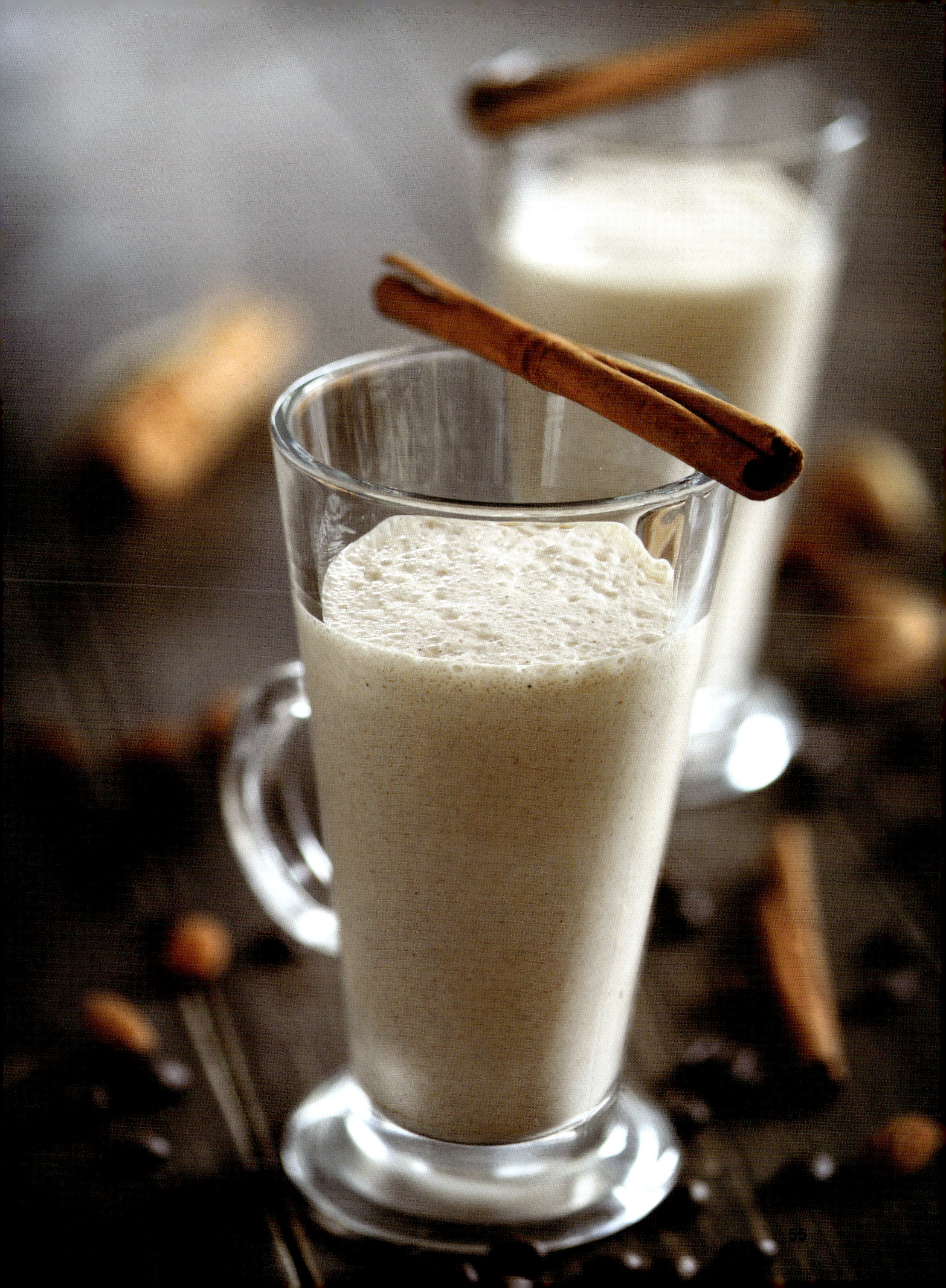

Parsley Yogurt Drink

250 g (9 oz) low fat yogurt
1 pink lady apple, peeled, cored and chopped
1 bunch of fresh parsley, (about 50 g/ 2 oz), stems and leaves finely chopped
2 celery stalks, chopped
fresh squeezed juice of 1 lime,
2 tablespoons honey
6 ice cubes
200 ml (6¾ fl oz) mineral water

Pour the yogurt into a blender and add the chopped apple, parsley, celery, lime juice, honey, ice cubes and mineral water. Blend for about 2 minutes until smooth. Serve cold!

Serves 4

Per serving
86 kcal, 0.8 g fat (0.4 g saturated), 3.6 g protein, 17.0 g carbs (17.0 g sugar), 1.6 g fibre, 0.1 g salt

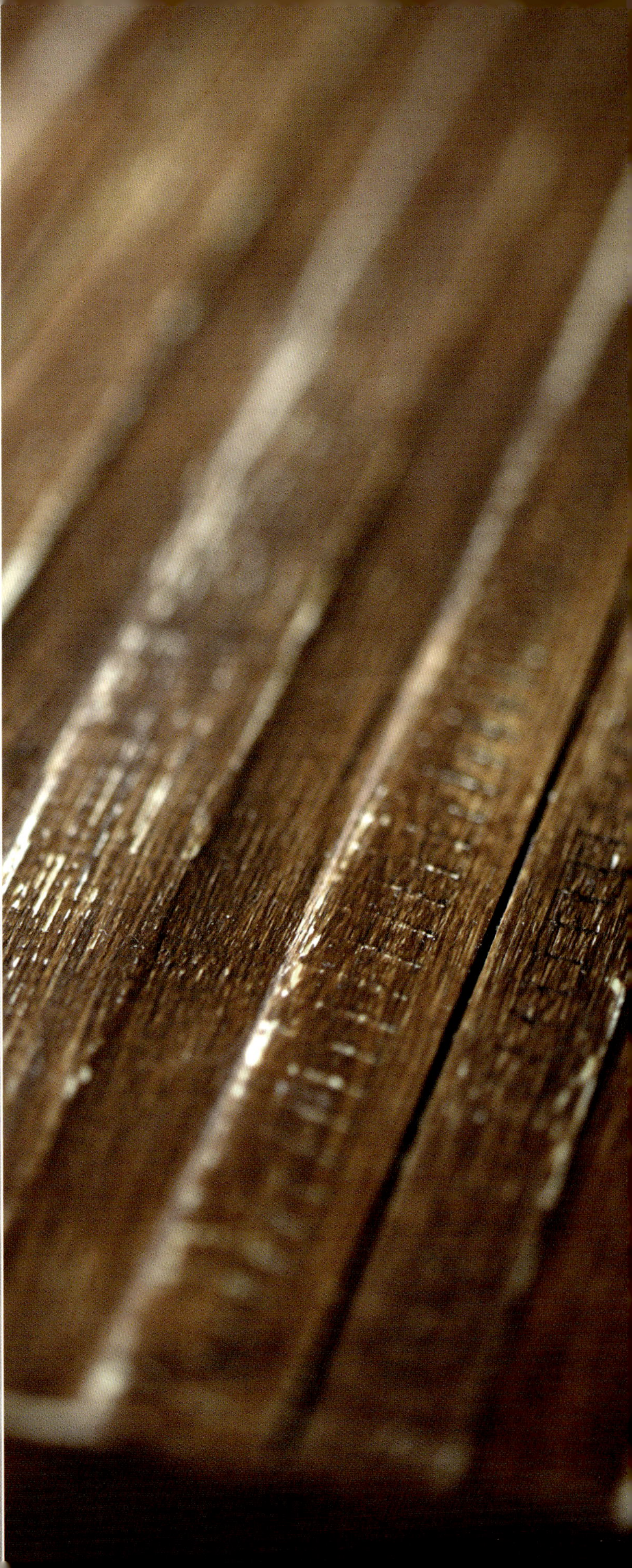

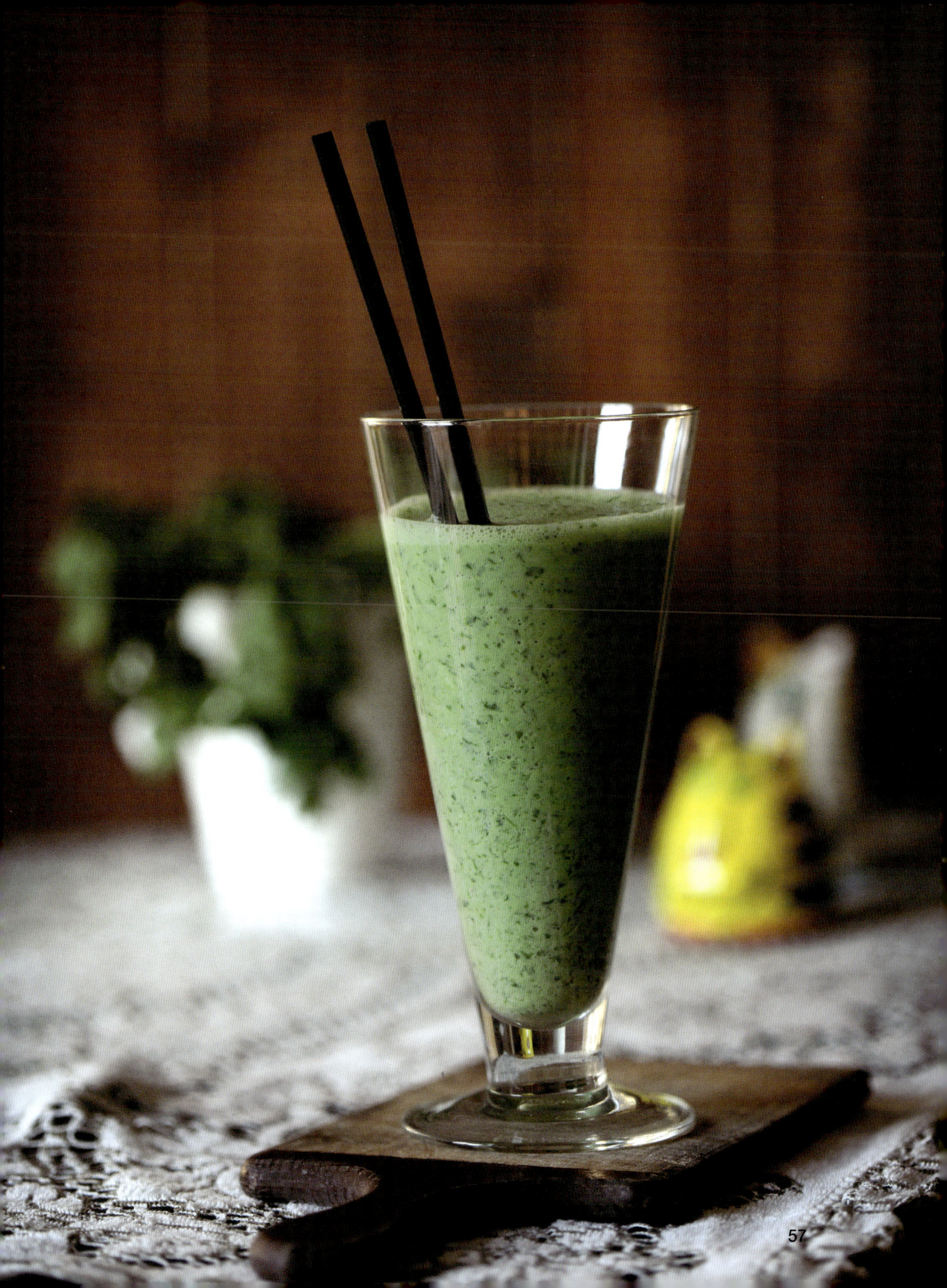

Pak Choi Yogurt Smoothie

2 small stalks pak choi
1 green apple, peeled, seeded and diced
1 banana, peeled and chopped
½ lemon, freshly squeezed juice
5 drops rum flavoring
5 ice cubes
250 g (9 oz) low fat yogurt
100 ml (3½ fl oz) semi-skimmed milk

Pour the semi-skimmed milk into the blender and add the yogurt, apple, pak choi, banana, lemon juice, ice cubes and rum flavoring. Then blend until smooth - about five minutes. Serve cold.

Serves 4

Per serving
80 kcal, 1 g fat (1 g saturated), 4 g protein, 14 g carbs (13 g sugar), 0.9 g fibre, 0.1 g salt

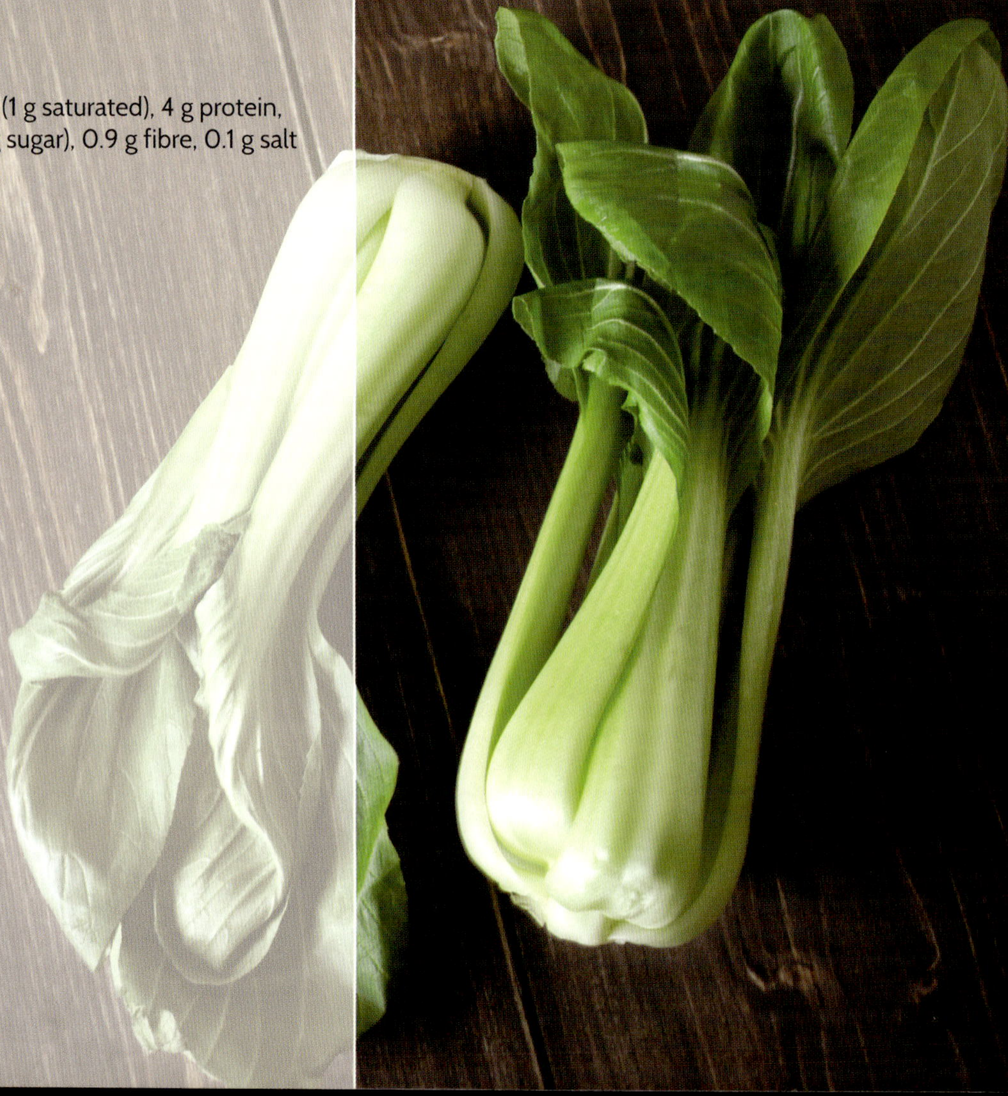

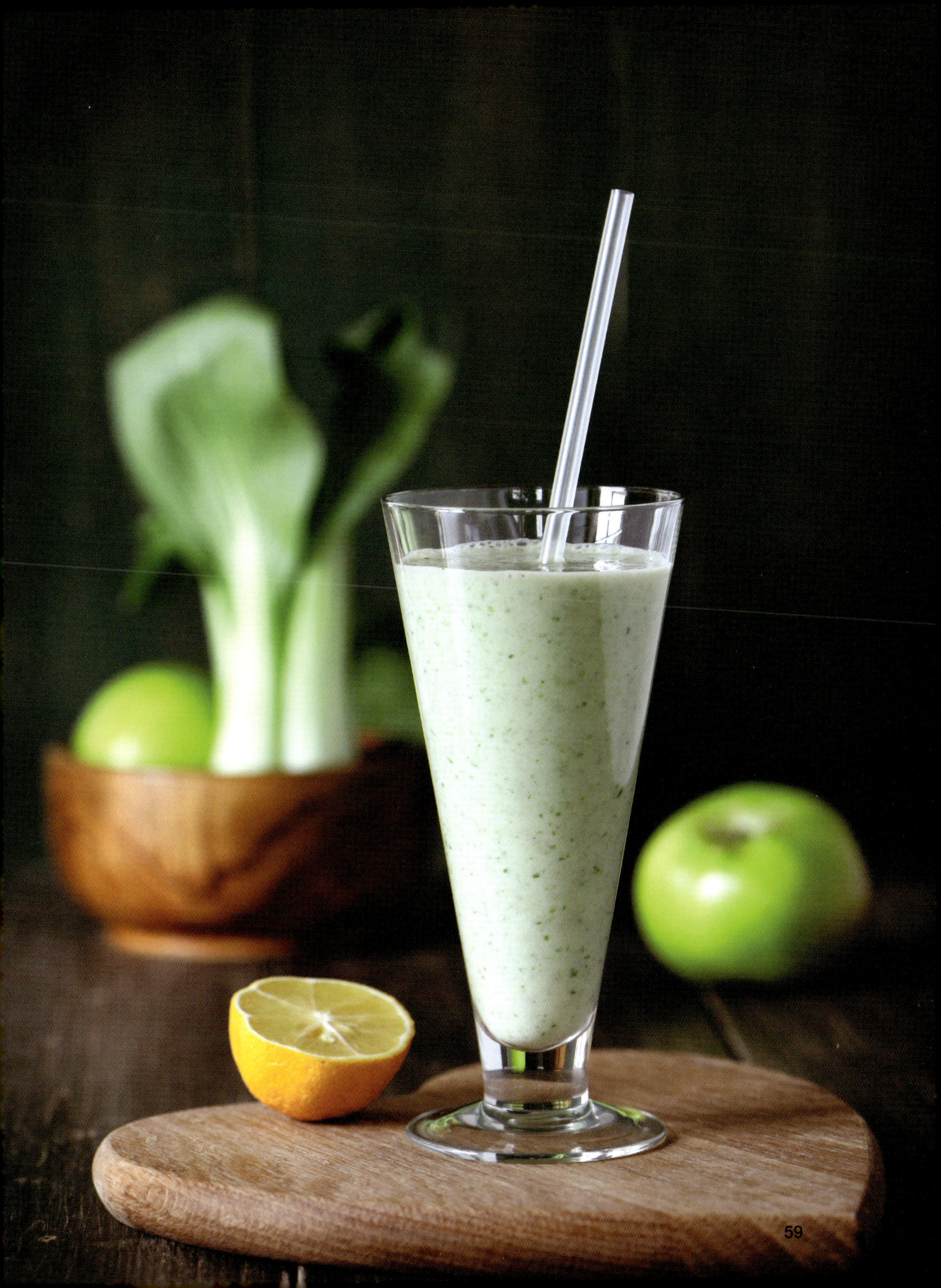

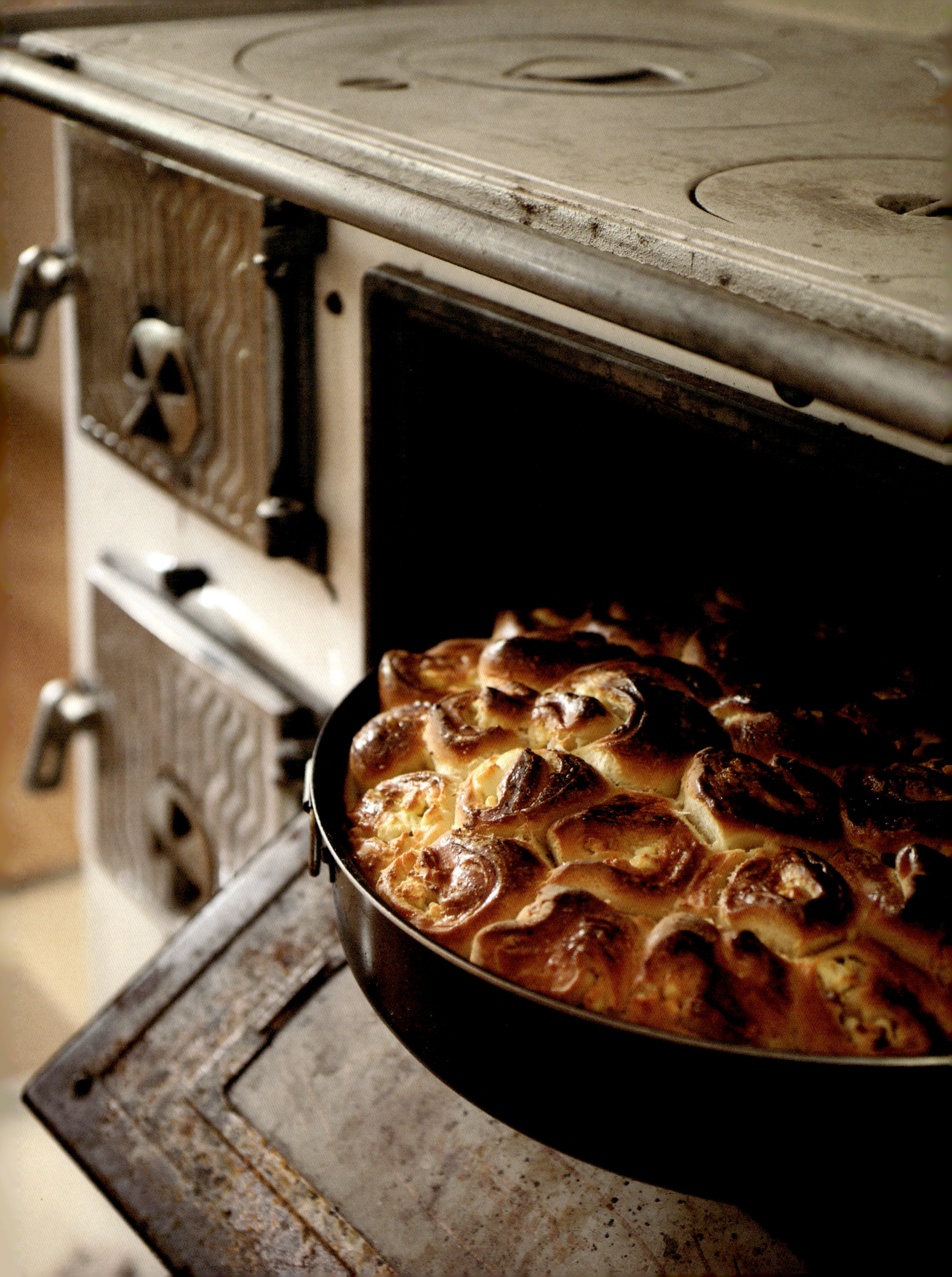

Bake and Breakfast

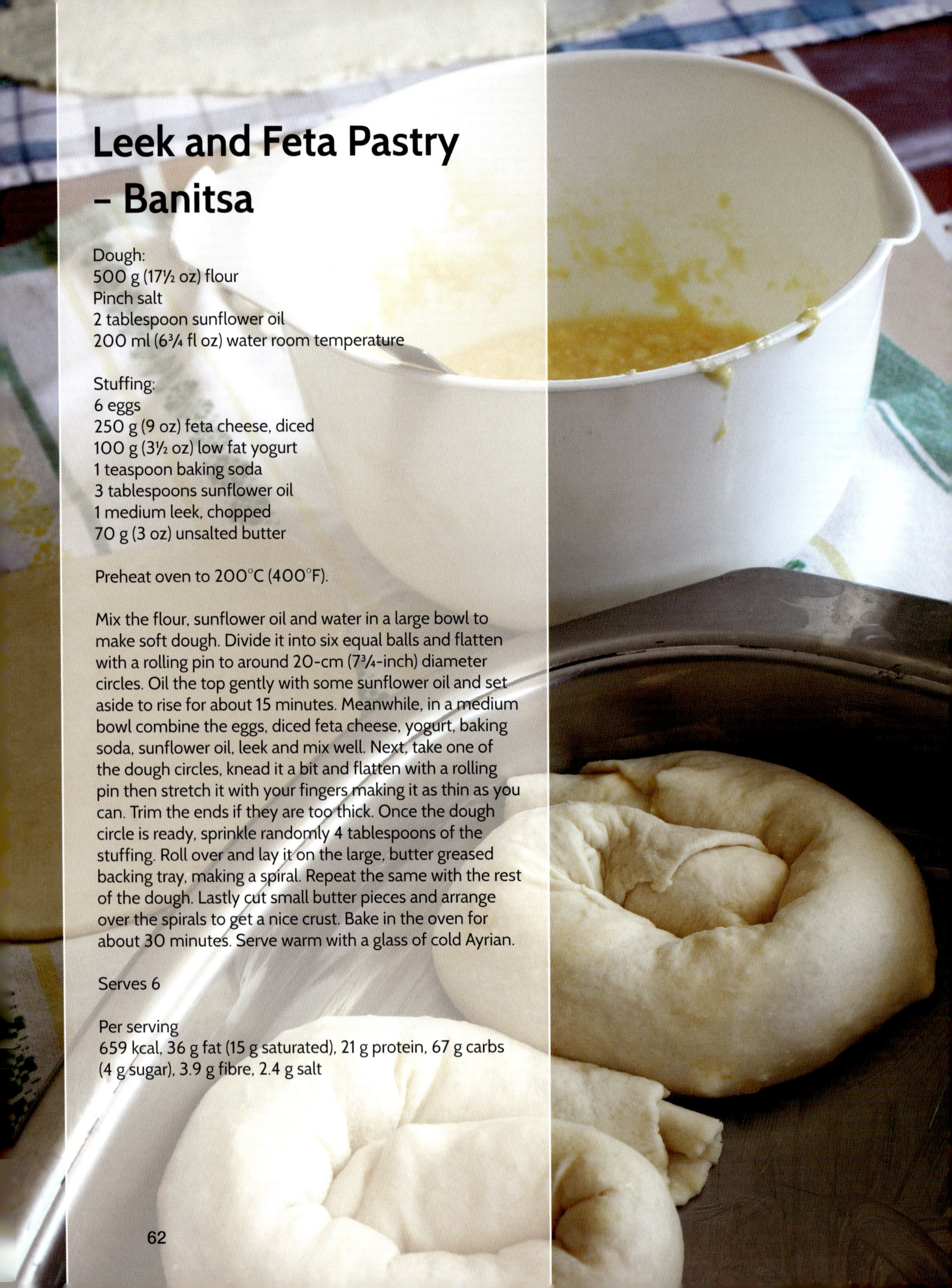

Leek and Feta Pastry – Banitsa

Dough:
500 g (17½ oz) flour
Pinch salt
2 tablespoon sunflower oil
200 ml (6¾ fl oz) water room temperature

Stuffing:
6 eggs
250 g (9 oz) feta cheese, diced
100 g (3½ oz) low fat yogurt
1 teaspoon baking soda
3 tablespoons sunflower oil
1 medium leek, chopped
70 g (3 oz) unsalted butter

Preheat oven to 200°C (400°F).

Mix the flour, sunflower oil and water in a large bowl to make soft dough. Divide it into six equal balls and flatten with a rolling pin to around 20-cm (7¾-inch) diameter circles. Oil the top gently with some sunflower oil and set aside to rise for about 15 minutes. Meanwhile, in a medium bowl combine the eggs, diced feta cheese, yogurt, baking soda, sunflower oil, leek and mix well. Next, take one of the dough circles, knead it a bit and flatten with a rolling pin then stretch it with your fingers making it as thin as you can. Trim the ends if they are too thick. Once the dough circle is ready, sprinkle randomly 4 tablespoons of the stuffing. Roll over and lay it on the large, butter greased backing tray, making a spiral. Repeat the same with the rest of the dough. Lastly cut small butter pieces and arrange over the spirals to get a nice crust. Bake in the oven for about 30 minutes. Serve warm with a glass of cold Ayrian.

Serves 6

Per serving
659 kcal, 36 g fat (15 g saturated), 21 g protein, 67 g carbs (4 g sugar), 3.9 g fibre, 2.4 g salt

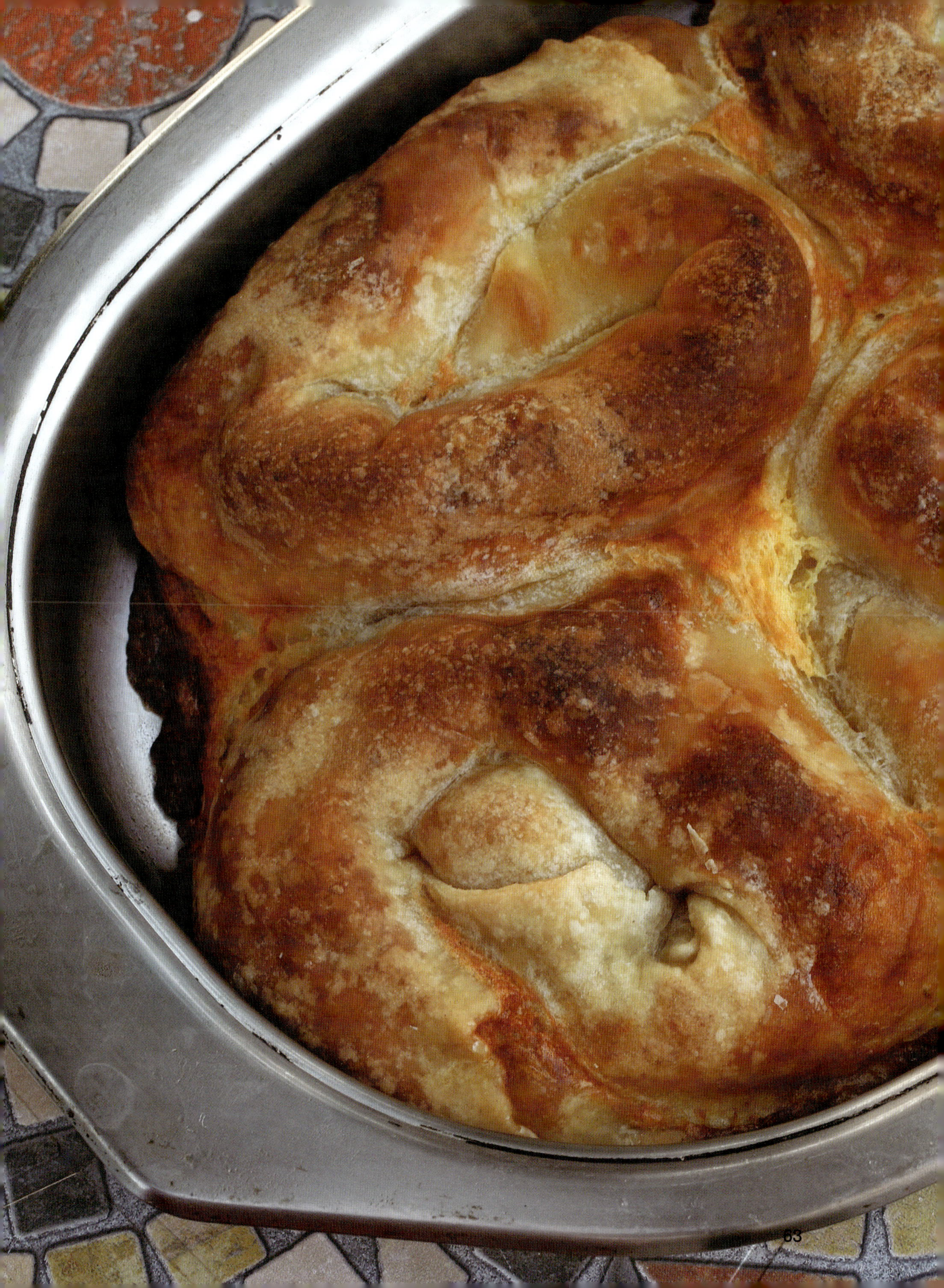

Strandja Bread Balls

200 g (7 oz) low fat yogurt
200 g (7 oz) feta cheese, finely crushed
1 teaspoon, baking soda
350 g (12 oz) wholemeal flour
70 g (3 oz) butter, melted
1 teaspoon caraway seeds
1 tablespoon linseeds seeds
1 teaspoon poppy seeds
1 egg yolk

Preheat the oven 180-200°C (350-400°F). Squash the feta cheese in a large bowl using a fork then add the yogurt and melted butter and mix well. Next add the wholemeal flour, baking soda, caraway seeds, linseeds and make a dough. Divide the dough into 6 balls and arrange them on a parchment-lined baking tray. Meanwhile, whisk the yolk of 1 egg and using a kitchen brush smear the egg yolk over the balls and sprinkle some poppy seeds on top. Bake in the oven for about 20 minutes until golden. Once baked, leave them to rest for another 15 minutes out of oven covered with kitchen towel.

Serves 6

Per serving
391 kcal, 20.3 g fat (11.4 g saturated), 15.5 g protein, 40.6 g carbs (4.3 g sugar), 7.5 g fibre, 1.6 g salt

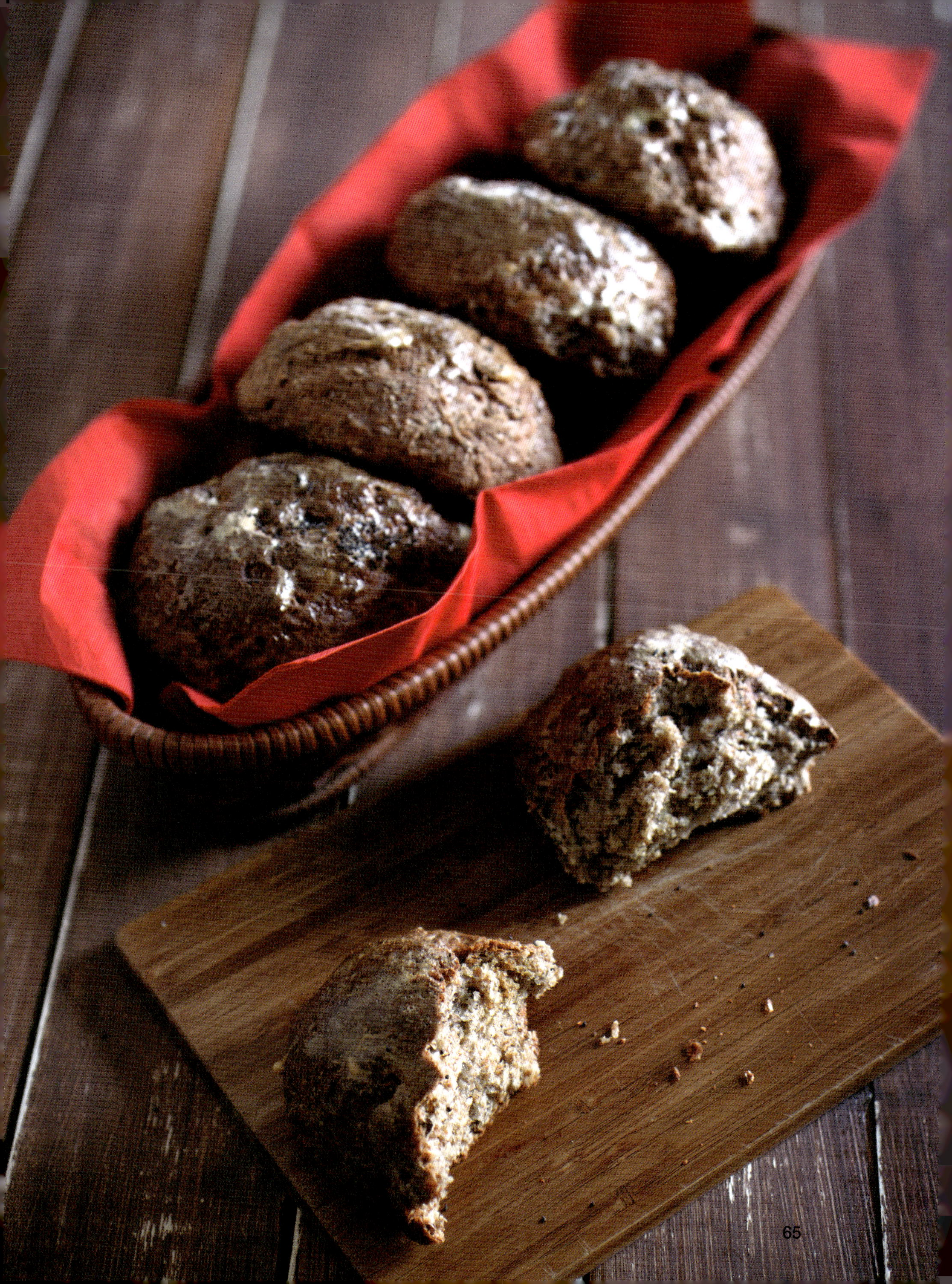

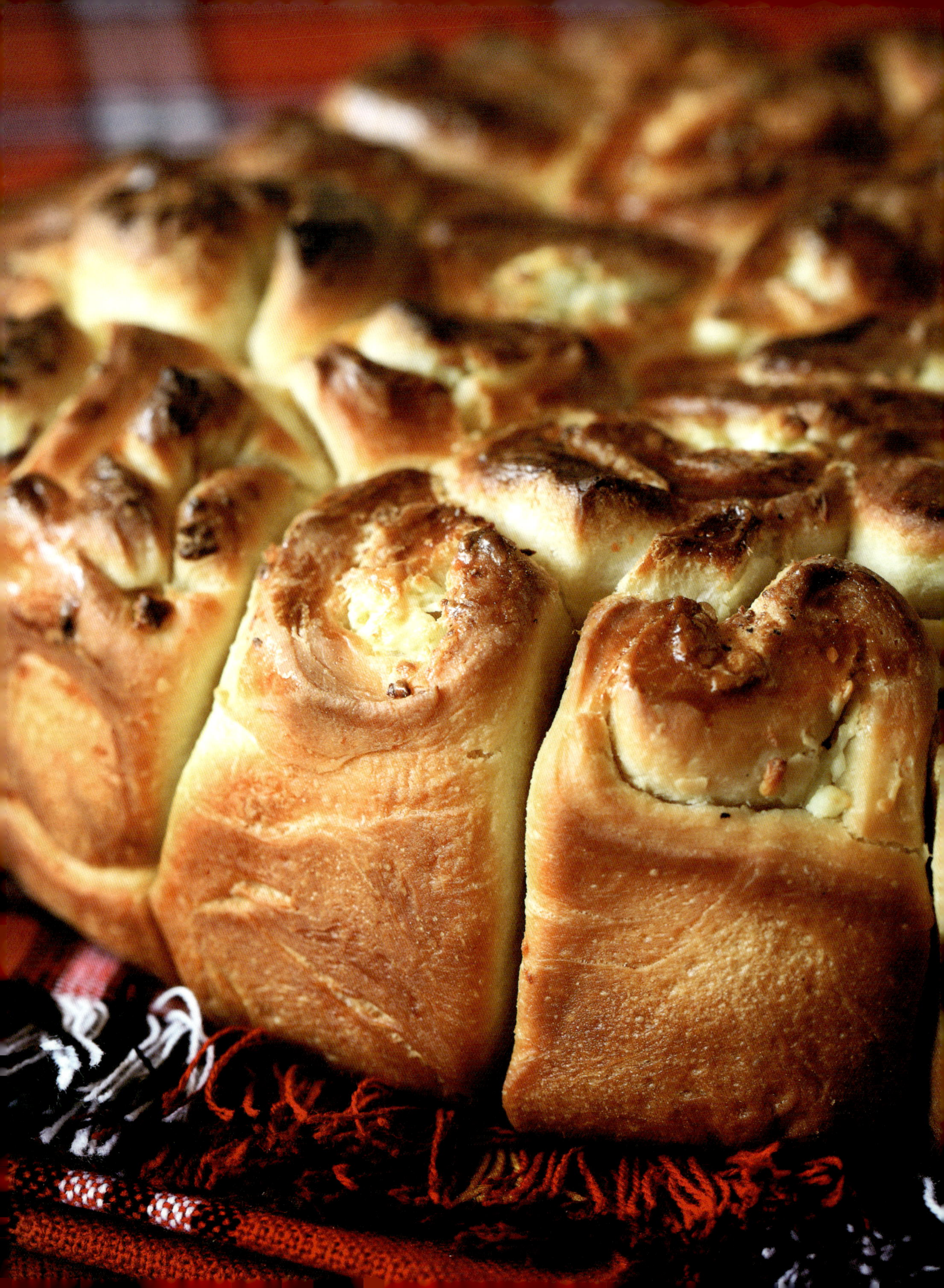

Festive Sunny Bread

400 g (14 oz) low fat yogurt
1 teaspoon baking soda
4 eggs
2 teaspoon dry yeast
1 tablespoon salt
1 teaspoon sugar
350 g (12 oz) room temperature water
150 g (5 oz) butter
400 g (14 oz) feta cheese, diced
1.5 kg (3.3 lb) wheat flour

Preheat the oven to 150-180°C (300-350°F). In a medium bowl mix together the yogurt and the baking soda. Leave to rest for a few minutes while you separate the yolk from the white of one egg. Put the egg yolk into a small glass for finishing egg wash and set aside.
To make the dough, dissolve 2 teaspoons of dry yeast in 100ml (3½ fl oz) of warm water and put aside. Put 1 kg (2.2 lb) wheat flour in a large baking tray and add salt, sugar and the dissolved yeast and mix well. Next add the rest of the eggs and the white of the one already separated from the yolk and mix well. Then add the yogurt mixture, mix again and knead to make a soft dough. Lay the dough on a chopping board, cover with kitchen towel and leave to rise for 30 minutes in a warm place at 25-30°C (75-80°F).
Knead the dough, adding about 300 g (10½ oz) more flour to make a soft non-sticky dough. Separate the dough into 5 similar balls, cover with kitchen towel and leave them to rise again for another 30 minutes at 25-30°C (75-80°F). Then roll out with a rolling pin each ball to make a long rectangle base around 5 mm (¼ inch) thick, 15 cm (6 inches) wide and 30 cm (12 inches) long. Grease the dough base with soft butter and sprinkle over some diced feta cheese. Then roll over the base to make 30 cm (12 inch) long roll and cut it in 5 cm (2-inch) pieces. Grease a large backing tray with soft butter and arrange the pieces in a sun shape. Cover with kitchen towel once again and leave to rise for another 30 minutes in a warm place at 25-30°C (75-80°F). Once it has risen, quickly and gently brush the egg wash over the top and bake in the oven for 30 minutes.

Serves 12 or more

Per serving
657 kcal, 21.4 g fat (12.5 g saturated), 21.2 g protein, 100.9 g carbs (5.5 g sugar), 5.2 g fibre, 2.9 g salt

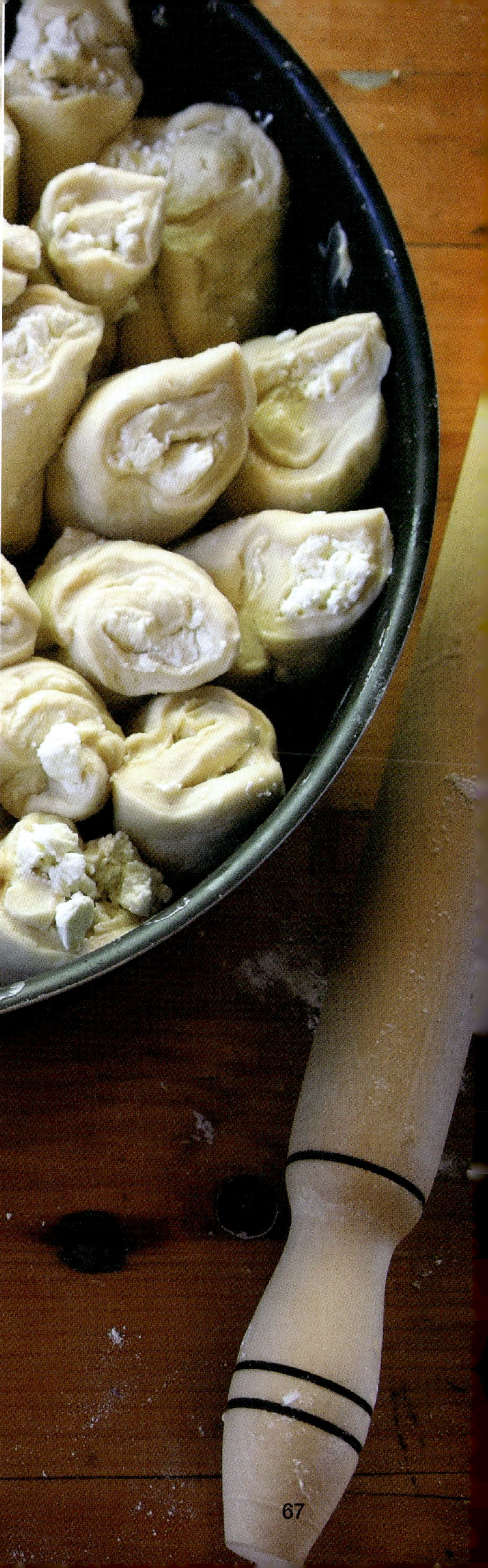

Monkey Bread

100 g (3½ oz) low fat yogurt
2 ripe bananas, peeled
1 orange, peeled
70 ml (2¼ fl oz) sunflower oil
2 eggs
300 g (10½ oz) wholemeal flour
30 g (1 oz) sesame seeds
30 g (1 oz) linseeds
1 teaspoon baking powder
2 teaspoons baking soda
1 teaspoon cinnamon, grounded
1 teaspoon ginger, grounded
1 teaspoon nutmeg, grounded

Preheat oven to 180°C (350°F). Throw into a blender the peeled orange and bananas and blend until smooth. Then pour in the yogurt, sunflower oil and add the eggs and blend again to remove any bits. Set aside for a moment. Meanwhile in a large bowl combine the wholemeal flour, sesame seeds, lean seeds, baking powder, backing soda, cinnamon, ginger, nutmeg and mix well. Then pour in the banana yogurt mixture and mix well again. Oil the inside of a bread-baking tin 10 x 26 x 6 cm (4 x 10 x 3 inches) and pour the mixture in. Finally sprinkle some sesame seeds over and bake the monkey bread in the oven for about 45 minutes. Once ready remove from the oven, take it out of the baking tin and cover with a kitchen towel for about 15 minutes to rest. The monkey bread is ready to be sliced and served.

Serves 8

Per serving
300 kcal, 15.7 g fat (2.3 g saturated), 10.2 g protein, 31.2 g carbs (7.1 g sugar), 6.3 g fibre, 0.6 g salt

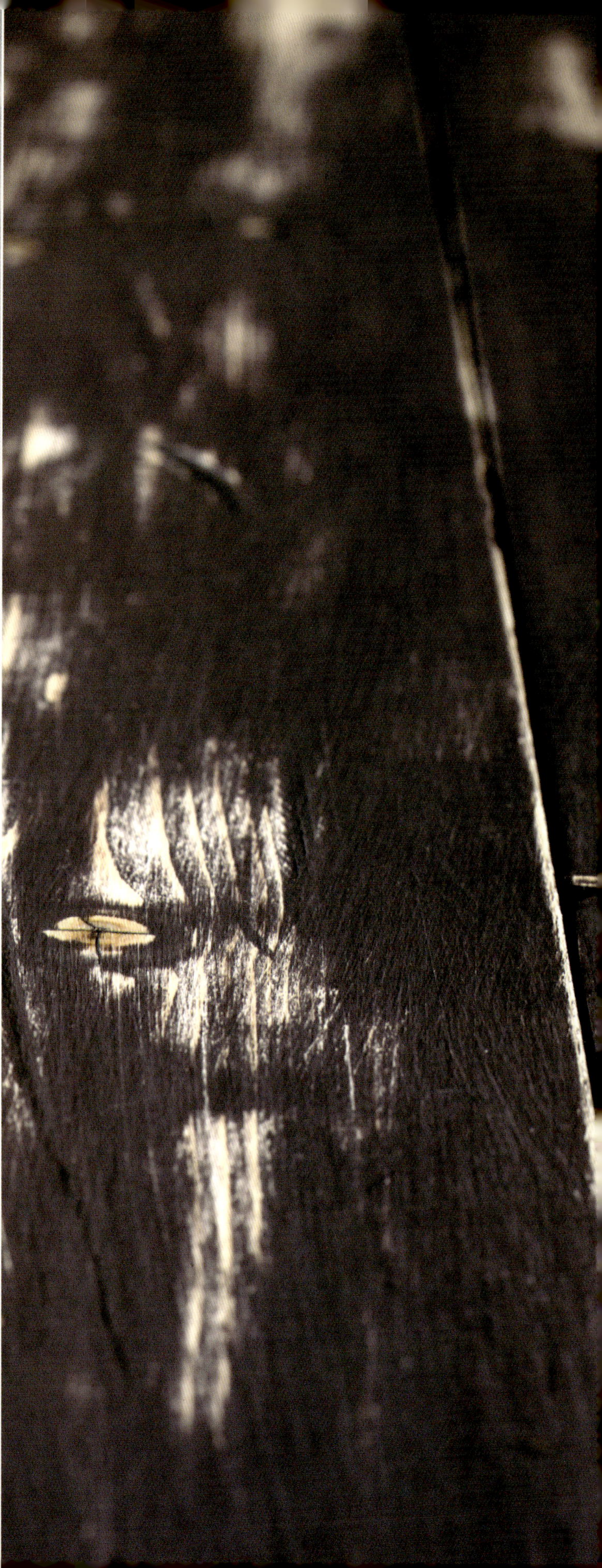

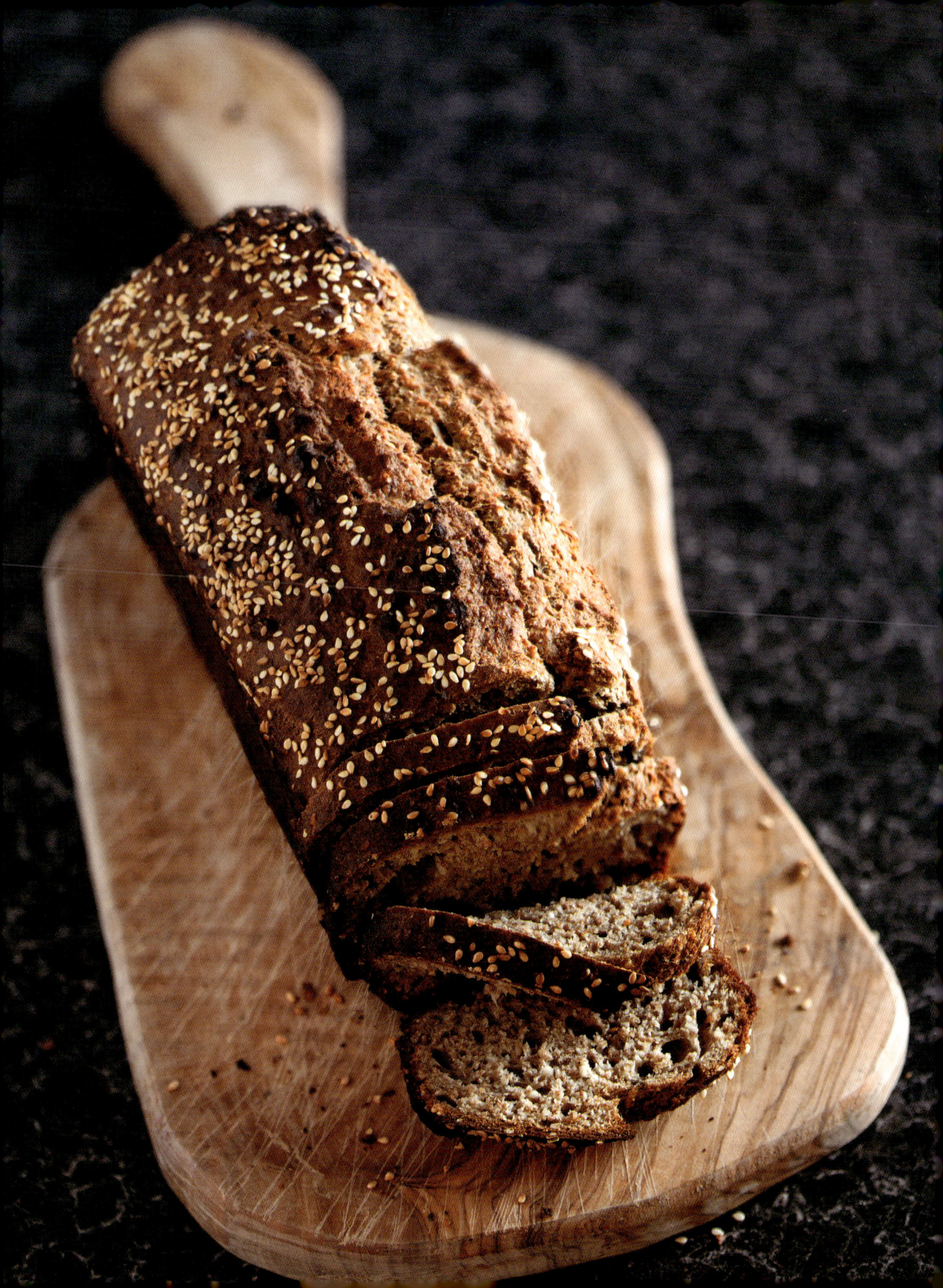

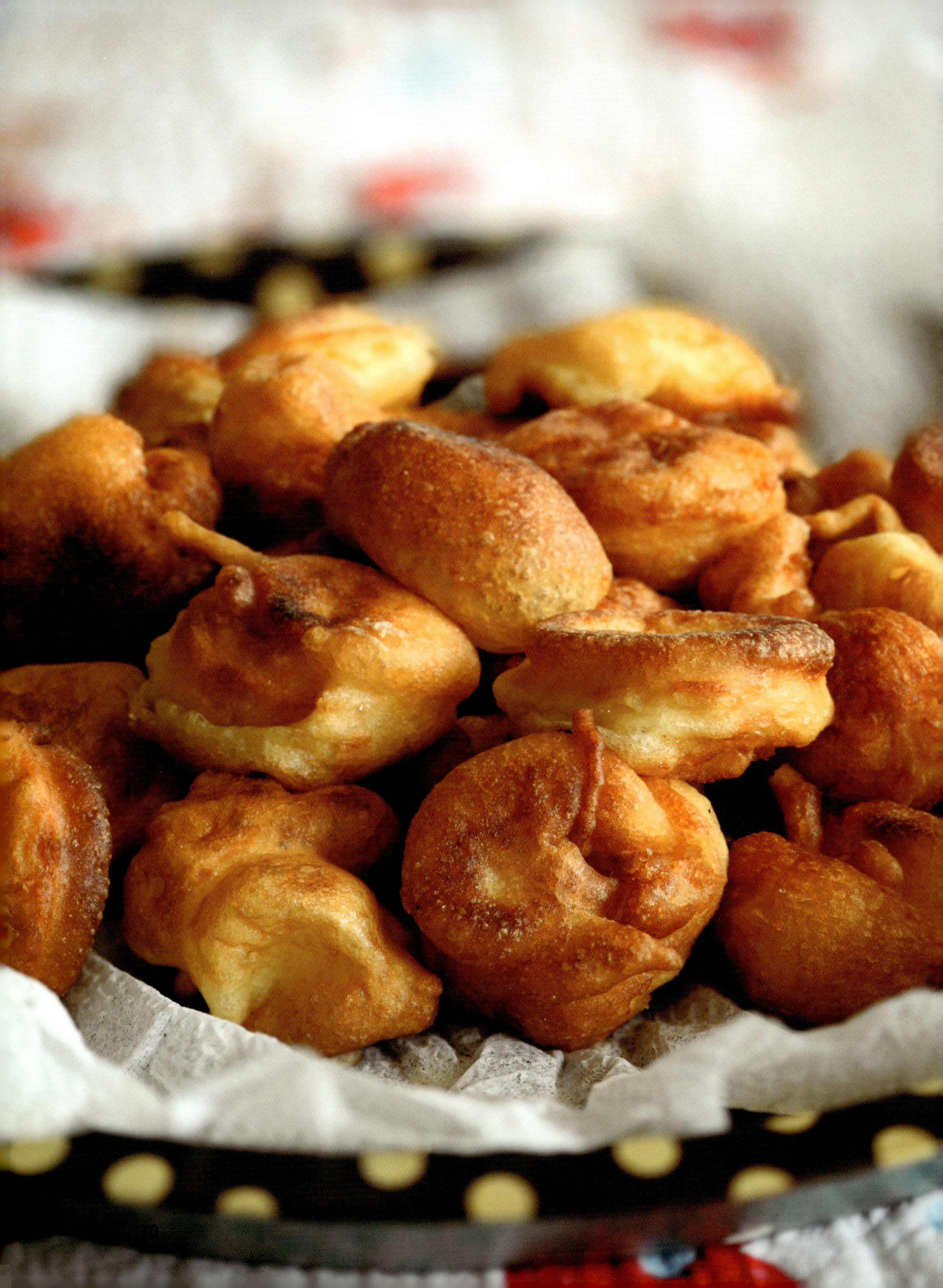

Yogurt Puffs
Buhti

200 g (7 oz) yogurt
3 eggs
50 ml (1½ fl oz) olive oil
1 teaspoon baking soda
200 g (7 oz) flour
½ teaspoon cardamom, grounded
pinch of salt
200 ml (6¾ fl oz) vegetable oil for frying

Whip the eggs with yogurt and olive oil in a small bowl and set aside. In a large bowl combine the flour, baking soda, ground cardamom, pinch of salt and mix well. Add the yogurt mixture to the flour and beat the mixture well. Preheat the oil to a medium heat and drop a tablespoon of the prepared mixture into the hot oil in batches and fry for about 2 minutes, or until golden. Remember to turn them over in the pan to cook both sides. They will rise on top of the oil and puff up. Once ready, remove from the oil and leave to drain on kitchen paper. Serve warm with some icing sugar on top or honey or even melted chocolate.

Serves 6

Per serving
552 kcal, 45.8 g fat (6.6 g saturated), 8.2 g protein, 28.8 g carbs (3.1 g sugar), 1.4 g fibre, 1.1 g salt

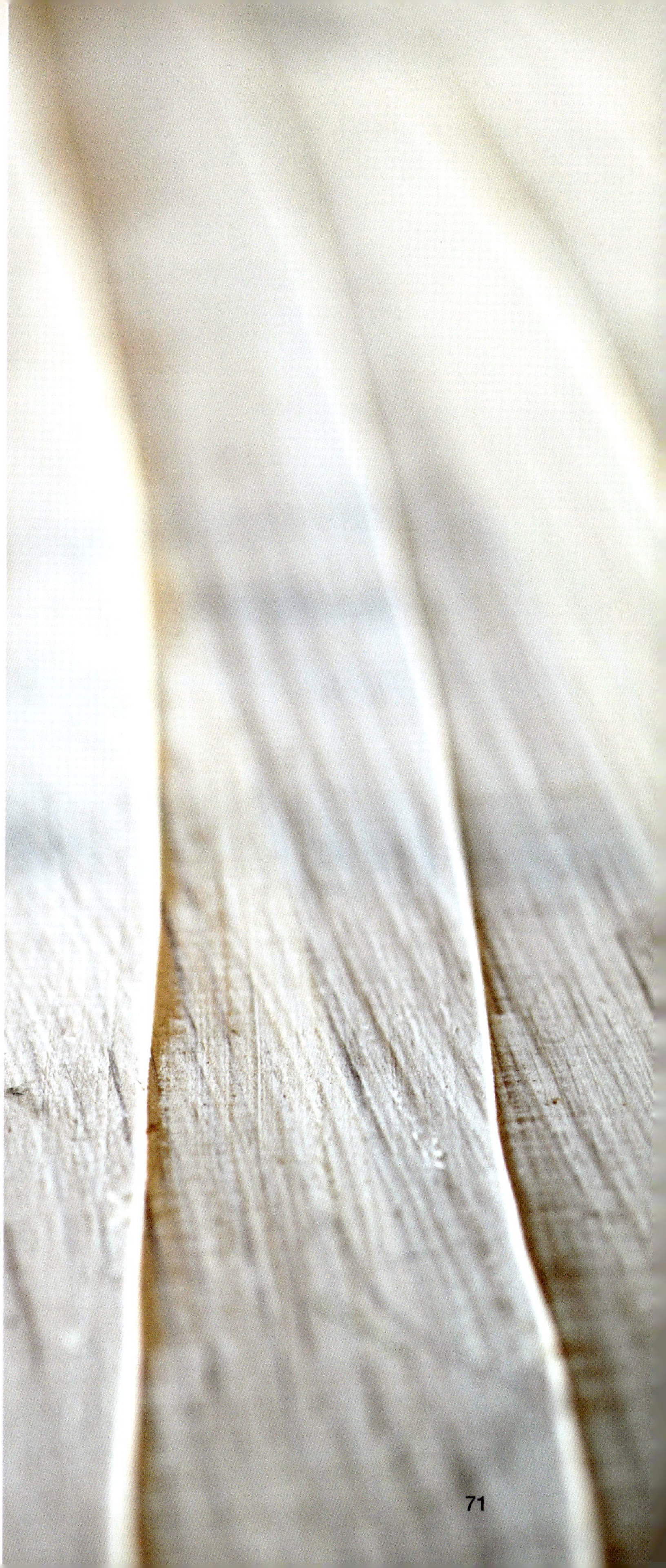

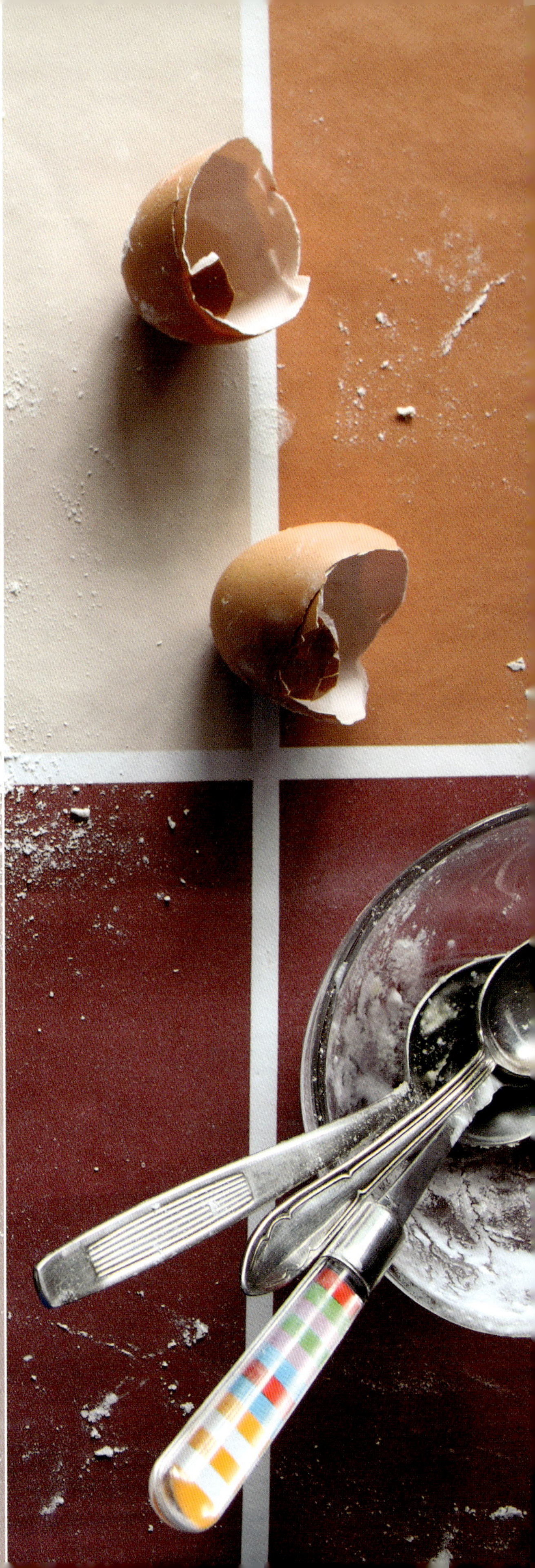

Fried Dough Pastry Mekitzi

500 g (17½ oz) flour
400 g (14 oz) low fat yogurt
2 eggs
50 ml (1½ fl oz) olive oil
1 teaspoon baking soda
pinch of salt
200 ml (6¾ fl oz) vegetable oil for frying

Beat the eggs, yogurt and olive oil together in a small bowl and set aside. In a large bowl combine the flour, baking soda, and a pinch of salt and mix well. Next gradually stir in the yogurt and eggs mixture to the flour until a dough is formed. Allow the dough to rest for about 2 hours at room temperature or overnight in the refrigerator. Once ready, knead the dough again and divide it into balls, the size of an egg. Stretch the balls with your fingers to make a circle piece no more than 2mm thick and about 14 cm (5½ inches) diameter. Preheat the oil on medium heat. Deep fry the dough in hot oil until golden on both sides for about 2 minutes. Then remove from the oil and leave to drain on kitchen paper. Serve warm together with any marmalade or, as I prefer, with some feta cheese and honey.

Serves 6

Per serving
722 kcal, 45.2 g fat (6.2 g saturated), 13.2 g protein, 70.0 g carbs (6.2 g sugar), 3.4 g fibre, 1.1 g salt

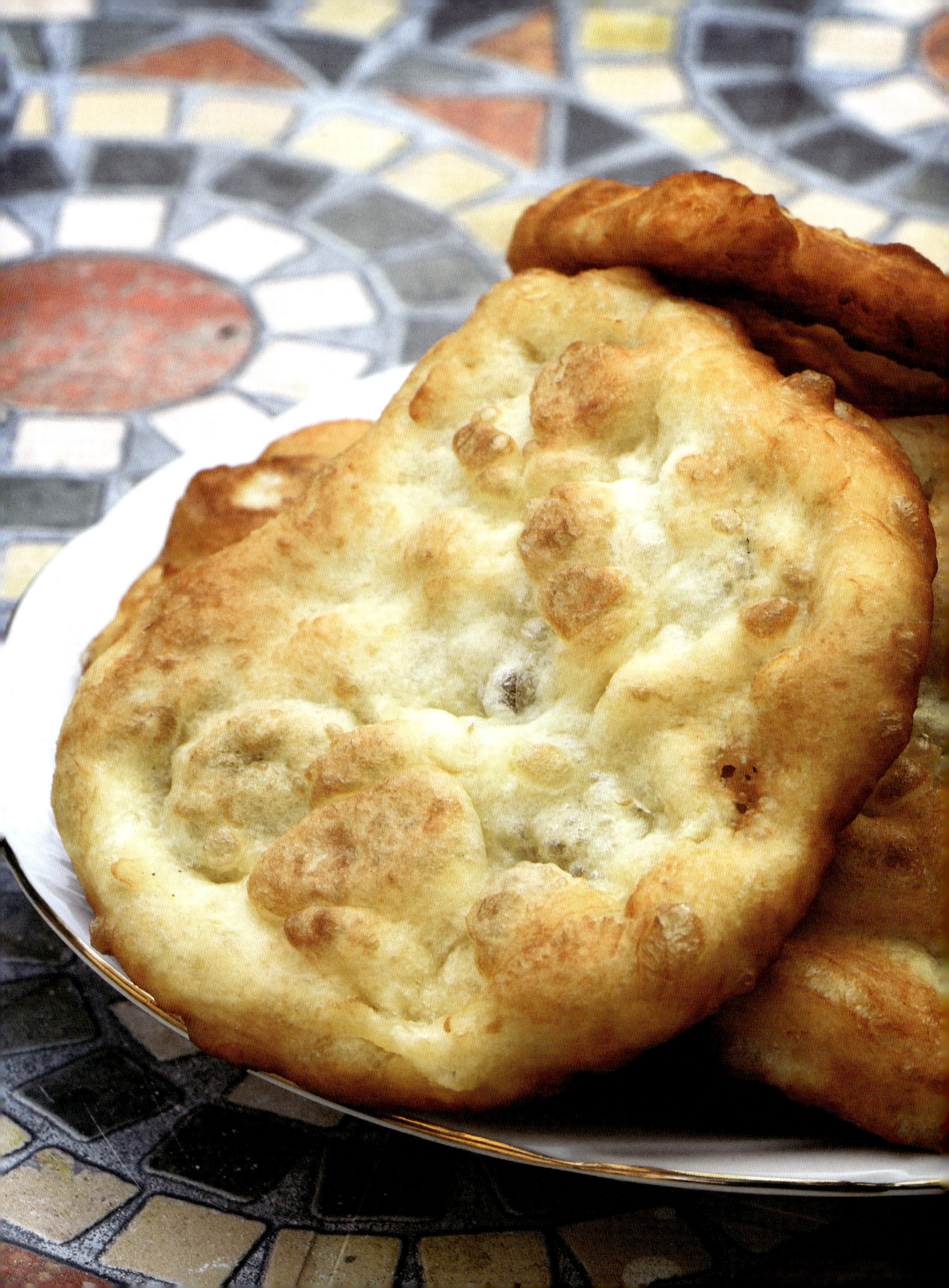

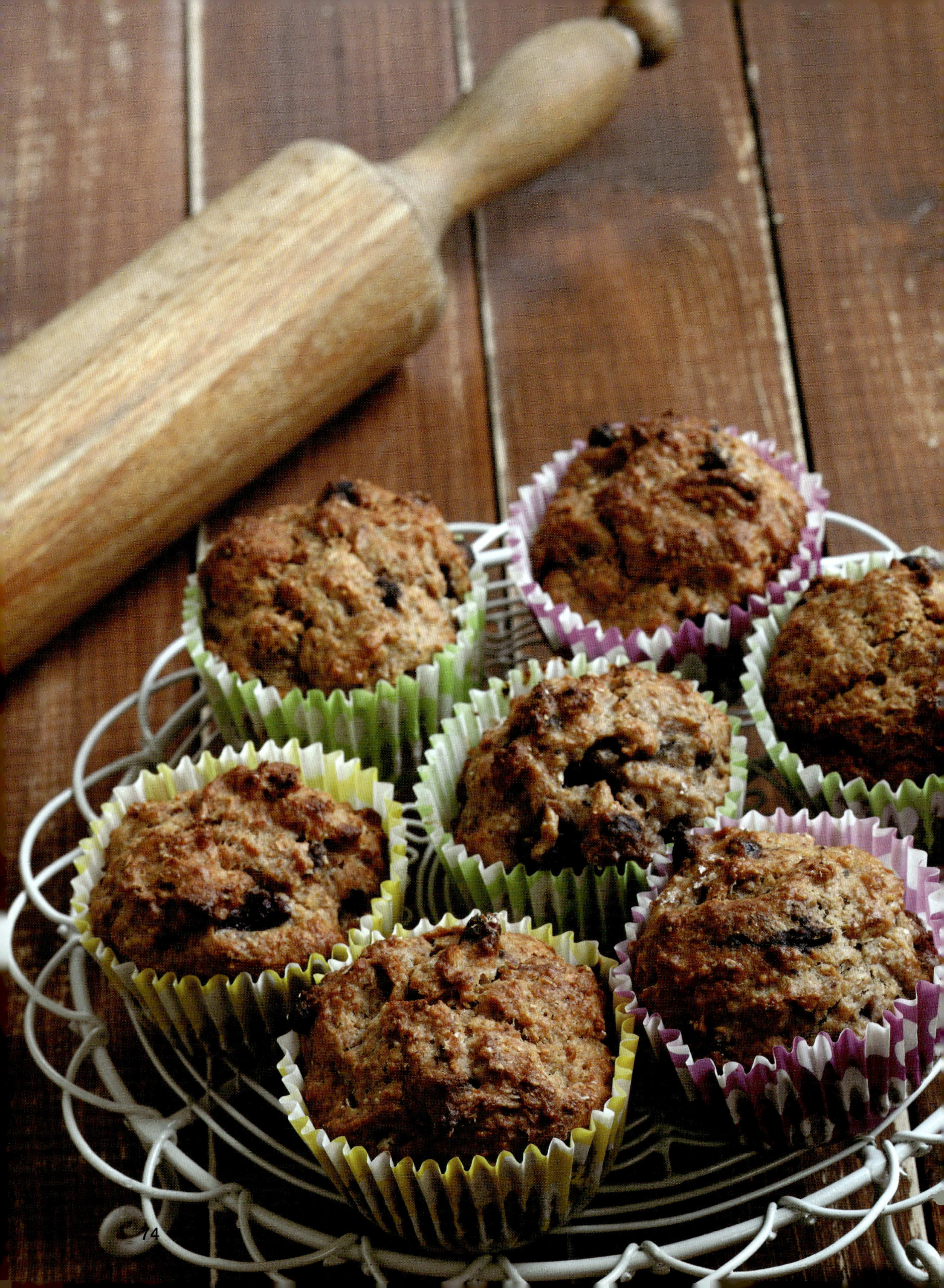

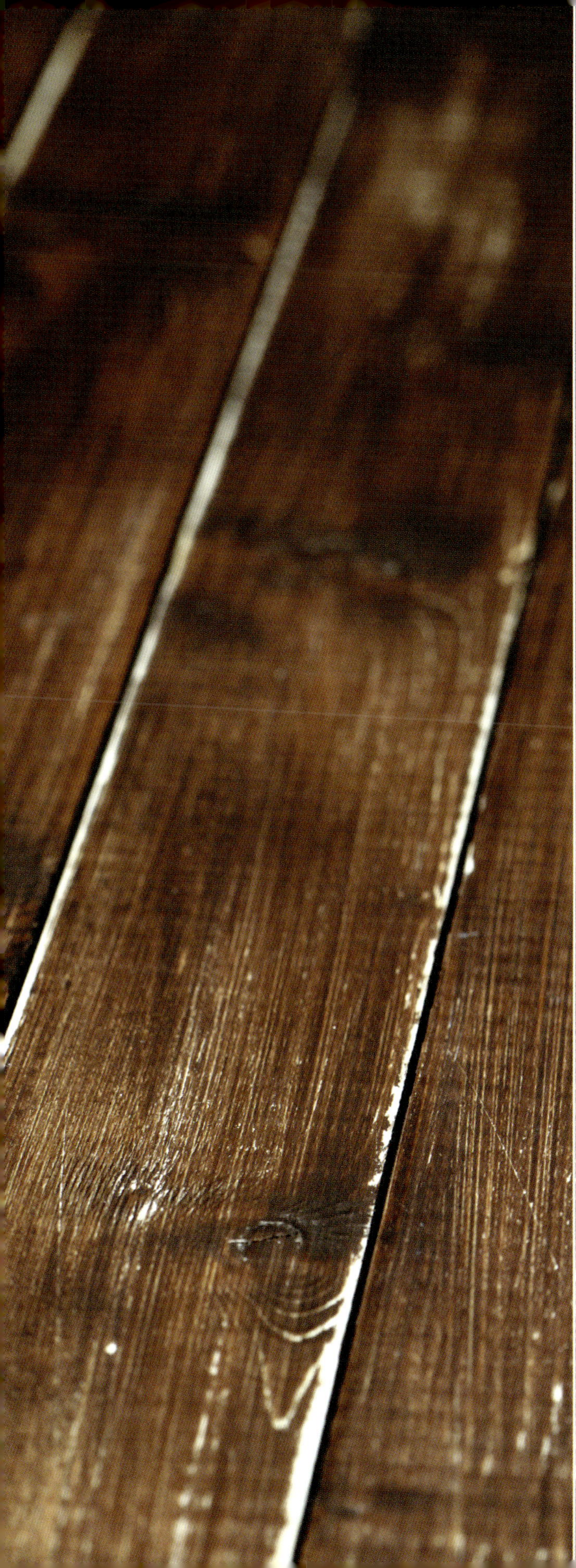

Plum Cupcakes

300 g (10½ oz) wholemeal flour
100 g (3½ oz) golden syrup
2 eggs
50 g (2 oz) butter
150 g (5 oz) yogurt
100 g (3½ oz) plums
1 teaspoon backing soda
40 g (1½ oz) walnuts chopped

Preheat oven to 180°C (350°F).
Put the flour, golden syrup, baking soda, softened butter, yogurt, eggs and chopped walnuts in a large bowl. Whisk to blend thoroughly, then add the chopped plums, stir again.
Spoon into the prepared cupcake cases and bake for 20 to 25 minutes.
Cool on a rack. Serve when cooled completely.

Makes 12 cupcakes

Per cupcake
189 kcal, 8.4 g fat (3.6 g saturated), 5.5 g protein, 24.2 g carbs (8.5 g sugar), 3.3 g fibre, 0.3 g salt

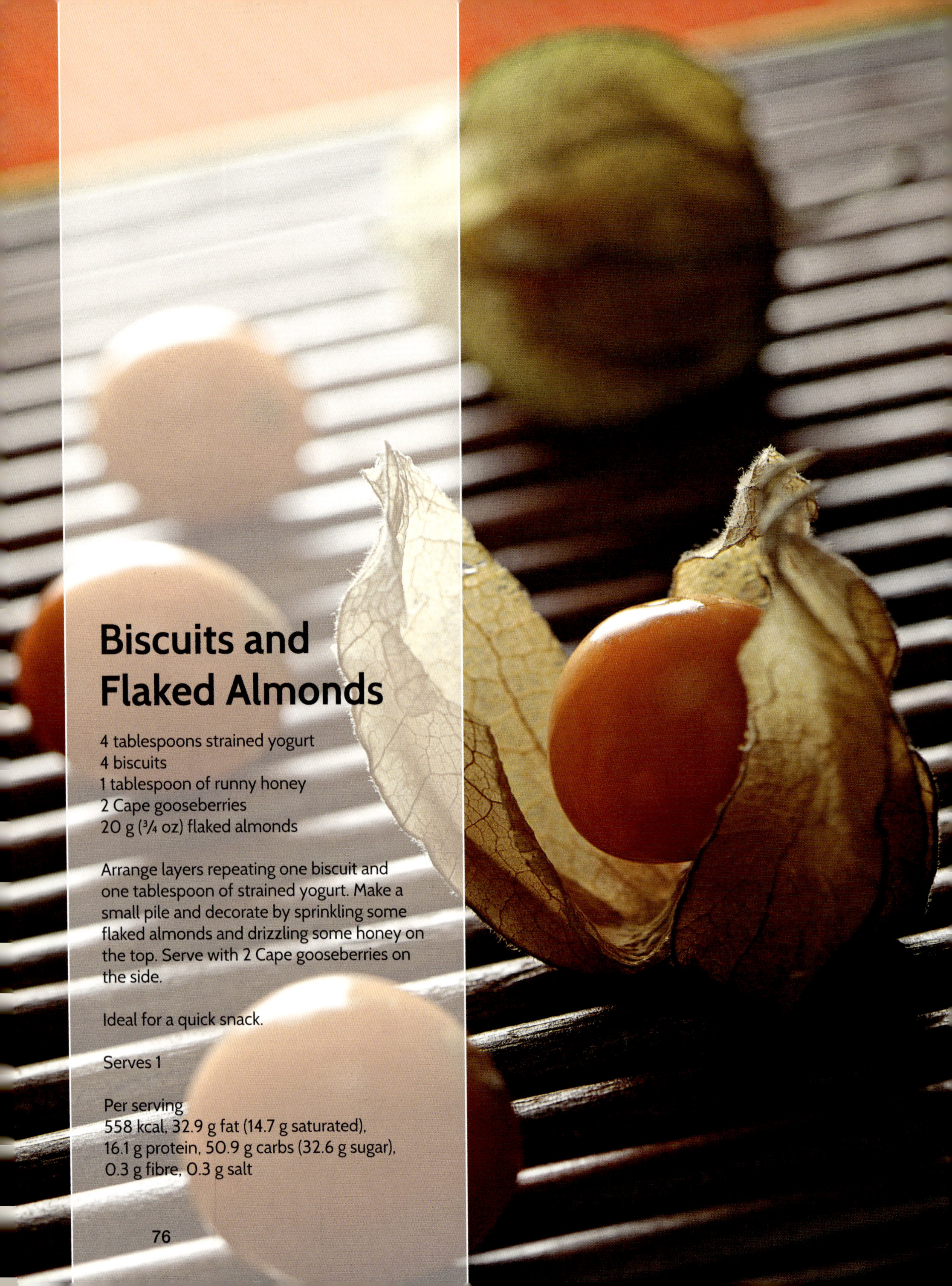

Biscuits and Flaked Almonds

4 tablespoons strained yogurt
4 biscuits
1 tablespoon of runny honey
2 Cape gooseberries
20 g (¾ oz) flaked almonds

Arrange layers repeating one biscuit and one tablespoon of strained yogurt. Make a small pile and decorate by sprinkling some flaked almonds and drizzling some honey on the top. Serve with 2 Cape gooseberries on the side.

Ideal for a quick snack.

Serves 1

Per serving
558 kcal, 32.9 g fat (14.7 g saturated), 16.1 g protein, 50.9 g carbs (32.6 g sugar), 0.3 g fibre, 0.3 g salt

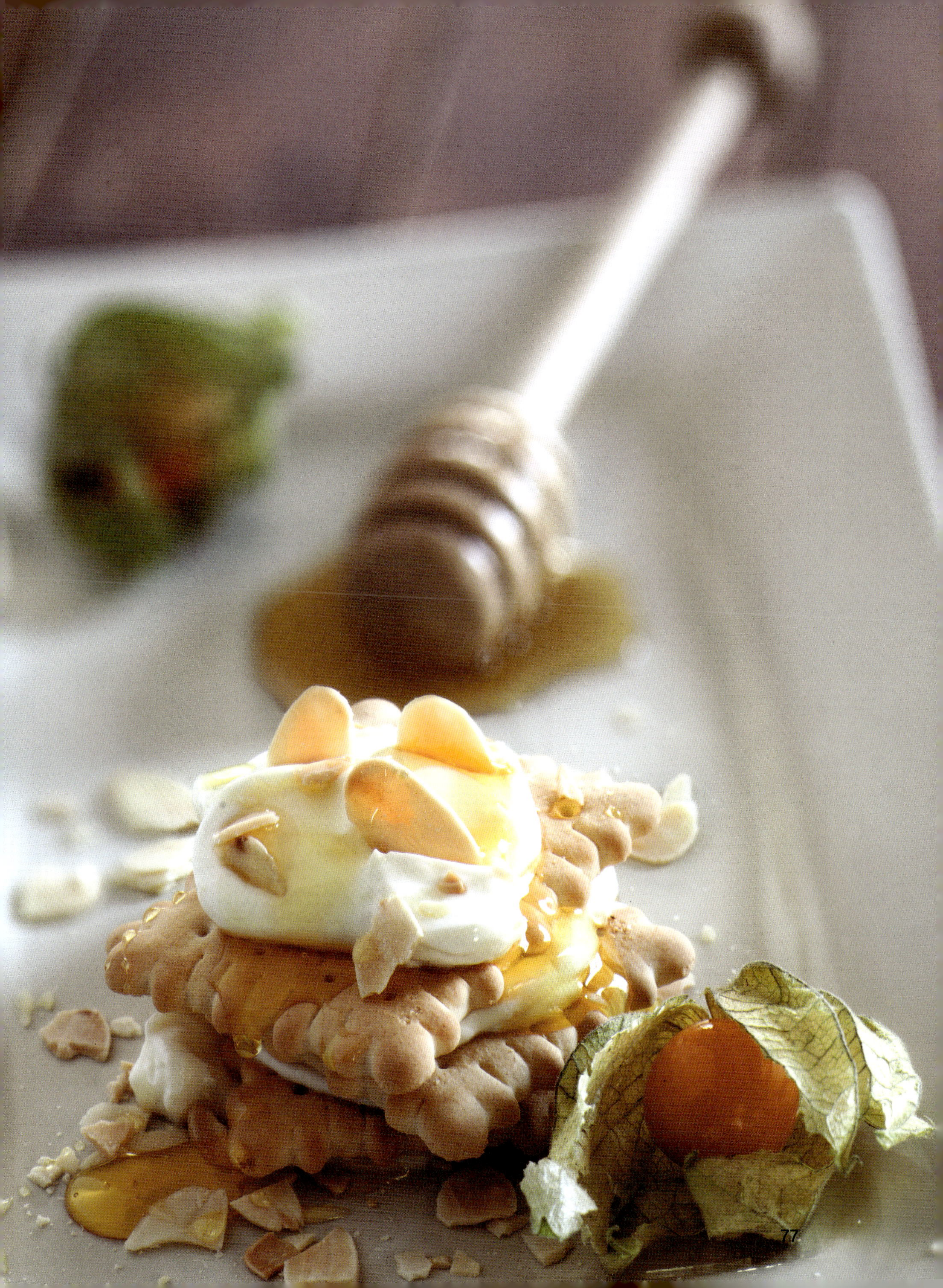

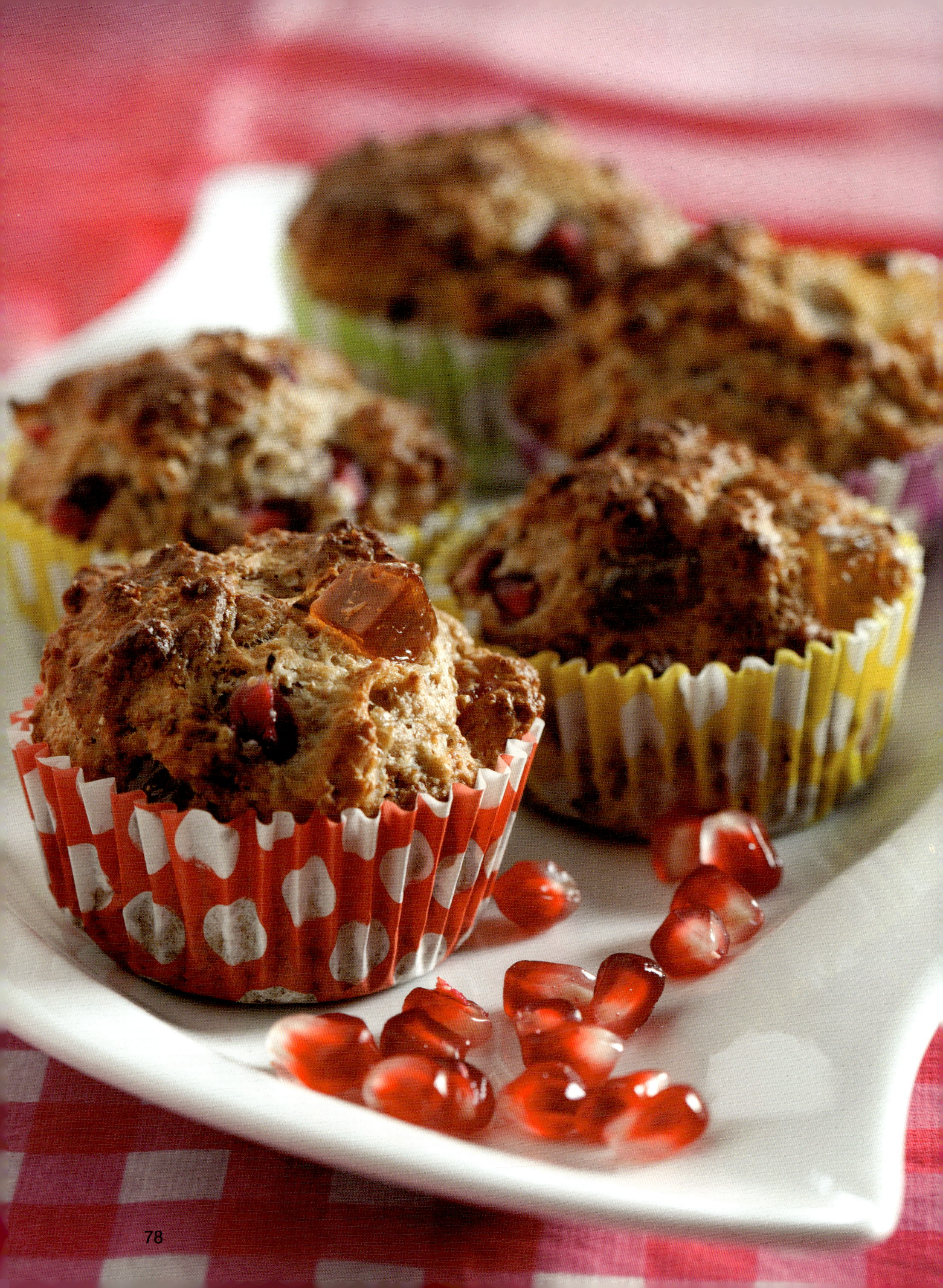

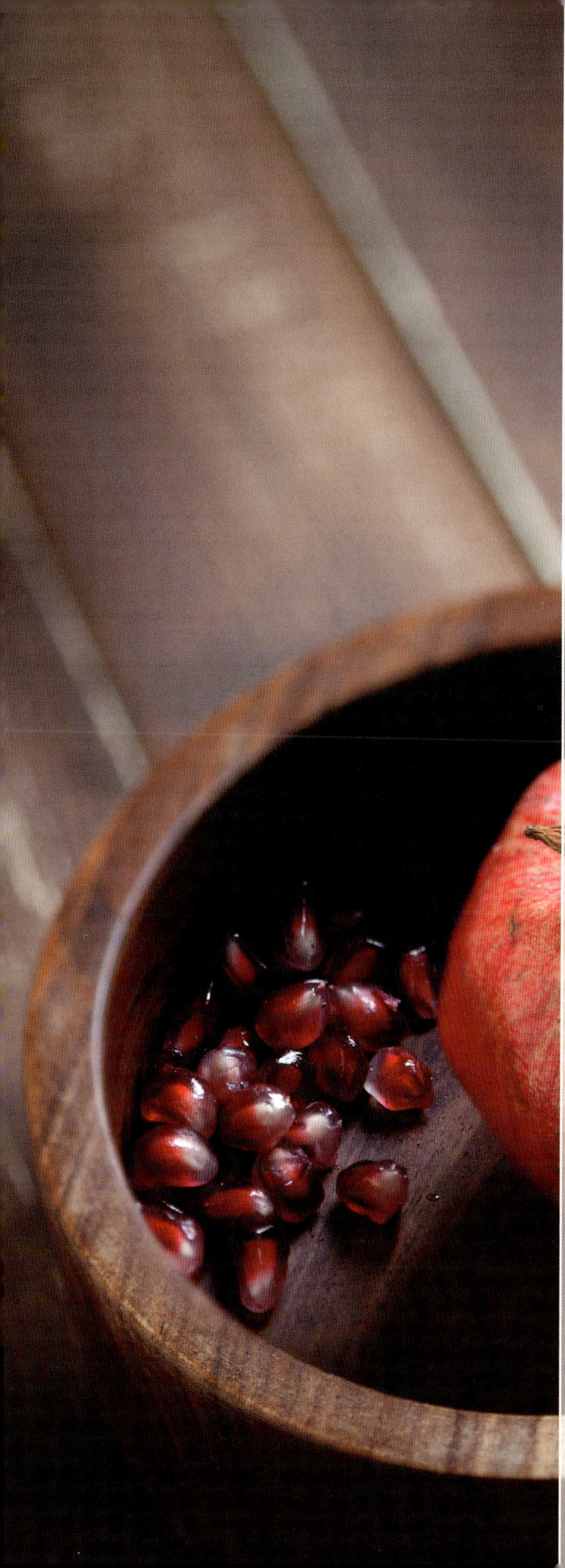

Turkish Delight and Pomegranate Cupcakes

300 g (10½ oz) wholemeal flour
1 egg
300 g (10½ oz) low fat yogurt
50 ml (1½ fl oz) sunflower oil
10 g (½ oz) baking soda
140 g (5 oz) Turkish delight, diced
100 g (3½ oz) pomegranate seeds

Preheat oven to 180°C (350°F). Cut the Turkish Delight into small pieces and throw them into a large bowl. Then add the pomegranate seeds, egg, yogurt, oil, wholemeal flour and baking soda. Gently mix well and pour into the cupcake cases until half full. Place into cupcake tray and bake in the oven for about 25 minutes. Once baked, leave them to cool at room temperature and serve.

Makes 12 cupcakes

Per cupcakes
175 kcal, 5.4 g fat (0.9 g saturated), 5.1 g protein, 28.2 g carbs (11.4 g sugar), 3.4 g fibre, 0.3 g salt

Scones

300 g (10½ oz) wheat flour
200 g (7 oz) rye flour
100 g (3½ oz) butter, softened
250 ml (8½ fl oz) semi-skimmed milk
50 g (2 oz) brown sugar
3 eggs
3 teaspoons baking soda
1 teaspoon carom seeds
pinch of rock salt

For serving:
20 g (¾ oz) butter
10 teaspoons jam
100 g (3½ oz) low fat yogurt, strained

Preheat oven to 220°C (425°F). Put the flour and butter into a large bowl and rub together to make a breadcrumb mixture. Add the sugar, two eggs, carom seeds and baking soda and keep rubbing in, make sure all the ingredients are well mixed. Next, gently pour in the milk and keep mixing to make a soft and sticky dough. If needed, you can add a bit more flour. Then sprinkle some flour on the work surface, tip out the dough and knead to make a smooth dough. Using a rolling pin, roll up the dough to make about 2.5 cm (1 inch) thick base and leave the dough to rest for a couple of minutes. Then using a pastry cutter, cut rounds from the dough and arrange them over a lightly greased baking tray. Meanwhile, beat the last egg and using a pastry brush, glaze the scones and sprinkle over some rock salt. Then transfer the tray to the oven and bake for about 20 minutes or until the scones are golden brown. Leave them to cool and serve halved with some softened butter, a teaspoon of jam and tablespoon of strained low fat yogurt.

Serves 8

Per serving
421 kcal, 16 g fat (9 g saturated), 10 g protein,
64 g carbs (16 g sugar), 5.5 g fibre, 2.0 g salt

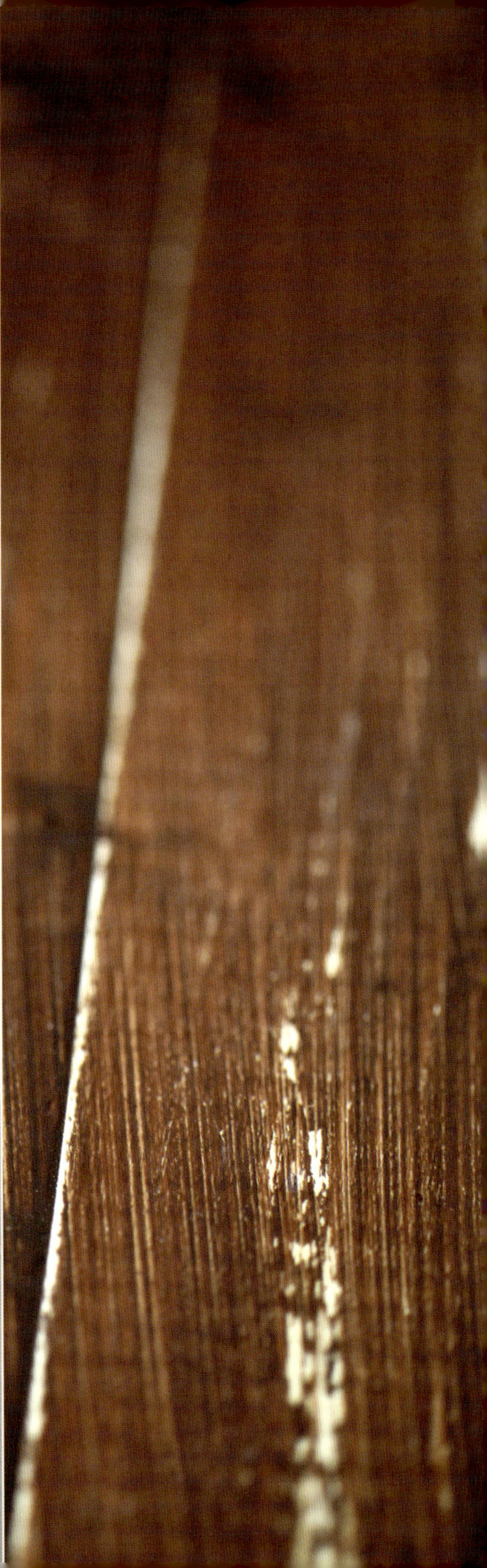

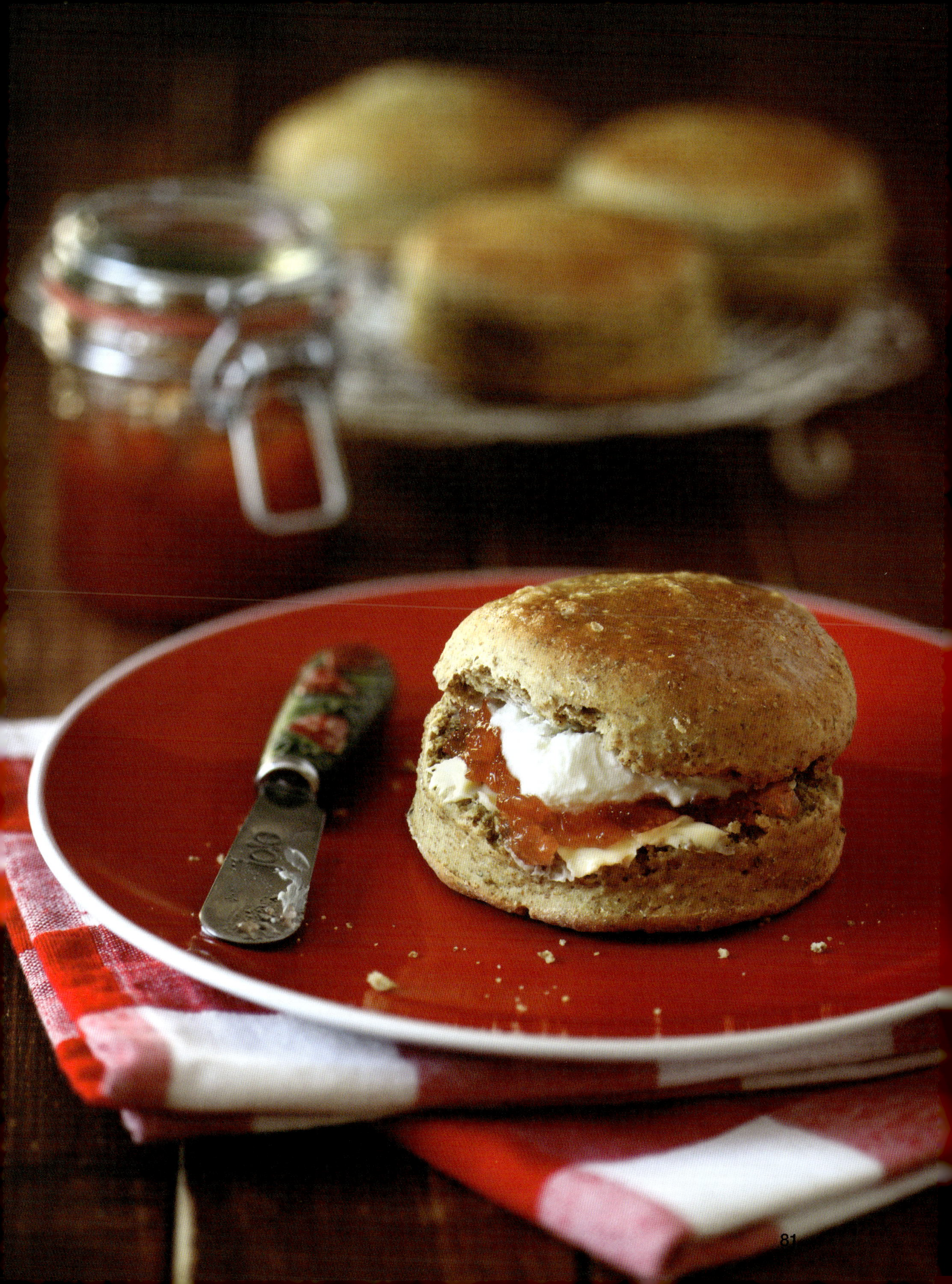

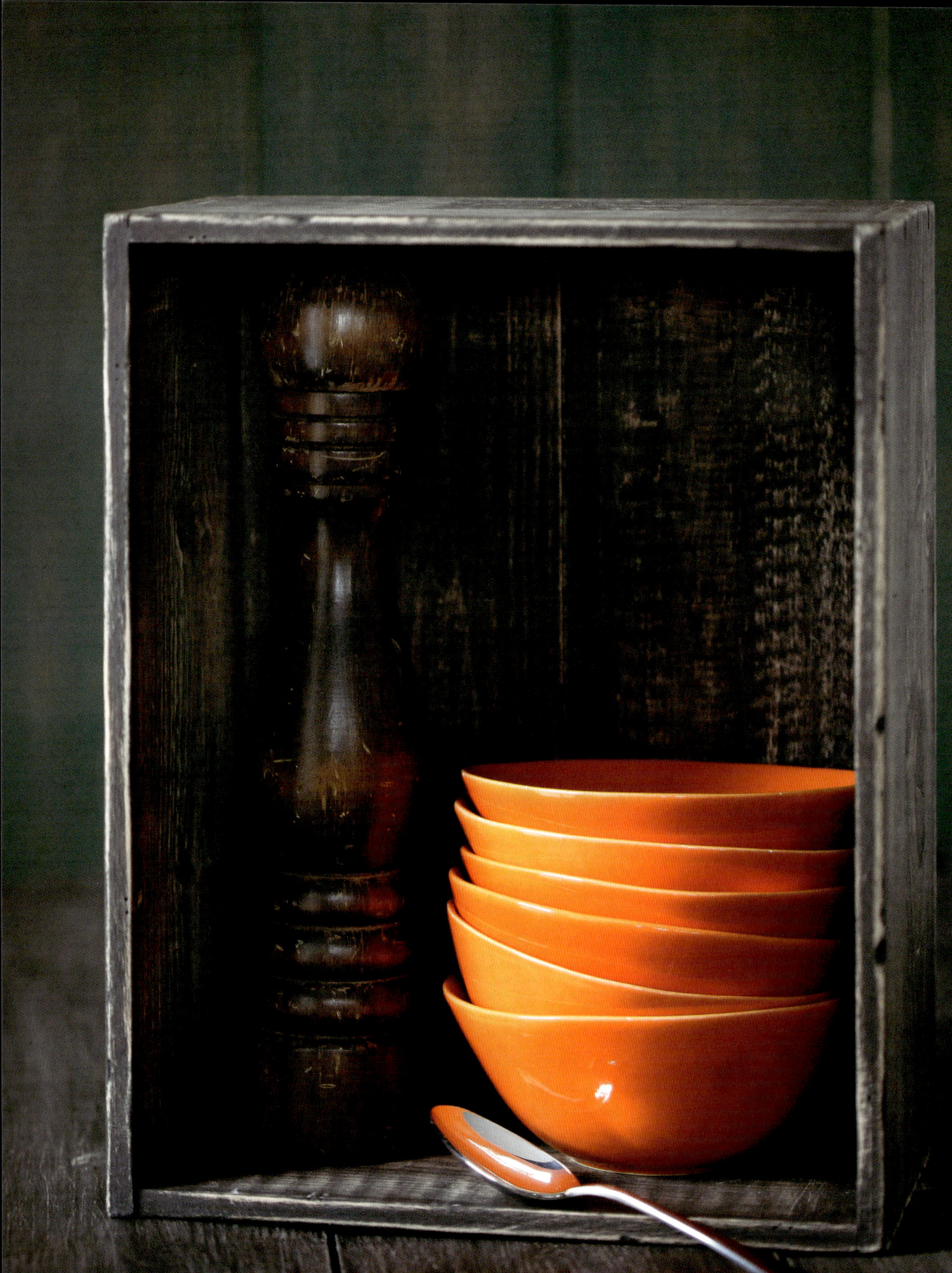

Soups

Carrot Tarator

250 ml (8½ fl oz) yogurt
250 ml (8½ fl oz) water
2 carrots, sliced into 3 mm thickness
handful chopped dill
1 tablespoon extra virgin olive oil
1 garlic clove, chopped
pinch of sugar
pinch of salt
50 g (2 oz) walnuts, roasted and chopped

Mix together the yogurt and water in a large bowl. Add the sliced carrots, dill, olive oil, garlic, sugar and salt. Leave it to rest in the refrigerator for 30 minutes before serving with chopped walnuts on the top of each bowl.

Serves 4

Per serving
213 kcal, 17.8 g fat (5.6 g saturated), 5.8 g protein, 7.7 g carbs (7.0 g sugar), 0.9 g salt, 1.9 g fibre

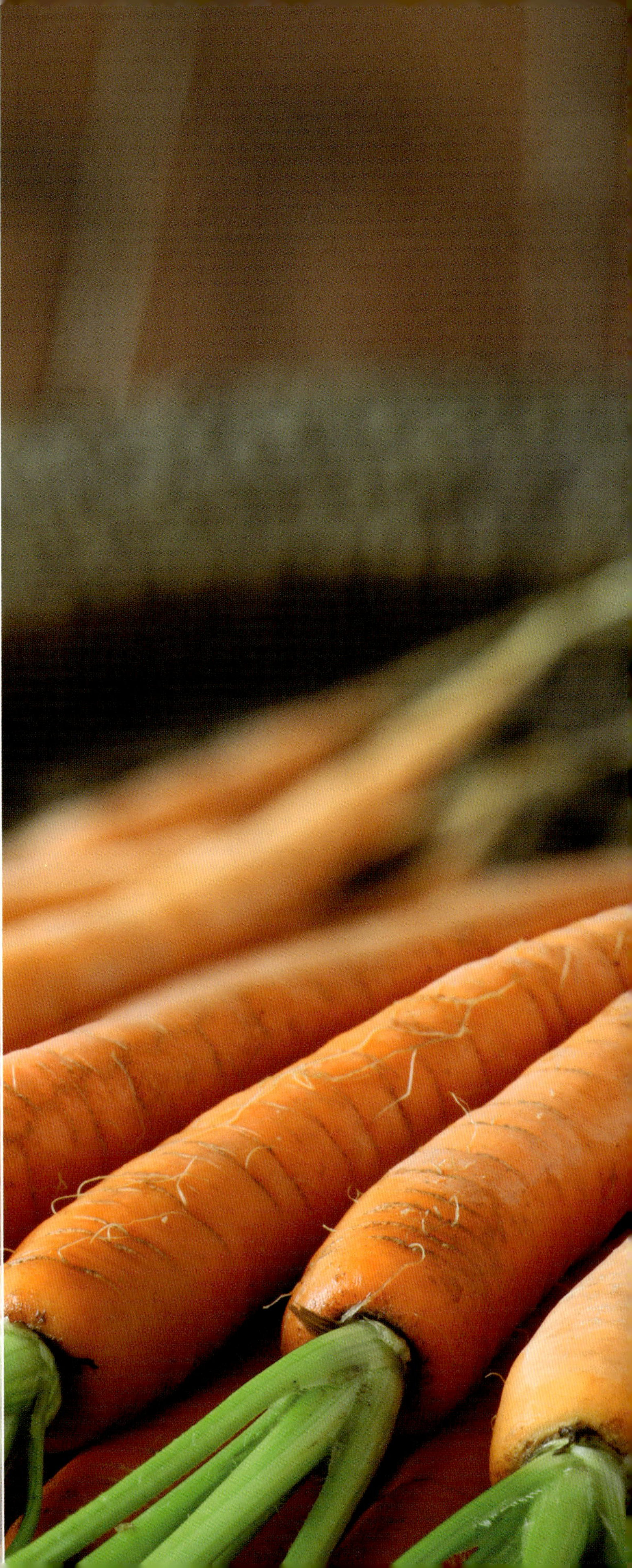

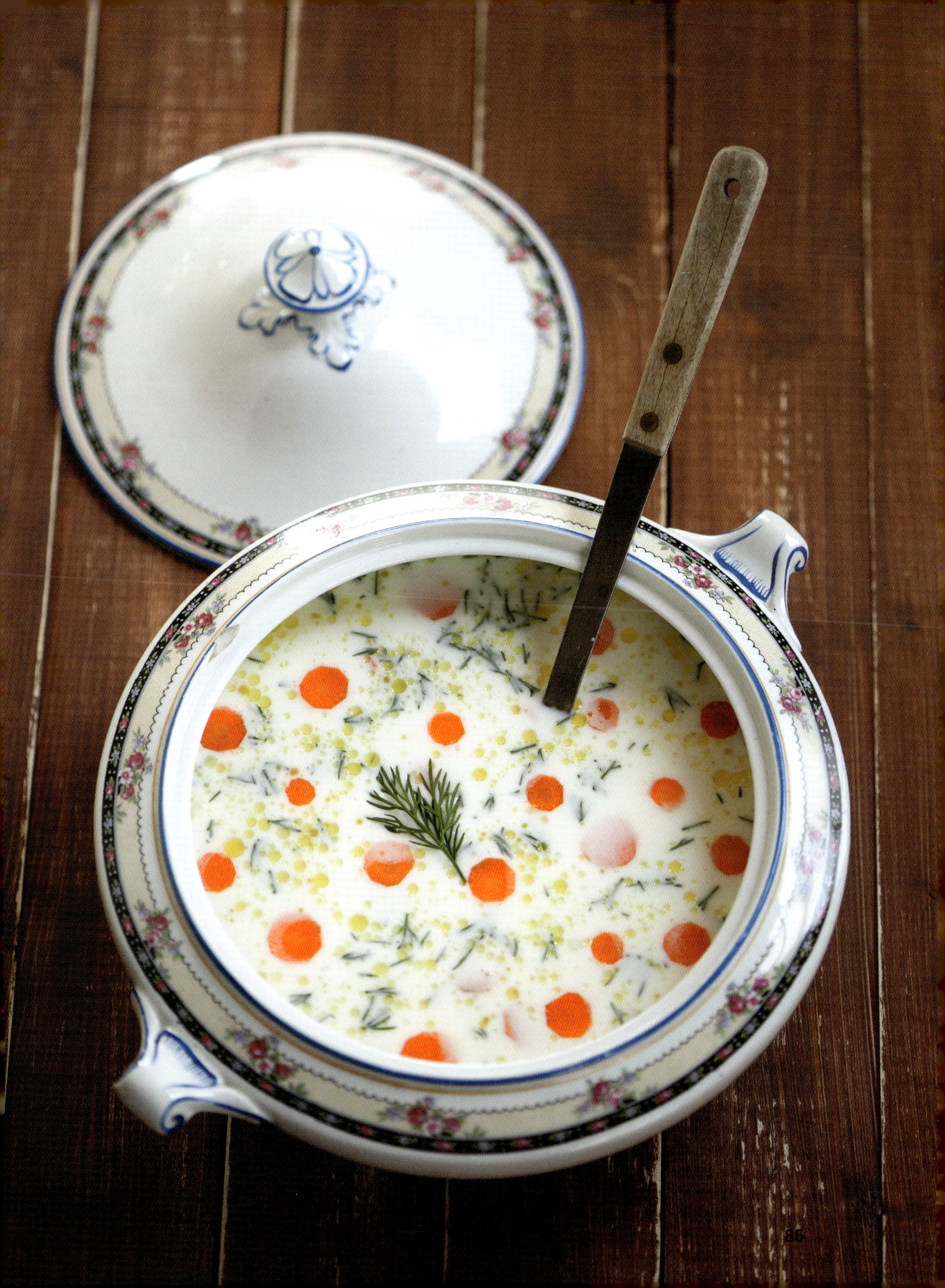

Baked Potato and Pepper Soup

1 kg (2.2 lb) potato (skin intact)
1 red pepper, finely chopped
1 onion, finely chopped
1 litre (2 pints) homemade chicken stock or vegetable stock
100 ml (3½ fl oz) semi-skimmed milk
70 g (3 oz) butter
1 garlic clove
½ tablespoon dry rosemary
pinch of salt
6 tablespoons plain yogurt
2 tablespoons finely chopped chives
2 tablespoons chopped walnuts

Preheat the oven to 200°C (400°F). Wash the potatoes well, dry and prick several times with a fork. Bake them for about 45 minutes in the oven. Once cooked, chop the potatoes in their skins into large cubes.
In a deep saucepan throw the butter, 100 ml (3½ fl oz) of stock, chopped onion and red pepper. Sauté over a low heat for about 5 minutes. Add the rest of the stock and stir well. Add the milk, garlic, rosemary and salt. Cook for a further 10 minutes. Then, add the potatoes in the same saucepan and blend together using a hand held blender.
Serve warm with tablespoon of plain yogurt, some chopped walnuts and finely chopped chives sprinkled over.

Serves 6

Per serving
321 kcal, 16.7 g fat (8.7 g saturated), 7.5 g protein, 37.5 g carbs (6.1 g sugar), 0.8 g salt, 4.7 g fibre

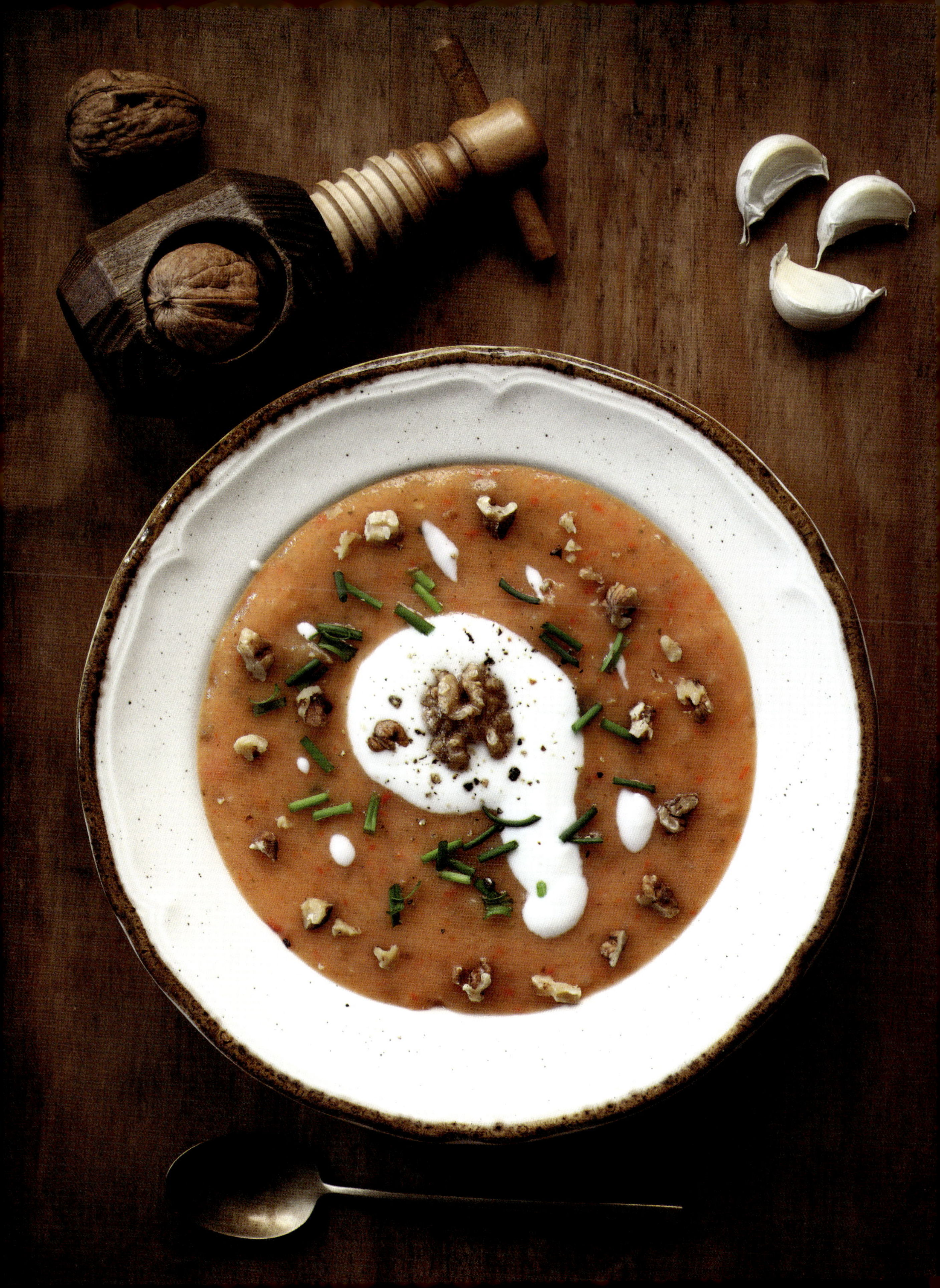

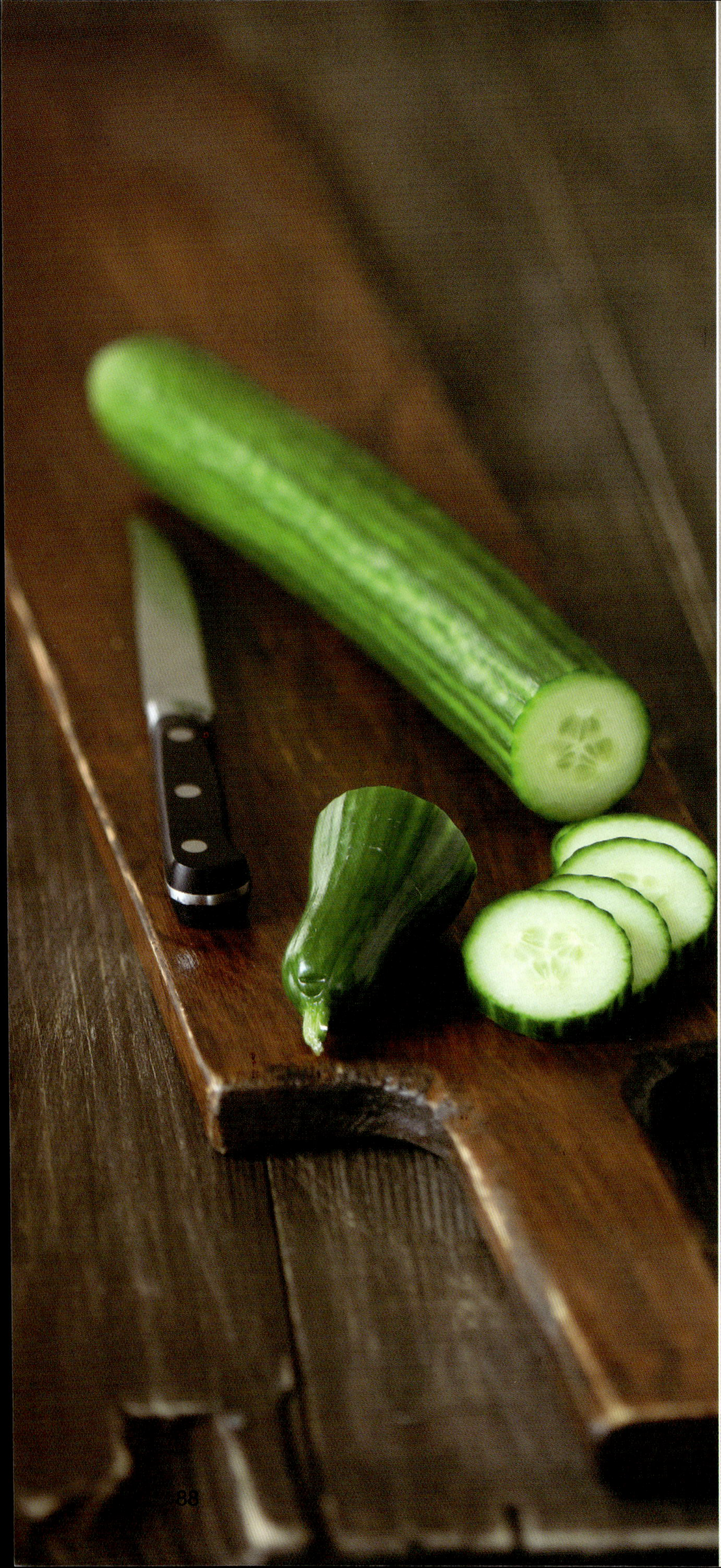

Tarator

1 cucumber
250 ml (8½ fl oz) yogurt
250 ml (8½ fl oz) water
1 tablespoon olive oil
1 clove garlic
pinch of sugar
pinch of salt
dill
2 walnuts, roasted and chopped

In a large bowl, stir the yogurt and water then add finely chopped cucumber, chopped dill, olive oil, chopped garlic, sugar and salt. Leave it to rest for 30 minutes in to the fridge and serve with chopped walnuts on the top of each bowl.

Serves 4

Per serving
145 kcal, 11.7 g fat (4.9 g saturated), 4.9 g protein, 5.3 g carbs (4.8 g sugars), 0.9 g salt, 1.0 g fibre

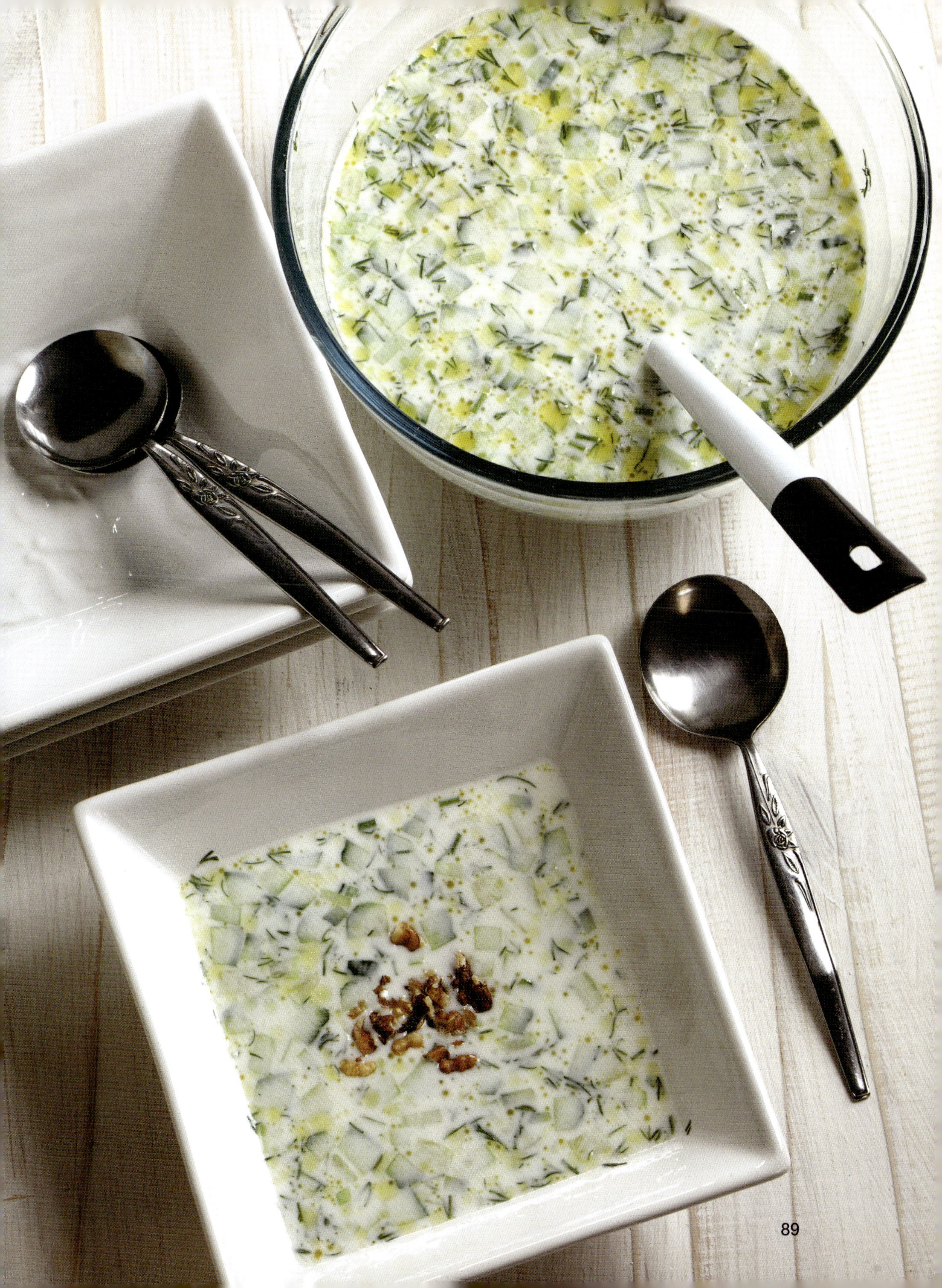

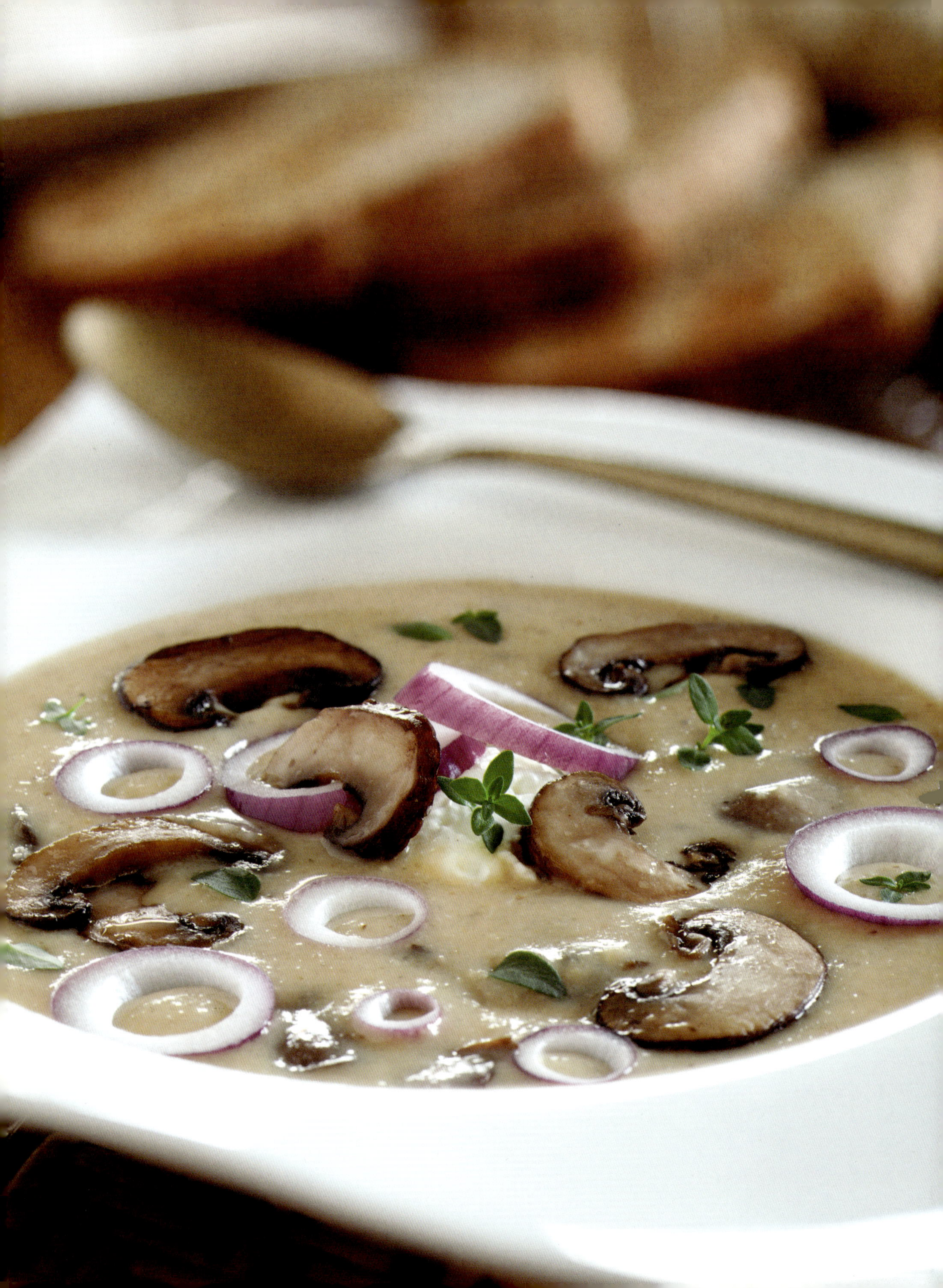

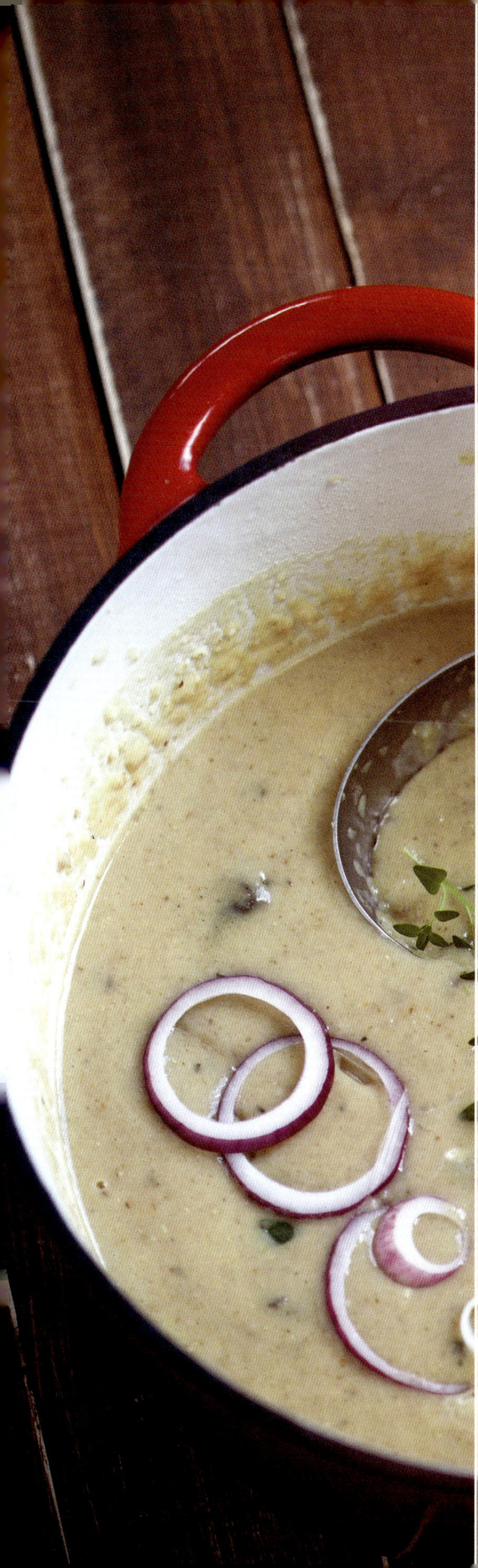

Mushroom and Caraway Seeds Soup

1 tablespoon caraway seeds, toasted
4 tablespoons olive oil
1.5 litres (2½ pints) mineral water
1 leek, finely chopped
3 carrots, diced
1 parsnip, diced
2 tablespoons oat bran
pinch of freshly ground black pepper
pinch of sea salt
300 g (10½ oz) chestnut mushrooms, sliced
6 tablespoons strained yogurt
pinch of fresh thyme
1 small red onion, sliced

Put the caraway seeds in a small frying pan and dry cook over a medium heat for 3-4 minutes, until the seeds start to burst.
Meanwhile, heat 2 tablespoons of olive oil and 100ml (3½ fl oz) of the mineral water in a large saucepan over a high heat. Throw the leek, carrots and parsnips into the saucepan and cook for about 5 minutes, until the leek is translucent. Add the toasted caraway seeds, oat bran, the rest of the mineral water, the black pepper and salt and leave the mixture to boil for another 10-15 minutes until the vegetables are softened. Turn the heat off and blend with a hand-held blender for couple of minutes until smooth.
Heat the remaining 2 tablespoons of oil in a medium pan over a high heat, add a pinch of salt and cook the sliced mushrooms for about 5 minutes until they turn golden. Add half of the mushrooms to the soup and the rest you can use to decorate the soup.
Serve warm with a tablespoon of strained yogurt and a garnish of some cooked mushrooms, thyme leaves and red onion rings.

Serves 6

Per serving
158 kcal, 10 g fat (2.1 g saturated), 5.4 g protein, 11.8 g carbs (8.2 g sugar), 4.9 g fibre, 0.61 g salt

Butter Bean Yogurt Soup

500 g (17½ oz) low fat yogurt
500 ml (17 fl oz) vegetarian broth
1 800 g (28 oz) tin butter beans, drained
2 tablespoons olive oil
125 g (4½ oz) spring onions, finely chopped
1 green bell pepper, finely chopped
2 garlic cloves, crushed
1 teaspoon ground cumin
1 teaspoon dry mint
pinch of salt
2 tablespoons chopped fresh mint leaves

In a large saucepan throw the finely chopped spring onions, finely chopped green pepper, crushed garlic, cumin, dry mint, pinch of salt, olive oil and 50 ml (1¾ fl oz) water. Cook on medium heat for about 5 minutes while stirring. Then add half of the drained butter beans and vegetarian broth, reduce heat to low and simmer, covered for another 10 minutes. Transfer into a blender bowl and leave to cool for about 15 minutes then add the yogurt and blend. Finally add the rest of the drained butter beans and the chopped mint and serve.

Serves 4

Per serving
244 kcal, 7.7 g fat (1.8 g saturated), 15.6 g protein, 30.1 g carbs (12.4 g sugar), 10 g fibre, 2.5 g salt

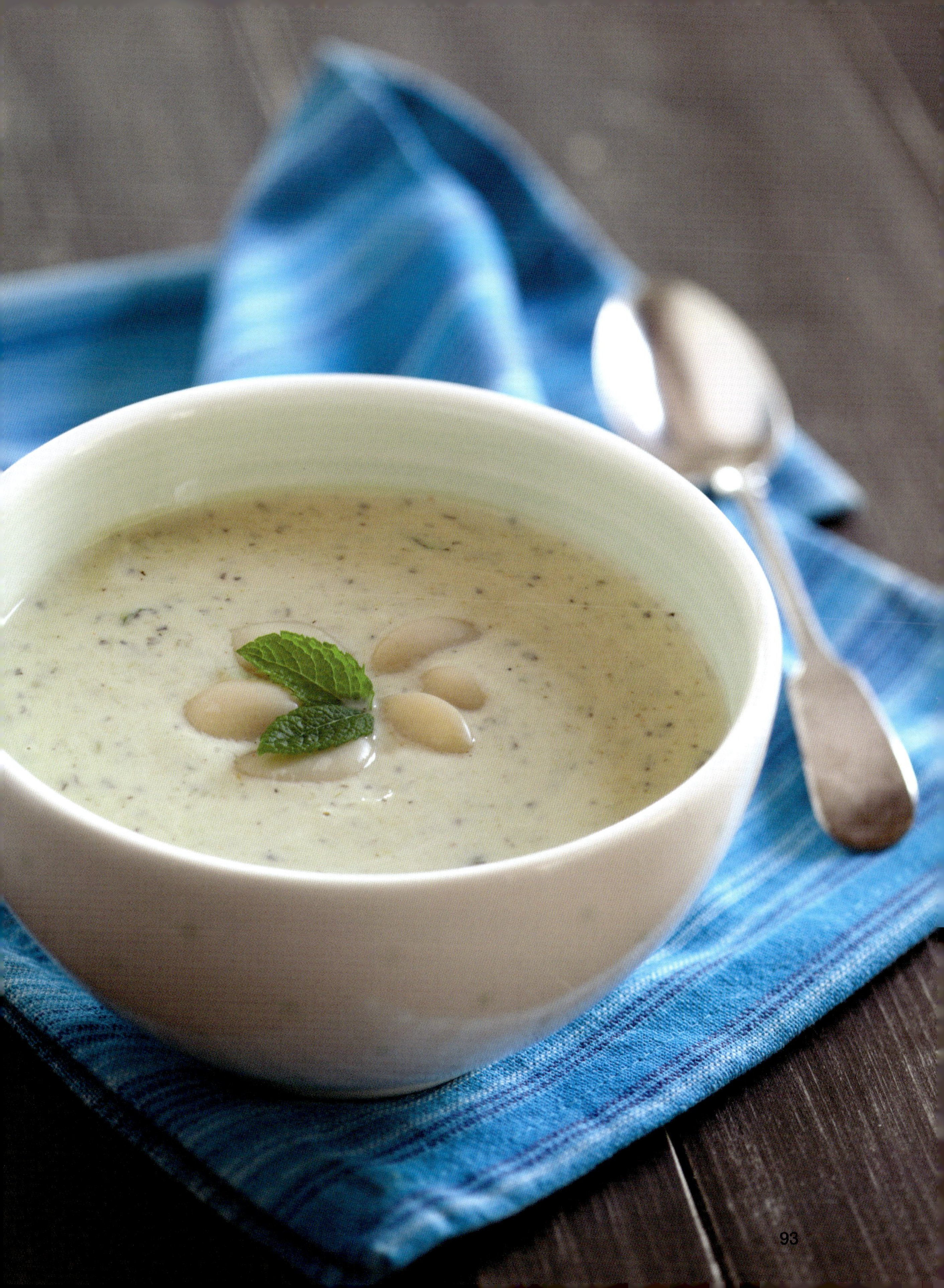

Meatball Soup

Meatballs:
250 g (9 oz) beef mince
50 g (2 oz) basmati rice
1 teaspoon dried thyme
1 teaspoon ground cumin
1 teaspoon black pepper
1 egg white
50 g (2 oz) white flour

Broth:
50 g (2 oz) basmati rice
1 tablespoon olive oil
3 medium potatoes, diced
1 medium onion, finely chopped
1 medium carrot, sliced into coins
1 medium red pepper, chopped
1 medium vine tomato, shredded
pinch of salt

Liaison:
100 g (3½ oz) yogurt
1 egg yolk
1 tablespoon fresh parsley

In a medium bowl combine the beef mince, rice, dried thyme, ground cumin, black pepper and egg white. Knead and form into small balls (whole walnut size). Gently roll them in flour and arrange next to each other on a plate. Then make the soup broth. In a large saucepan throw the finely chopped onion, sliced carrots, chopped red pepper, shredded vine tomato, pinch of salt and add 2 litres (4¼ pints) boiling water. Then gently add the meatballs one by one. Boil on a high heat for about 15 minutes then add the diced potatoes and basmati rice, reduce to a medium heat and simmer for another 20 minutes. When the soup is ready turn the heat off. In a small bowl, mix together the yogurt and egg yolk and carefully add the mix to the hot but not boiling soup, stirring well. Finally sprinkle chopped fresh parsley and leave it for couple minutes to cool and serve.

Serves 6

Per serving
294 kcal, 11.7 g fat (4.6 g saturated), 13.9 g protein, 34.2 g carbohydrates (5.5 g sugar), 2.8 g fibre, 0.7 g salt

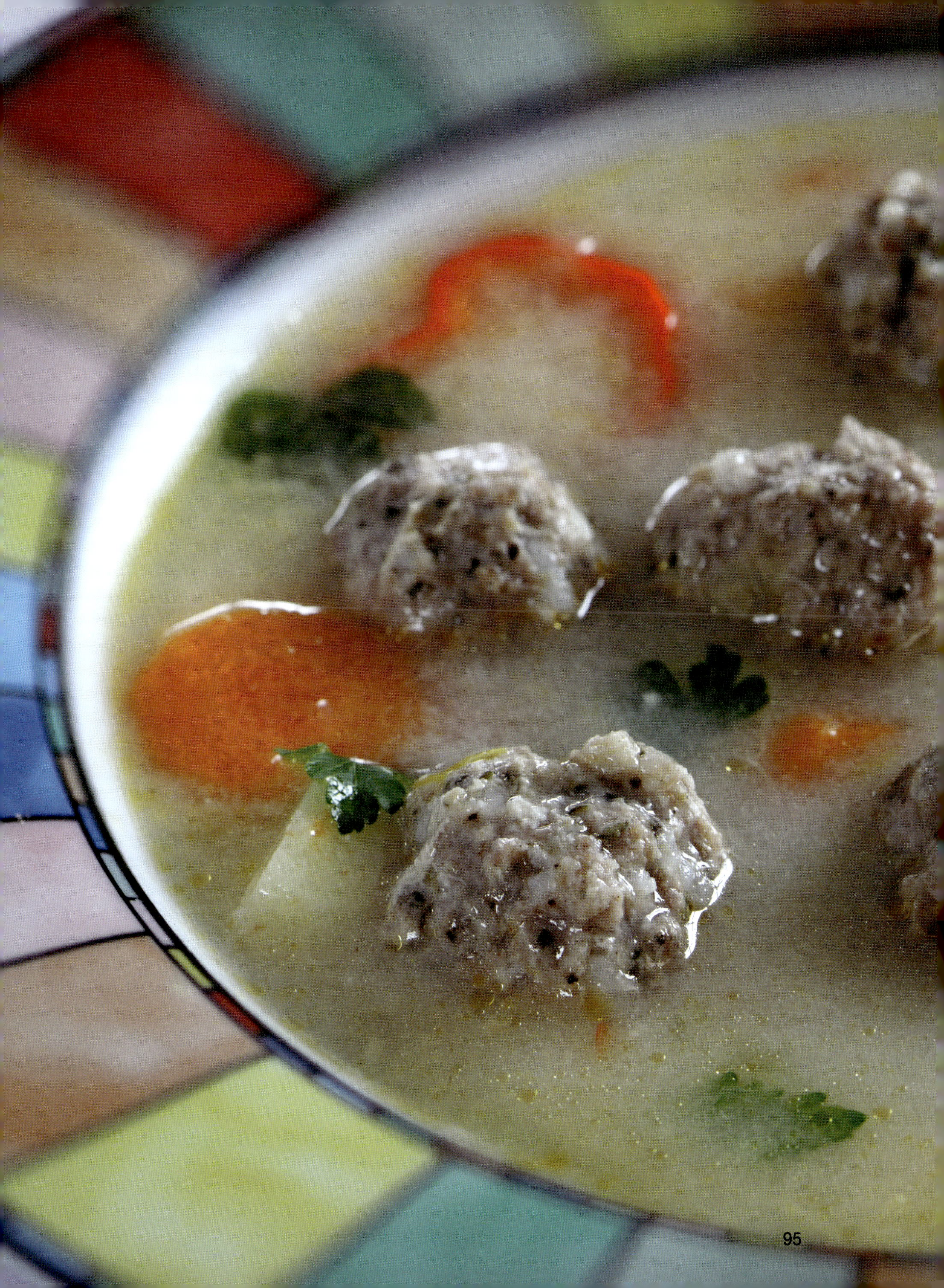

Lamb Soup

600 g (21 oz) fresh lamb leg steak, diced
2 wine tomatoes, chopped
2 medium onions, peeled and chopped
2 medium carrots, peeled and chopped
100 g (3½ oz) celeriac, diced
1 tablespoon rice, washed
1 teaspoon black pepper grains
1 egg
2 tablespoons yogurt
pinch of salt, optional
chili pepper, chopped (optional)

Throw the lamb cubes into a large saucepan, add black pepper and 2.5 litres (5¼ pints) boiling water and boil for about 30 minutes on medium heat,regularly removing the foam. Then add the chopped carrots, onions and celeriac and boil for another 10 minutes. Afterwards, add rice and chopped tomatoes and boil for another 15 minutes. When the soup is ready turn the heat off. In a small bowl mix together the yogurt and egg and carefully add the mix to the hot but not boiling soup stirring well. Finally sprinkle chopped fresh parsley and leave it for a couple of minutes to cool, then serve.

Serves 6

Per serving
248 kcal, 12.8 g fat (5.7 g saturated), 22.7 g protein, 11.1 g carbs (7 g sugar), 3.0 g fibre, 0.8 g salt

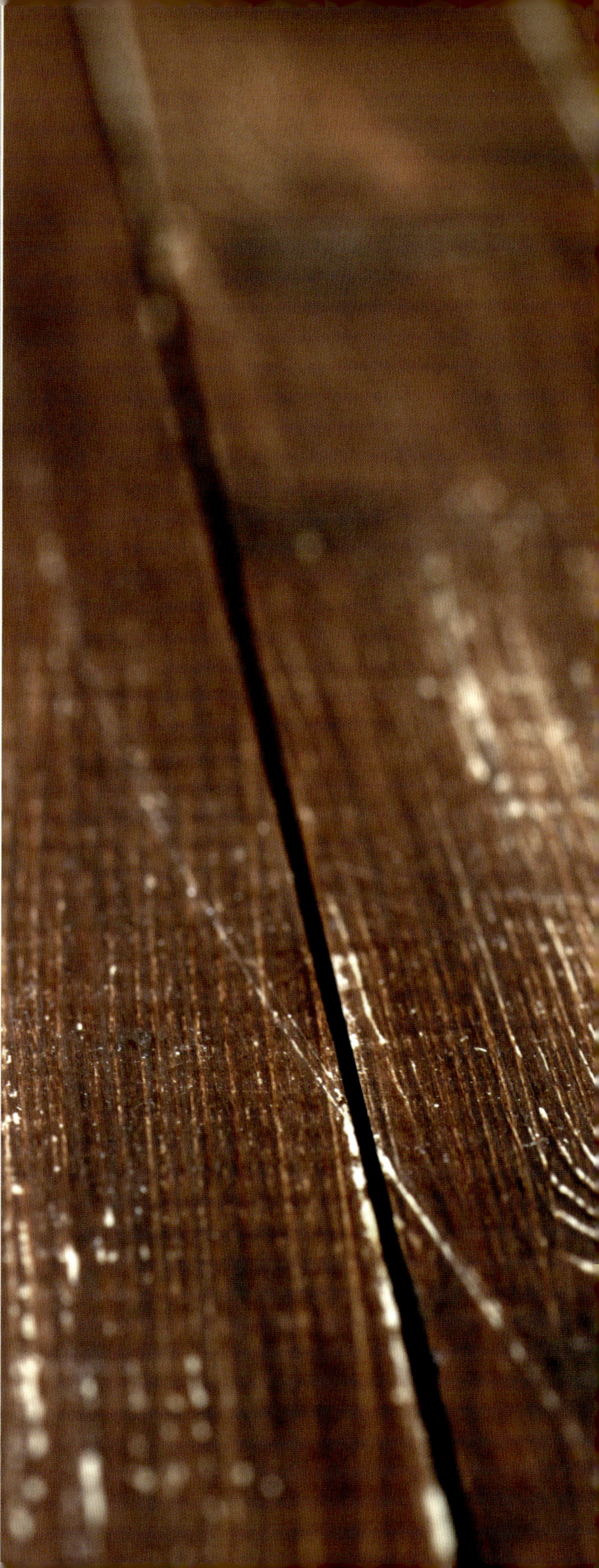

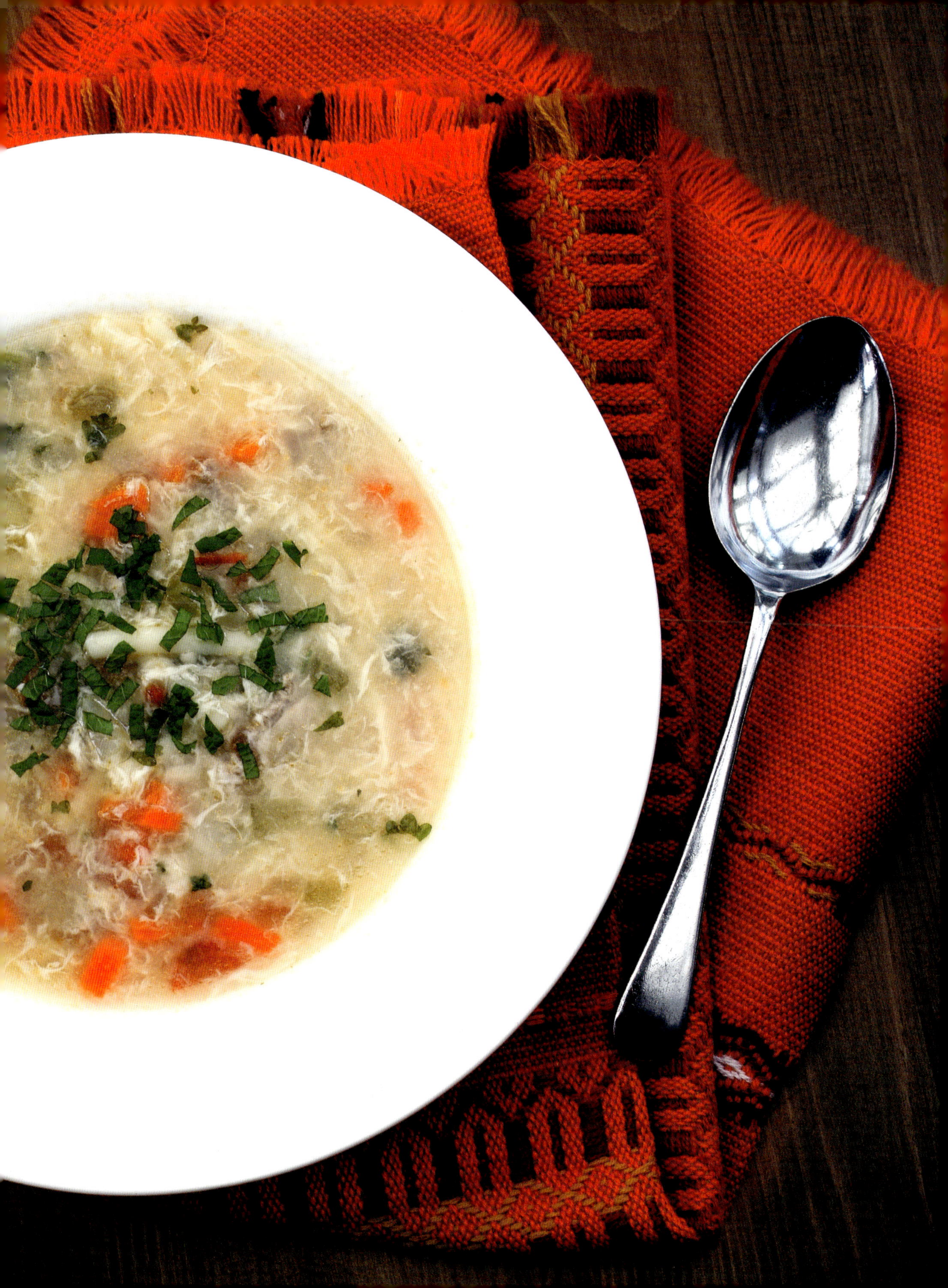

Chicken Soup

350 g (12 oz) chicken, skinned, boned
1 medium leek, chopped
1 parsnip, peeled and chopped
2 medium carrots, peeled and chopped
50 g (2 oz) vermicelli, broken
handful freshly chopped parsley
pinch of salt, optional
1 egg
2 tablespoons yogurt
chili pepper, chopped (optional)

Put the skinned chicken in a large saucepan and add 2 litres (4¼ pints) of boiling water and boil for about 30 minutes. Carefully take the chicken out of the pan and leave it to cool. Add to the boiling bullion the chopped leek, parsnip, carrots, vermicelli and pinch of salt and boil for another 10 minutes. Meanwhile, chop the chicken and add it back into the soup. When the soup is ready turn the heat off. In a small bowl mix together the yogurt and egg and carefully add to the hot but not boiling soup, stirring well. Finally sprinkle chopped fresh parsley and leave it for 10 minutes to cool and then serve.

Serves 6

Per serving
172 kcal, 4.4 g fat (0.6 g saturated),
20.7 g protein, 12.5 g carbs (4.5 g sugar),
2.8 g fibre, 0.7 g salt

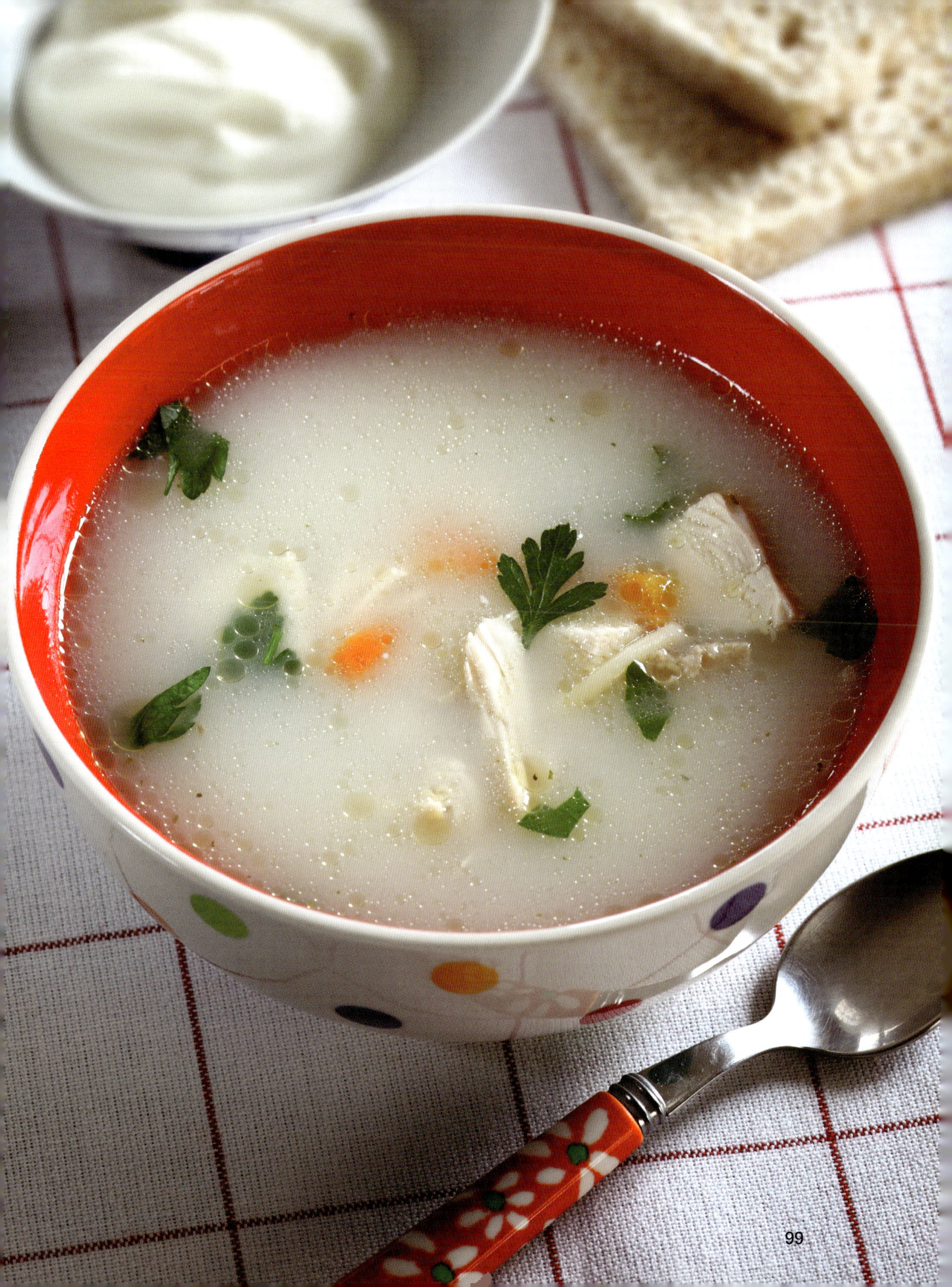

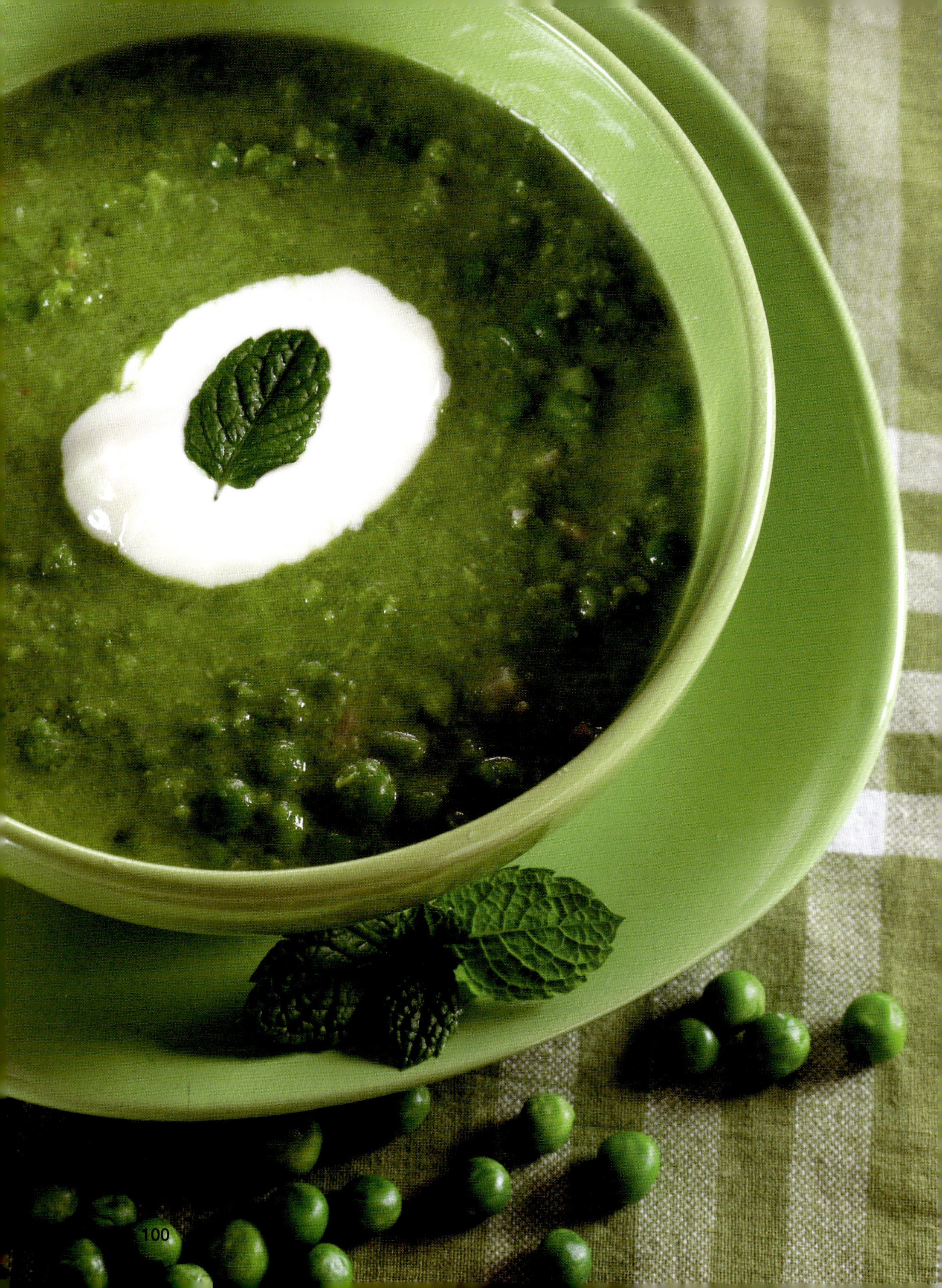

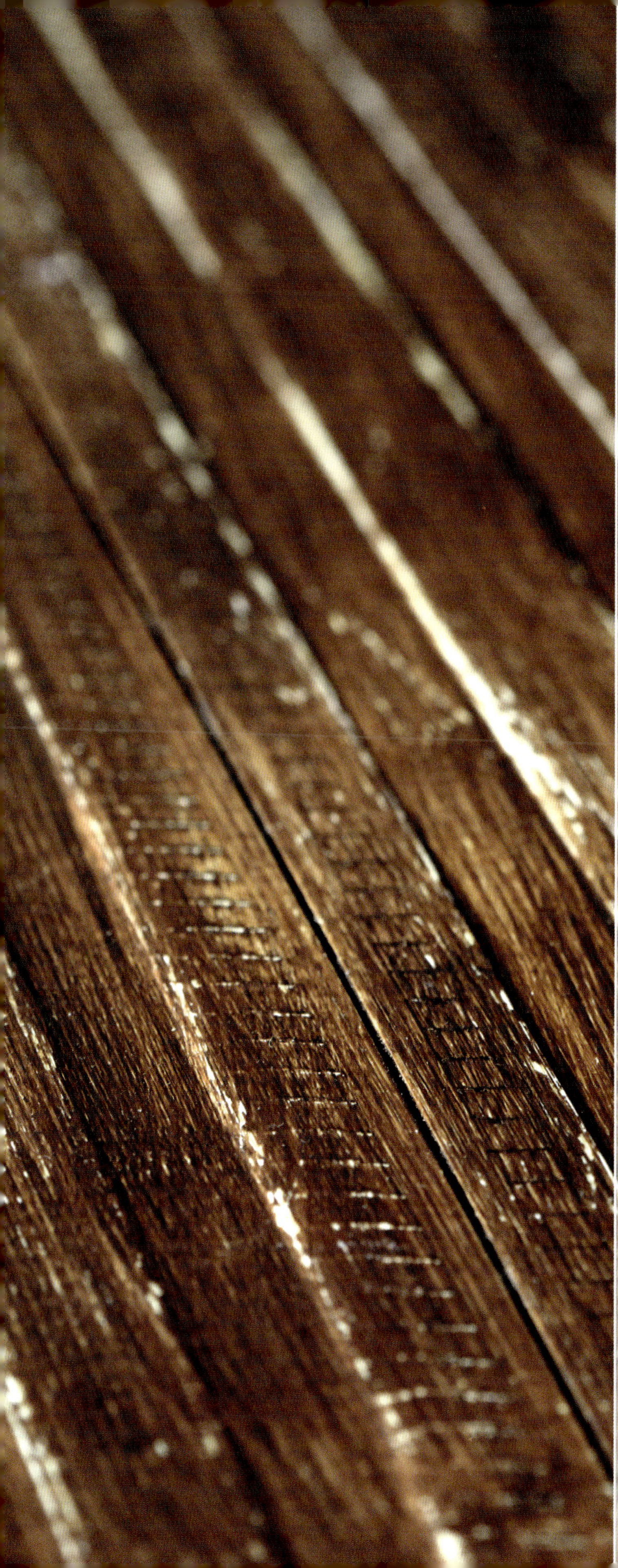

Pea Soup

750 g (26½ oz) garden peas, frozen
1 large leek, chopped
50 g (2 oz) butter
150 g (5 oz) yogurt
75 g (2½ oz) mint leaves, roughly chopped
200 g (7 oz) bacon, baked
2 garlic cloves, peeled and minced

Preheat oven to 250°C (480°F). Spread the bacon on a baking sheet and bake for about 25 minutes. In a large saucepan melt the butter and add the leek, garlic, 100ml (3½ fl oz) water, pinch of salt and cook for 3 minutes. Then add 2 litres (4¼ pints) water and the peas and boil for 15 minutes. Separate one ladle of peas and set aside in separate small bowl. Then using a hand blender blend the soup. Once blended you then add the separated whole peas from the small bowl. Roughly chop the bacon and add to the soup and mix well. Serve with a good tablespoon of yogurt on the top and some fresh mint.

Serves 6

Per serving
258 kcal, 15.6 g fat (7.5 g saturated),
14.8 g protein, 15.4 g carbs (5.9 g sugar),
9.5 g fibre, 1.4 g salt

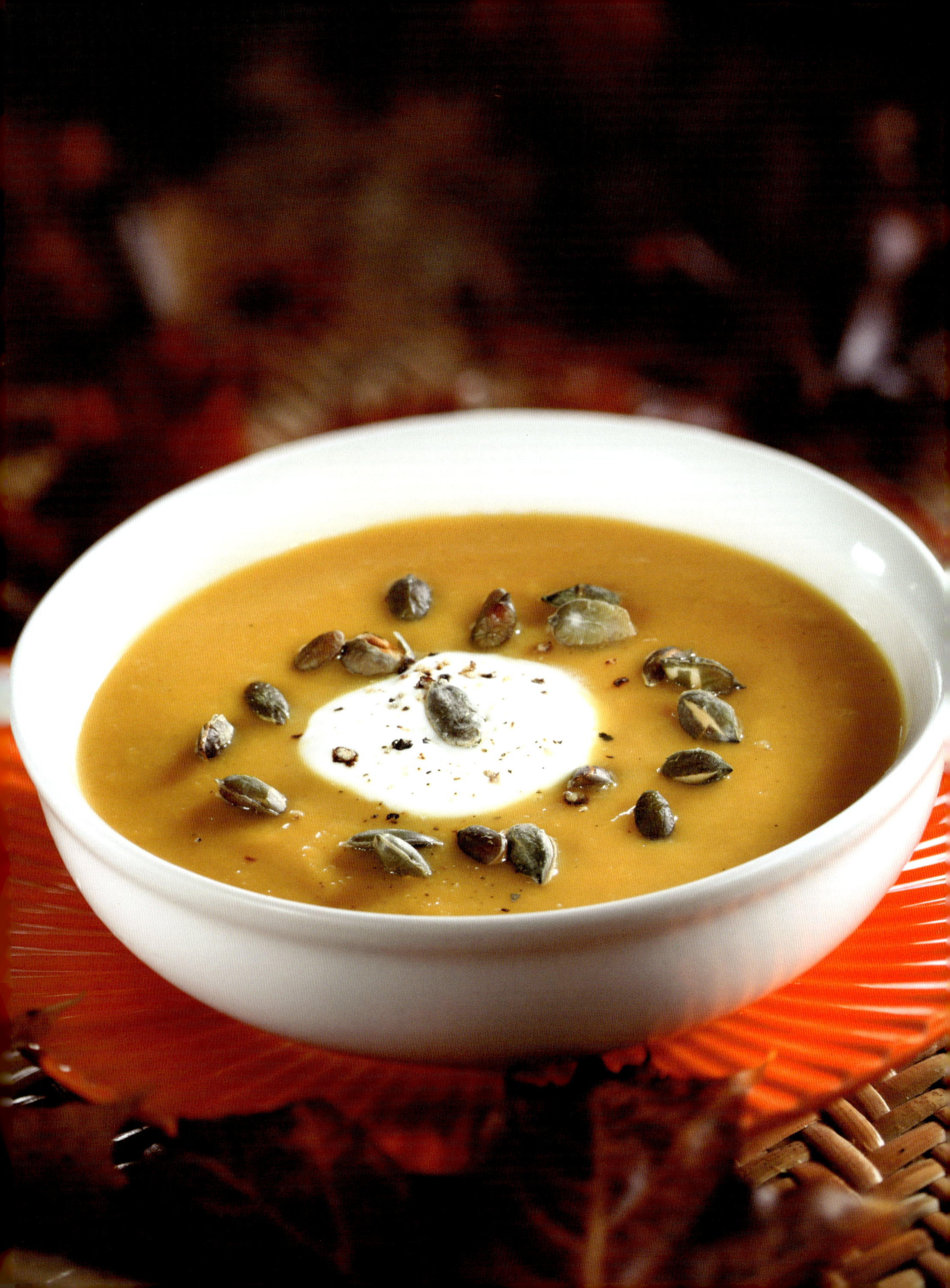

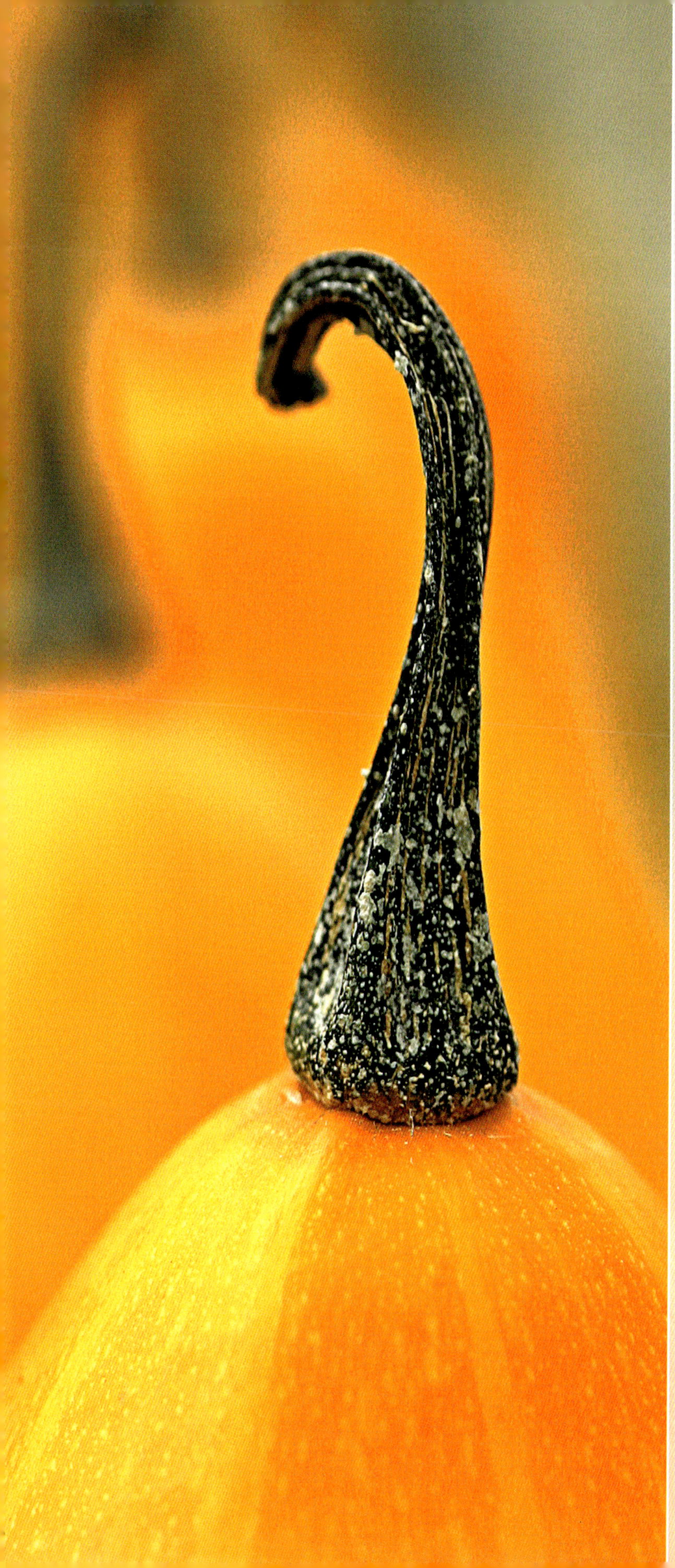

Squash Soup

1.5 kg (3.3 lb) squash
50 g (2 oz) butter
1 leek, chopped
25 ml (3/4 fl oz) water
1 carrot, chopped
1 apple, peeled and chopped
1.2 litres (2½ pints) vegetable stock
1 cinnamon stick
100 ml (3½ fl oz) double cream
25 ml (3/4 fl oz) (5 teaspoons) sherry
pinch of salt
200 g (7 oz) low fat yogurt
pumpkin seeds, toasted

Using a sharp knife, peel the skin and cut the squash into chunks. Using a spoon, carefully hollow out the squash, removing the flesh. Finally cut the squash into 2.5 cm (1 inch) cubes. In a large saucepan, melt the butter and add the chopped leek. Add the water and cook over a medium heat for about 3 minutes. Add the squash cubes, chopped carrot, apple, vegetable stock and cinnamon stick. Cook for 25-30 minutes, stirring occasionally to prevent the base from burning. Remove from the heat and take out the cinnamon stick. Add the double cream, sherry and pinch of salt. Using a hand-held blender, blend until smooth and creamy.
Serve warm with a large tablespoon of yogurt and sprinkle some toasted pumpkin seeds around.

Serves 6

Per serving
256 kcal, 16.2 g fat (9.9 g saturated), 3.5 g protein, 24.8 g carbs (15.1 g sugar), 6.6 g fibre, 0.7 g salt

Lentil Soup

3 tablespoons sunflower oil
2 medium onions, roughly chopped
1 medium carrot, roughly chopped
1 tablespoon caraway seeds, toasted and finely ground
2 large cloves garlic, cut in half
1.5 litres (2½ pints) vegetable stock
200 g (7 oz) red lentils, rinsed and drained
pinch of salt

200 g (7 oz) low fat yogurt
3 tablespoons fresh mint, finely chopped
handful of homemade croutons
chili pepper, chopped (optional)

In a large saucepan warm the oil and add the chopped onions, then 25 ml (¾ fl oz) water and cook for around 3 minutes until the onions start going transparent. Then add the carrot, garlic, vegetable stock, lentils and cook for about 30-35 minutes, stirring occasionally to prevent the base from burning. Meanwhile in a small saucepan toast the caraway seeds for about 3-5 minutes and grind with a mortar. Remove the vegetables from the heat, add the grounded caraway seeds and salt. Using a hand blender blend all until smooth and creamy.
Serve warm with a tablespoon of yogurt, chopped fresh mint leaves and chili pepper.

Serves 4

Per serving
316 kcal, 10.0 g fat (1.5 g saturated), 16.5 g protein, 43.4 g carbs (11 g sugar), 5.6 g fibre, 1.0 g salt

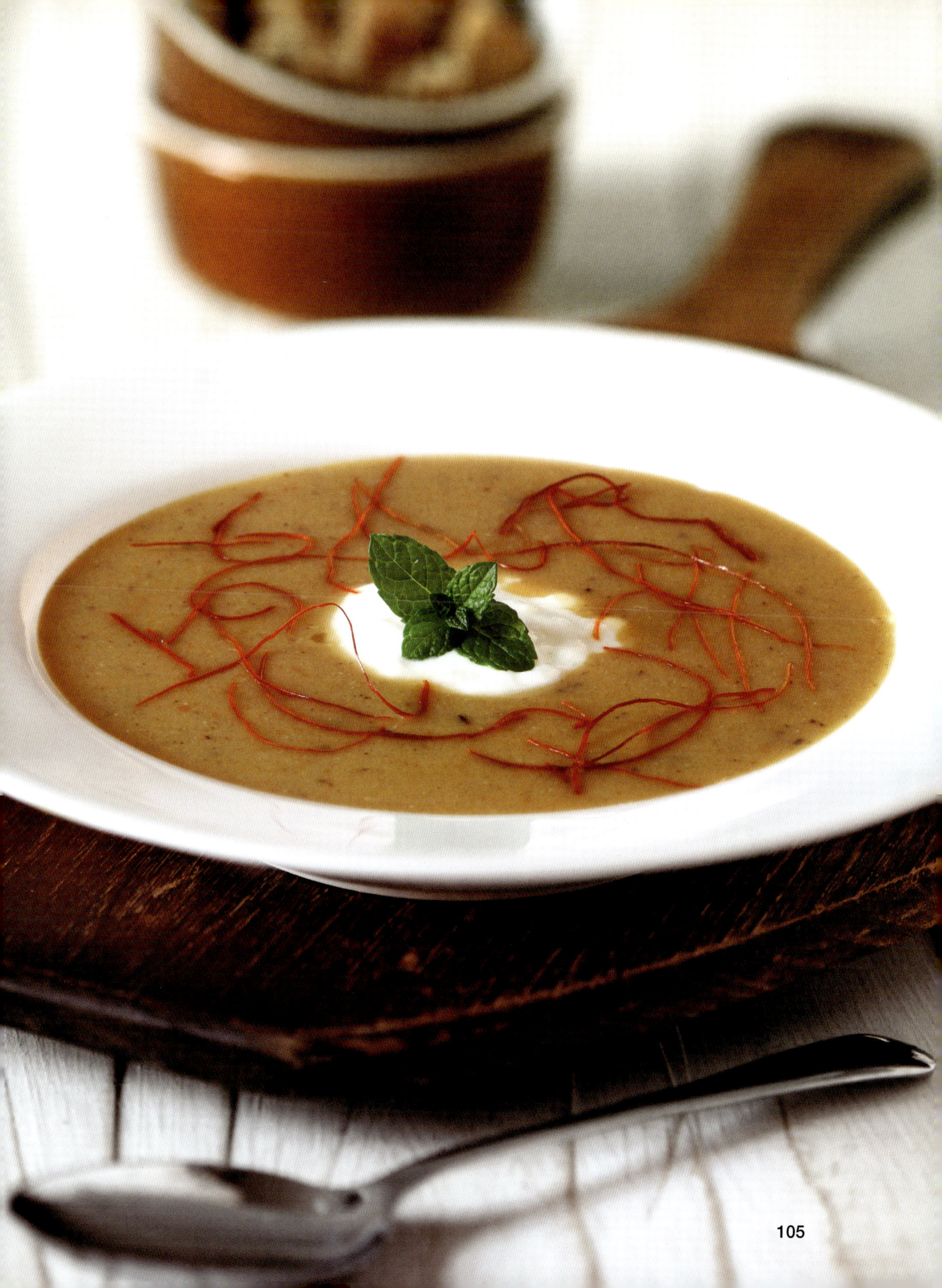

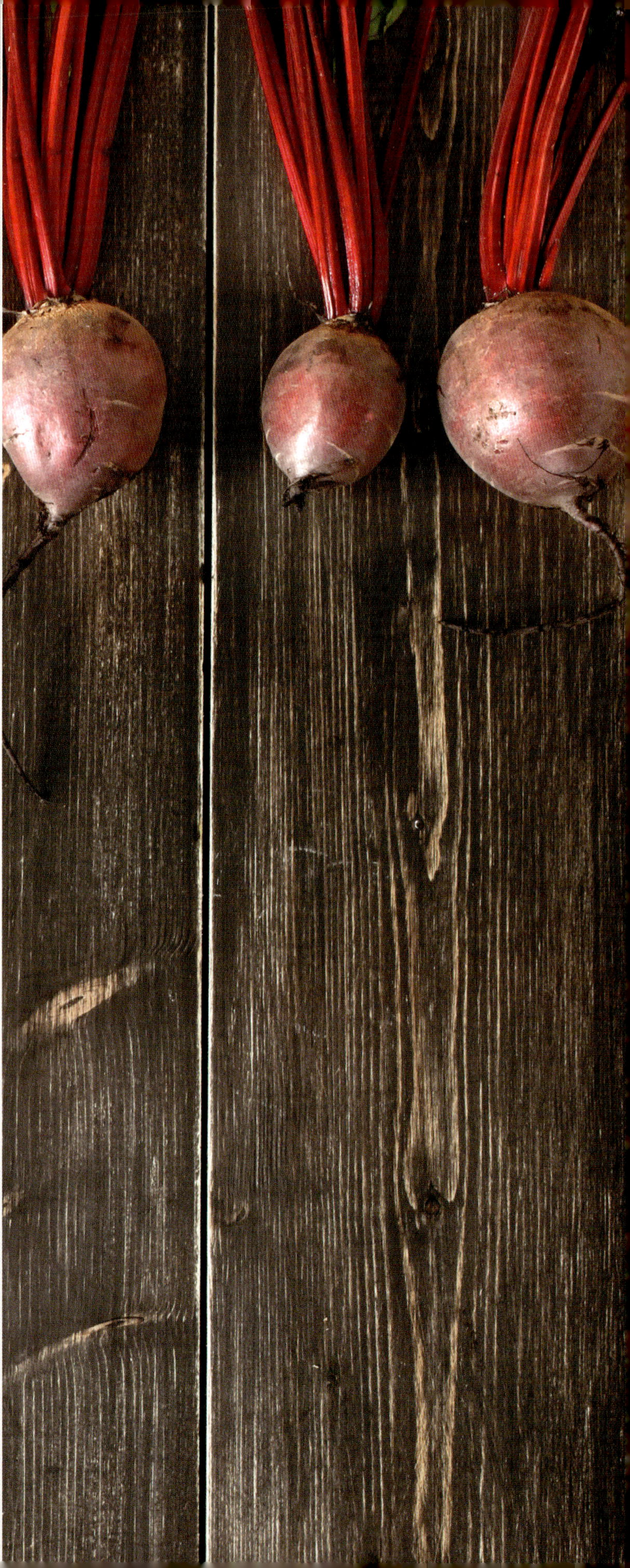

Beetroot Yogurt Soup

500 g (17½ oz) beetroot
350 g (12 oz) low fat yogurt
1 handful fresh dill, washed and chopped
1 lemon freshly squeezed juice
1 teaspoon cardamom seeds, crushed
pinch of salt
6 ice cubes
150 g (5 oz) low fat yogurt for serving
2 tablespoons pistachios, chopped

Peel and cut beetroot into chunks, using latex gloves to protect your hands from beet ink. Arrange beetroot on a parchment-lined baking tray and put in the oven to roast at around 180°C (350°F) for 40 minutes, or until just tender.

In a blender, combine the baked beetroot chunks, yogurt, dill, lemon juice, ground cardamom, and salt, blend on high speed until smooth. Serve cold with a tablespoon of yogurt on the top and chopped pistachios.

Serves 4

Per serving
191 kcal, 8.3 g fat (1.8 g saturated), 10.5 g protein, 20.0 g carbs (18.7 g sugar), 4.3 g fibre, 0.6 g salt

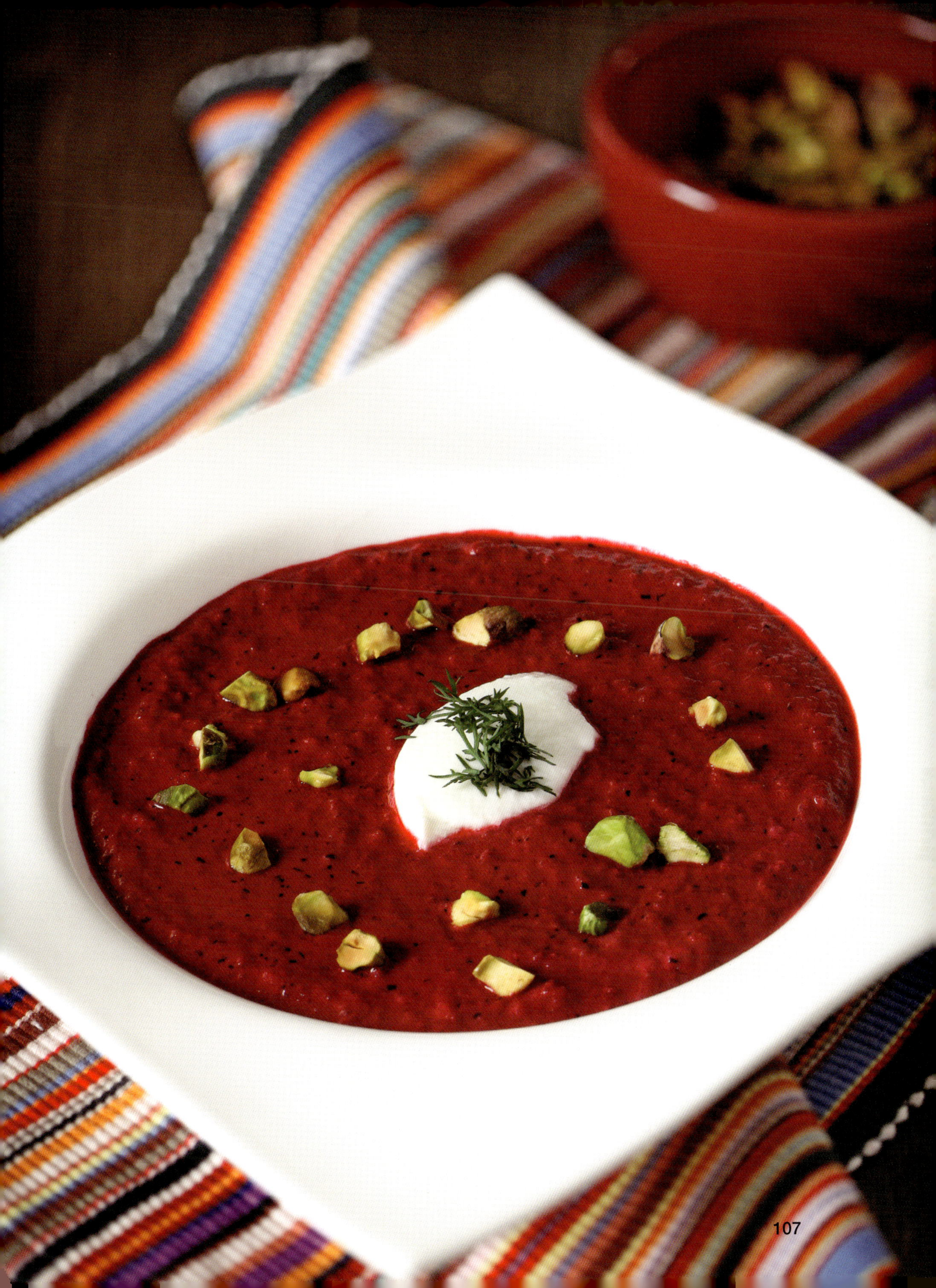

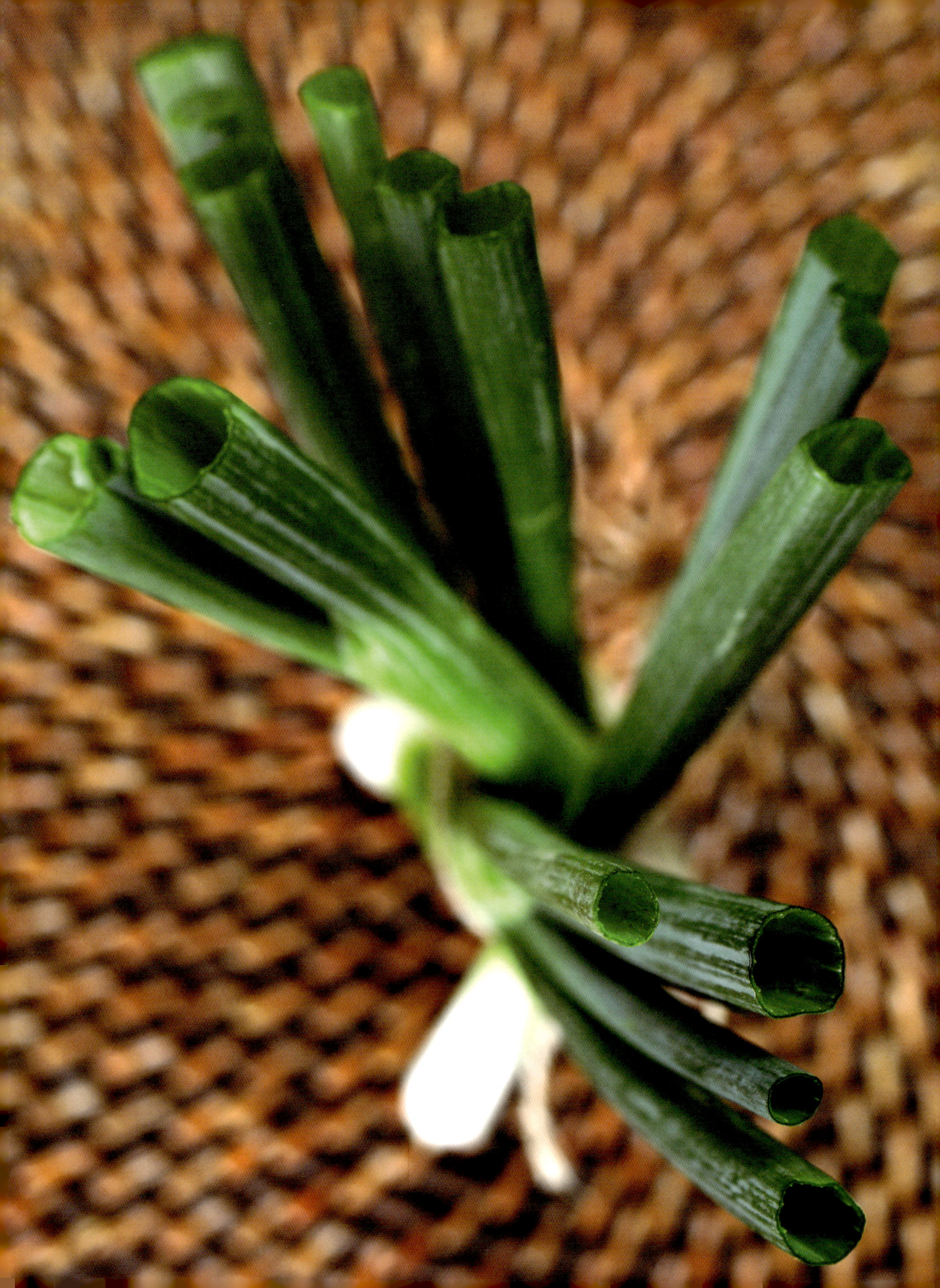

Salads

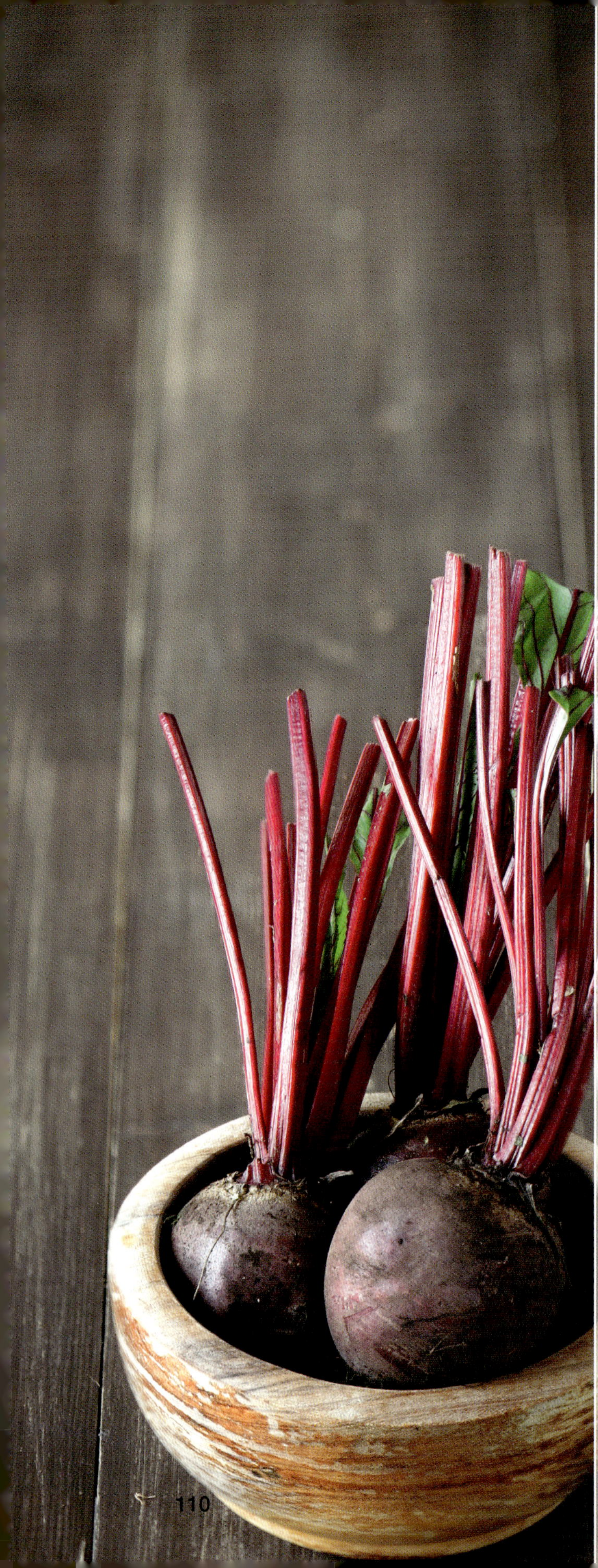

Beetroot Salad and Yogurt Dressing

Salad:
300 g (10½ oz) raw beetroot, peeled and grated
2 tablespoons sultanas
handful of chives, coarsely chopped
handful of fresh mint
½ lemon, freshly squeezed juice
1 tablespoon extra virgin olive oil
pinch of salt
tablespoon flaked almonds

Grate the raw beetroot and put into a medium bowl. Add a pinch of salt, mix, cover with kitchen foil and leave to rest in the refrigerator for 30 minutes. Then strain the beetroot, add the lemon juice, the oil and mix well. Finally add the sultanas, chopped chives, mint and mix again gently. Sprinkle the almond flakes on top and pour over the yogurt dressing.

Dressing:
250 g (9 oz) yogurt
1 clove garlic, crushed
1 teaspoon sumac
pinch of salt

Crush the garlic clove. Pour the yogurt Into a small bowl and add the garlic, sumac and a pinch of salt. Mix well and garnish with some more sumac.

Serves 6 to share

Per serving
140 kcal, 8.1 g fat (3.2 g saturated), 4.4 g protein, 13.3 g carbs (12.5 g sugar), 1.1 g salt, 1.6 g fibre

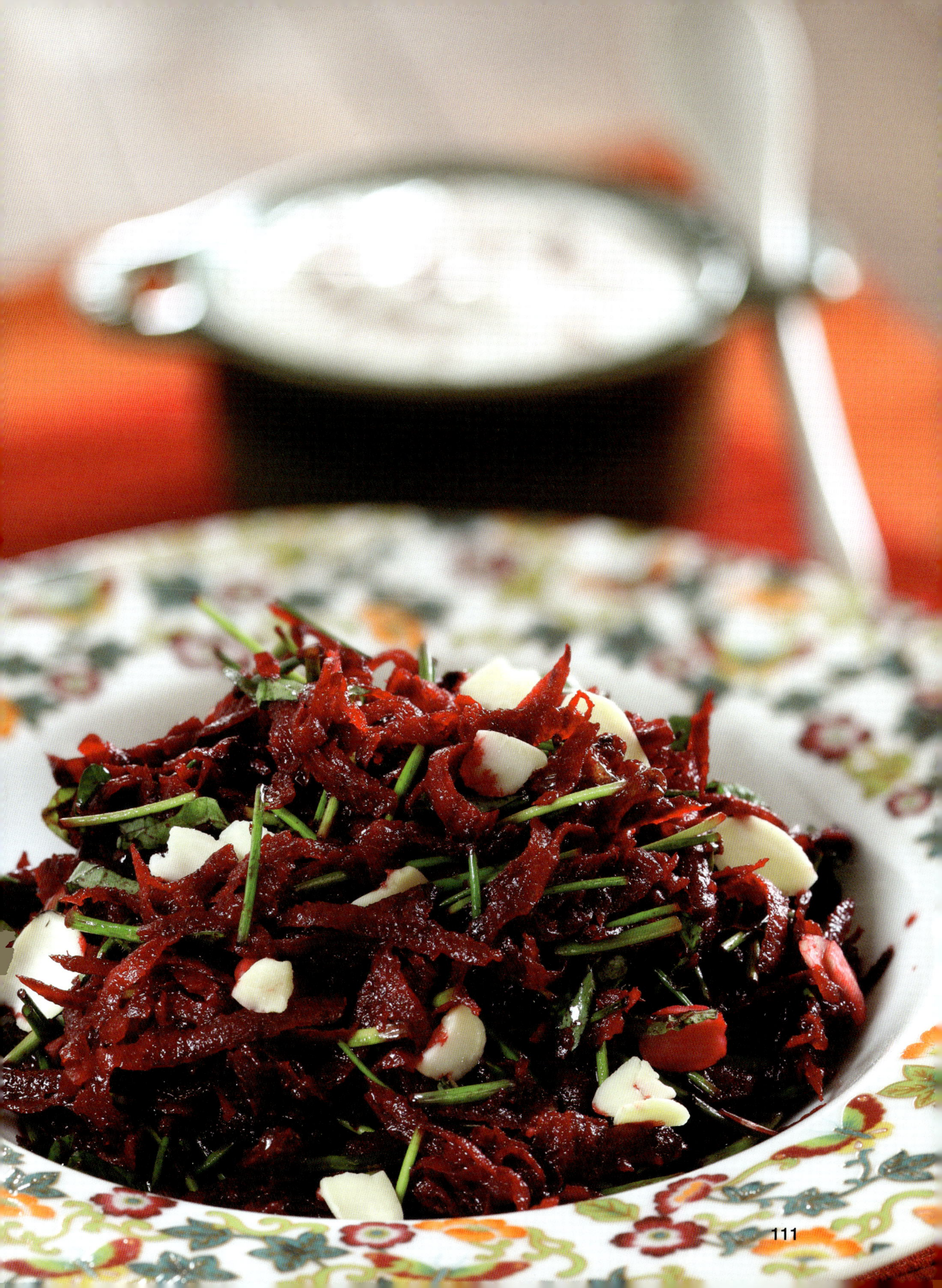

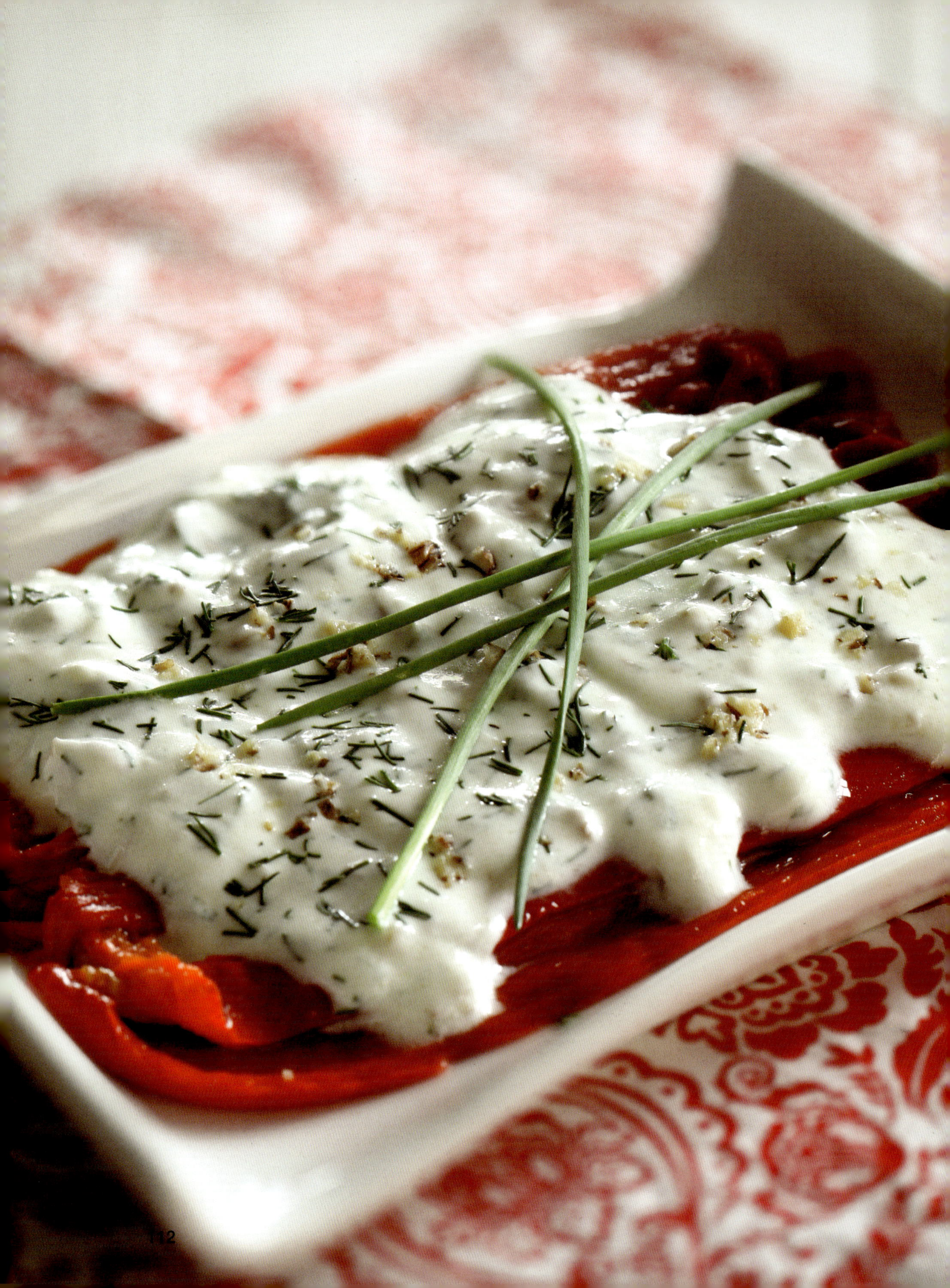

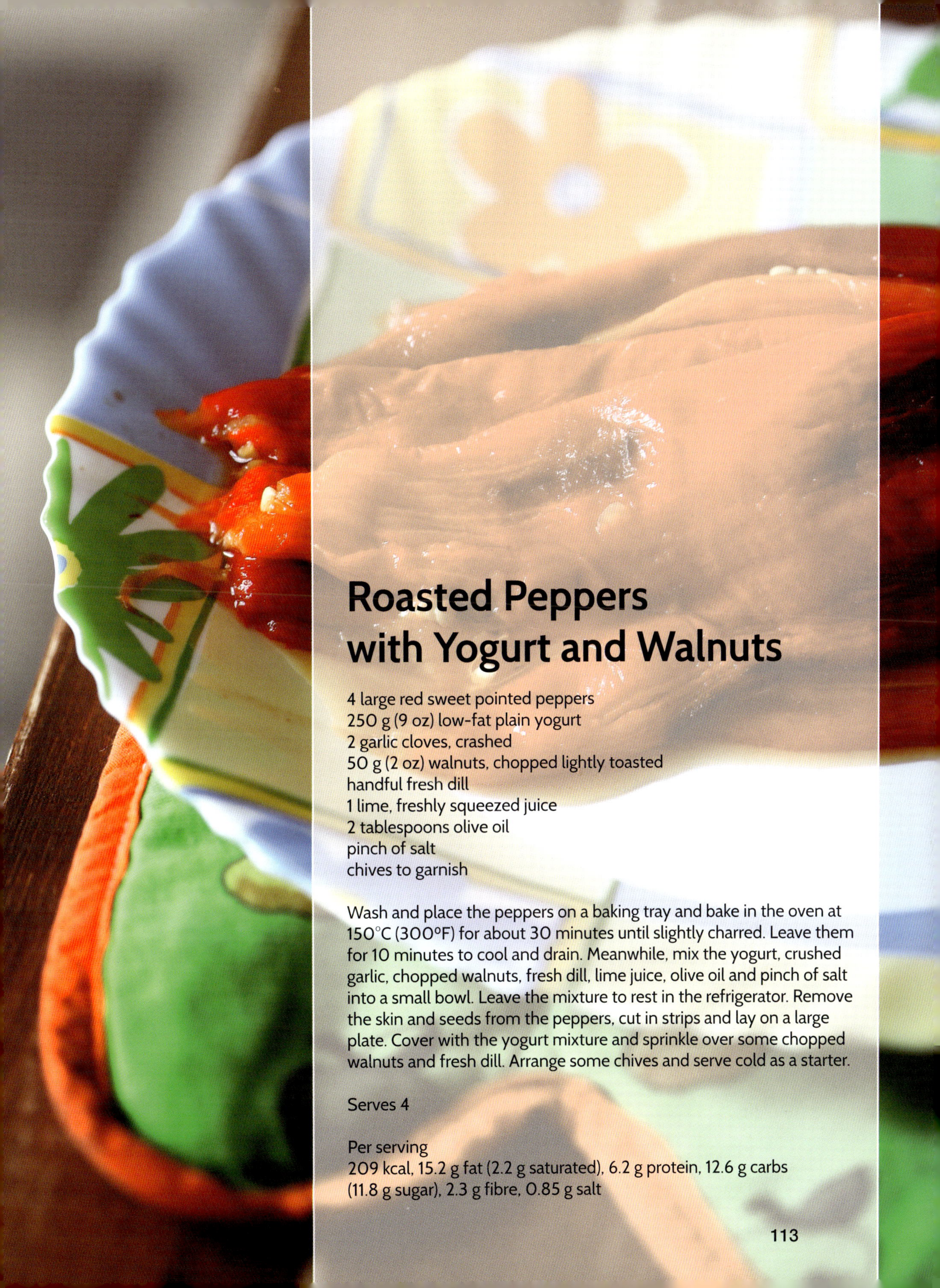

Roasted Peppers with Yogurt and Walnuts

4 large red sweet pointed peppers
250 g (9 oz) low-fat plain yogurt
2 garlic cloves, crashed
50 g (2 oz) walnuts, chopped lightly toasted
handful fresh dill
1 lime, freshly squeezed juice
2 tablespoons olive oil
pinch of salt
chives to garnish

Wash and place the peppers on a baking tray and bake in the oven at 150°C (300°F) for about 30 minutes until slightly charred. Leave them for 10 minutes to cool and drain. Meanwhile, mix the yogurt, crushed garlic, chopped walnuts, fresh dill, lime juice, olive oil and pinch of salt into a small bowl. Leave the mixture to rest in the refrigerator. Remove the skin and seeds from the peppers, cut in strips and lay on a large plate. Cover with the yogurt mixture and sprinkle over some chopped walnuts and fresh dill. Arrange some chives and serve cold as a starter.

Serves 4

Per serving
209 kcal, 15.2 g fat (2.2 g saturated), 6.2 g protein, 12.6 g carbs (11.8 g sugar), 2.3 g fibre, 0.85 g salt

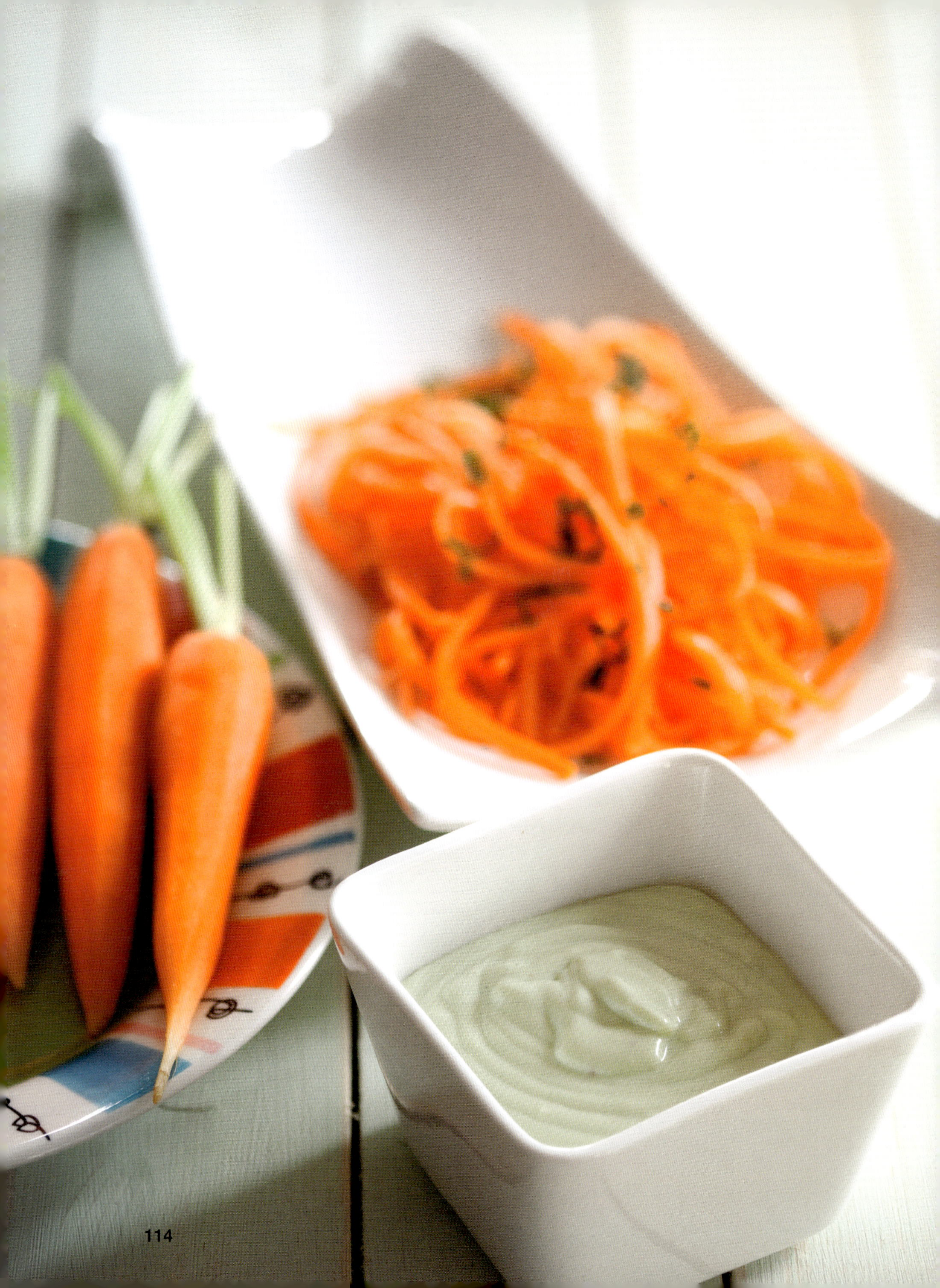

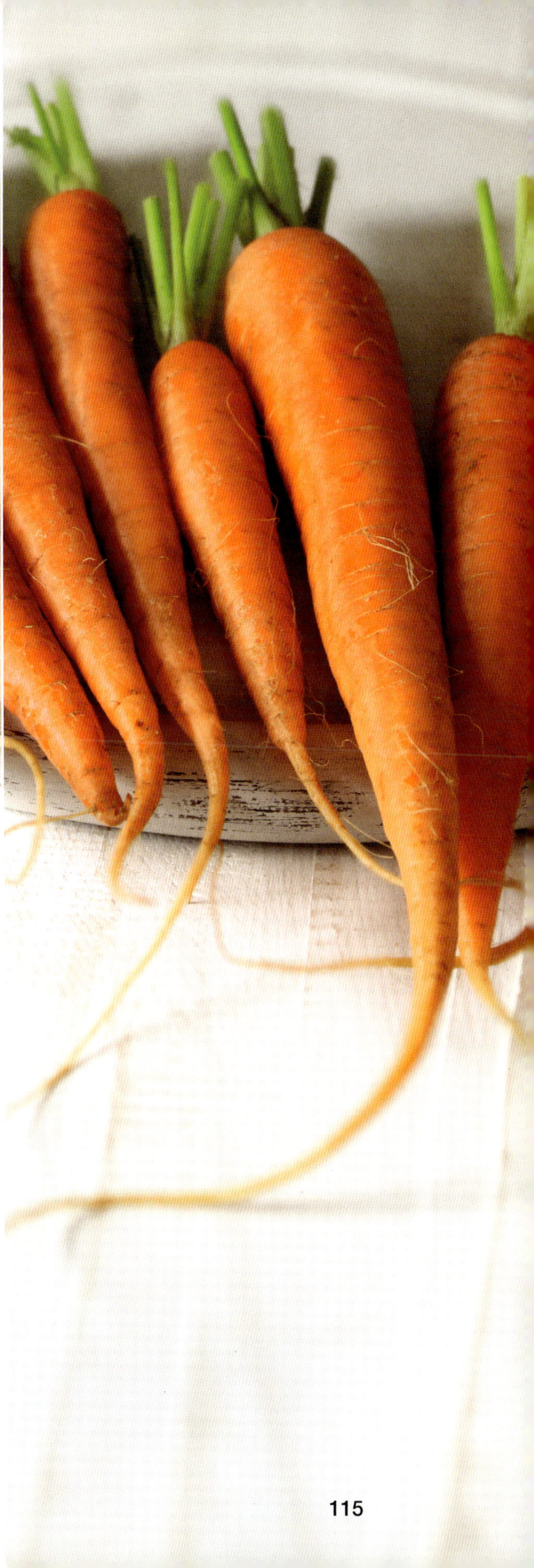

Avocado and Blue Cheese Topping

300 g (10½ oz) low fat yogurt
1 avocado
50 g (2 oz) blue cheese
1 teaspoon horseradish sauce
1 teaspoon caster sugar
pinch of salt and black pepper

Throw all the ingredients into the blender, blend well until smooth. Transfer to a serving bowl and leave for 30 minutes in the refrigerator to rest. This topping is suitable to be served with vegetable salads like – carrot, cucumbers or turnip.

Serves 6

Per serving
107 kcal, 7.7 g fat (2.9 g saturated), 4.6 g protein, 5.1 g carbohydrate (4.7 g sugar), 1.1 g fibre, 0.9 g salt

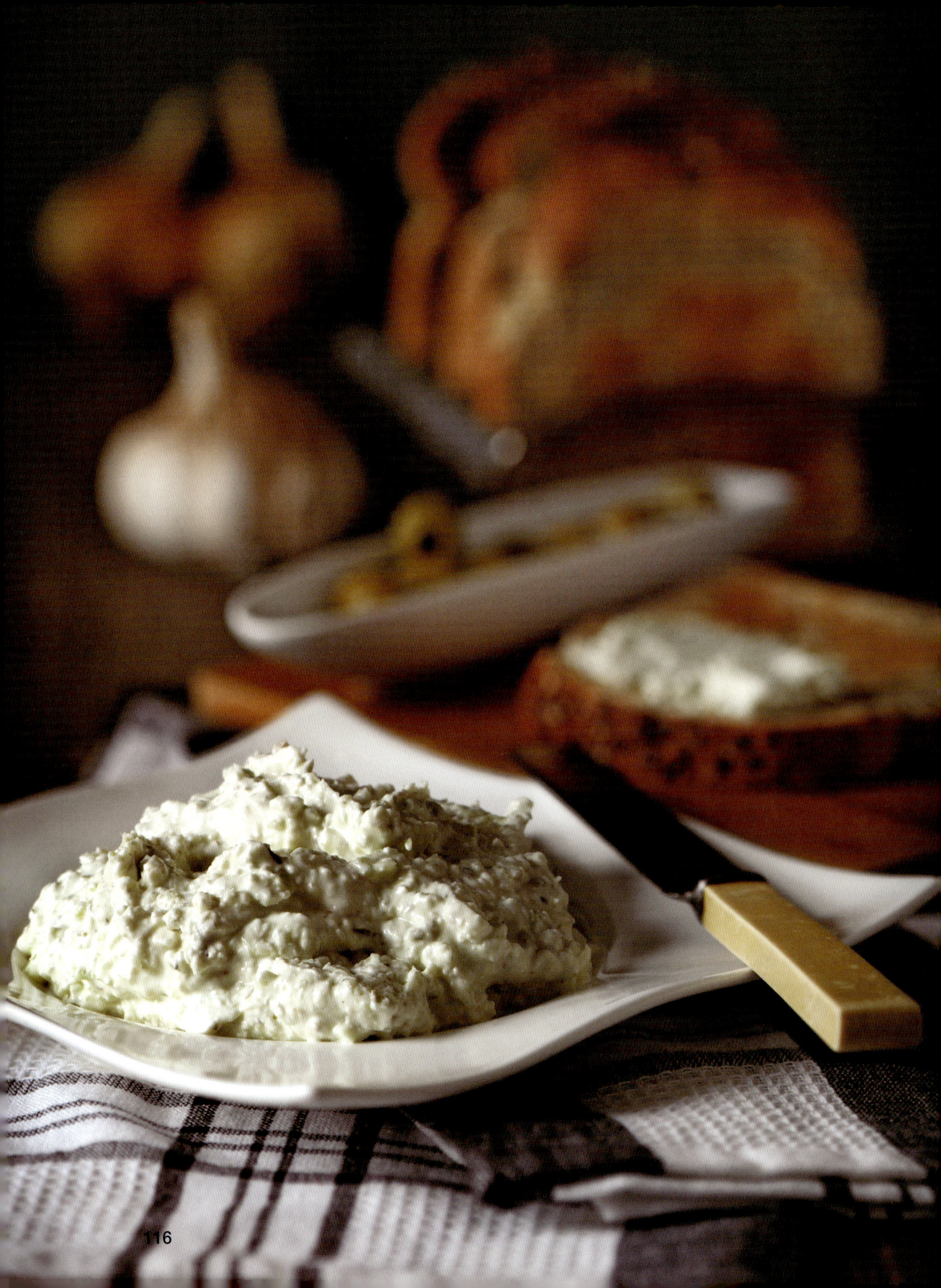

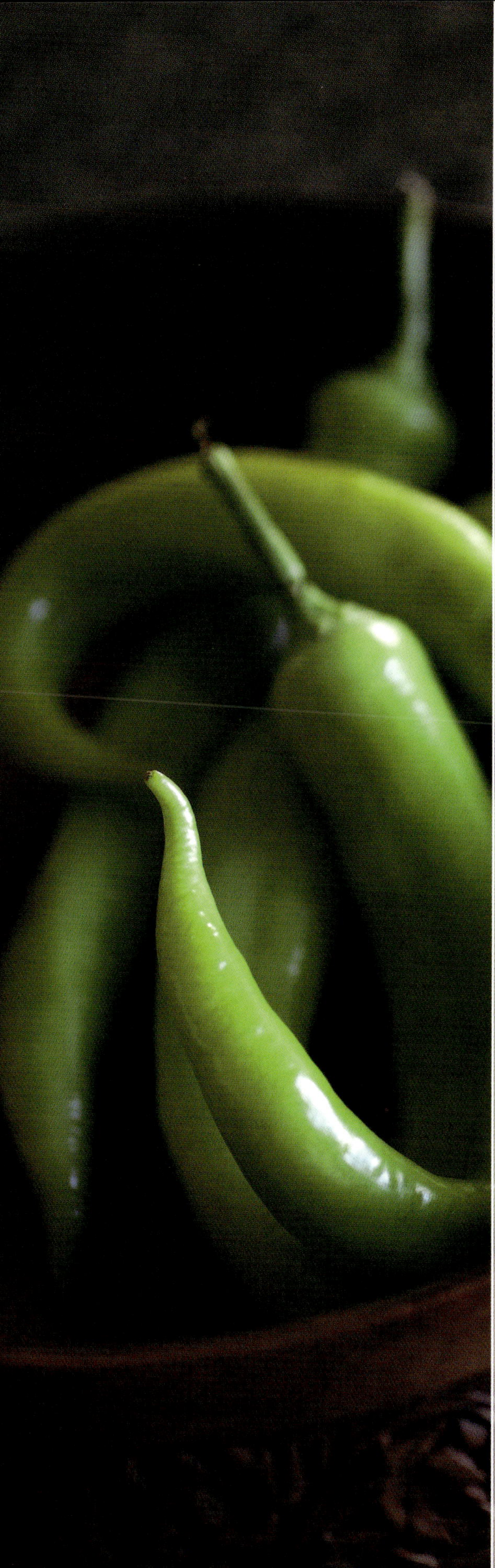

Tiro salad

250 g (9 oz) feta cheese, diced
2 pepperoncini, seeded and chopped
1 small dried red chili pepper, seeded and chopped
1 lemon, freshly squeezed juice
2 tablespoons extra virgin olive oil
2 tablespoons low fat yogurt
2 tablespoon dried oregano
2 cloves garlic, crushed

Blend together the pepperoncini, diced feta chees, yogurt, crushed garlic, lemon juice, olive oil, dried red chili pepper and dried oregano. Blend until smooth. Serve with sliced toasted bread or savoury biscuits and some olives.

Serves 6

Per serving
245 kcal, 20.5 g fat (12.0 g saturated), 13.3 g protein, 1.9 g carbs (1.6 g sugar), 0.1 g fibre, 3.1 g salt

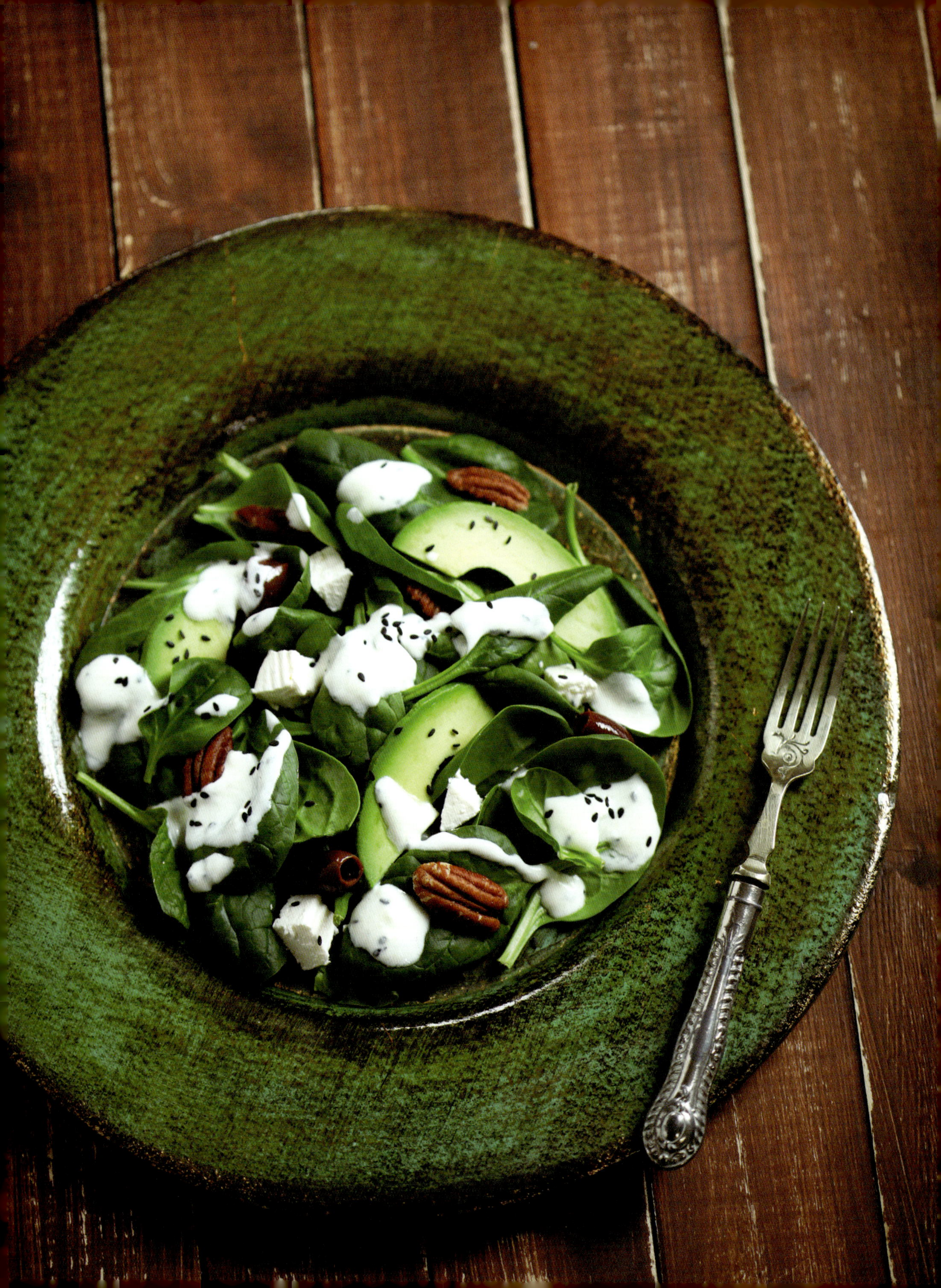

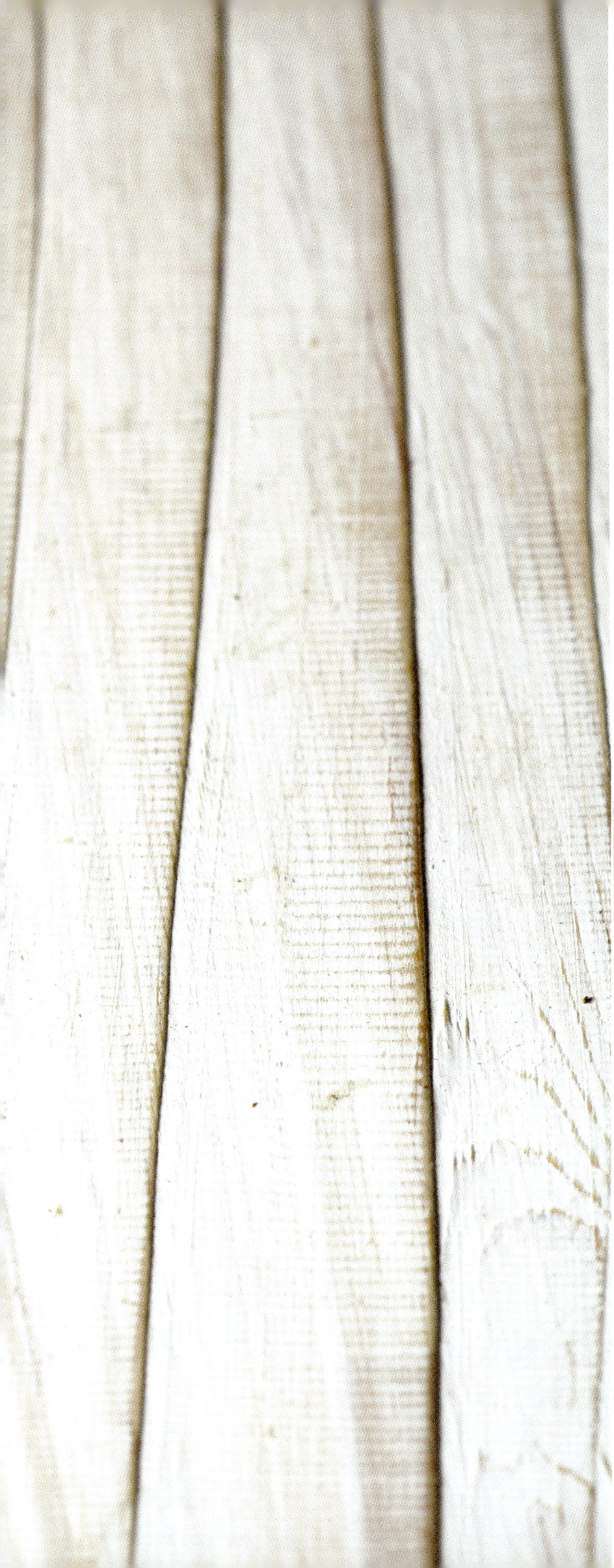

Spinach Salad

250 g (9 oz) young spinach
50 g (2 oz) pecans, chopped
100 g (3½ oz) kalamata olives
200 g (7 oz) feta cheese, diced
1 avocado, sliced
200 g (7 oz) low fat yogurt
1 clove garlic, crushed
1 lemon freshly squeezed juice
2 tablespoons extra virgin olive oil
1 tablespoon black sesame seeds
pinch of salt

Combine the yogurt, garlic, lemon juice, extra virgin olive oil and a pinch of salt In a medium bowl and mix well. Wash the young spinach and then divide and arrange onto four plates. Throw over some kalamata olives, pecans, sliced avocado and diced feta cheese. Pour over yogurt dressing and sprinkle with some black sesame seeds.

Serves 4

Per serving
416 kcal, 36.6 g fat (10.9 g saturated), 14.6 g protein, 7.3 g carbs (6.3 g sugar), 5.5 g fibre, 4.2 g salt

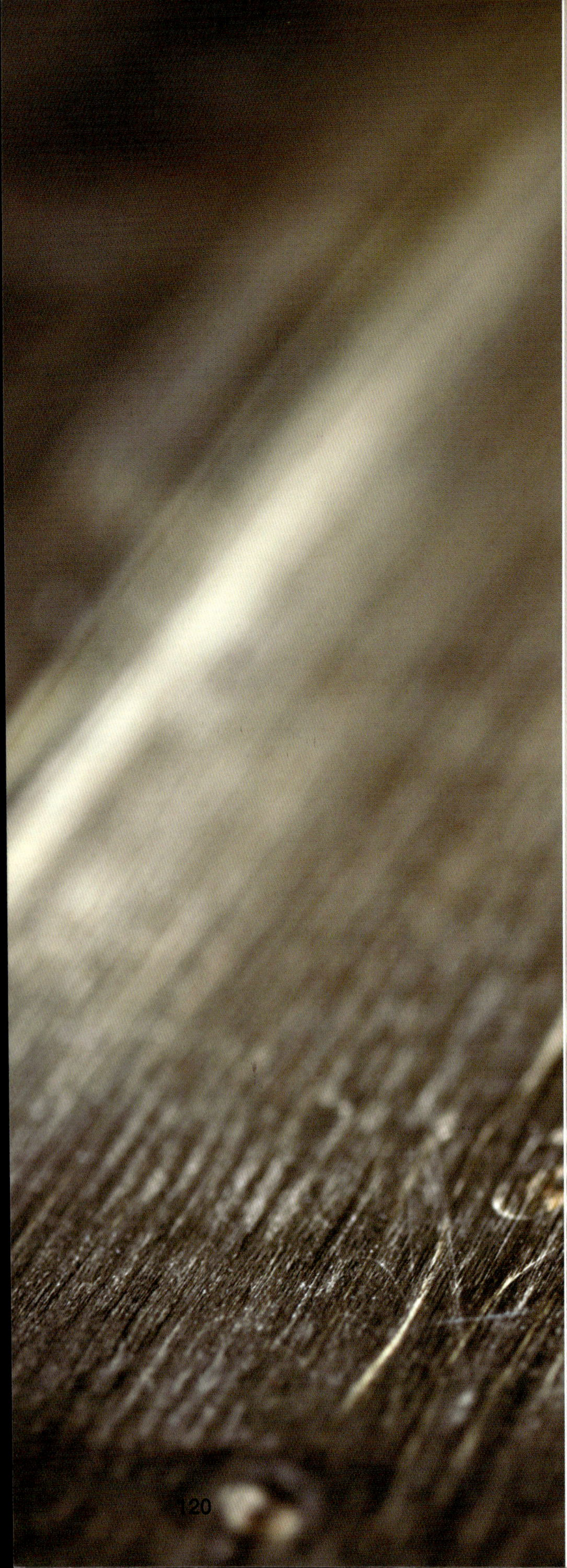

Green Salad with Mustard Yogurt Dressing

200 g (7 oz) young leaf salad
150 g (5 oz) pancetta, diced
2 boiled eggs, peeled and sliced
100 g (3½ oz) low fat yogurt
1 teaspoon mustard
1 teaspoon mustard seeds
1 tablespoon runny honey
1 lime, fresh squeezed juice
1 tablespoon extra virgin olive oil
pinch of salt
handful homemade croutons

Combine the low fat yogurt, mustard, mustard seeds, runny honey, lime juice, olive oil and a pinch of salt in a small bowl and mix well. Set aside to rest. In a small pan boil the eggs for about 8 minutes, leave to cool for a couple of minutes in cold water and then peel and slice. Meanwhile throw the pancetta into a small frying pan and cook over high heat for about 5 minutes. Wash the young leaf salad in a colander and leave to drain for a few minutes. Divide the salad onto 4 large plates. On top arrange the sliced eggs and the cooked pancetta. Serve with 3–4 spoons of the yogurt mustard dressing and some croutons.

Serves 4

Per serving
193 kcal, 13.8 g fat (4.1 g saturated), 11.2 g protein, 7.7 g carbs (5.3 g sugar), 0.8 g fibre, 2.4 g salt

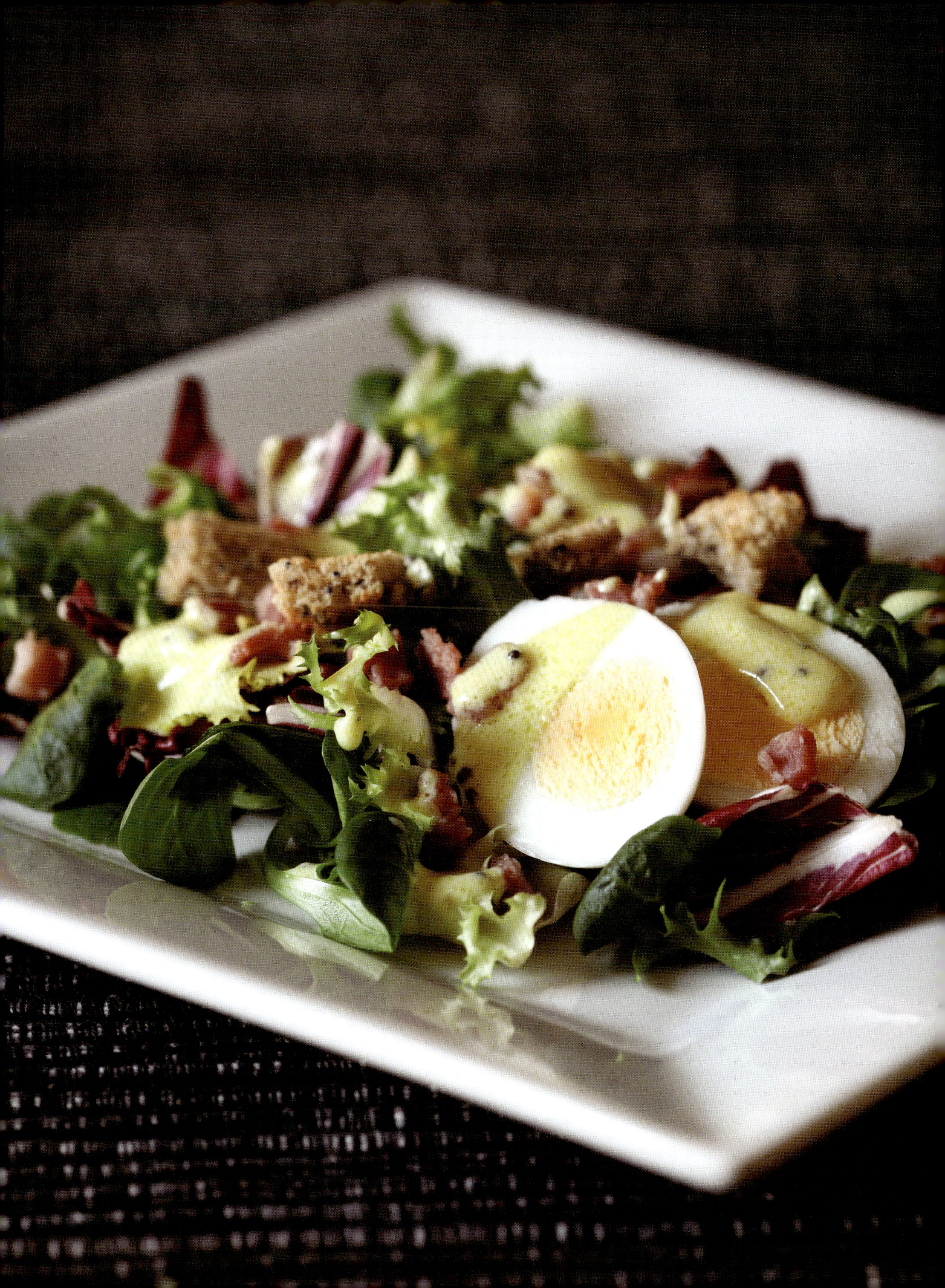

Kumquats Green Salad with Yogurt Dressing

Salad:
2 gem hearts or any other green salad, washed and chopped
4 spring onions
2 tablespoons of toasted almond, slices
6 kumquats, washed and sliced

Throw the chopped green salad and spring onions in a large bowl and mix. Just before serving the salad, arrange the kumquat slices on top and pour over the dressing. Finally sprinkle some toasted almond slices.

Dressing:
250 g (9 oz) low fat yogurt
1 lime, fresh juice
2 tablespoons extra virgin olive oil
1 teaspoon dried dill
1 teaspoon dried oregano
1 clove garlic, crashed
a pinch of salt

Combine the yogurt, lime juice and olive oil in a medium bowl, mix well. Add the dried dill, oregano, crushed garlic, a pinch of salt and mix again. Leave it to rest in the refrigerator for a couple of minutes and the salad is ready to serve.

Serves 4

Per serving
140 kcal, 9.3 g fat (1.5 g saturated), 4.9 g protein, 9.7 g carbs (9.2 g sugar), 3.0 g fibre, 0.9 g salt

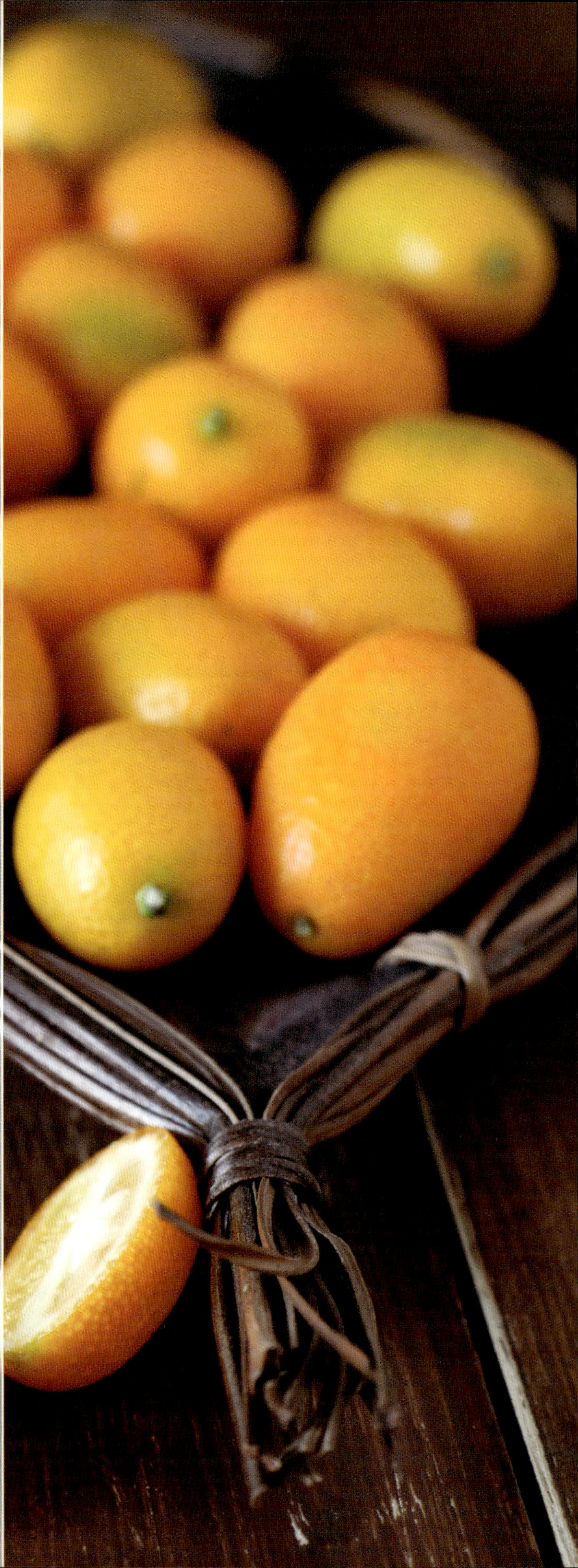

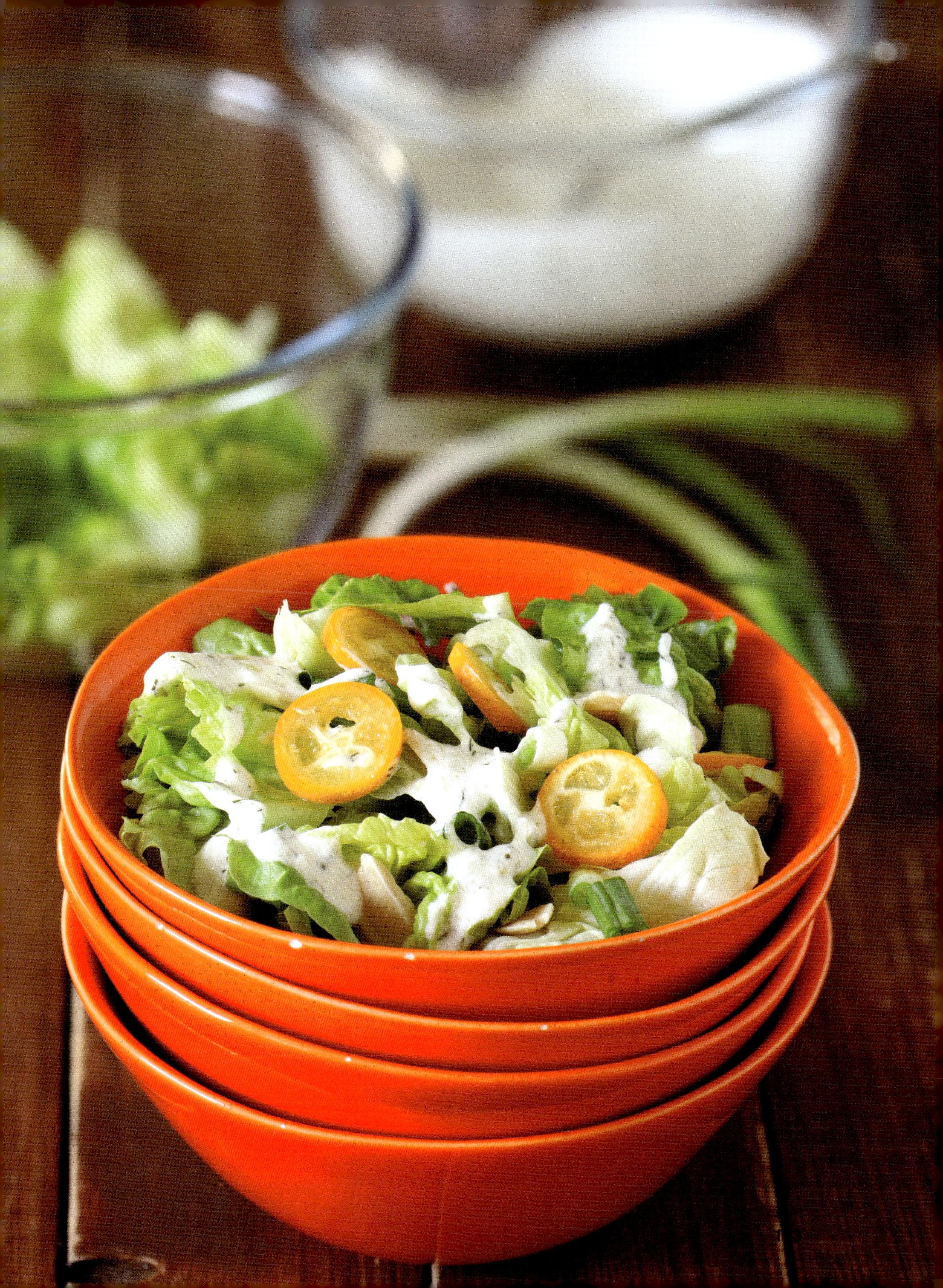

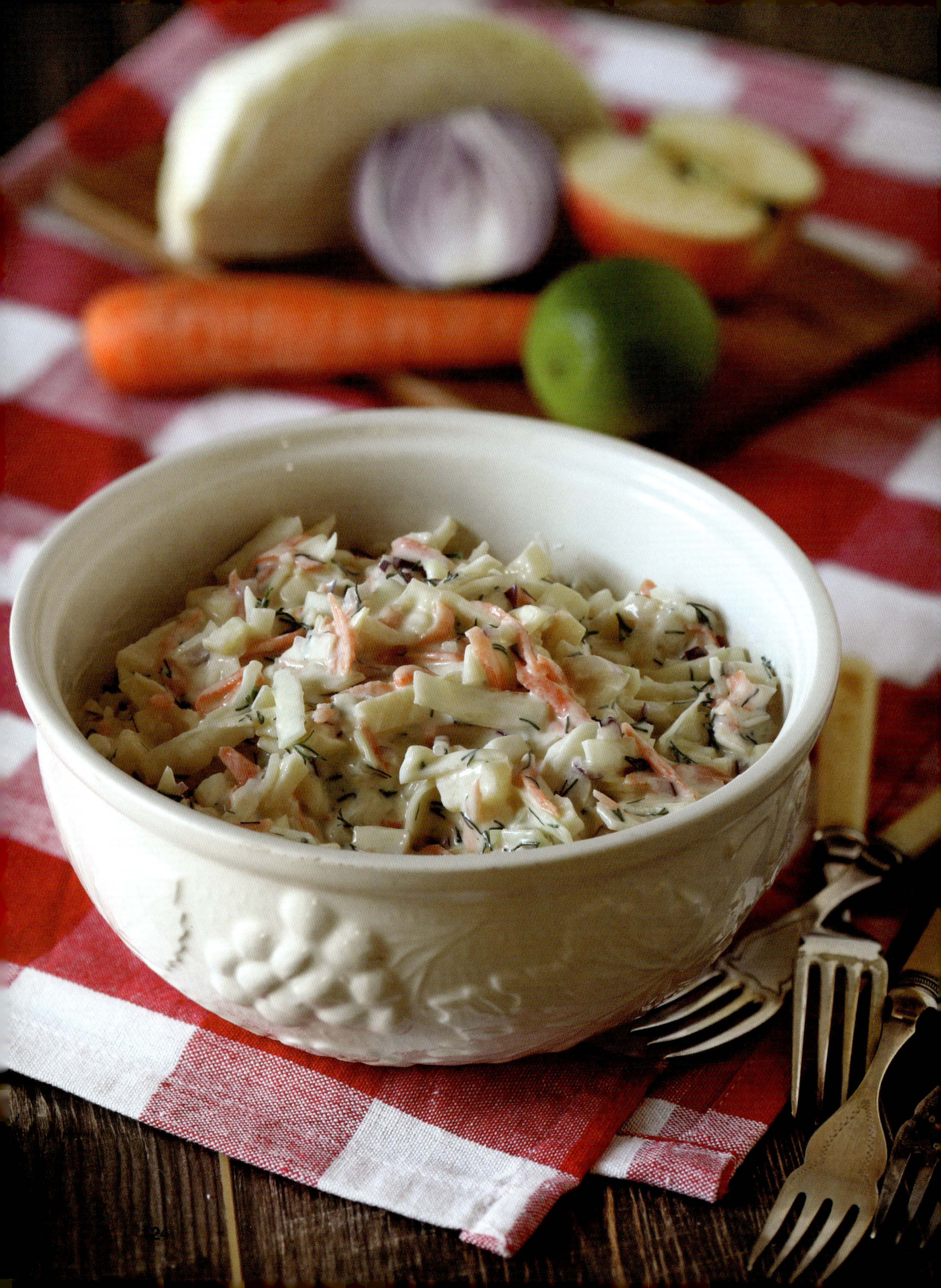

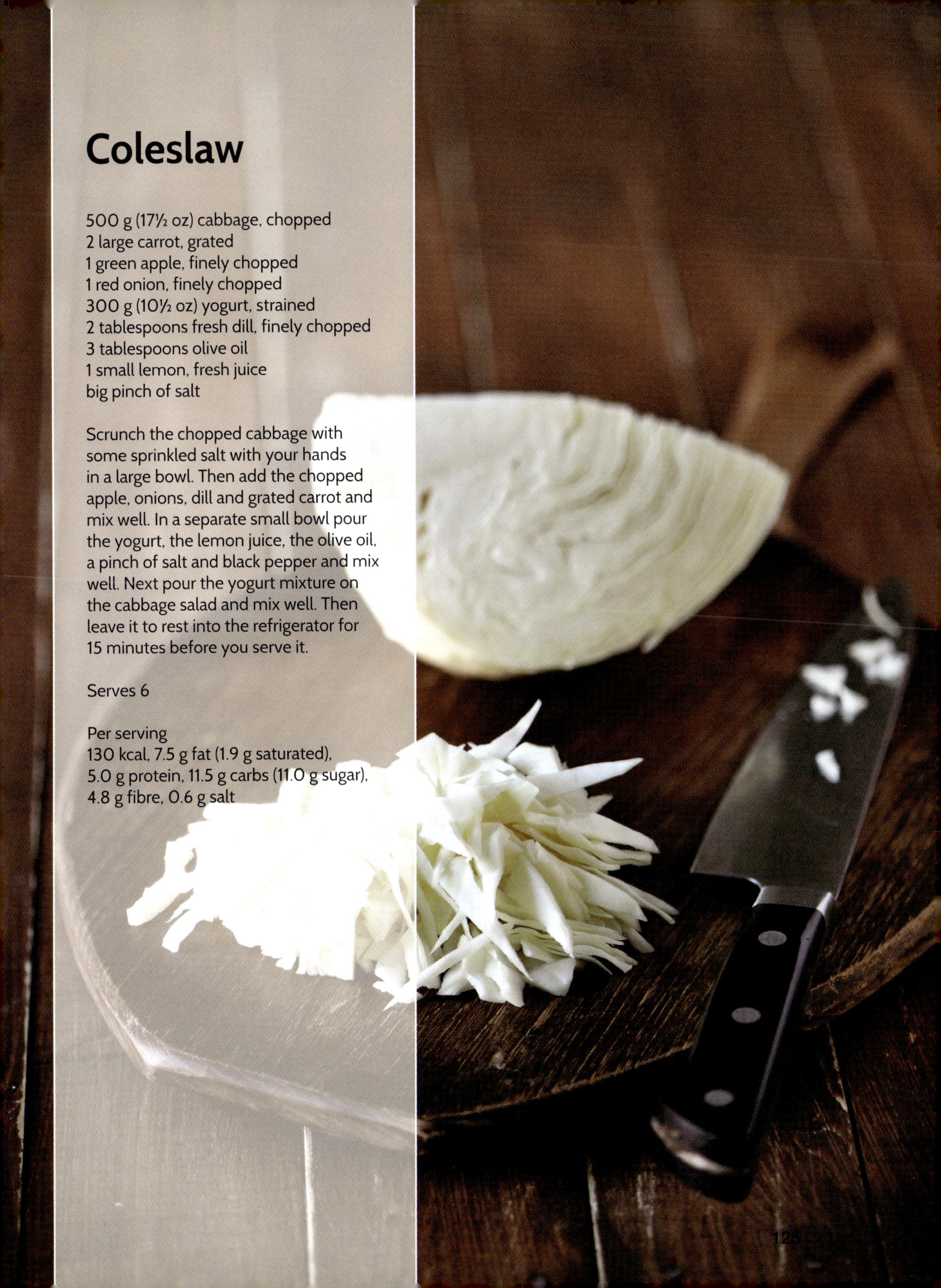

Coleslaw

500 g (17½ oz) cabbage, chopped
2 large carrot, grated
1 green apple, finely chopped
1 red onion, finely chopped
300 g (10½ oz) yogurt, strained
2 tablespoons fresh dill, finely chopped
3 tablespoons olive oil
1 small lemon, fresh juice
big pinch of salt

Scrunch the chopped cabbage with some sprinkled salt with your hands in a large bowl. Then add the chopped apple, onions, dill and grated carrot and mix well. In a separate small bowl pour the yogurt, the lemon juice, the olive oil, a pinch of salt and black pepper and mix well. Next pour the yogurt mixture on the cabbage salad and mix well. Then leave it to rest into the refrigerator for 15 minutes before you serve it.

Serves 6

Per serving
130 kcal, 7.5 g fat (1.9 g saturated),
5.0 g protein, 11.5 g carbs (11.0 g sugar),
4.8 g fibre, 0.6 g salt

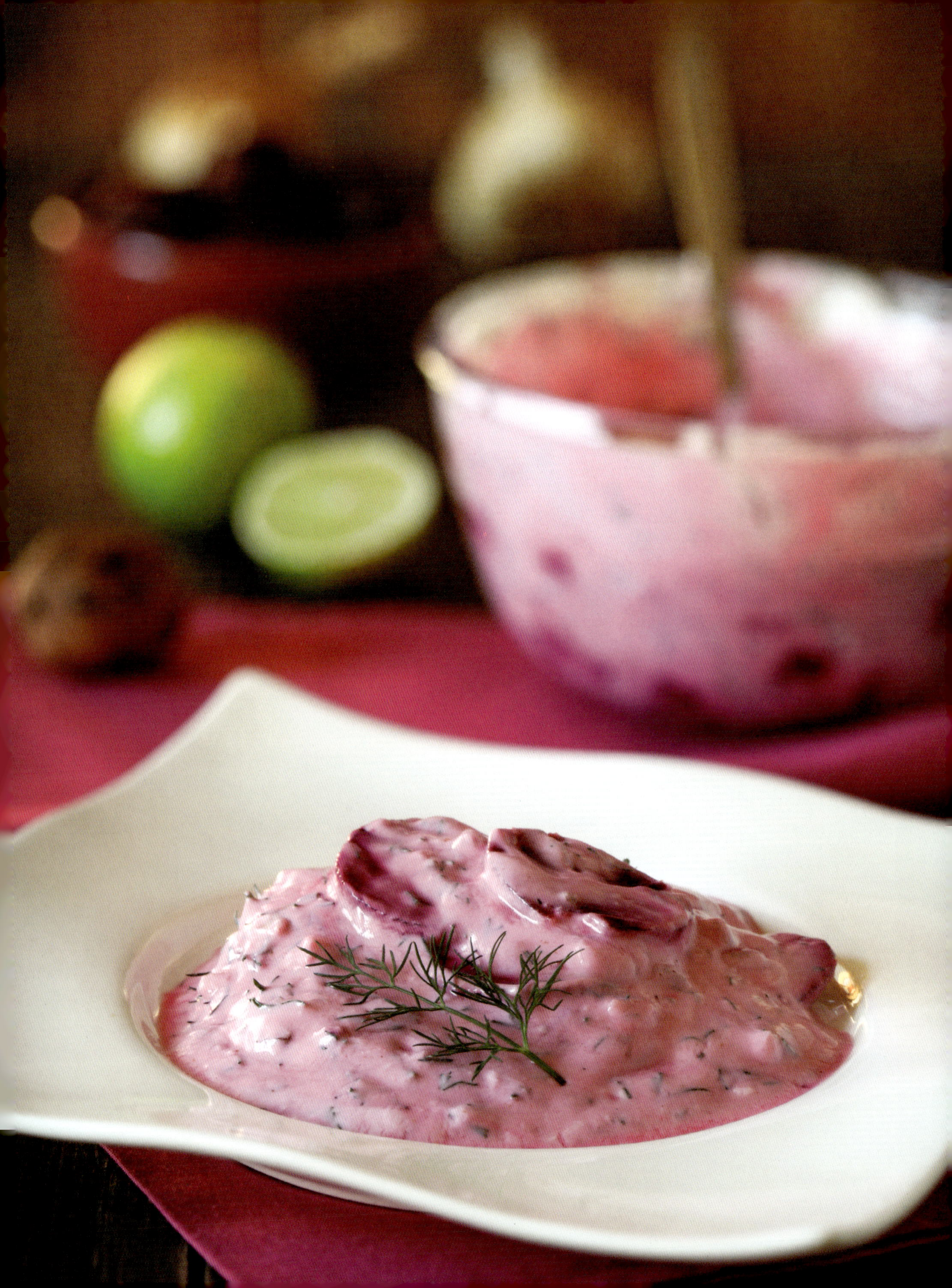

Beetroot and Yogurt Salad

200 g (7 oz) beetroot
250 g (9 oz) low fat yogurt
2 garlic cloves, crushed
1 teaspoon ground coriander
1 teaspoon ground cumin
freshly squeezed juice of 1 lime
2 tablespoons chopped dill
2 tablespoon extra virgin olive oil
1 tablespoon toasted walnuts, chopped
pinch of salt

Wearing latex gloves to protect your hands from beet ink, wash, peel and slice the beetroots. Fill the bottom of a steamer with 5 cm (2 inches) of water and bring to the boil. Place the sliced beetroots on the second floor of the steamer, cover and steam for about 25 minutes. The beetroots are cooked when you can easily insert a fork into the slice. Drain into a colander and leave to cool. Meanwhile, in a large bowl, combine the yogurt, garlic, cardamom, cumin, freshly squeezed lime juice, chopped dill, olive oil, chopped walnuts and a pinch of salt and mix well. Finally add the drained, sliced beetroots and mix again. The yogurt mixture will turn into a pretty pink cream. Leave the salad in the refrigerator for about 30 minutes or longer and serve cold.

Serves 4

Per serving
142 kcal, 9.8 g fat (1.6 g saturated),
4.8 g protein, 9.2 g carbs (8.5 g sugar),
1.7 g fibre, 0.9 g salt

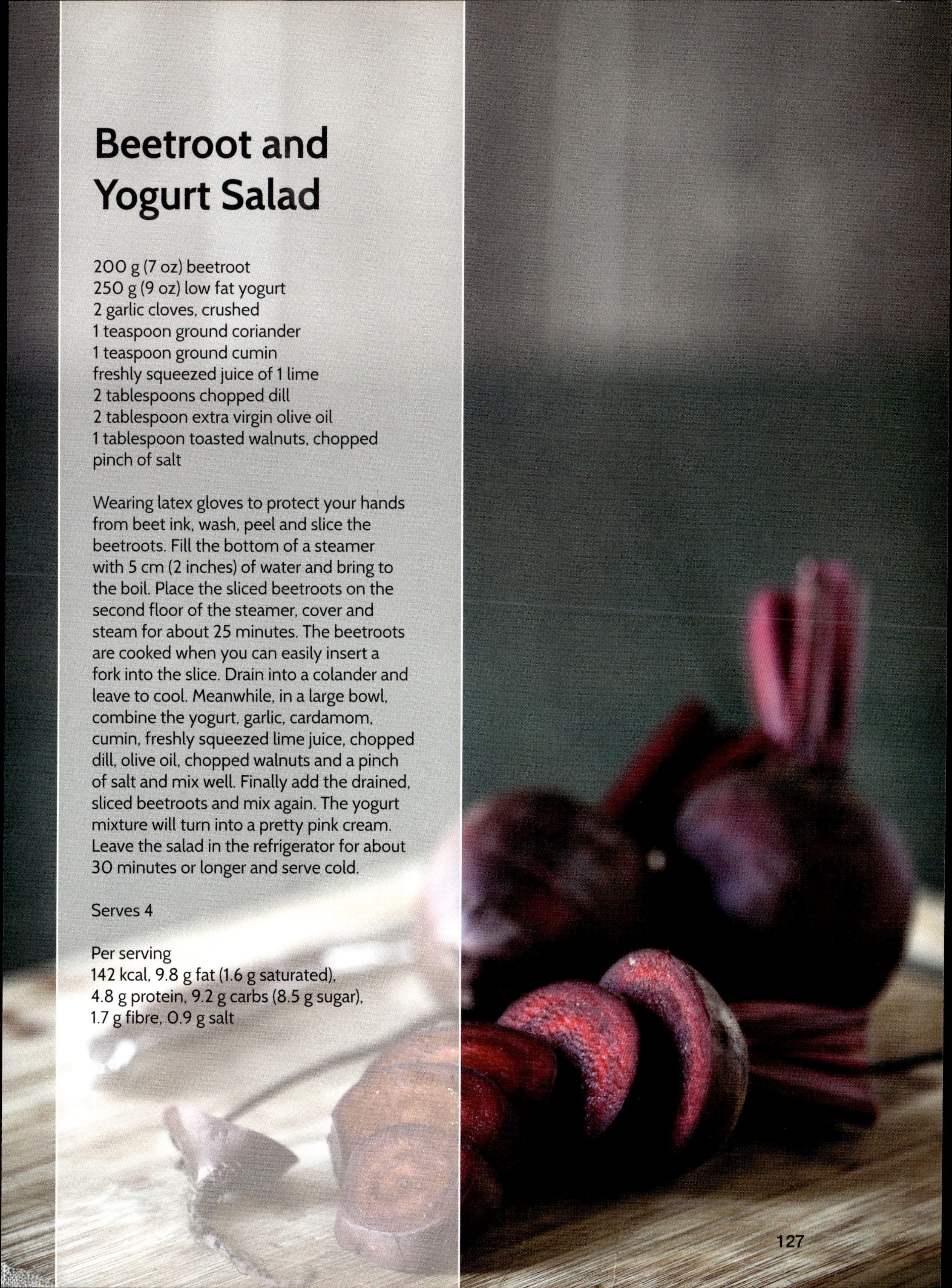

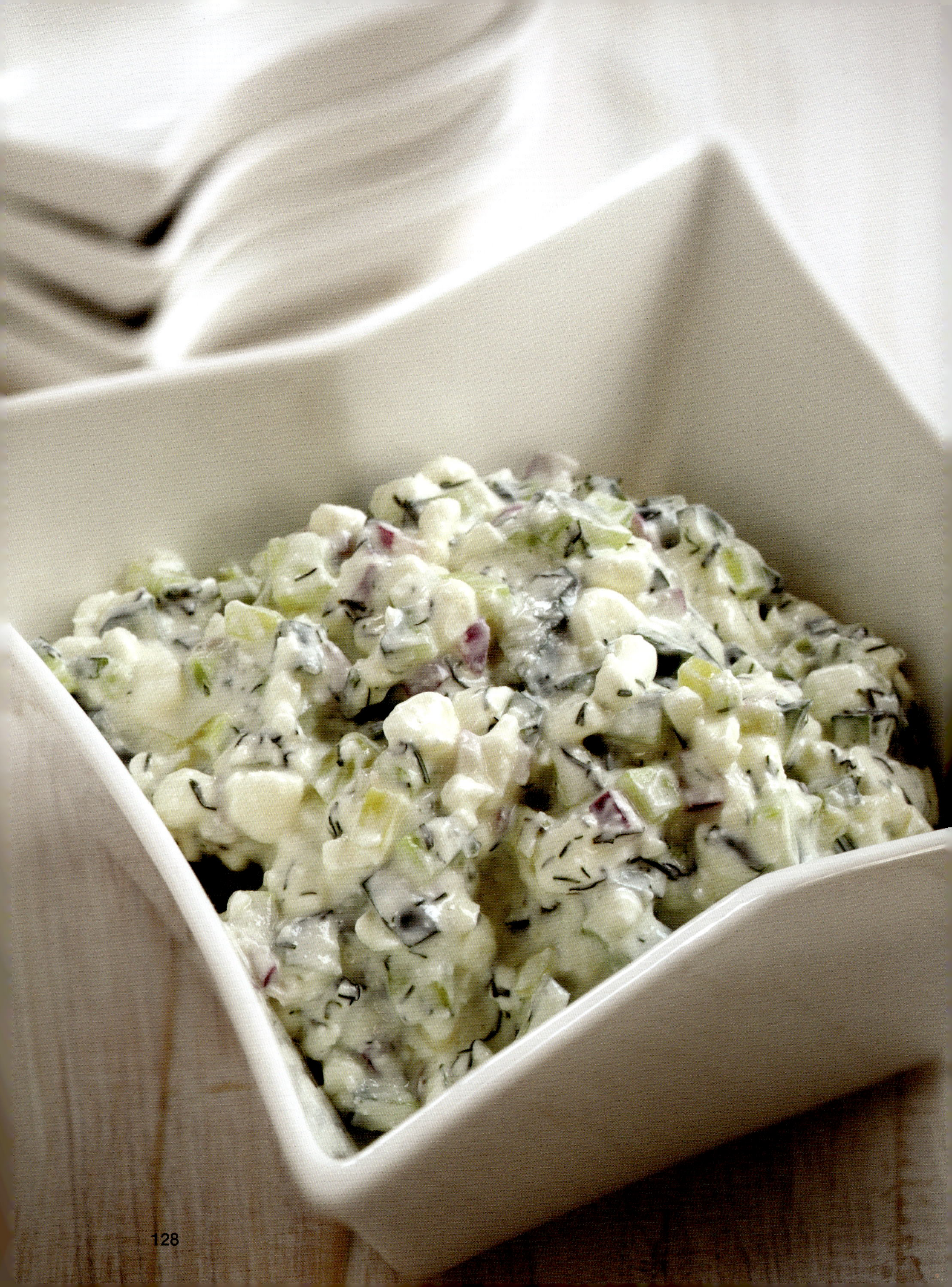

Cucumber and Cottage Cheese Starter

1 medium cucumber, finely diced
250 g (9 oz) cottage cheese
1 red onion, finely chopped
100 g (3½ oz) low fat yogurt
2 tablespoons fresh dill, chopped

In a large bowl combine the chopped in cucumber (5mm cubes), finely chopped onion, dill, cottage cheese and the low fat yogurt, mix well. Leave to rest for about 15 minutes in the refrigerator and serve cold as a starter together with savoury biscuits or sliced bread.

Serves 4

Per serving
95 kcal, 3.1 g fat (1.6 g saturated), 9.9 g protein, 7.3 g carbs (6.4 g sugar), 1.1 g fibre, 0.5 g salt

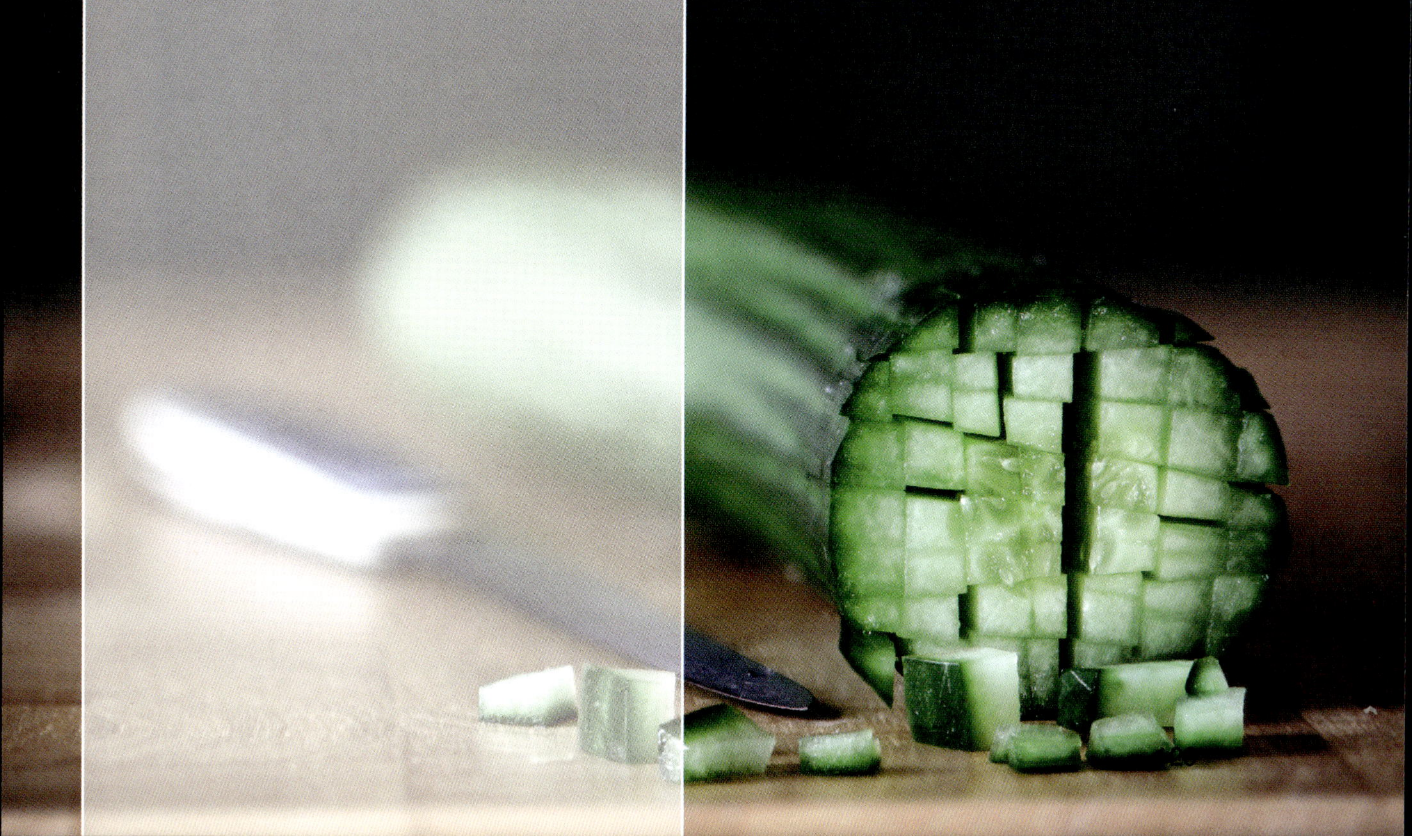

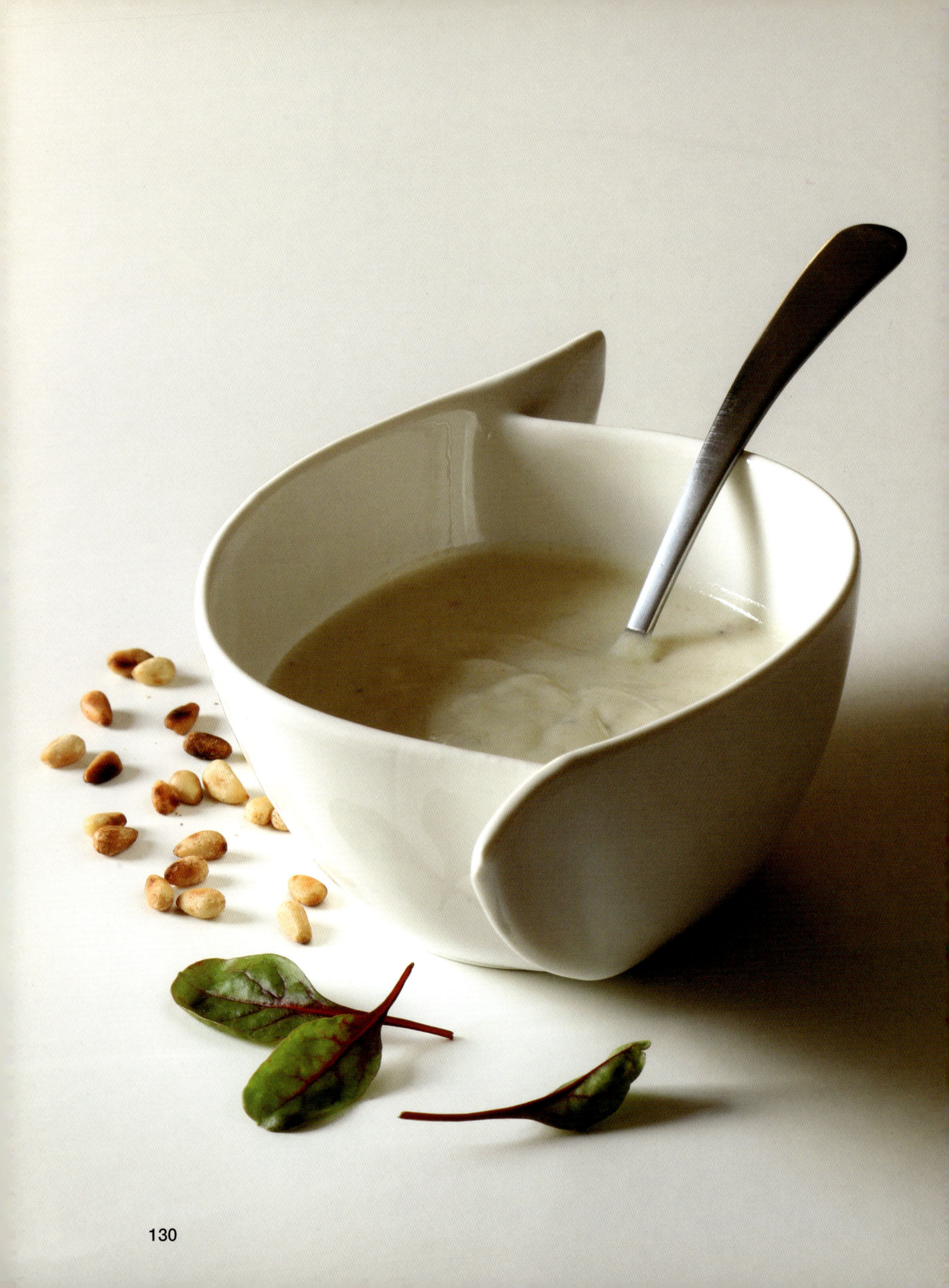

Green Leaf Salad and Ginger Yogurt Dressing

70 g (3 oz) flat egg noodles, fried
100 ml (3½ oz) sunflower oil
200 g (7 oz) low fat yogurt
1 teaspoon ground ginger
freshly squeezed juice of 1 lime
1 tablespoon extra virgin olive oil
pinch of freshly ground black pepper
pinch of salt
200 g (7 oz) green leaf salad
100 g (3½ oz) feta cheese, diced
2 tablespoons pine nuts, toasted

Soak the egg noodles in a small bowl of boiling water for 2 minutes and then drain for a couple of minutes. Heat the oil in a small frying pan and fry the noodles for 5 minutes. Drain on a plate lined with kitchen paper and set aside. Meanwhile, in a small bowl combine the yogurt, ginger, lime juice, olive oil, black pepper and salt. Mix well and leave to rest in the refrigerator. Finally, in a large bowl mix the salad leaves with the feta cheese and pine nuts. Divide onto 4 plates, arrange some fried egg noodles on top and pour over some ginger yogurt dressing.

Serves 4

Per serving
429 kcal, 40.7 g fat (7.8 g saturated), 8.2 g protein, 8.2 g carbs (5.7 g sugar), 1.0 g fibre, 1.7 g salt

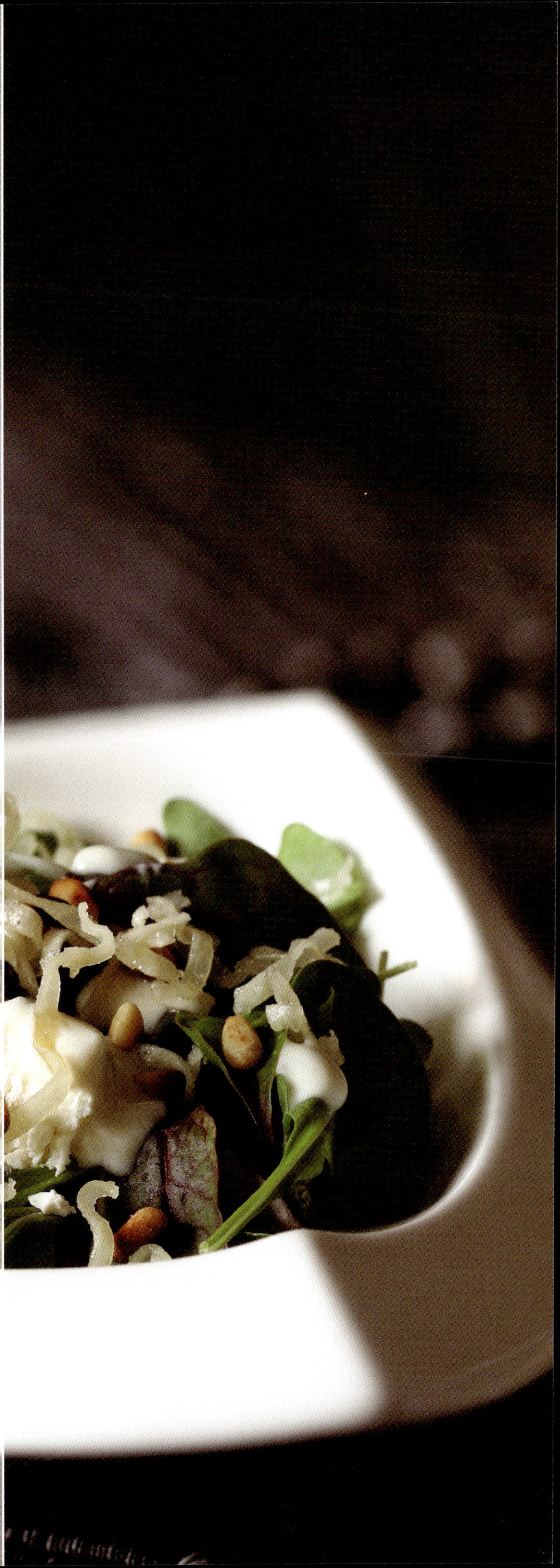

Iceberg Salad and Horseradish Yogurt Dressing

200 g (7 oz) low fat yogurt
1 small lemon freshly squeezed juice
1 tablespoon fresh dill, chopped
1 tablespoon horseradish
1 tablespoon extra virgin oil
pinch of salt
1 Iceberg lettuce
100 g (3½ oz) radish, sliced
20 g (¾ oz) wild arugula (rocket) salad
30 g (1 oz) parmesan cheese

In a small bowl combine the yogurt, freshly squeezed lemon juice, chopped fresh dill, horseradish, extra virgin oil, pinch of salt and mix well. Leave into the refrigerator to rest for about 15 minutes. Meanwhile tear up the iceberg lettuce into small pieces with hands and throw in a large bowl. Slice the radishes and add to the iceberg salad together with the arugula salad. Mix well and divide the salad onto 4 plates. Pour over some spoonfuls of the horseradish yogurt dressing and grate some parmesan cheese over the top.

Serves 4

Per serving
101 kcal, 5.8 g fat (2.2 g saturated), 6.2 g protein, 6.5 g carbs (6.3 g sugar), 1.4 g fibre, 1.0 g salt

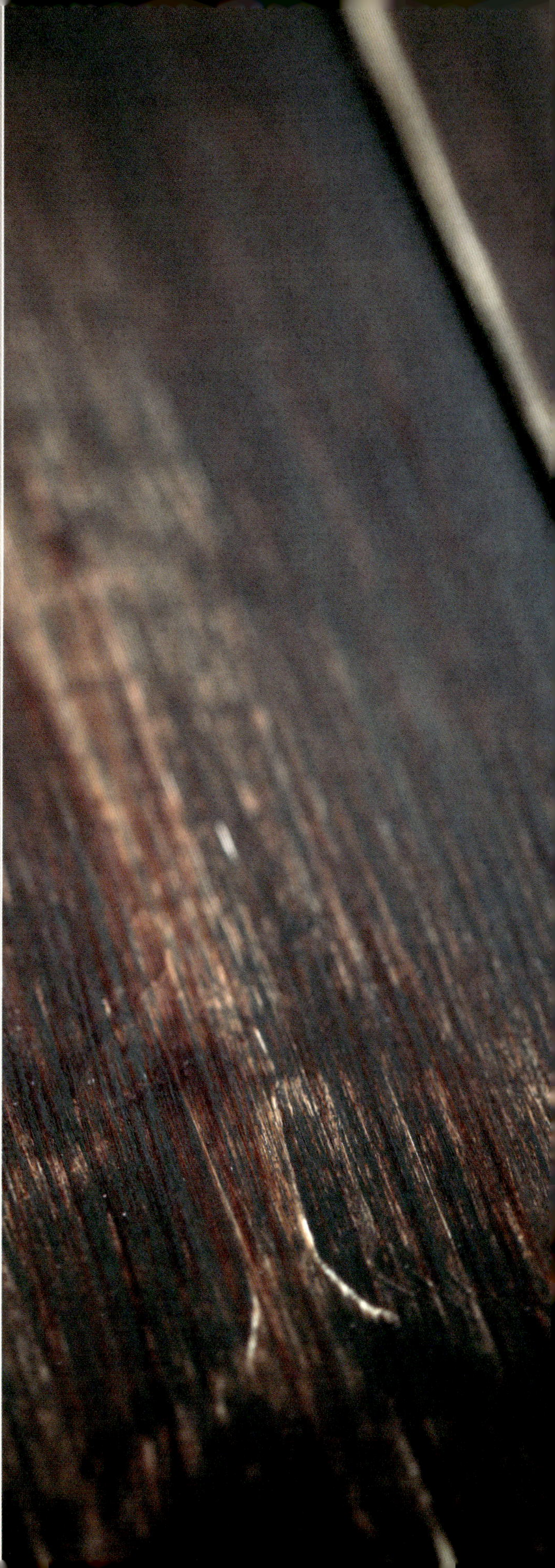

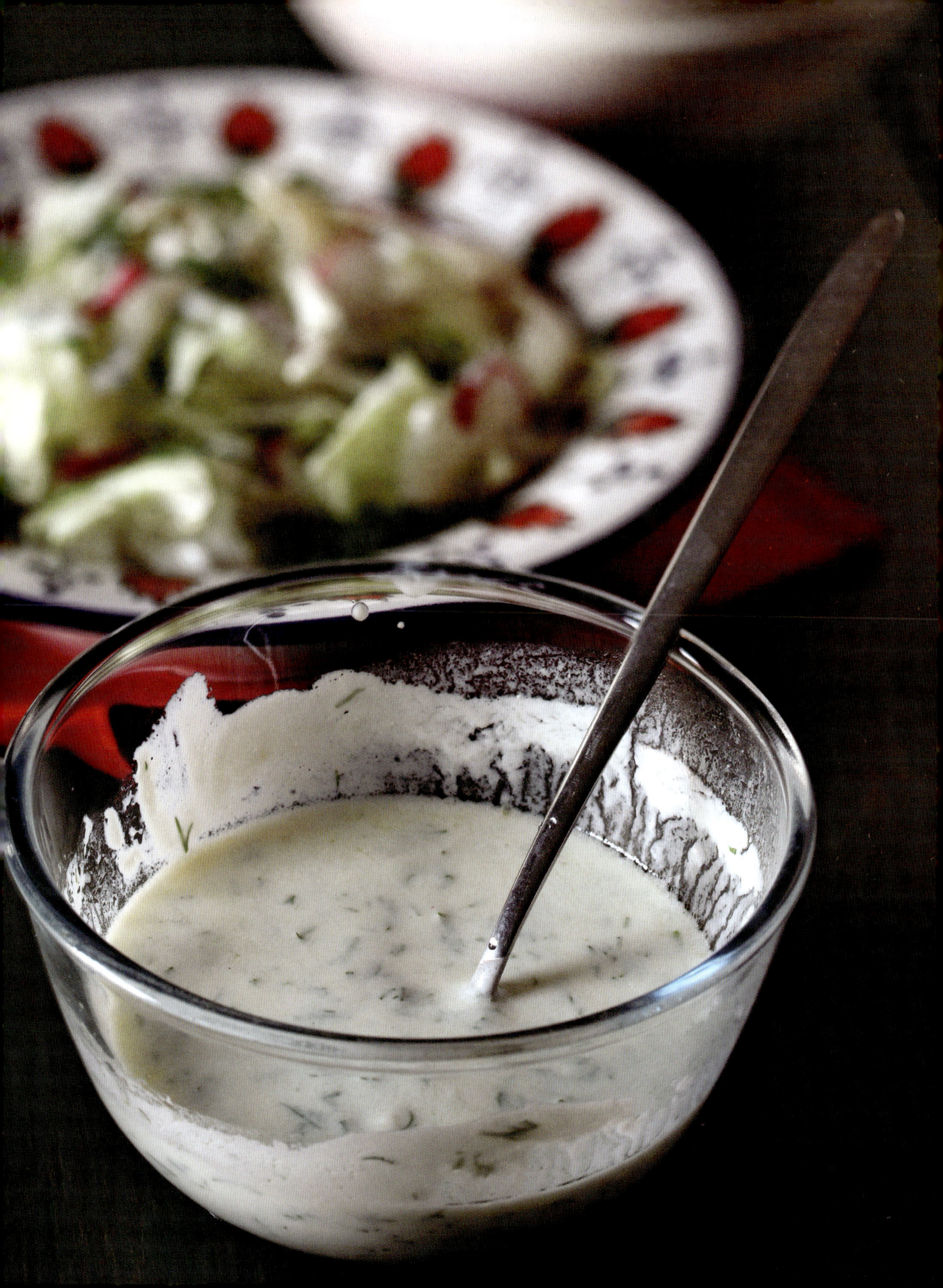

Olivier Salad

500 g (17½ oz) jacket potatoes, boiled, peeled and diced
200 g (7 oz) pickled gherkins, diced
150 g (5 oz) frozen garden peas
2 large carrots, peeled and diced
1 small red onion, finely chopped
1 small pink lady apple, seeded and finely diced
4 boiled eggs
300 g (10½ oz) ham or boiled chicken breast, diced
300 g (10½ oz) light mayonnaise
200 g (7 oz) low fat yogurt
1 large lemon freshly squeezed juice
pinch of salt

Wash the potatoes well and cut them in half or quarters, if quite large. Throw the potato pieces into a large pot and add cold water to cover them. Add a pinch of salt, cover the pot and bring the water to the boil over a high heat for about 20 minutes or until a fork pierces the potato easily. Then drain, leave to cool, peel and dice. Meanwhile in a medium pan add the diced carrots, garden peas, and water, bring to the boil over a high heat for about 5 minutes. Next in another small pan, boil the eggs for about 10 minutes then peel and dice. Finally in a large bowl combine the diced boiled potatoes, pickled gherkins, garden peas, boiled diced carrots, chopped onion, diced boiled eggs, diced ham, finely diced apple, yogurt, mayonnaise, lemon juice, pinch of salt and mix well. Leave the salad in the refrigerator to rest for about 15 minutes or more and serve cold with some olives. The salad can stay in the refrigerator overnight and can be served the next day.

Serves 8

Per serving:
274 kcal, 15.1 g fat (3.0 g saturated), 14.4 g protein, 21.5 g carbs (8.1 g sugar), 3.7 g fibre, 3.0 g salt

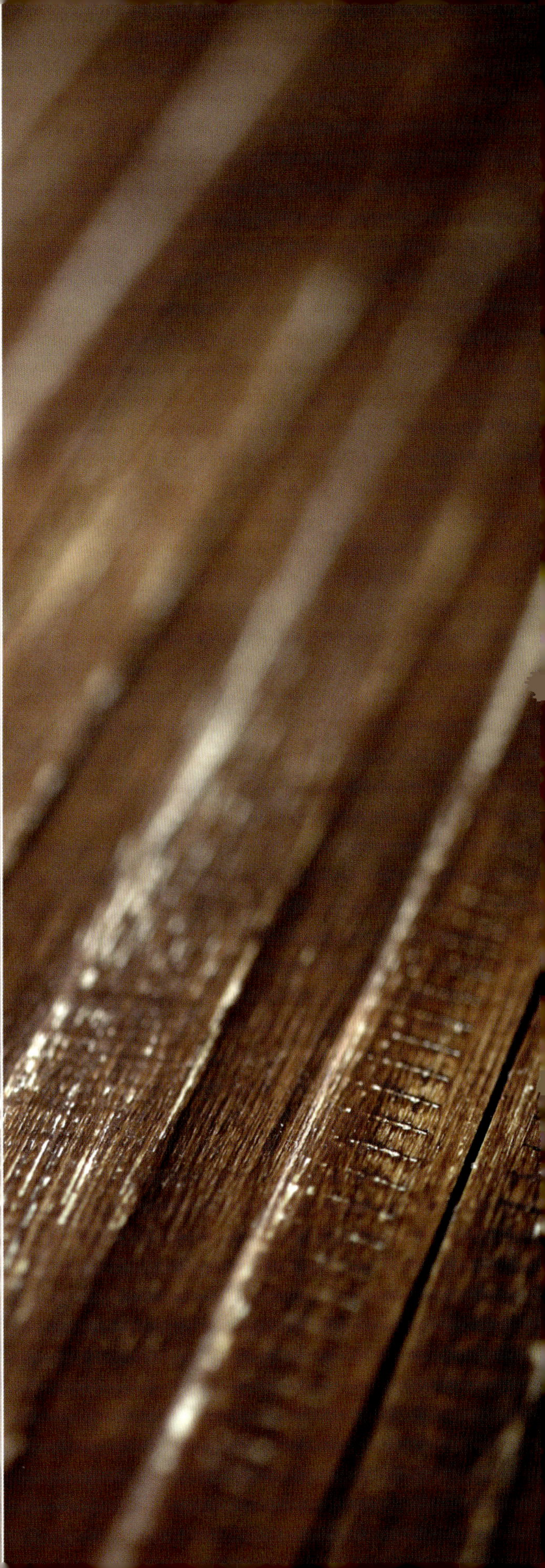

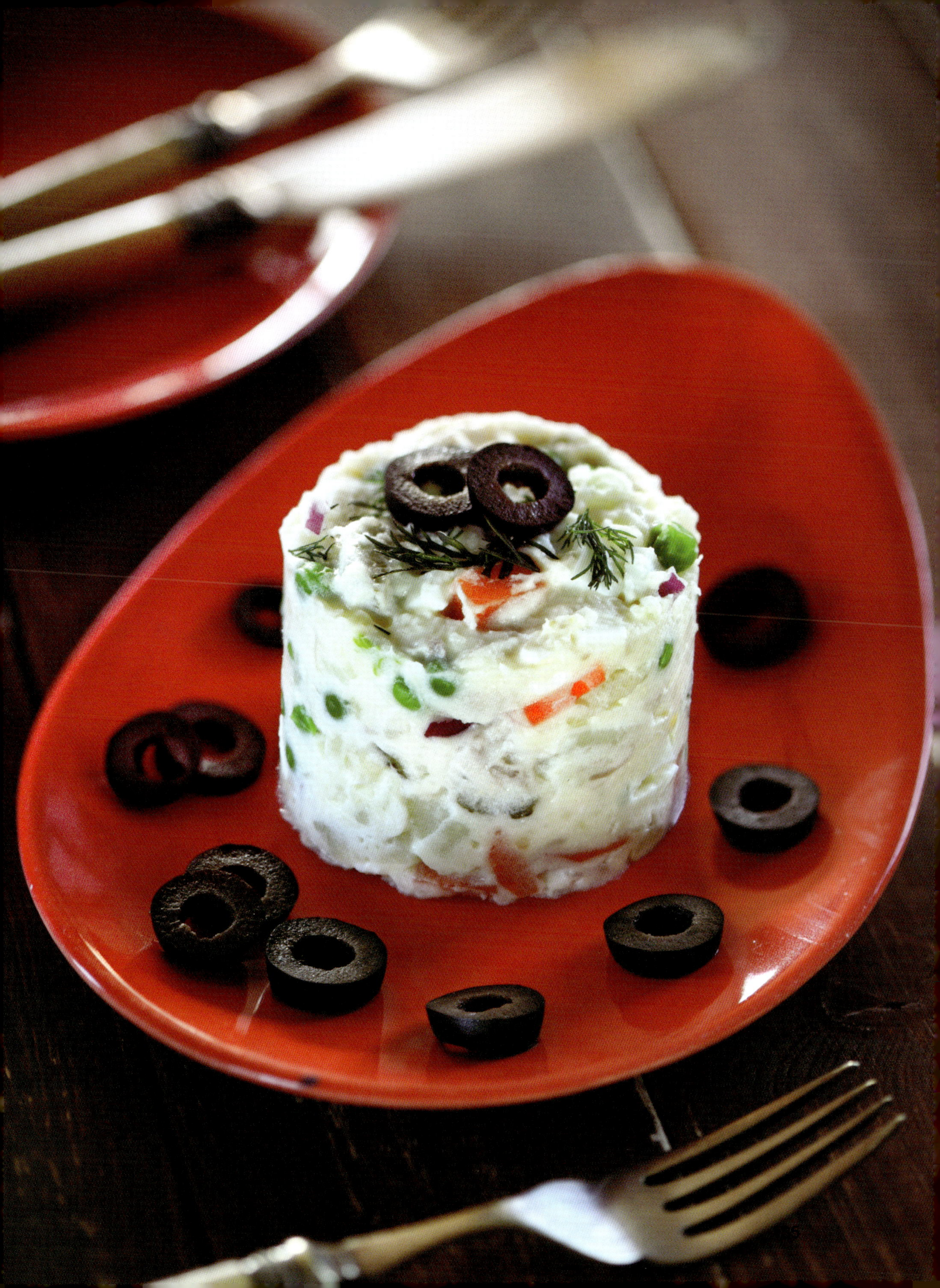

Snejanka Salad

500 g (17½ oz) low fat yogurt, strained
200 g (7 oz) pickled gherkins, diced
2 cloves garlic, crushed
2 tablespoons extra virgin olive oil
50 g (2 oz) walnuts, chopped
4 tablespoons fresh dill, chopped
pinch of salt

Combine the strained yogurt, diced pickled gherkins, crushed garlic, olive oil, chopped walnuts, chopped dill and a pinch of salt In a large bowl and mix well. Leave it to rest in the refrigerator for about 15 minutes and serve cold as a starter together with some savoury biscuits or toasted bread.

Serves 4

Per serving
216 kcal, 15.4 g fat (2.5 g saturated),
8.7 g protein, 11.5 g carbs (11.0 g sugar),
1.7 g fibre, 1.8 g salt

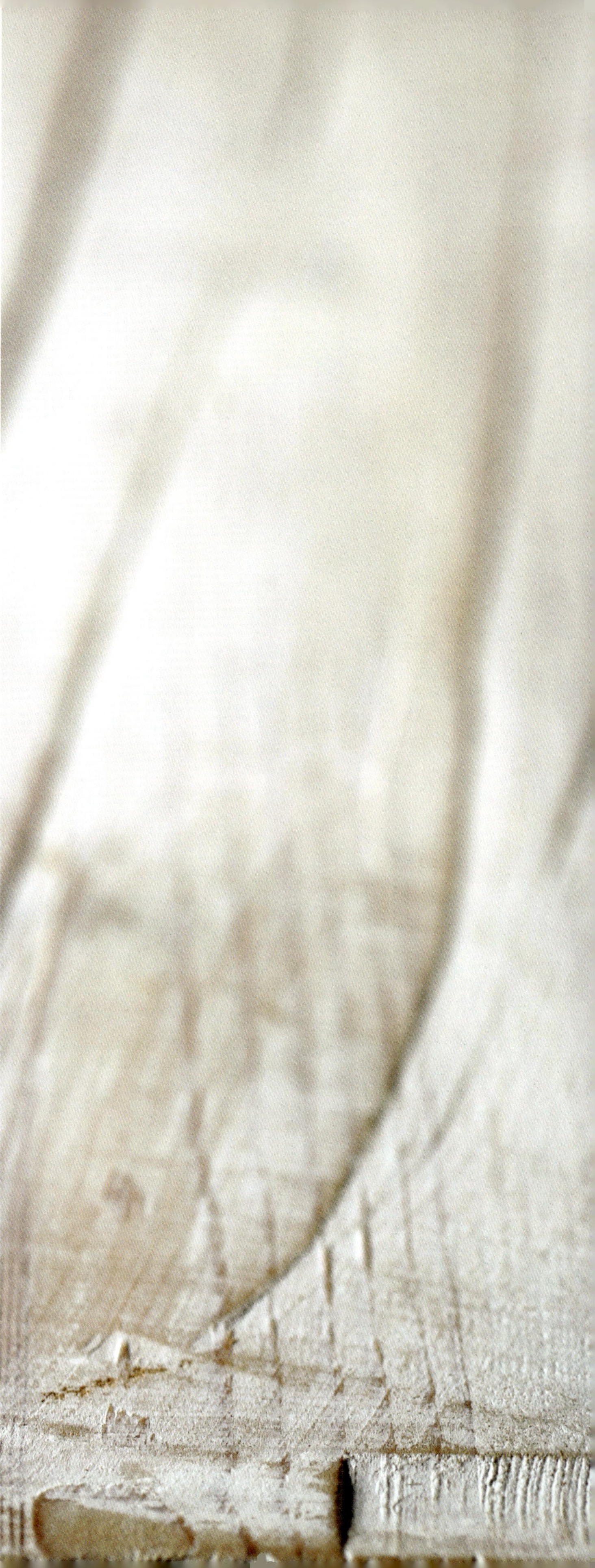

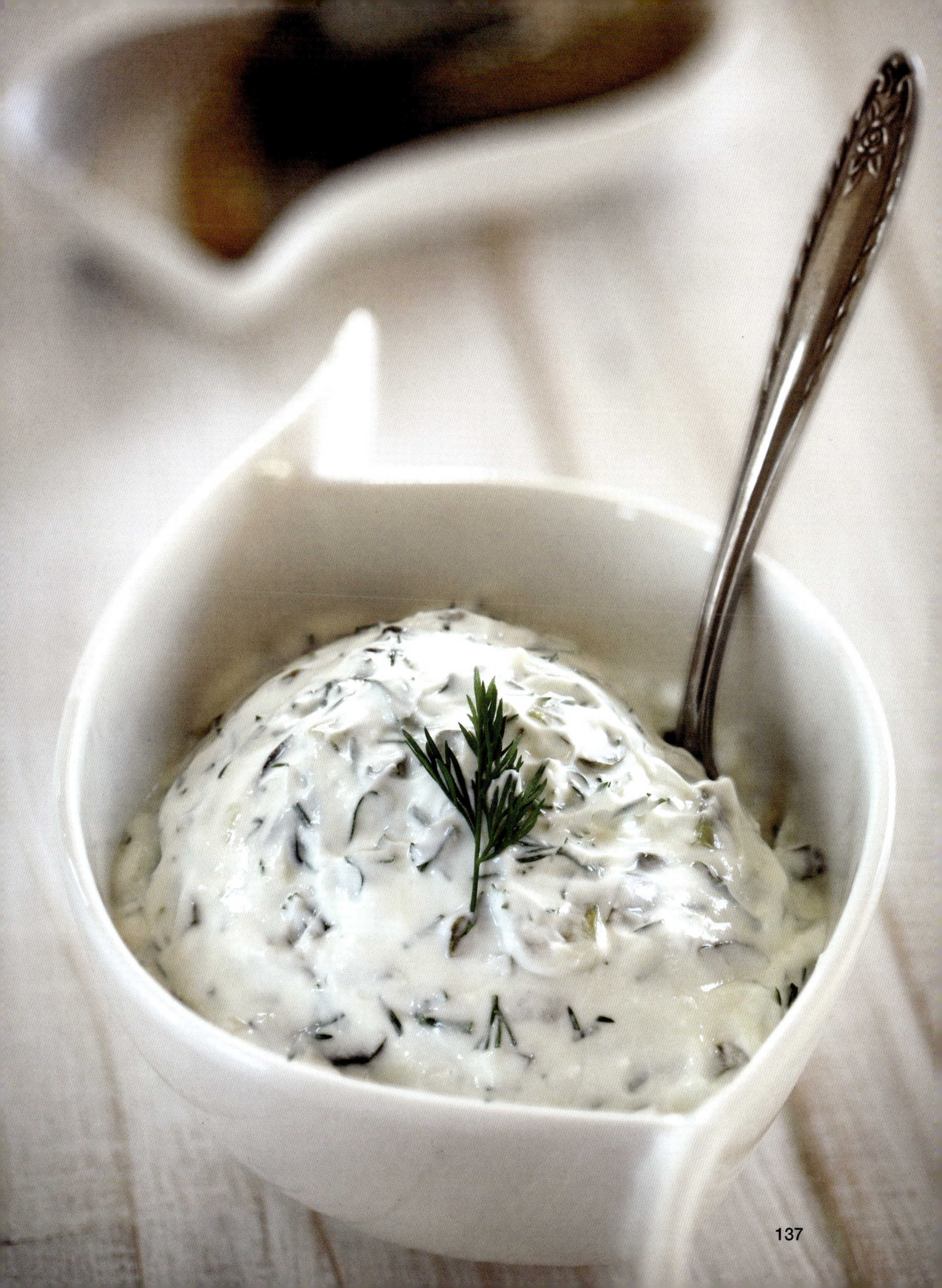

Artichoke and Spinach Salad

1 artichoke
a few grains allspice
2 bay leaves
2 garlic cloves, crushed

100 g (3½ oz) baby spinach, washed
4 spring onions, finely chopped
juice of 1 lime
2 tablespoons extra virgin olive oil
pinch of salt
2 garlic cloves, crushed
250 g (9 oz) low fat yogurt
100 g (3½ oz) feta cheese
1 teaspoon freshly ground black pepper
30 g (1 oz) pine nuts

Wash the artichoke and cut off the little thorns at the end of the leaves using kitchen scissors. Cut the tip and the stem of the artichoke and carefully remove the hairy choke in the middle. Put the artichoke in the pressure cooker, add 1 litre (1¾ pints) cold water, the allspice, bay leaves and garlic. Close the lid and cook for about 15 minutes under pressure. Once ready, remove from the heat and wait for a short time for the pressure cooker to release its pressure before opening the lid. Once opened, transfer the artichoke to a colander to drain and cool a little. Meanwhile, into a large bowl. Combine the spinach, spring onions, lime juice, olive oil, salt and garlic, stir and mash by hand. Using a tablespoon, scrape and remove the soft, pulpy, delicious part from the boiled artichoke petals, one by one, and add to the spinach. Add the yogurt, and feta cheese, breaking It up and squashing with a fork, and mix well. Finally sprinkle over some ground black pepper and the pine nuts to serve.

Serves 4

Per serving
224 kcal, 16.7 g fat (5.1 g saturated), 11.0 g protein, 8.8 g carbs (6.9 g sugar), 1.5 g fibre, 1.9 g salt

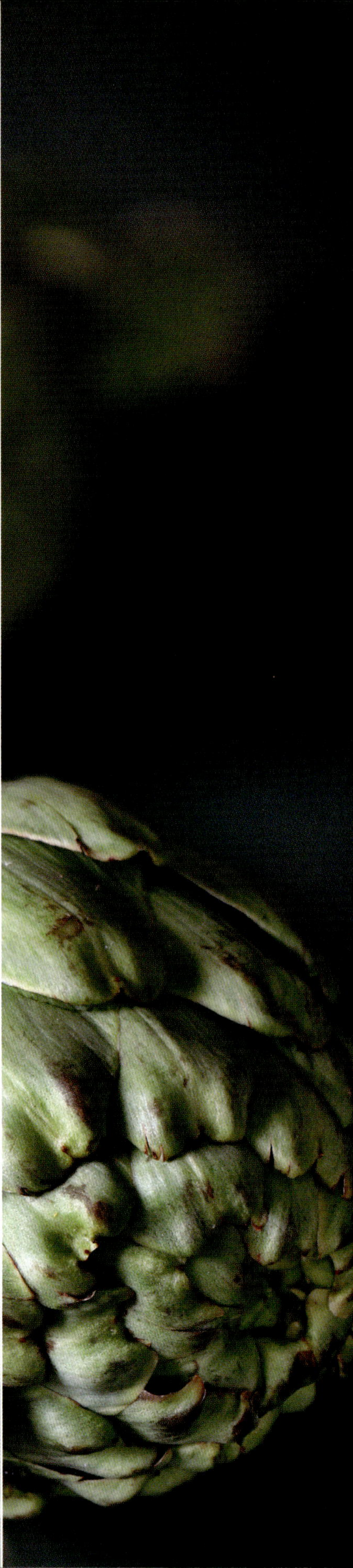

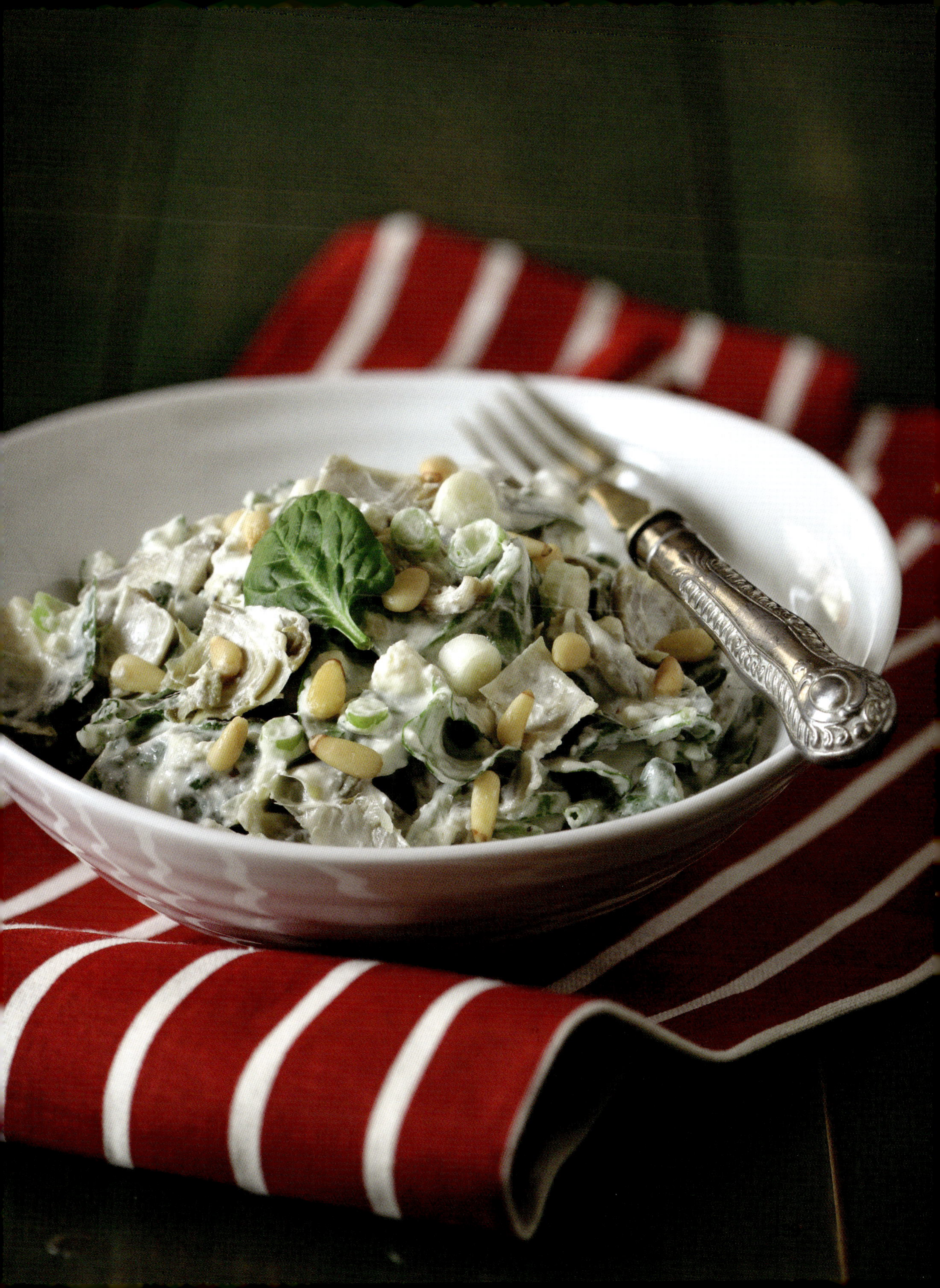

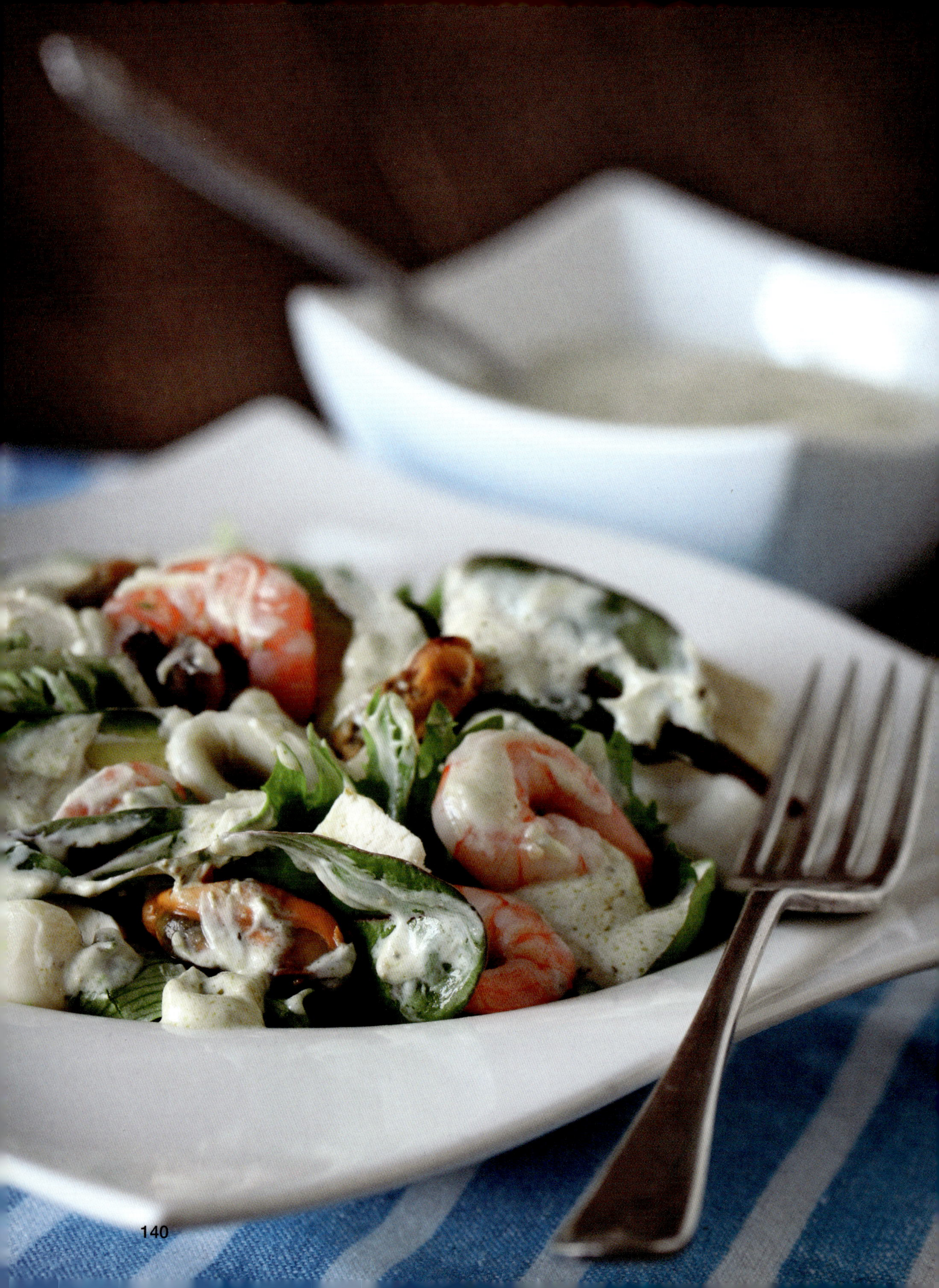

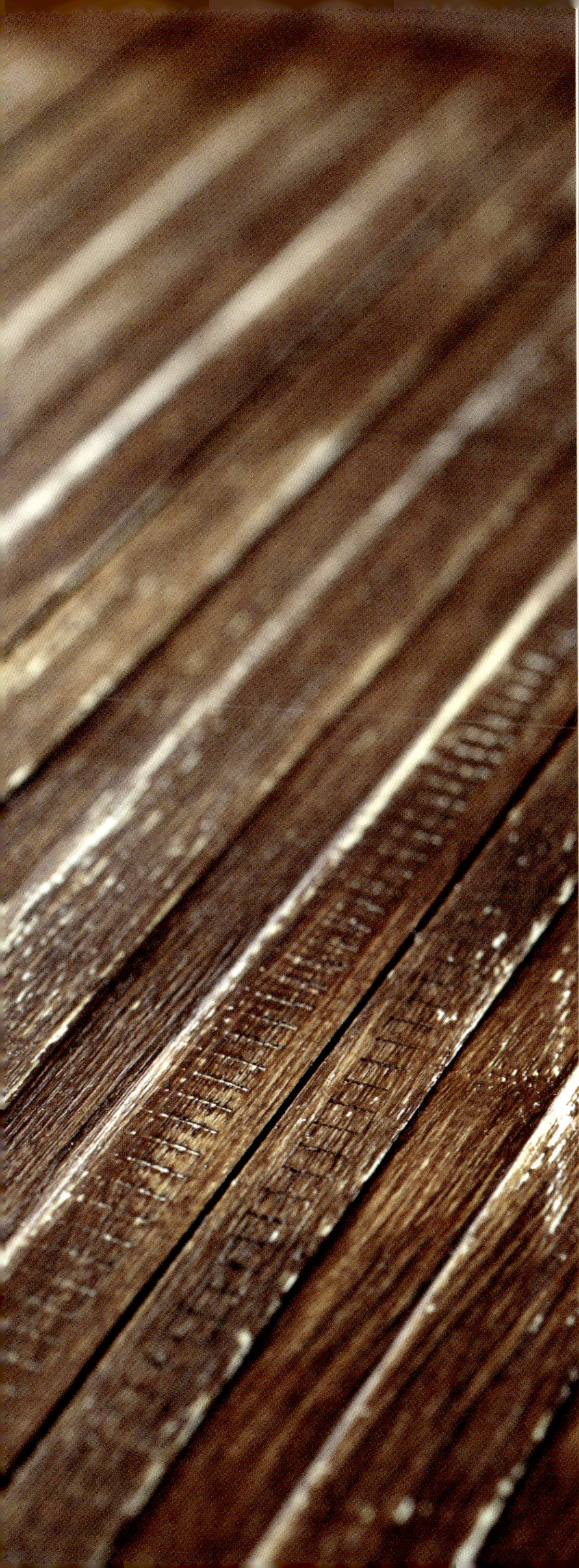

Basil Pesto Salad Dressing

150 g (5 oz) low fat yogurt
1 tablespoon basil pesto
freshly squeezed juice of 1 lime
1 tablespoon extra virgin olive oil
1 teaspoon brown sugar
200 g (7 oz) mixed green leaves
200 g (7 oz) seafood selection, cooked
100 g (3½ oz) feta cheese, diced
1 small avocado, sliced
a pinch of salt

Combine the yogurt, basil pesto, lime juice, extra virgin olive oil, sugar and salt In a small bowl and mix well. Leave it in the refrigerator for couple of minutes to rest. Meanwhile wash the green salad and leave it to drain for a couple of minutes. Divide it onto 4 plates and arrange over some cooked seafood, diced feta cheese, sliced avocado and pour over a few tablespoons of the basil pesto salad dressing.

Serves 4

Per serving
254 kcal, 18.4 g fat (6.0 g saturated), 16.4 g protein, 6.3 g carbs (5.6 g sugar), 2.4 g fibre, 2.0 g salt

Fennel and Cucumber Salad

150 g (5 oz) low fat yogurt
100 g (3½ oz) feta cheese, diced
2 fennel bulbs, sliced
1 cucumber, diced
1 red onion, finely chopped
2 celery ribs, chopped
1 lemon, freshly squeezed juice
2 tablespoons extra virgin olive oil
pinch of salt

In a small bowl combine the low fat yogurt, freshly squeezed lemon juice, extra virgin olive oil, a pinch of salt and mix well, set aside for a few minutes. Then in a large bowl add the cored and sliced fennel, diced cucumber, chopped celery ribs, finely chopped red onion, diced feta cheese and pour over the dressing, mix well and serve.

Serves 4

Per serving
156 kcal, 11.1 g fat (4.5 g saturated), 6.8 g protein, 7.6 g carbs (6.7 g sugar), 2.6 g fibre, 1.8 g salt

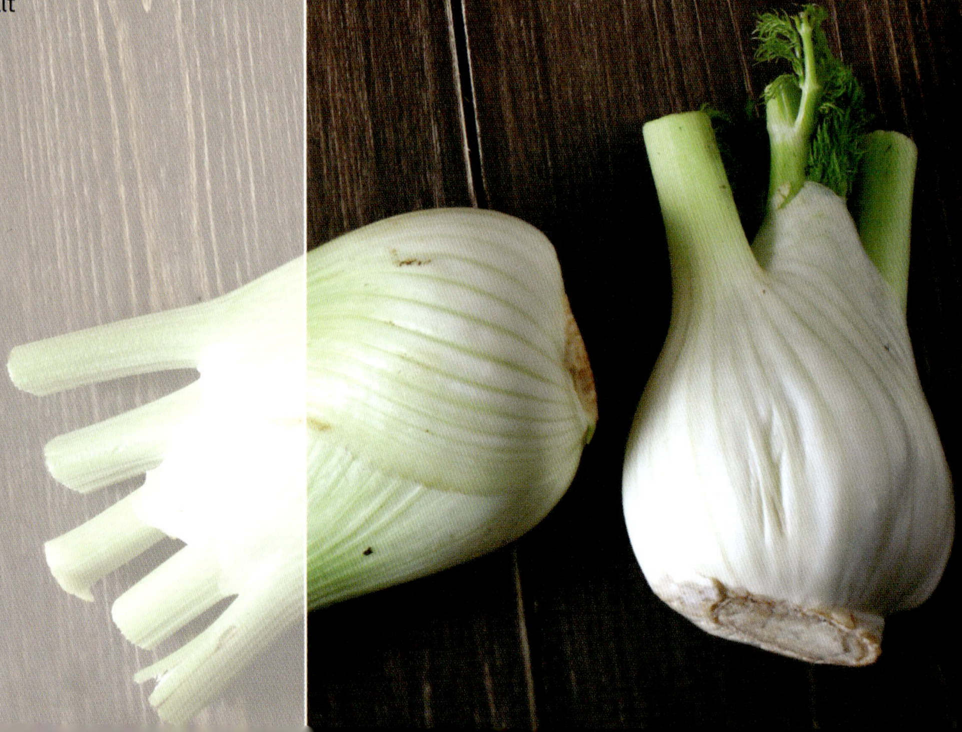

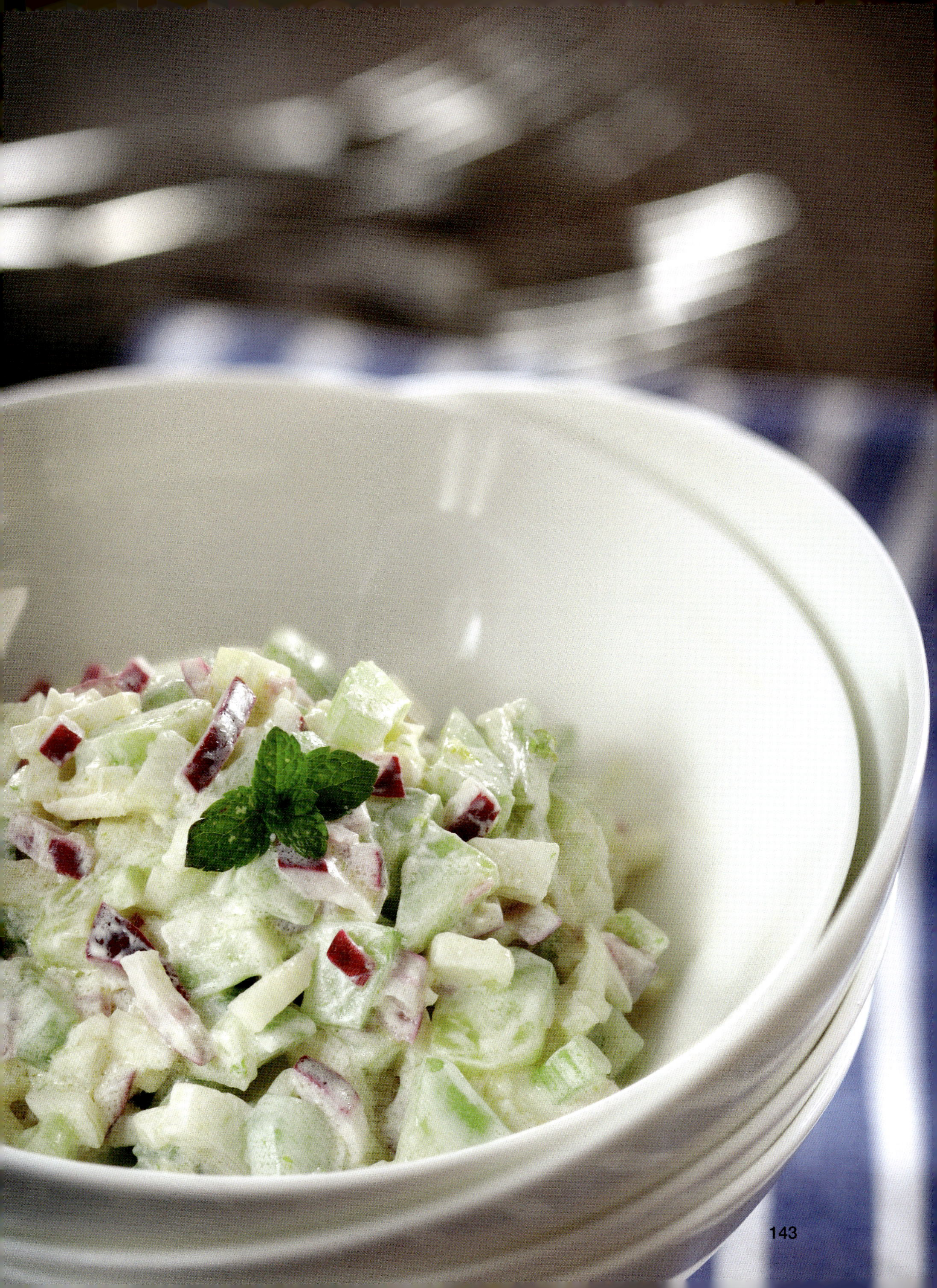

Swede and Fennel Salad

Half a 500 g (17½ oz) swede, peeled and shredded
2 small fennel bulbs, finely chopped
2 green apples, peeled and shredded
freshly squeezed juice of 1 lemon
4 tablespoons extra virgin olive oil
200 g (7 oz) low fat yogurt
1 teaspoon black sesame seeds
pinch of salt
1 handful fresh parsley, chopped
2 tablespoons pine nuts, toasted

Combine the swede, finely chopped fennel and apples in a large bowl. Pour in the lemon juice and mix well. Add the olive oil, yogurt, black sesame seeds and pinch of salt and mix again. Serve the salad with the toasted pine nuts and chopped parsley sprinkled over the top to garnish.

Serves 6

Per serving
148 kcal, 11 g fat (2 g saturated), 3 g protein, 10 g carbs (10 g sugar), 4.0 g fibre, 0.6 g salt

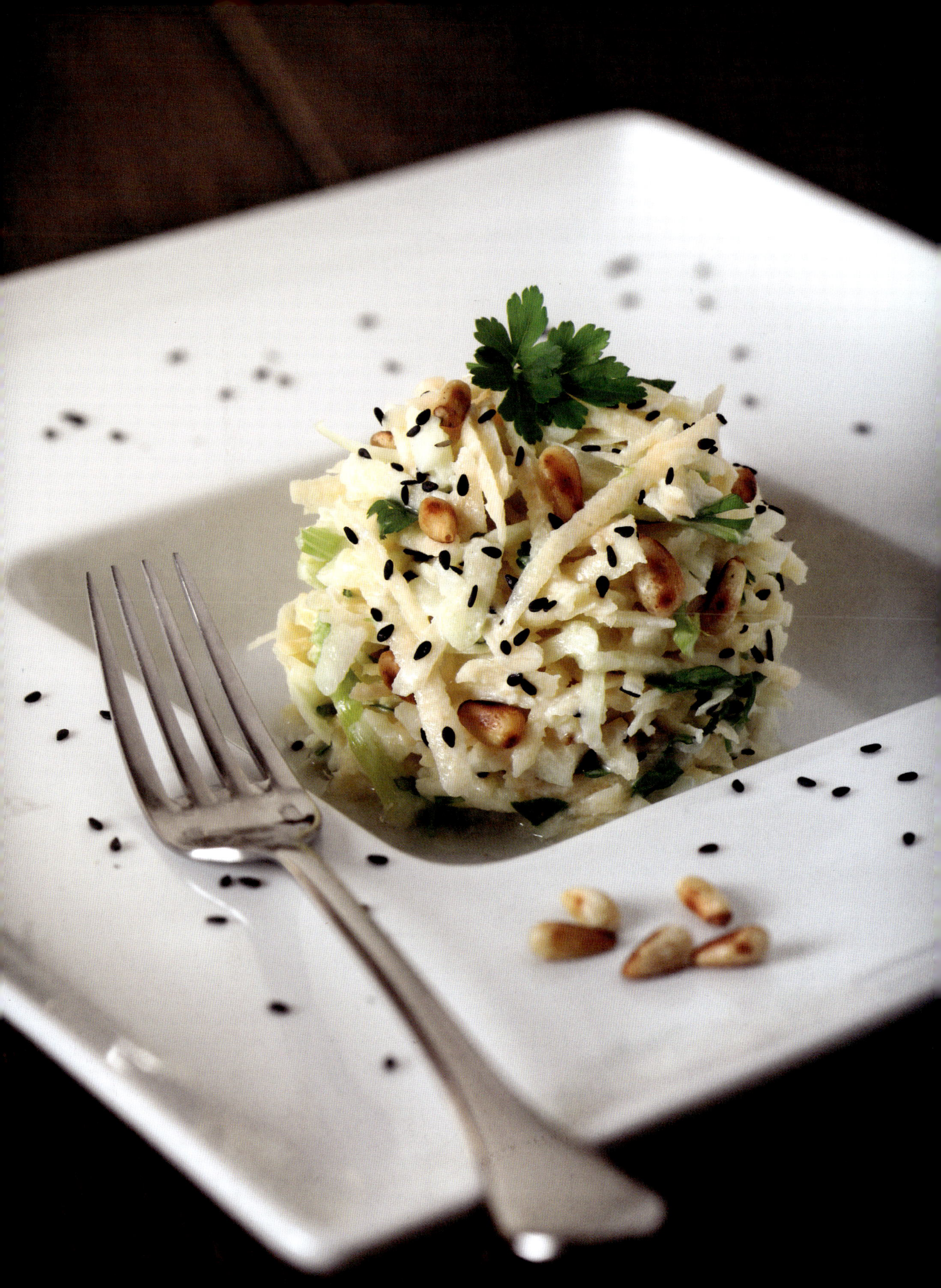

Curly Kale Salad

200 g (7 oz) curly kale, sliced, stems off
4 spring onions, finely chopped
2 tablespoons extra virgin olive oil
15 g (½ oz) capers
30 g (1 oz) almonds, flaked
50 g (2 oz) parmesan cheese, shaved

Throw the sliced curly kale into a large bowl and add the extra virgin olive oil, pinch of salt and mix well. Then sprinkle over the capers, flaked almonds and shaved parmesan. Serve with the yogurt mustard dressing.

Yogurt mustard dressing:
200 g (7 oz) low fat yogurt
½ lemon, freshly squeezed juice
1 tablespoon extra virgin olive oil
1 tablespoon wholegrain mustard
a pinch of salt

Pour the low fat yogurt into a small bowl and add the freshly squeezed lemon juice, extra virgin olive oil, wholegrain mustard and mix well.

Serves 4

Per serving
224 kcal, 18 g fat (4 g saturated), 11 g protein, 6 g carbs (5 g sugar), 2.5 g fibre, 1.7 g salt

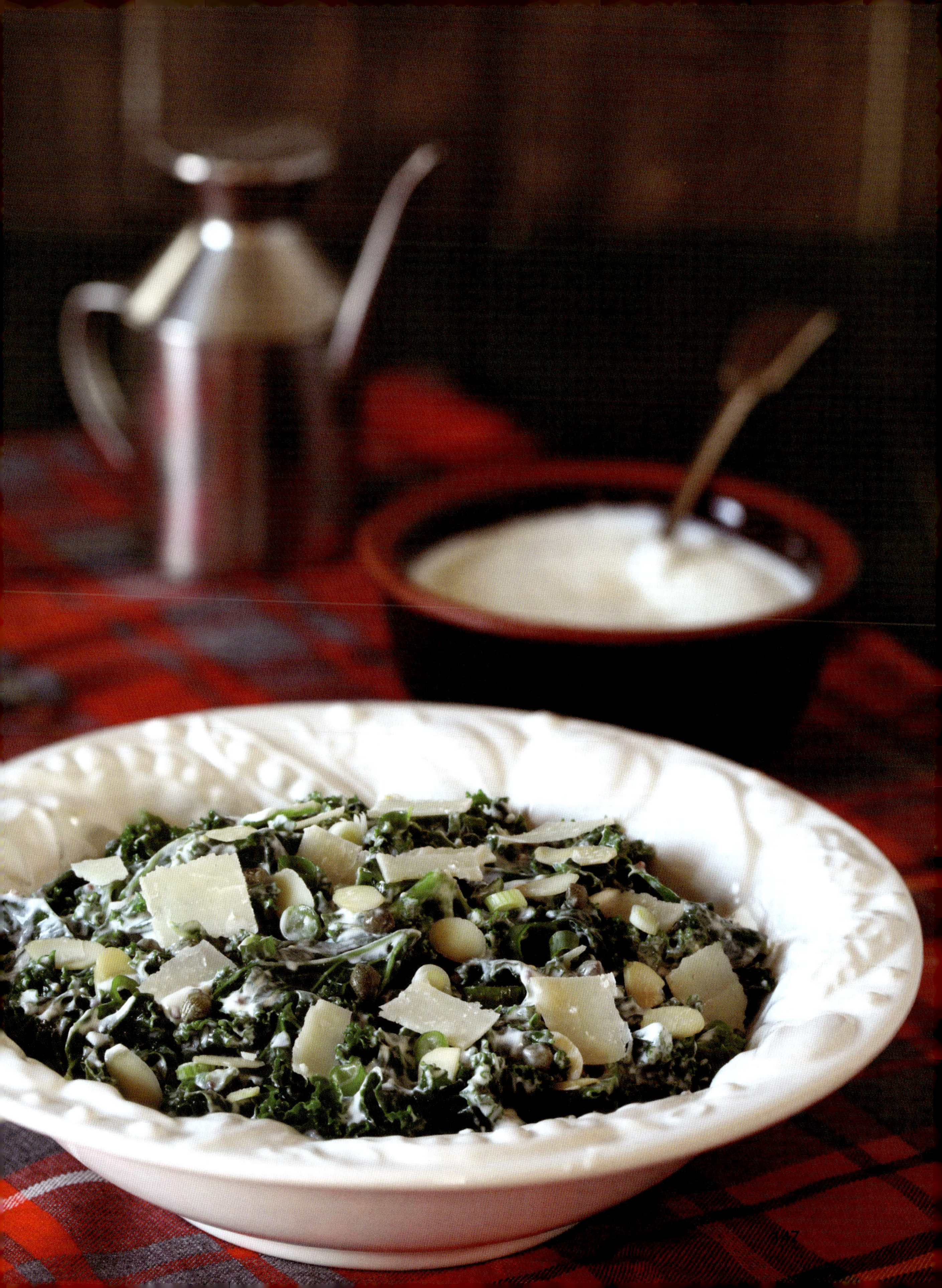

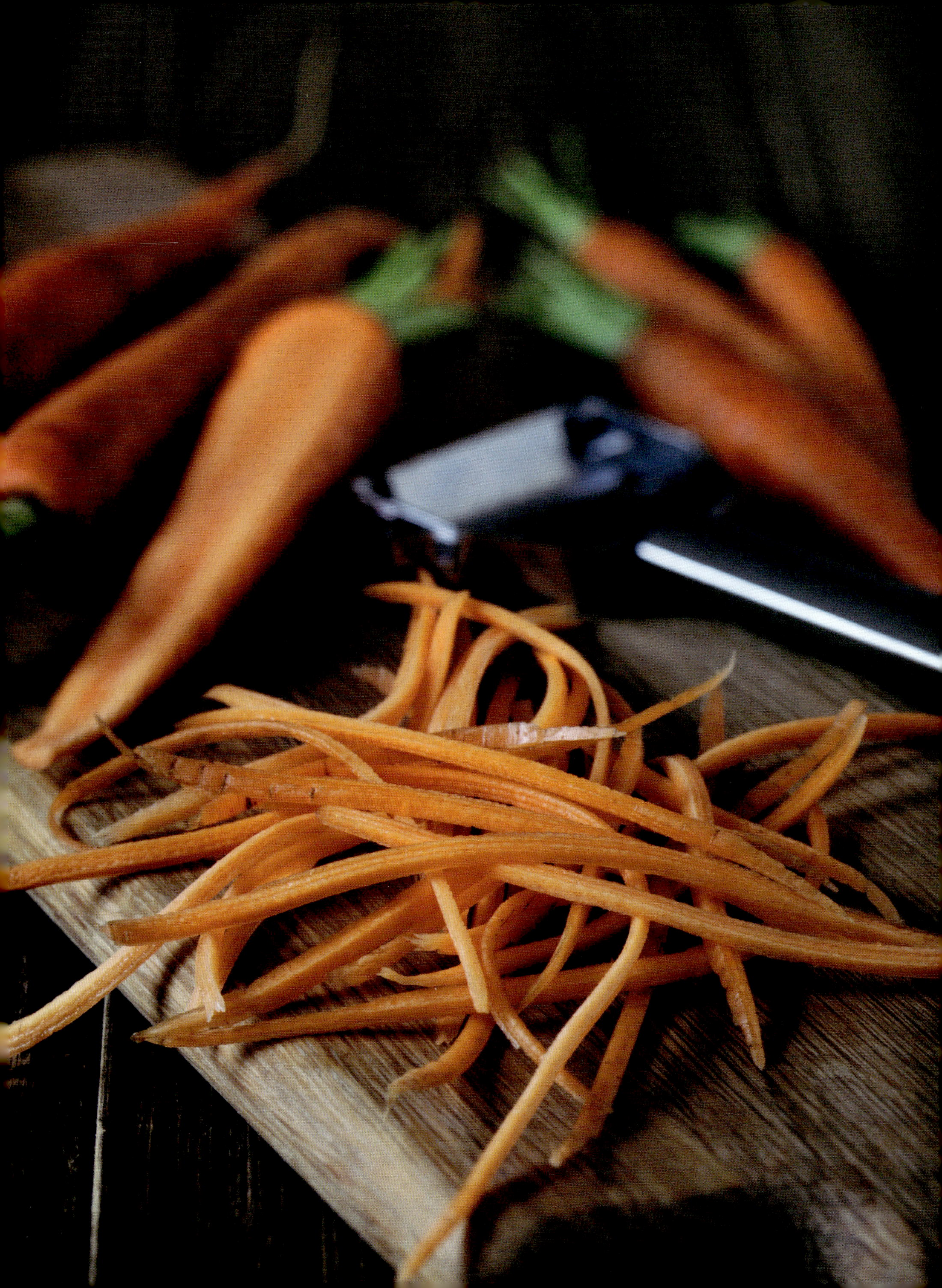

Starters

Bulgarian Eggplant Dip – Kyopolou

3 eggplants (aubergines)
3 color peppers
1 small tomato
100 g (3½ oz) low fat yogurt
1 clove of garlic
3 tablespoons extra virgin oil
a pinch of salt

Prick the skin of the raw eggplants with a fork a few times. Bake the eggplants, the peppers and the tomato in the oven for about 40 minutes at 220°C (425°F) until the skins are slightly charred. Leave to cool and then peel the skins of all the vegetables as much as you can, remove the stalk and seeds of the peppers, trim off the eggplant stalk and coarsely chop the flesh of the vegetables and put in a strainer for 5 minutes to drain. Transfer to a blender bowl and add the yogurt, garlic, olive oil and a pinch of salt and mix well with the blender.
Serve on a toast or biscuits together with feta cheese and olives. Sprinkle some parsley and red onion on top. Enjoy!

Serves 6

Per serving
176 kcal, 11 g fat (3.3 g saturated), 5.8 g protein, 14.3 g carbs (6.9 g sugars), 2.0g salt, 6.6 g fibre

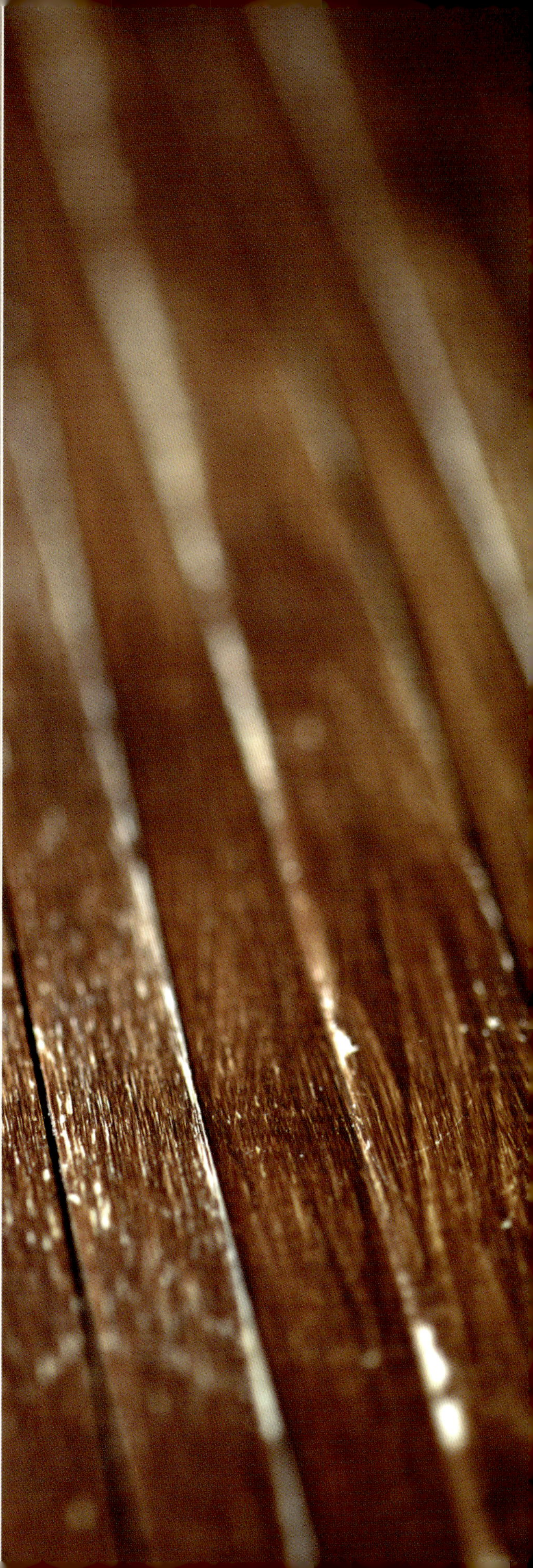

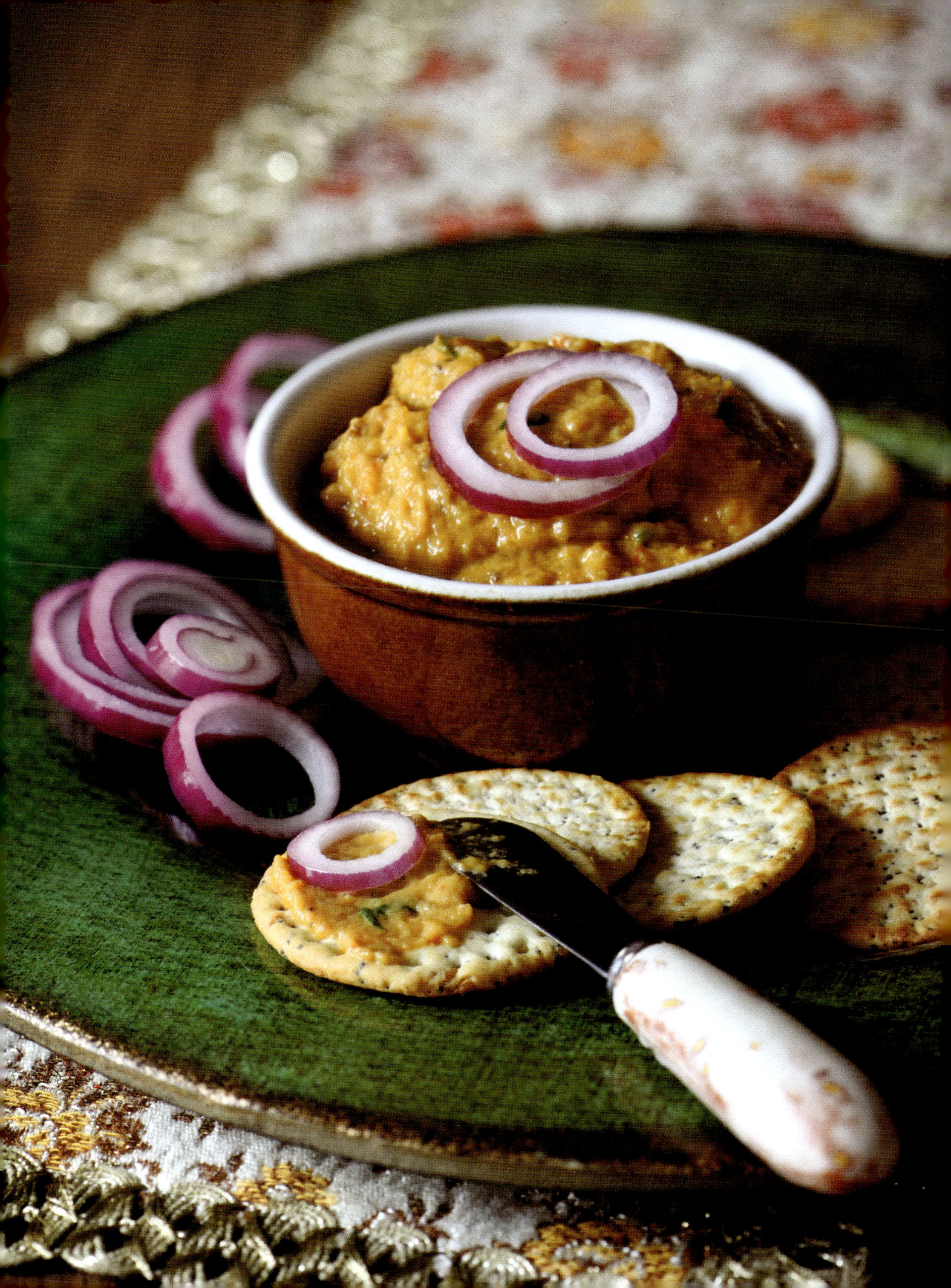

Eggplant and Yogurt Starter

2 medium eggplants (aubergines), for best result 'Listada de Gandia'
250 g (9 oz) yogurt
20 g (¾ oz) mint leaves
pinch of salt
2 tablespoons olive oil
20 g (¾ oz) dill

Dice the eggplants and place in a stir fry pan with the olive oil. Cook for about 10 minutes on a medium heat until the eggplant gets tender. Transfer it into a large bowl and leave it to rest. Meanwhile in a medium bowl combine the yogurt, chopped mint leaves, dill and salt, mix thoroughly. Pour the yogurt mixture over the eggplants and serve.

Serves 6

Per portion
106 kcal, 8.4 g fat (3.4 g saturated), 3.5 g protein, 4.4 g carbs (3.9 g sugars), 0.6 g salt, 2.8 g fibre

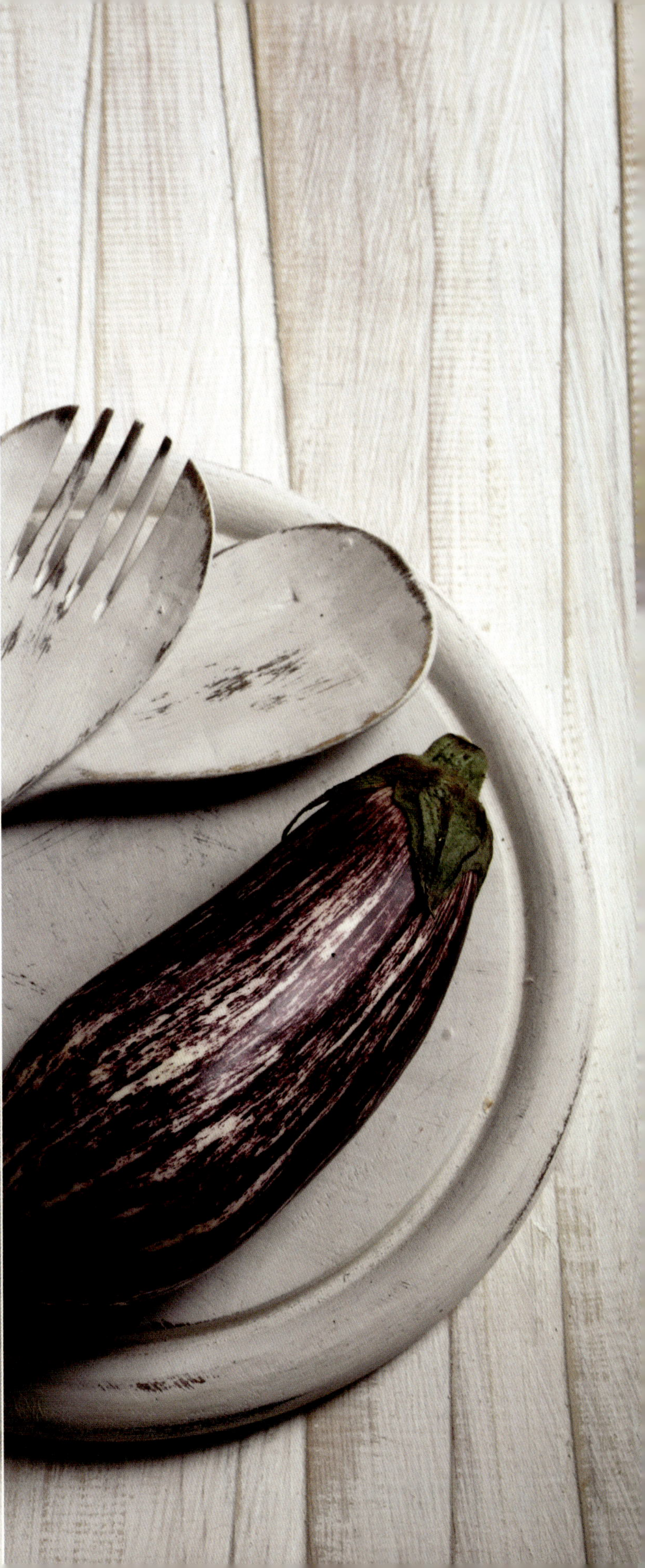

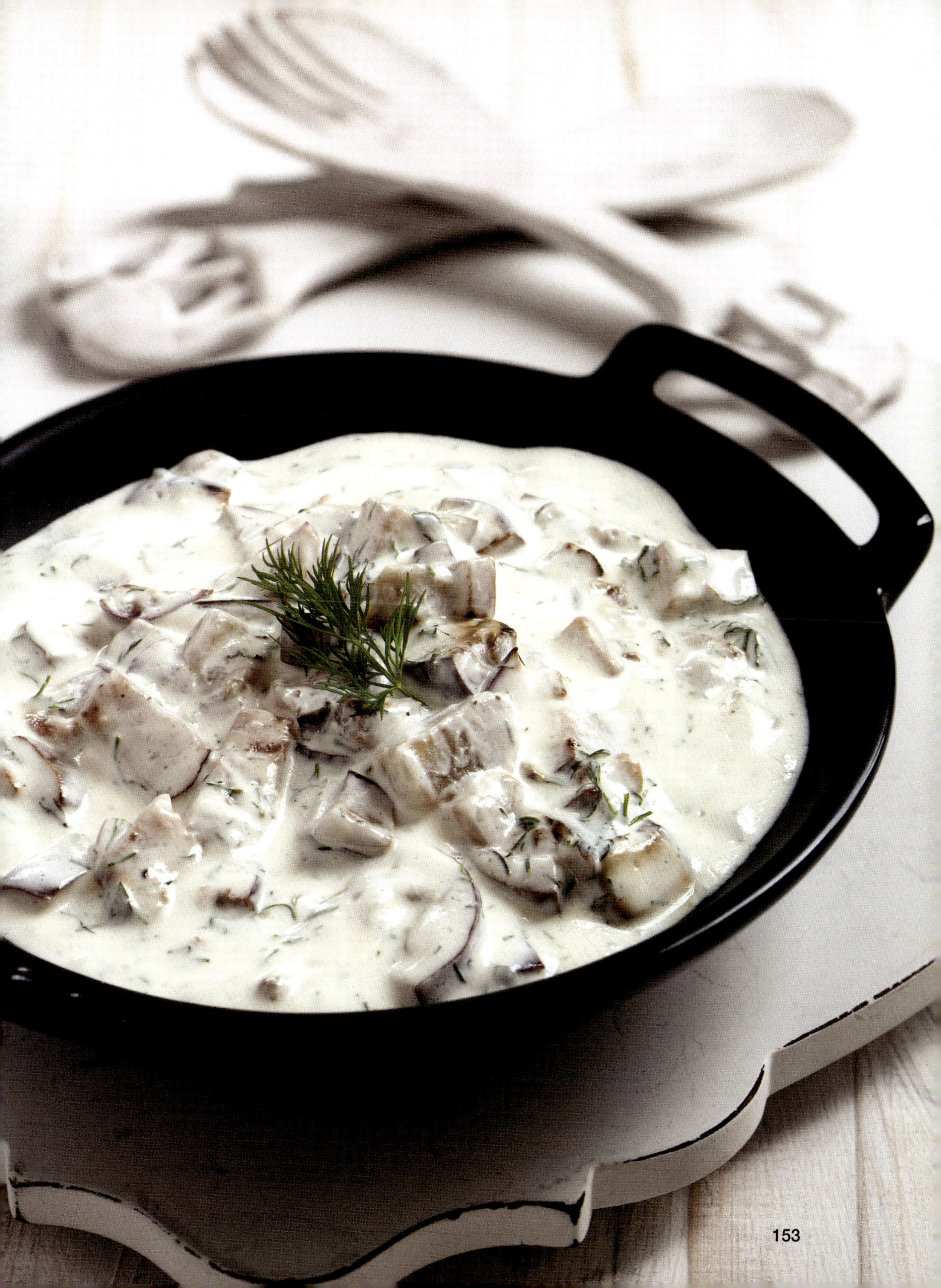

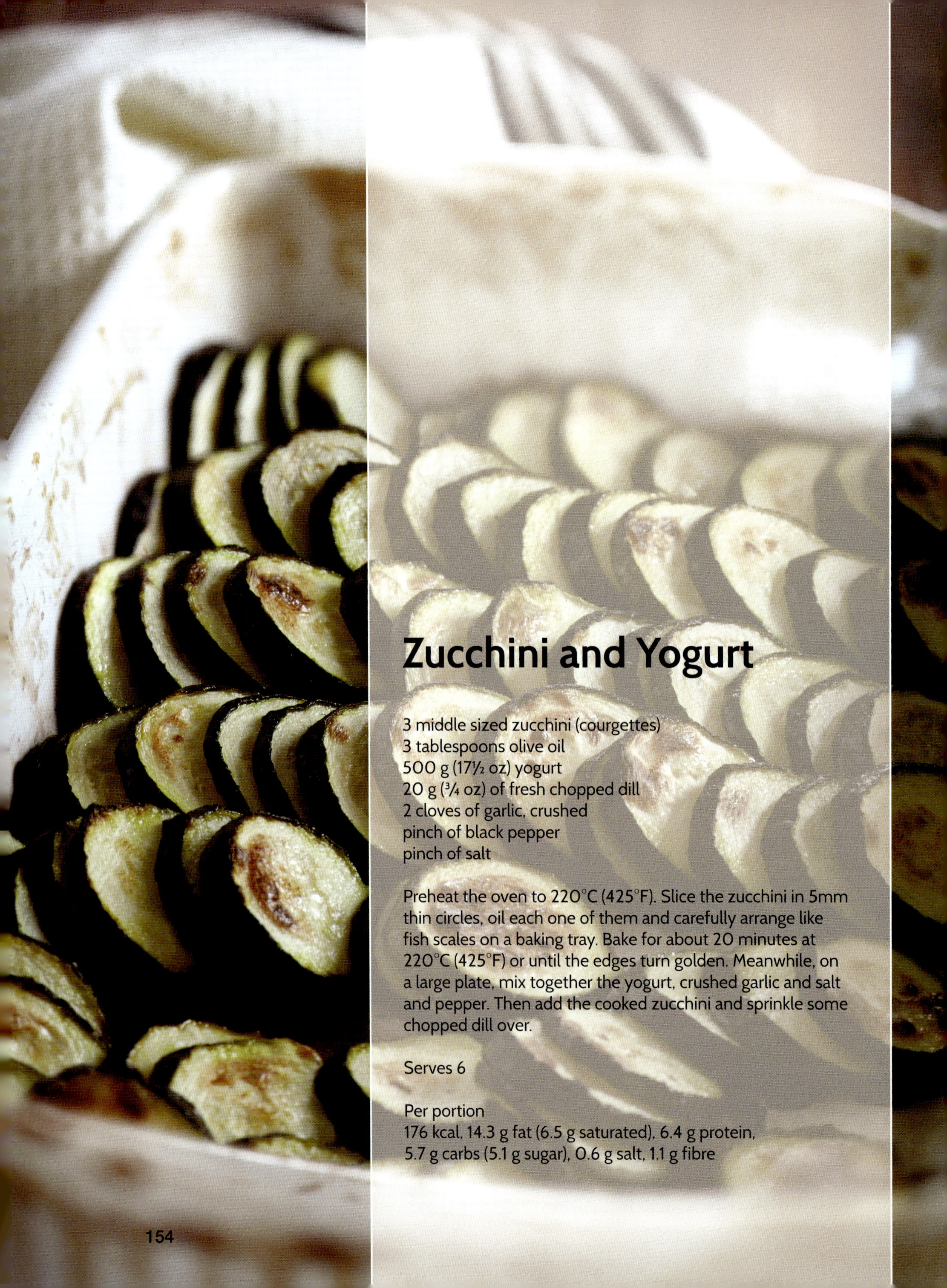

Zucchini and Yogurt

3 middle sized zucchini (courgettes)
3 tablespoons olive oil
500 g (17½ oz) yogurt
20 g (¾ oz) of fresh chopped dill
2 cloves of garlic, crushed
pinch of black pepper
pinch of salt

Preheat the oven to 220°C (425°F). Slice the zucchini in 5mm thin circles, oil each one of them and carefully arrange like fish scales on a baking tray. Bake for about 20 minutes at 220°C (425°F) or until the edges turn golden. Meanwhile, on a large plate, mix together the yogurt, crushed garlic and salt and pepper. Then add the cooked zucchini and sprinkle some chopped dill over.

Serves 6

Per portion
176 kcal, 14.3 g fat (6.5 g saturated), 6.4 g protein, 5.7 g carbs (5.1 g sugar), 0.6 g salt, 1.1 g fibre

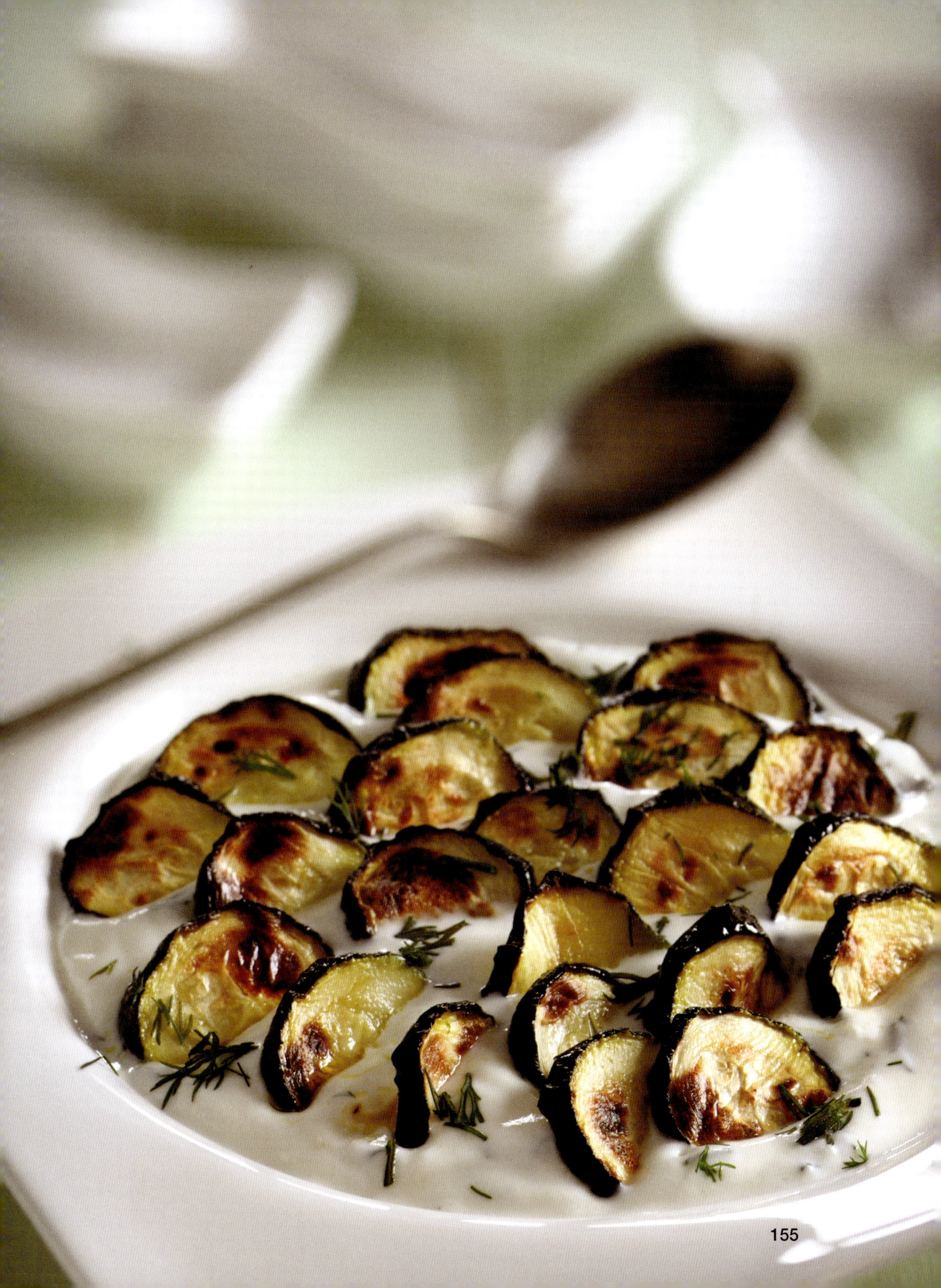

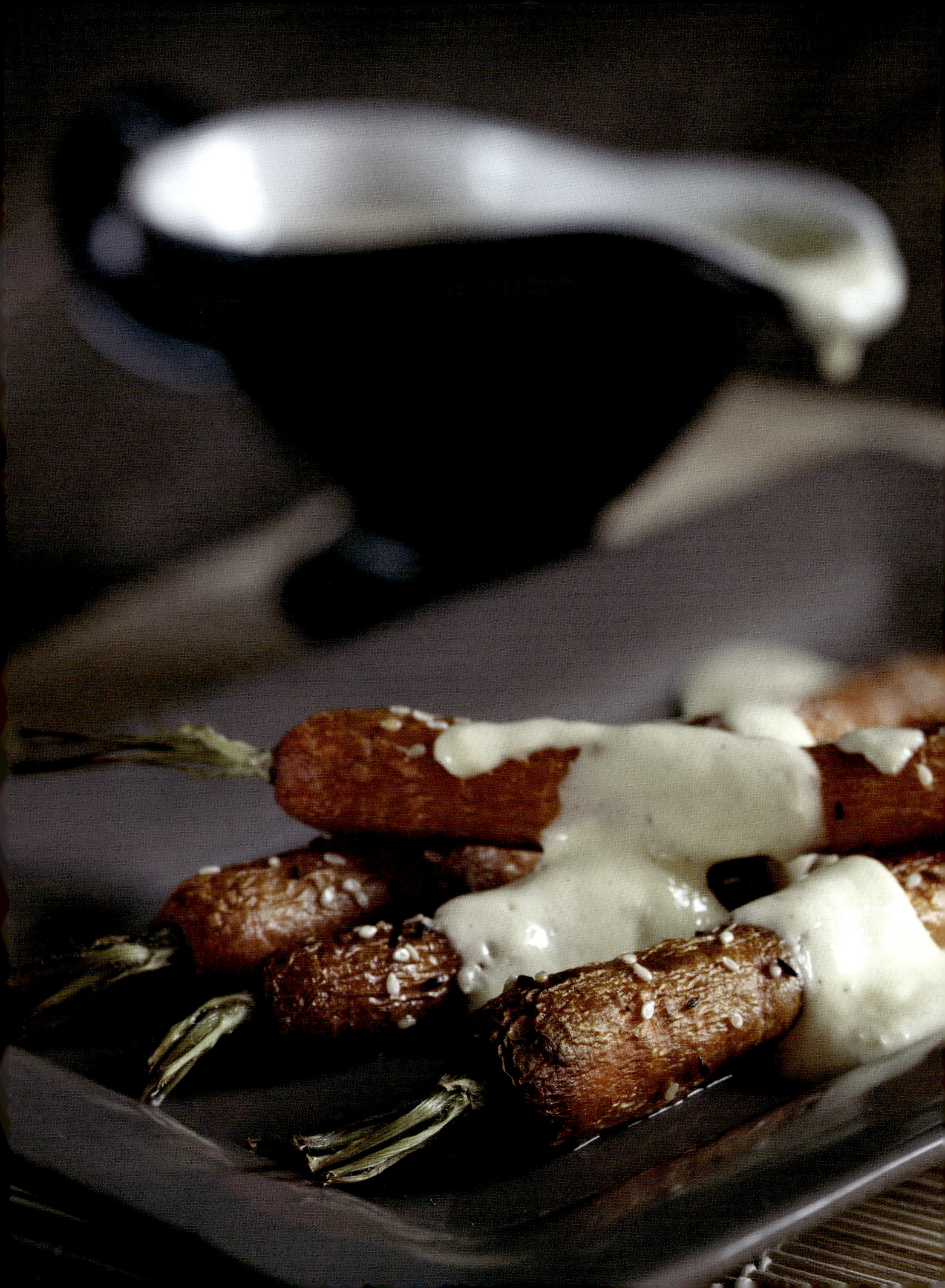

Caramelized Carrots and Mango Yogurt Sauce

8 medium young carrots
1 tablespoon vegetable oil
pinch of brown sugar
1 teaspoon sesame seeds
½ teaspoon caraway seeds

Preheat oven to 200°C (400°F). Wash 8 medium young carrots and oil with vegetable oil. Place the carrots on a baking tray, sprinkle some brown sugar, a pinch of sesame seeds and caraway seeds over each carrot and bake in the oven for about 20 minutes. Serve warm with the yogurt mango sauce.

Mango yogurt sauce:
half medium mango, diced
250 g (9 oz) low fat yogurt
1 teaspoon ground ginger
1 teaspoon allspice
pinch of salt

Put all the ingredients in a blender bowl and blend together until smooth.

Serves 4

Per serving
125 kcal, 5 g fat (1 g saturated), 4 g protein, 18 g carbs (16 g sugar), 5.0 g fibre, 0.9 g salt

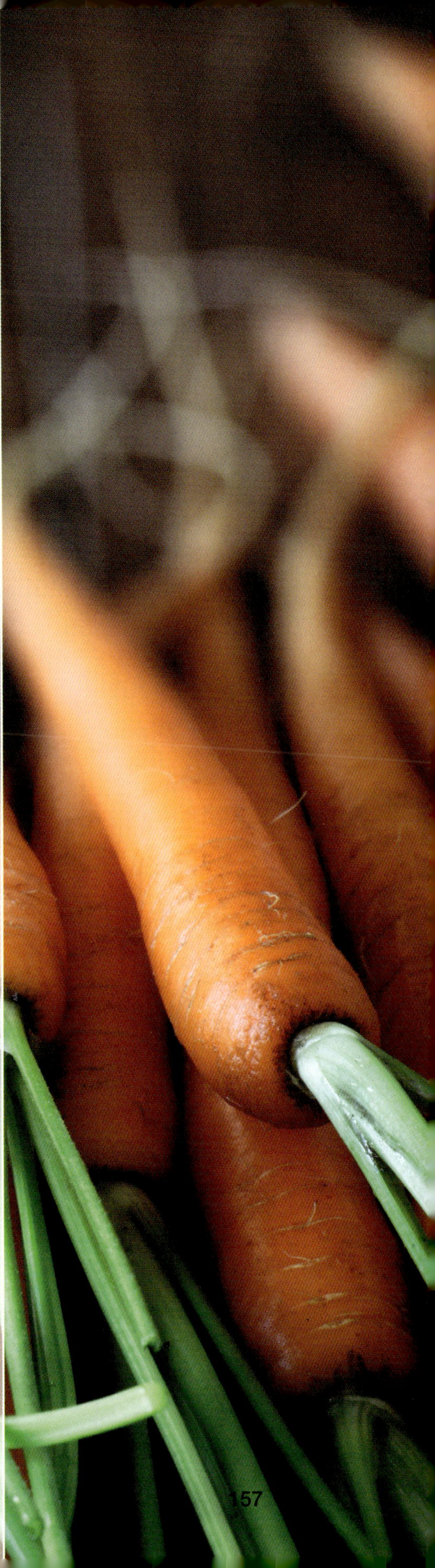

Chickpeas and Eggplant

2 eggplants (aubergines)
2 red onions
1 tablespoon extra virgin olive oil, plus extra for brushing
1 garlic clove
pinch of salt
400 g (14 oz) can chickpeas, drained
250 g (9 oz) full fat yogurt
a handful fresh mint, chopped
a handful fresh coriander, chopped

Place the eggplants on a baking tray. Skin and halve the onions, brush with oil and put next to the eggplants. Bake in the oven at 150°C (300°F) for about 30 minutes until slightly charred. Leave to cool for 15 minutes then remove the skin from the eggplants, coarsely chop and throw into a food processor. Add the onions, garlic, salt and olive oil and whiz until it becomes a paste. Transfer to a medium bowl, add the chickpeas, yogurt, mint and coriander. Mix well and serve cold on toasted bread or savory biscuits.

Serves 6

Per portion
152 kcal, 7.2 g protein, 7.9 g fat (3.3 g saturated), 13.8 g carbs (5.2 g sugar), 0.8 g salt, 5.7 g fibre

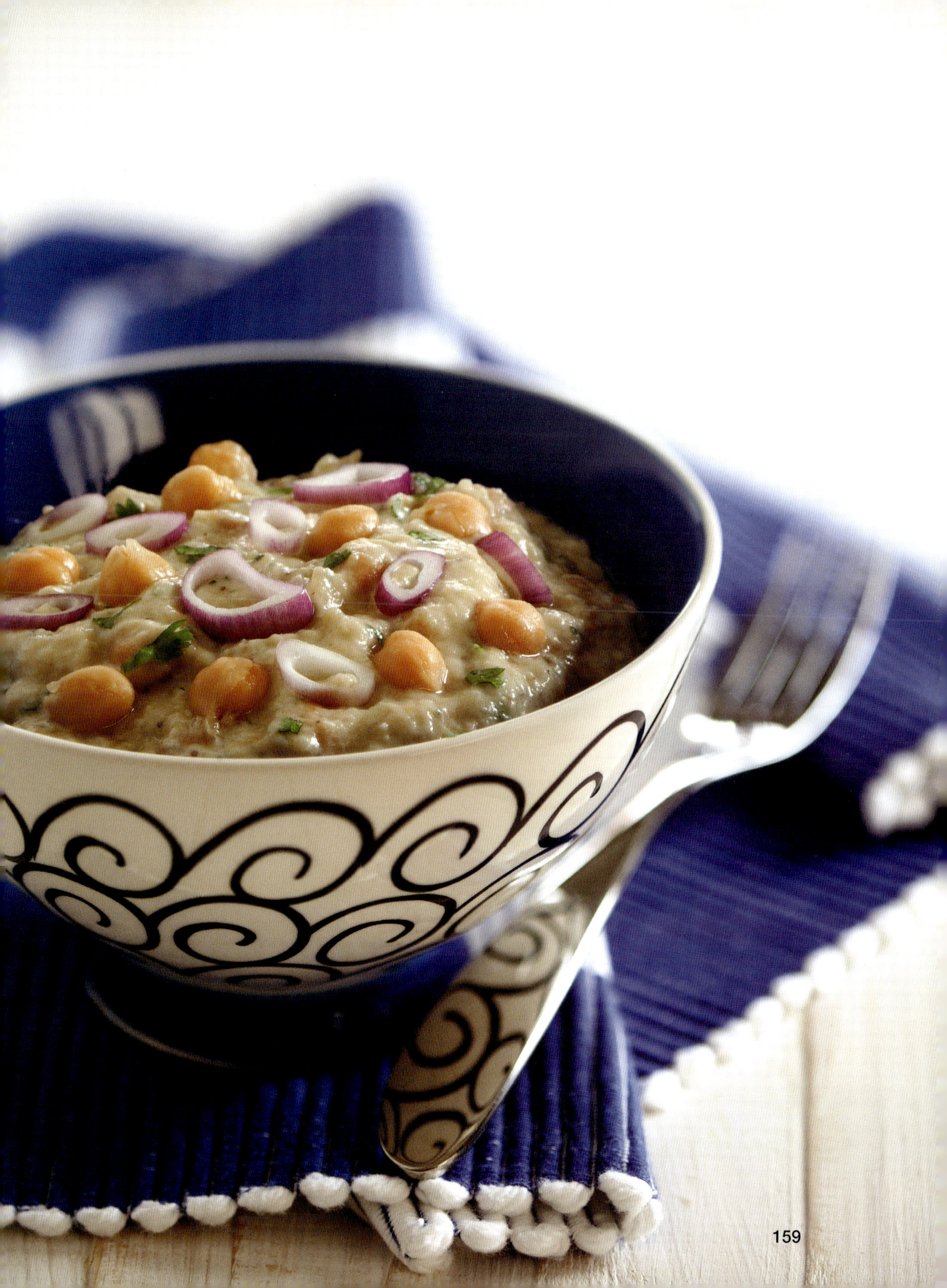

Roasted Pepper Dip

3 large Red Sweet Pointed Pepper
250 g (9 oz) low-fat plain yogurt
250 g (9 oz) feta cheese
1 garlic clove, crashed
50 g (2 oz) walnuts, chopped
1 lime, freshly squeezed juice
2 tablespoons olive oil
handful fresh dill, chopped
pinch of salt if needed

Wash and the peppers and then place them on a baking tray. Bake in the oven at 150°C (300°F) for about 30 minutes until slightly charred. Leave for 10 minutes to cool and drain. Remove the skin and seeds from the peppers. Throw all ingredients into a food processor bowl – roasted peppers, diced feta cheese, yogurt, crushed garlic, chopped walnuts, lime juice, olive oil and fresh dill. Blend until smooth. Taste and adjust seasonings, to taste. Serve with sliced toasted bread or savory biscuits.

Serves 4

Per serving
355 kcal, 27.7 g fat (10.8 g saturated), 15.6 g protein, 11.6 g carbs (11.1 g sugar), 2.5 g fibre, 3.1 g salt

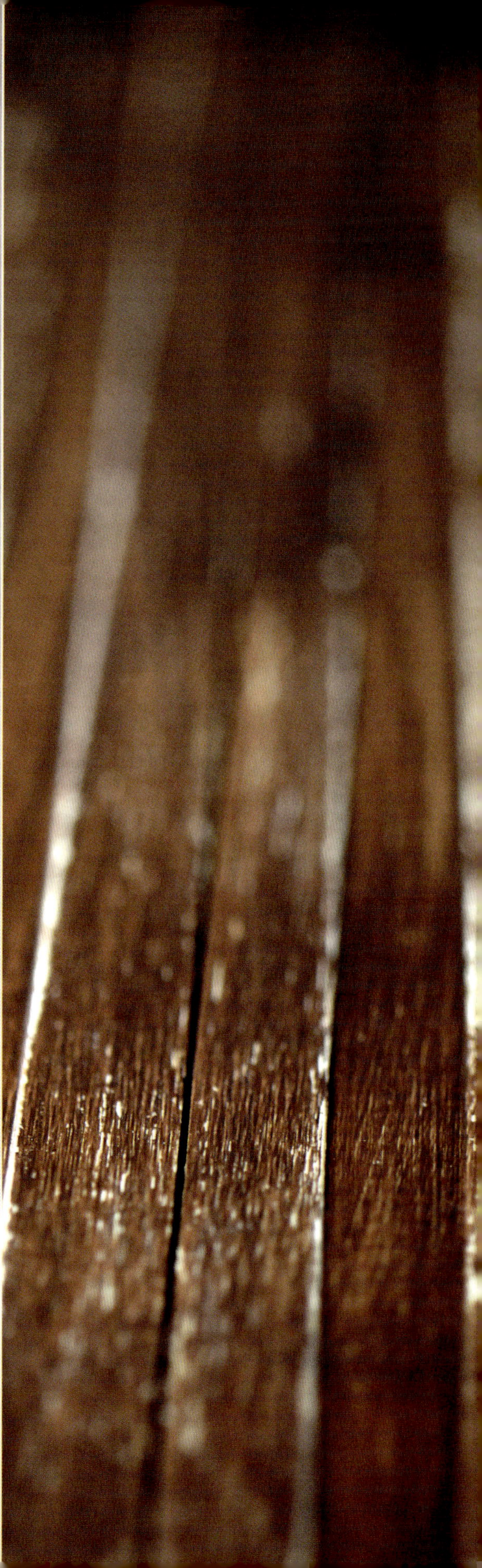

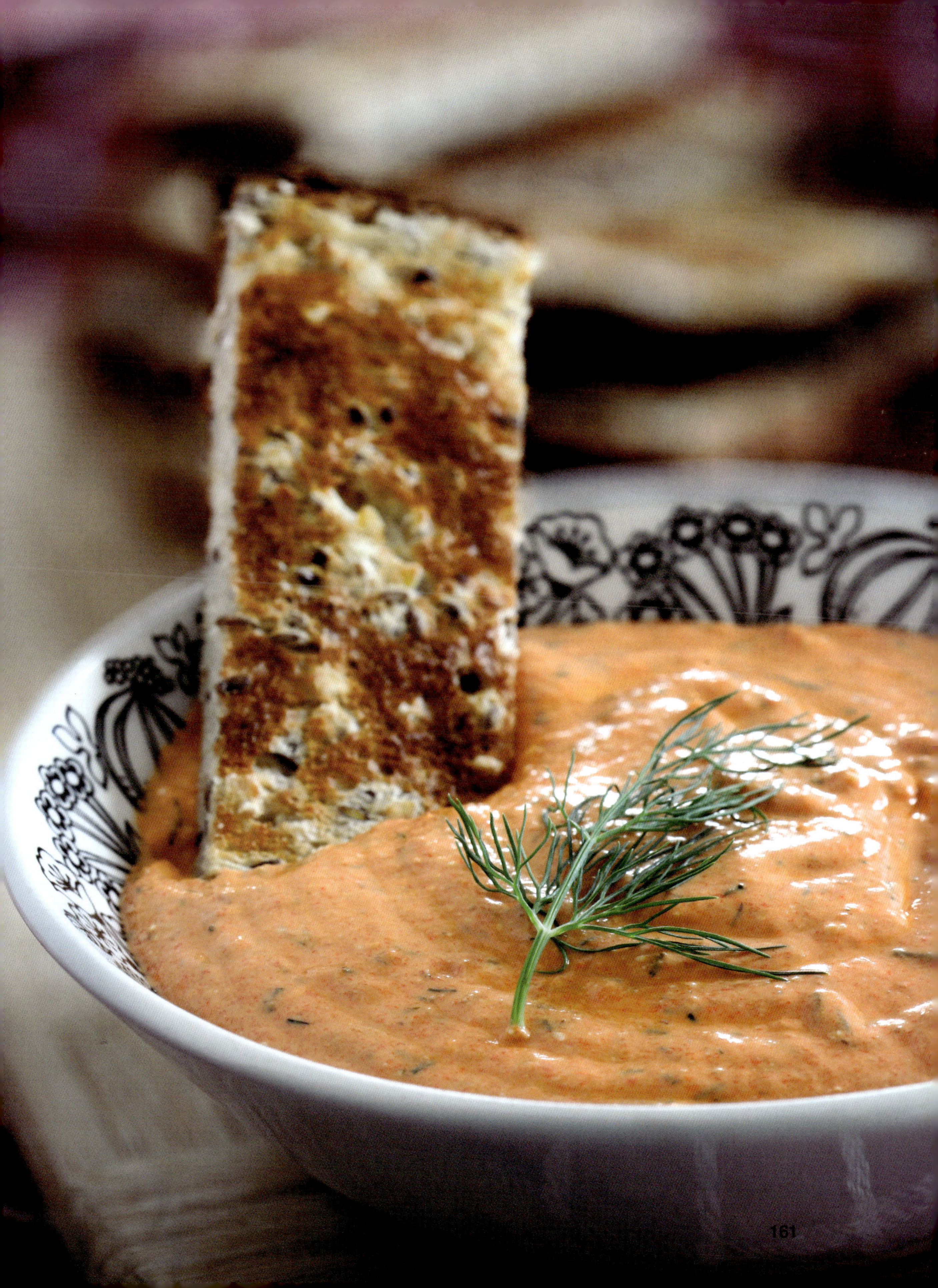

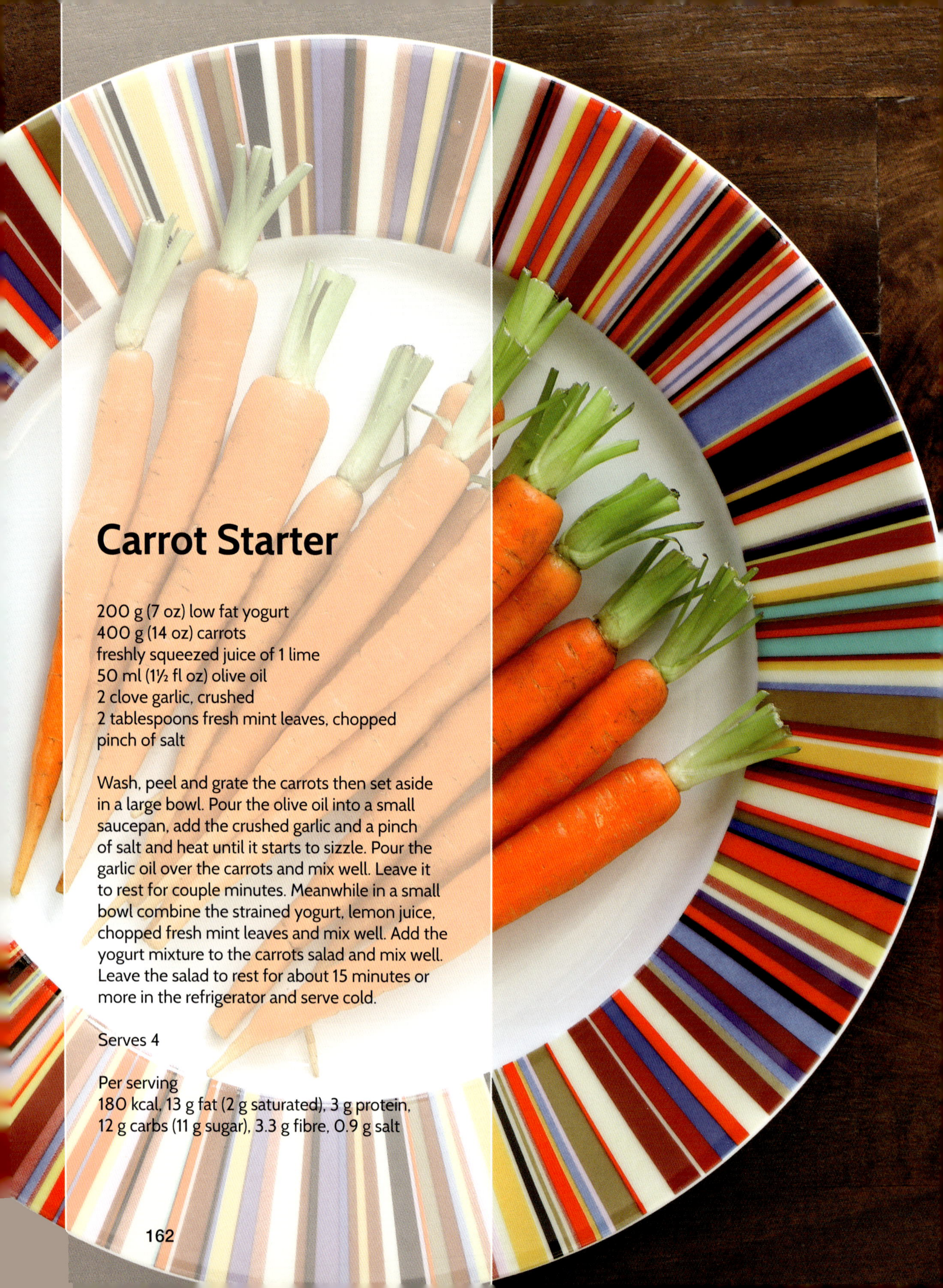

Carrot Starter

200 g (7 oz) low fat yogurt
400 g (14 oz) carrots
freshly squeezed juice of 1 lime
50 ml (1½ fl oz) olive oil
2 clove garlic, crushed
2 tablespoons fresh mint leaves, chopped
pinch of salt

Wash, peel and grate the carrots then set aside in a large bowl. Pour the olive oil into a small saucepan, add the crushed garlic and a pinch of salt and heat until it starts to sizzle. Pour the garlic oil over the carrots and mix well. Leave it to rest for couple minutes. Meanwhile in a small bowl combine the strained yogurt, lemon juice, chopped fresh mint leaves and mix well. Add the yogurt mixture to the carrots salad and mix well. Leave the salad to rest for about 15 minutes or more in the refrigerator and serve cold.

Serves 4

Per serving
180 kcal, 13 g fat (2 g saturated), 3 g protein, 12 g carbs (11 g sugar), 3.3 g fibre, 0.9 g salt

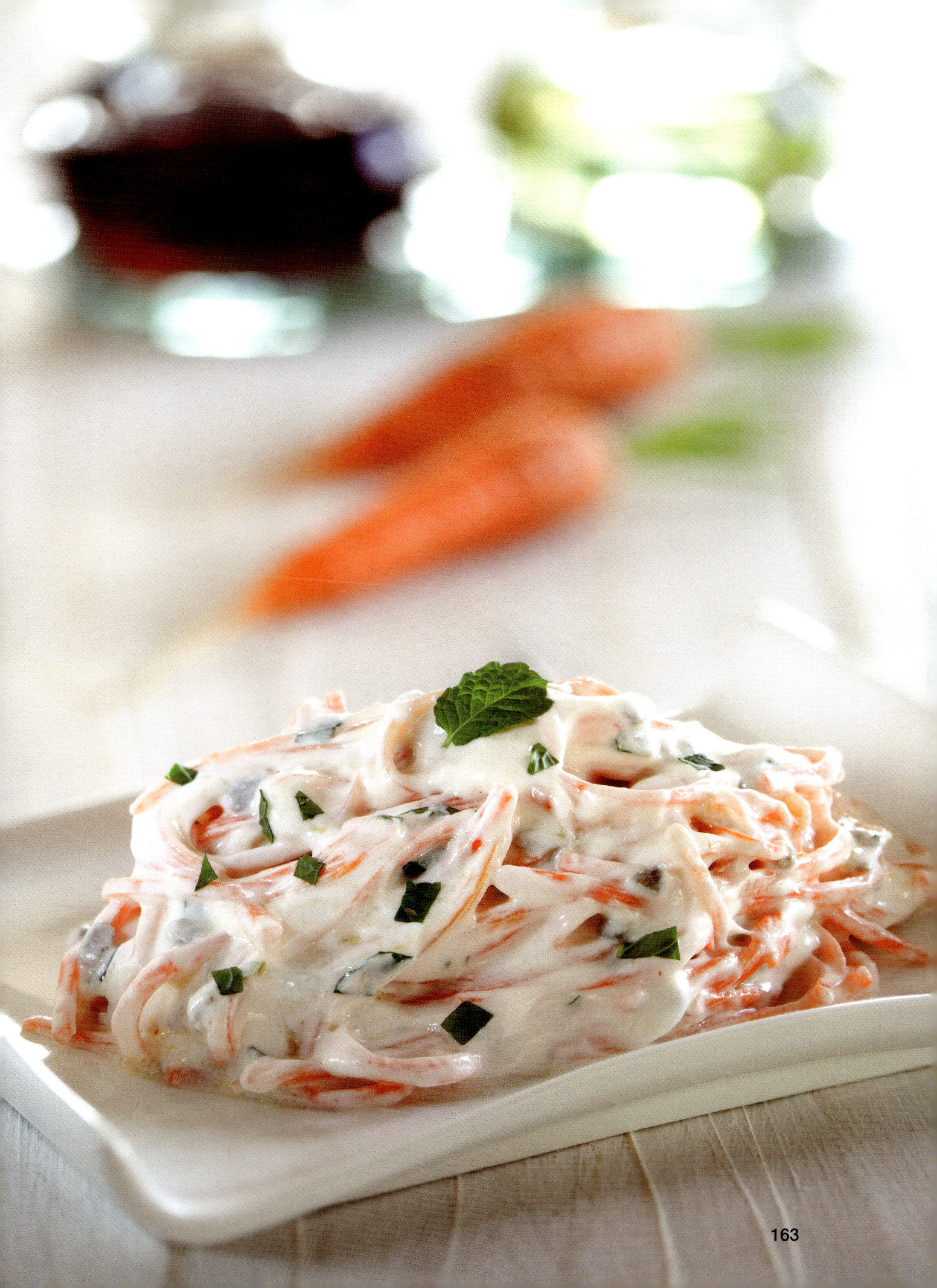

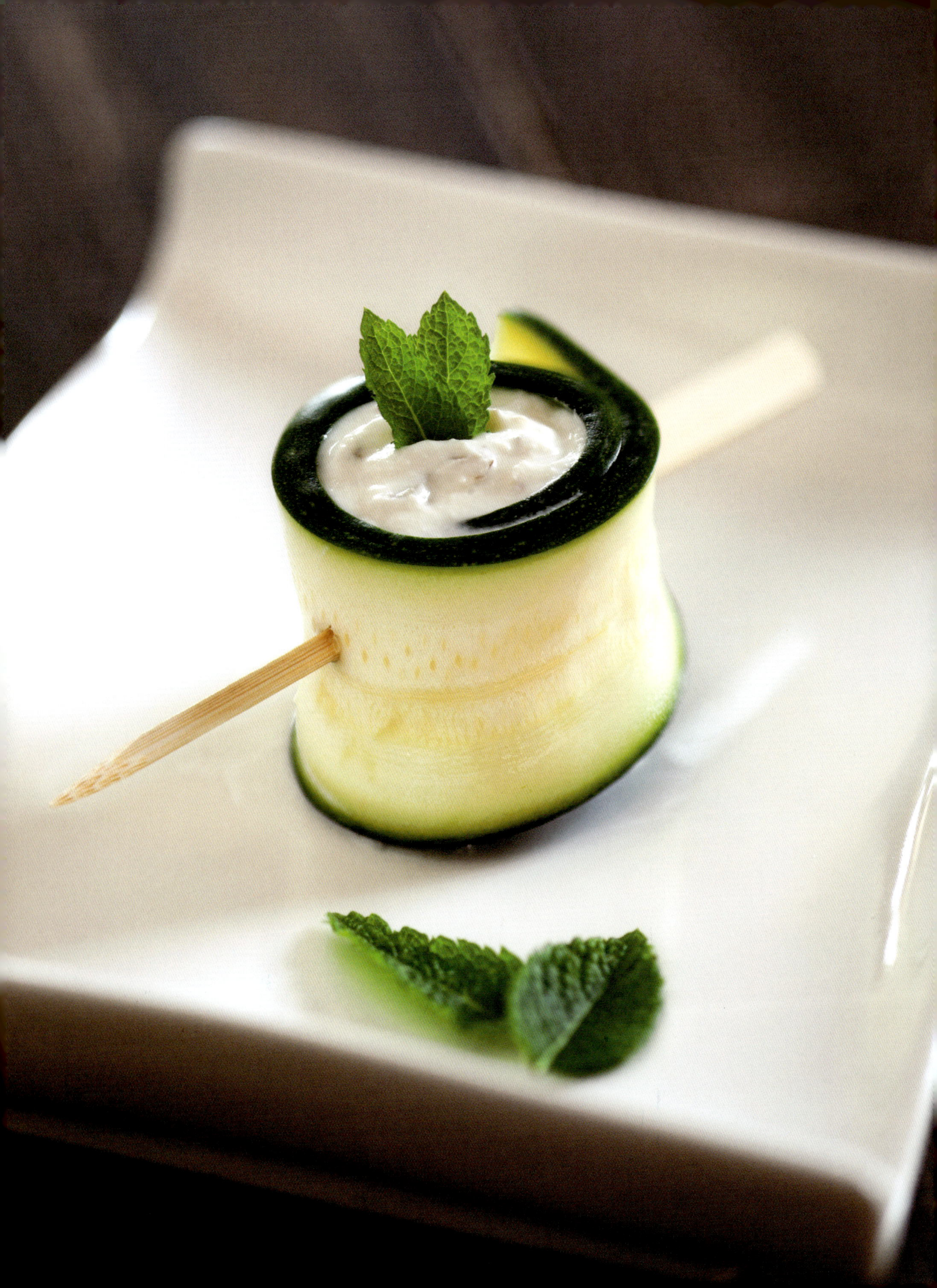

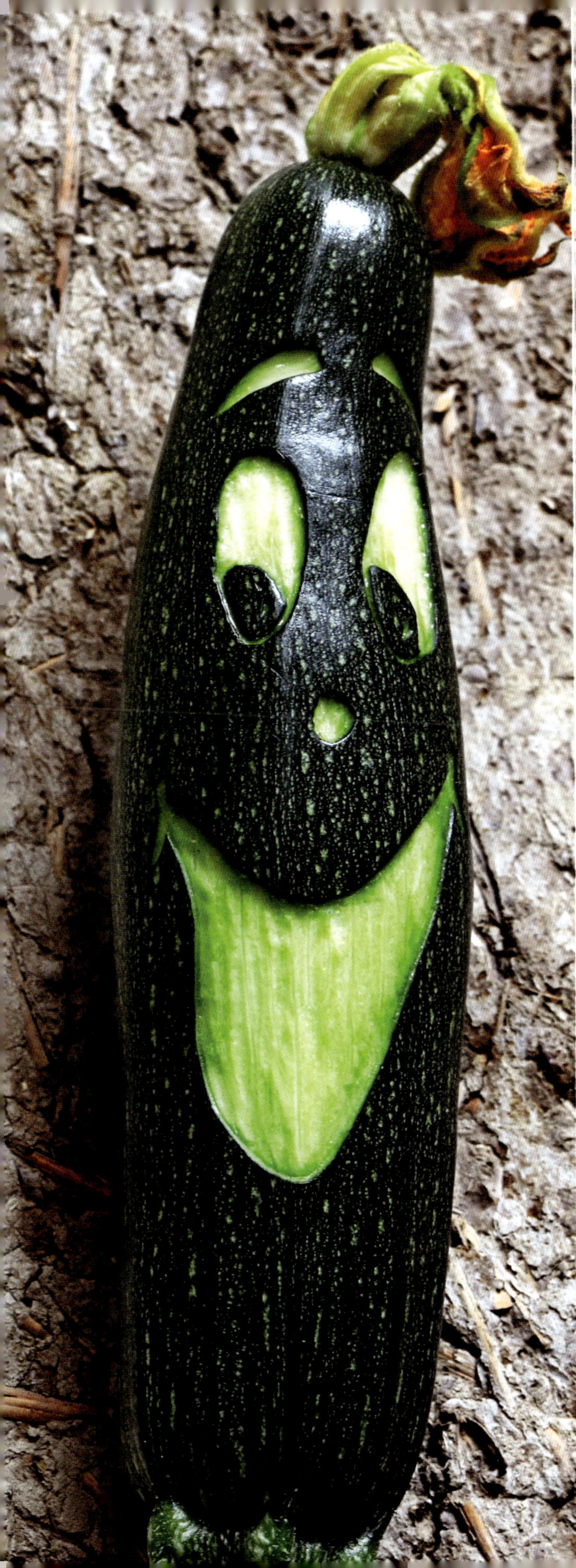

Zucchini Rolls

500 g (17½ oz) large zucchini (courgettes) (about 2)
pinch of salt
250 g (9 oz) strained yogurt
250 g (9 oz) ricotta cheese
50 g (2 oz) walnuts, finely chopped
1 garlic clove, finely chopped
1 tablespoon fresh mint leaves, finely chopped
1 tablespoon extra virgin olive oil
8 bamboo skewers

Cut the zucchini into 3mm thick slices. Sprinkle well with salt and leave in the refrigerator for 1 hour. Meanwhile, pour the strained yogurt into a medium bowl. Add the ricotta cheese, walnut, garlic, mint leaves, olive oil and a pinch of salt, mix all the ingredients together with a spoon. Once the zucchini have become flexible and easy to roll, lay one on a chopping board and roll it, making a tube no more than 5 cm (2 inches) in diameter. Lock it using a bamboo skewer and fill it with the yogurt mixture. Repeat with the rest of zucchini slices. You can serve immediately or store in the refrigerator.

Serves 8

Per serving
130 kcal, 9.7 g fat (3.1 g saturated), 6.6 g protein, 4.4 g carbs (4.2 g sugar), 1.1 g fibre, 0.5 g salt

Eggs and Yogurt Starter

2 large free-range eggs
pinch of salt
2 tablespoons light mayonnaise
1 garlic clove, crushed
500 g (17½ oz) low fat yogurt
1 teaspoon freshly ground black pepper
toast or savoury biscuits, to serve

Put the eggs in a small saucepan of cold water, bring to the boil then simmer for 10 minutes. Add a pinch of salt to the water while boiling to make shelling the eggs easier. Rinse the eggs under cold water to cool down for a couple of minutes. Gently crack the eggshells, shell the eggs and then cut into slices. Prepare the yogurt mixture by adding the mayo, garlic and a pinch of salt to the yogurt and mix well. Arrange the eggs on top of the yogurt mixture and sprinkle with the black pepper. Leave to rest in the refrigerator for 30 minutes before serving cold with toast or savoury biscuits.

Serves 4

Per serving
131 kcal, 5.9 g fat (2 g saturated), 10.3 g protein, 9.8 g carbohydrates (9.6 g sugar), 0 g fibre, 1.1 g salt

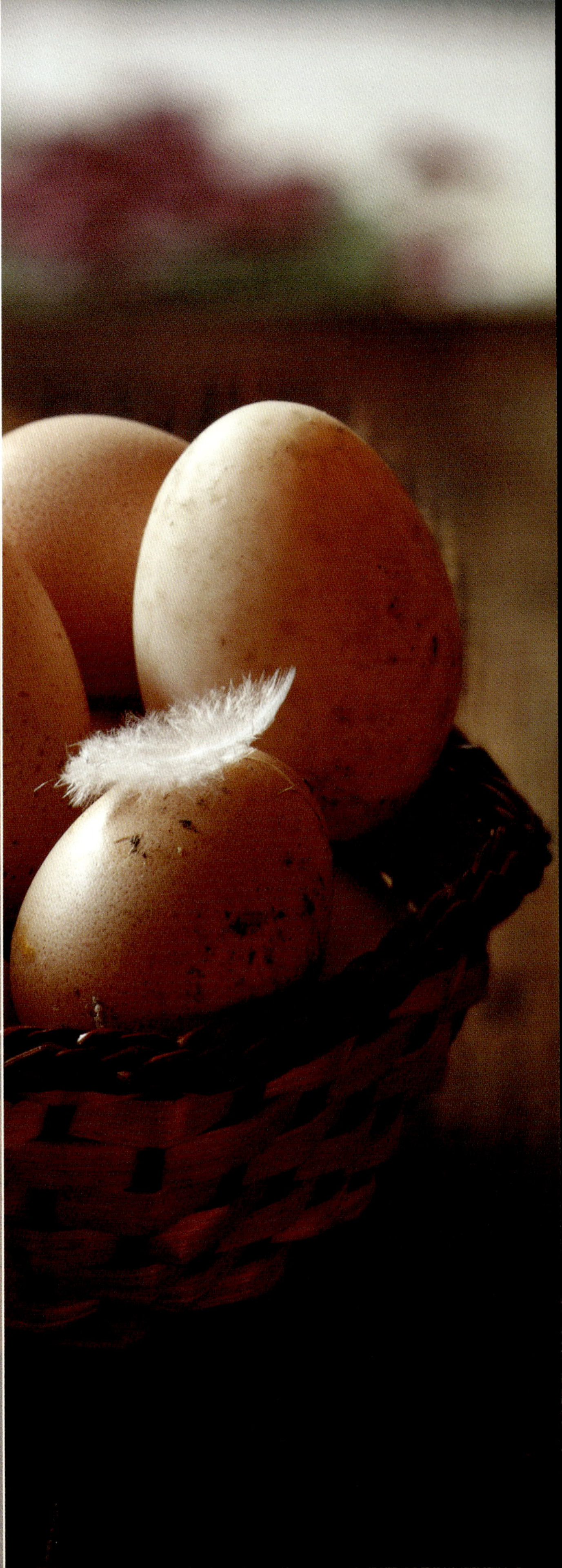

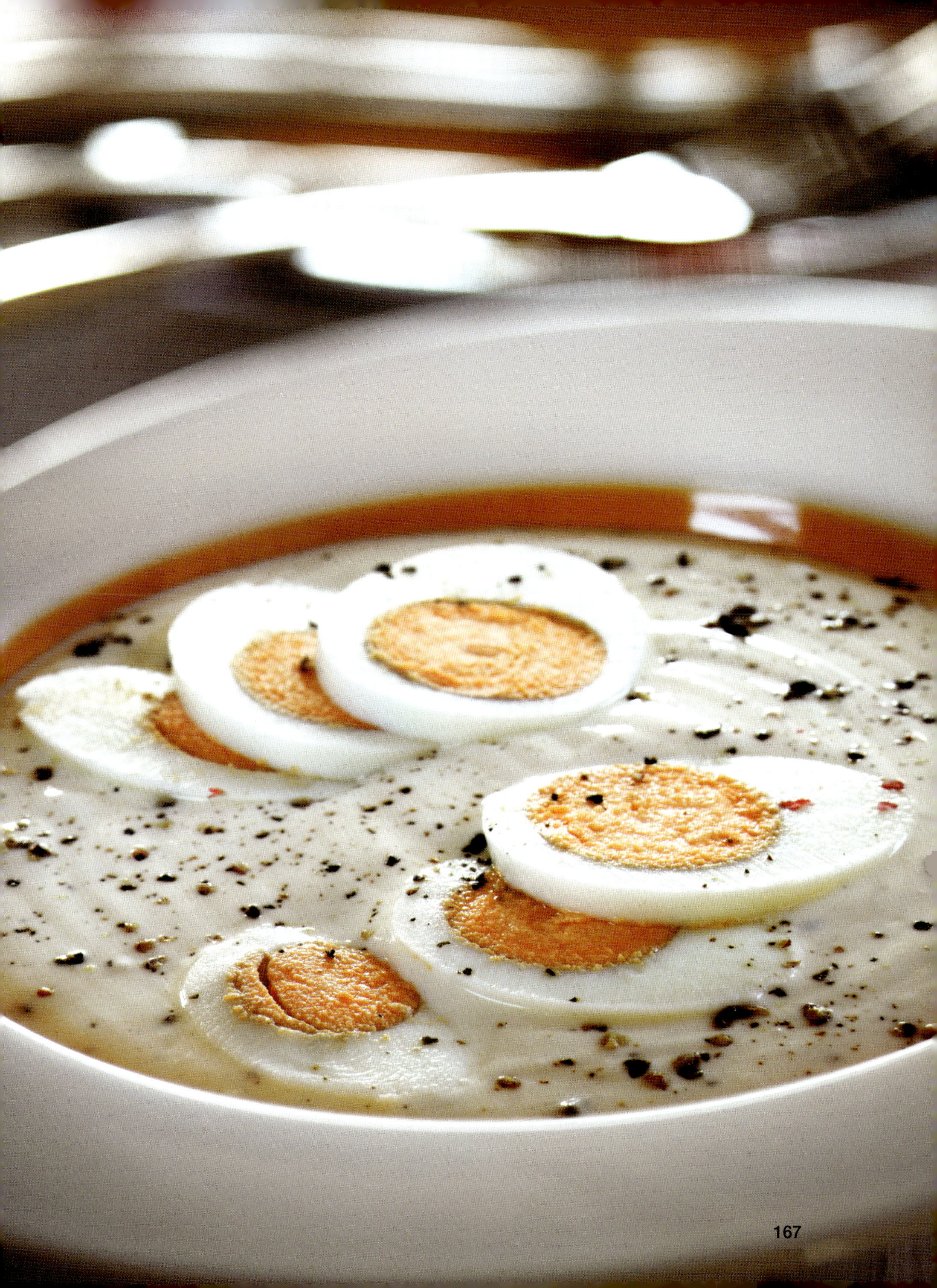

Yogurt Guacamole

250 g (9 oz) low fat yogurt
2 avocados, peeled, seeded, mashed
1 small vine tomato, finely chopped
1 lime, juice
1 shallot, finely chopped
2 spring onions
a pinch of ground chili pepper
a pinch of black pepper, ground

In the blender combine the yogurt, avocados, lime juice, shallot, spring onions, ground chili pepper, ground black pepper, salt and blend until smooth. Transfer the mixture into a medium bowl, add the finely chopped vine tomato and mix well with a spoon. It is ready to serve!

Serves 6

Per serving
118 kcal, 9.9 g fat (2.3 g saturated), 3.1 g protein, 4.6 g carbs (3.9 g sugar), 2.4 g fibre, 0.1 g salt

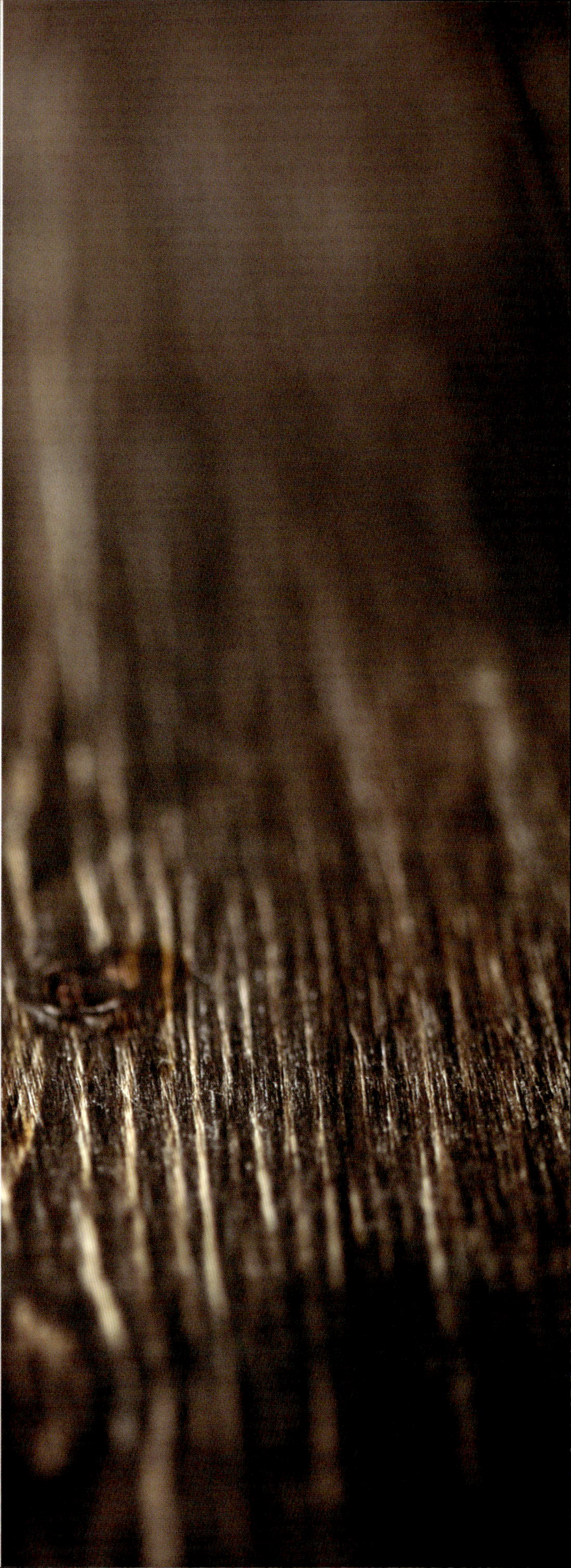

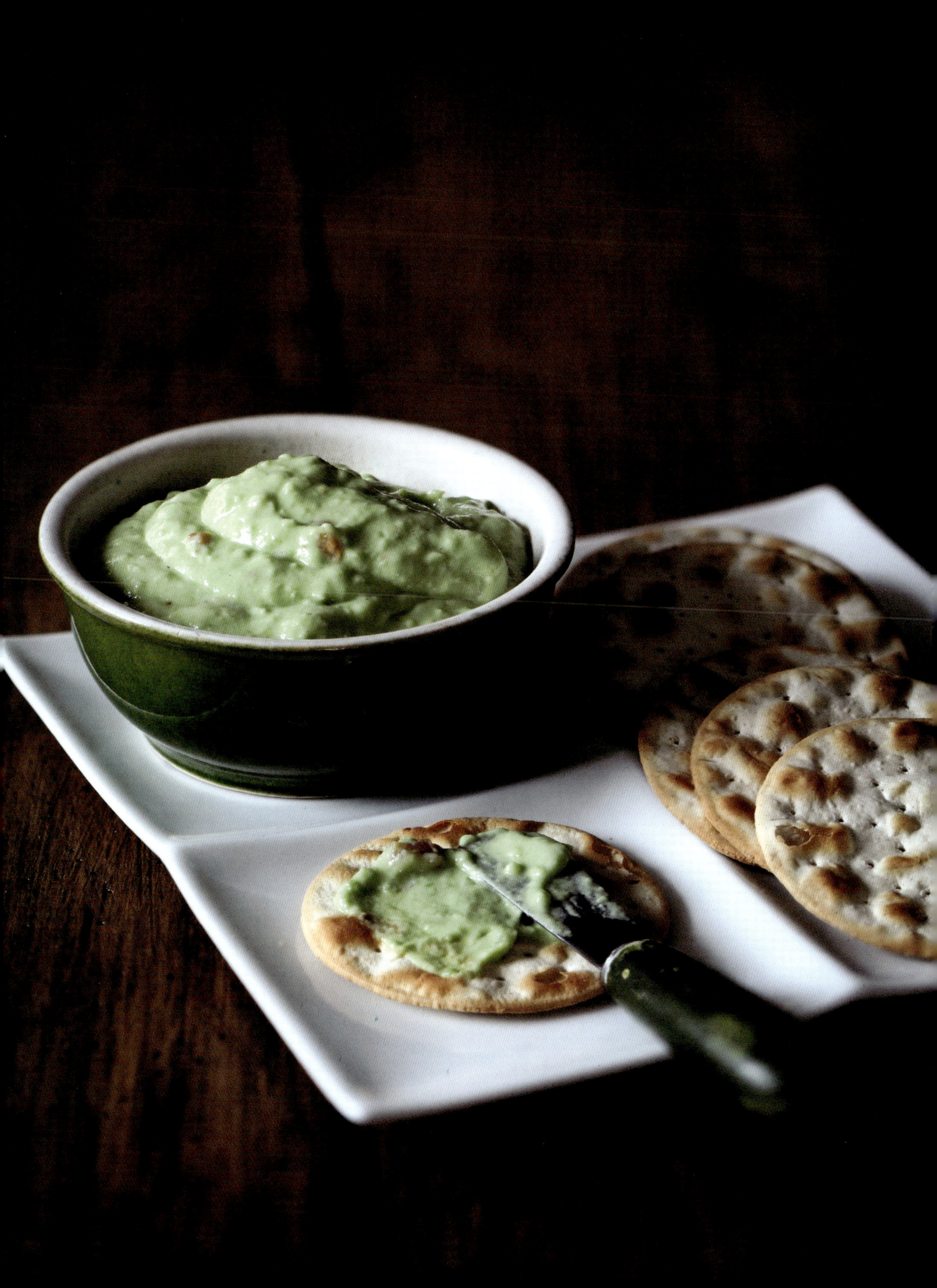

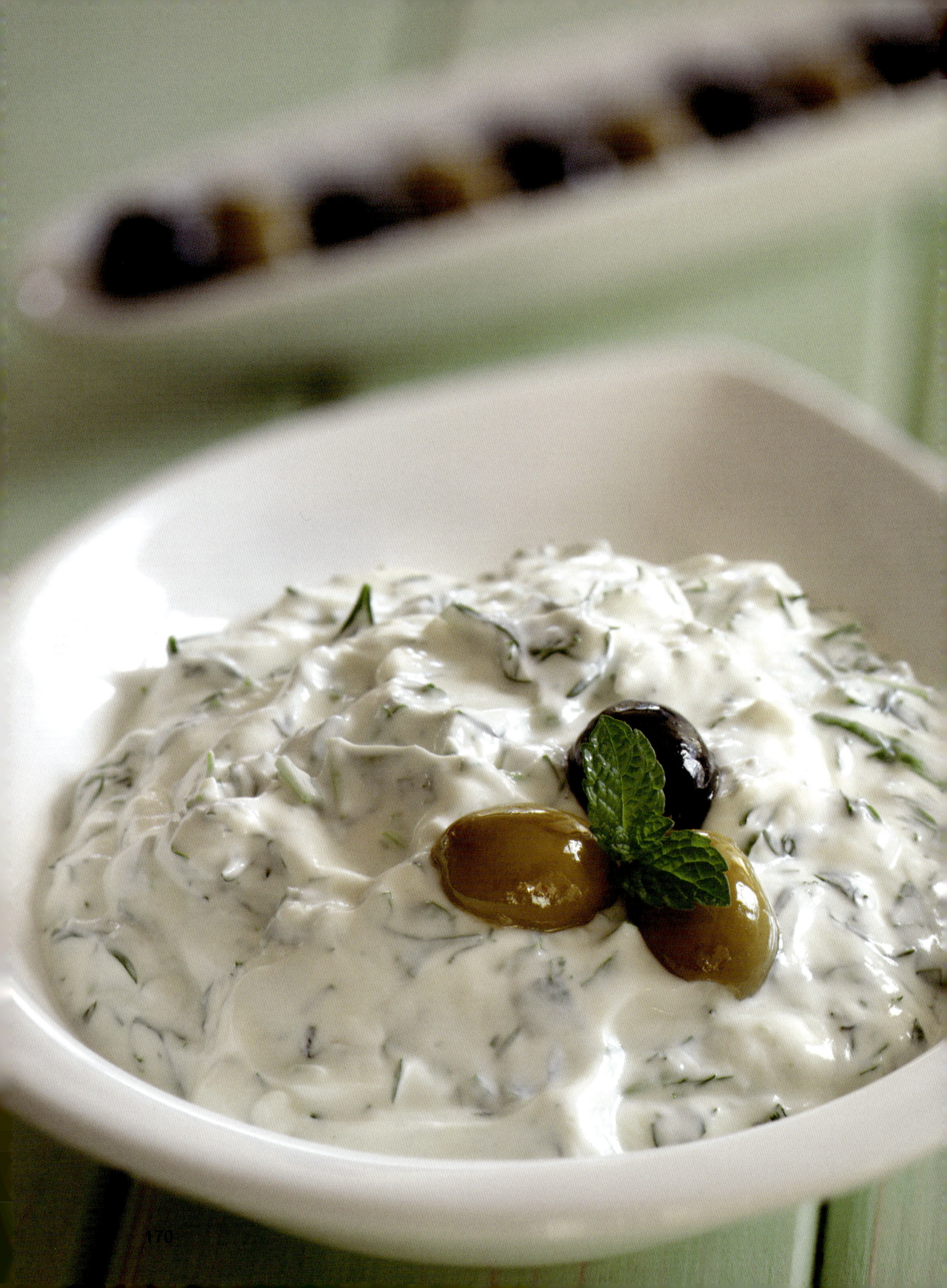

Tzatziki Yogurt Dip

250 g (9 oz) low fat yogurt, strained
3 tablespoons extra virgin olive oil
1 lemon, freshly squeezed juice
2 cloves garlic, finely minced
1 tablespoon fresh dill, chopped
2 tablespoons fresh mint leaves, finely chopped
1 tablespoon fresh parsley, finely chopped
pinch of salt
100 g (3½ oz) olives

Combine into a medium bowl the strained yogurt, minced garlic, dill, mint, parsley, lemon juice, olive oil and a pinch of salt. Mix well and serve with some olives.

Serves 4

Per serving
140 kcal, 11.7 g fat (2.0 g saturated), 3.7 g protein, 5.4 g carbs (4.9 g sugar), 1.3 g fibre, 2.2 g salt

Baked Potatoes with Yogurt Spread

500 g (17½ oz) small jacket potatoes
2 tablespoons sunflower oil
250 g (9 oz) strained yogurt
1 tablespoon fresh mint, finely chopped
1 small red onion, finely chopped
100 g (3½ oz) feta cheese, diced
30 g (1 oz) walnuts, chopped
1 teaspoon chilies crushed
1 teaspoon sumac
1 tablespoon extra virgin olive oil
pinch of salt

Preheat the oven to 220°C (425°F). Slice the potatoes in about 5 mm thick rings, oil and arrange over roaster tray grill rack. Bake for about 25 minutes until golden. Meanwhile in a medium bowl combine the chopped mint, onion, walnuts, chilies, sumac, salt and mix well. Next add the diced feta cheese, extra virgin olive oil and strained yogurt, mix again. Serve the potatoes warm with a tablespoon of yogurt spread over.

Serves 6

Per serving
225 kcal, 13.7 g fat (4.2 g saturated), 7.6 g protein, 18.8 g carbs (4.7 g sugar), 1.9 g fibre, 1.2 g salt

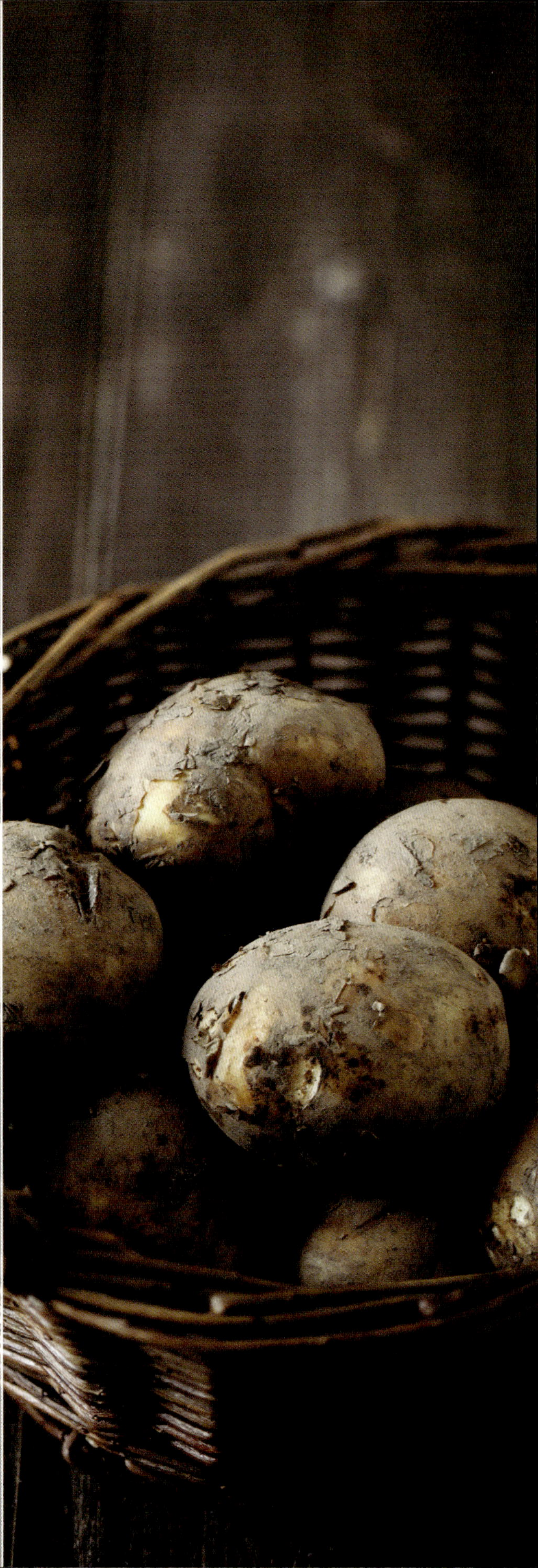

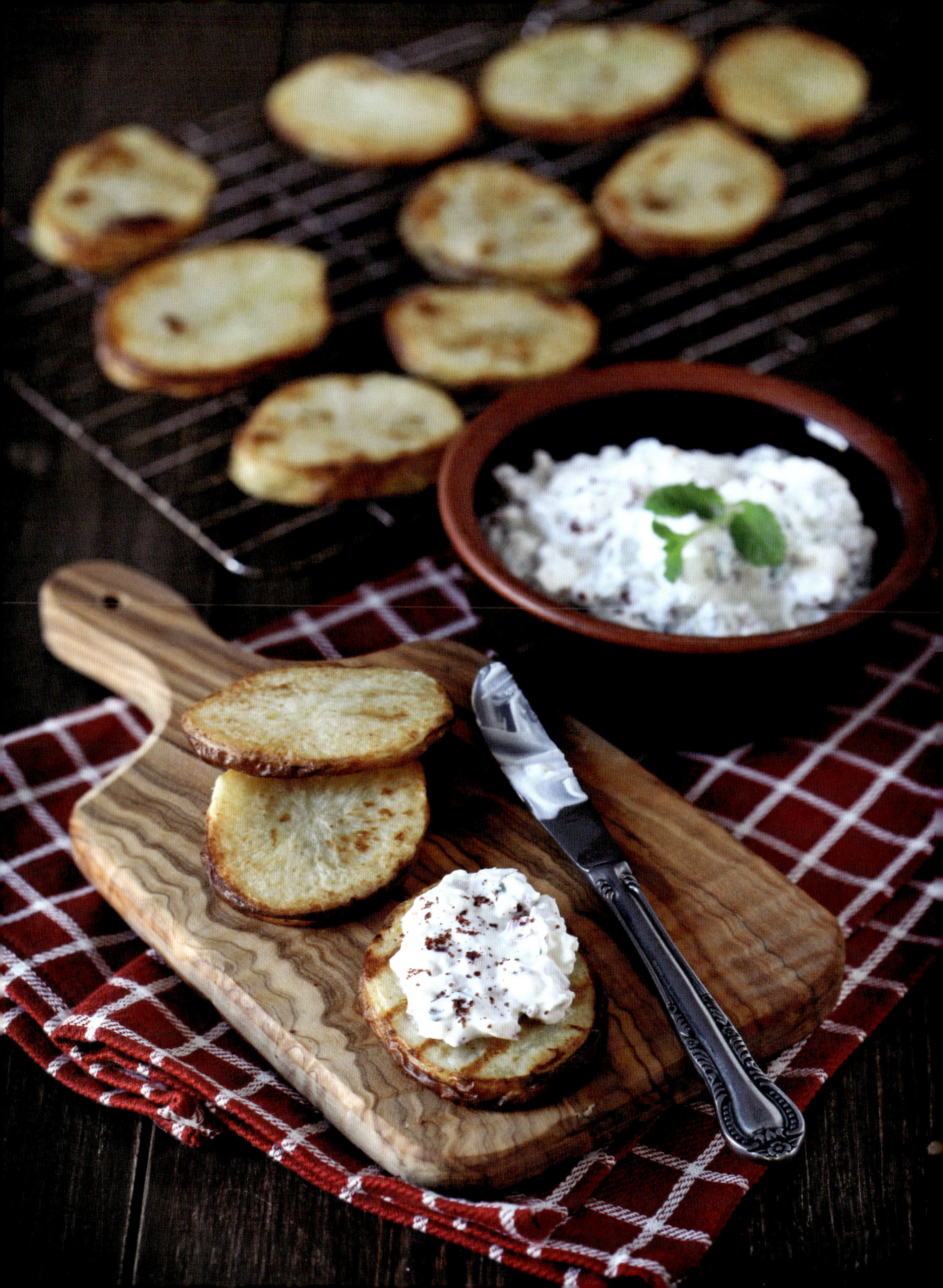

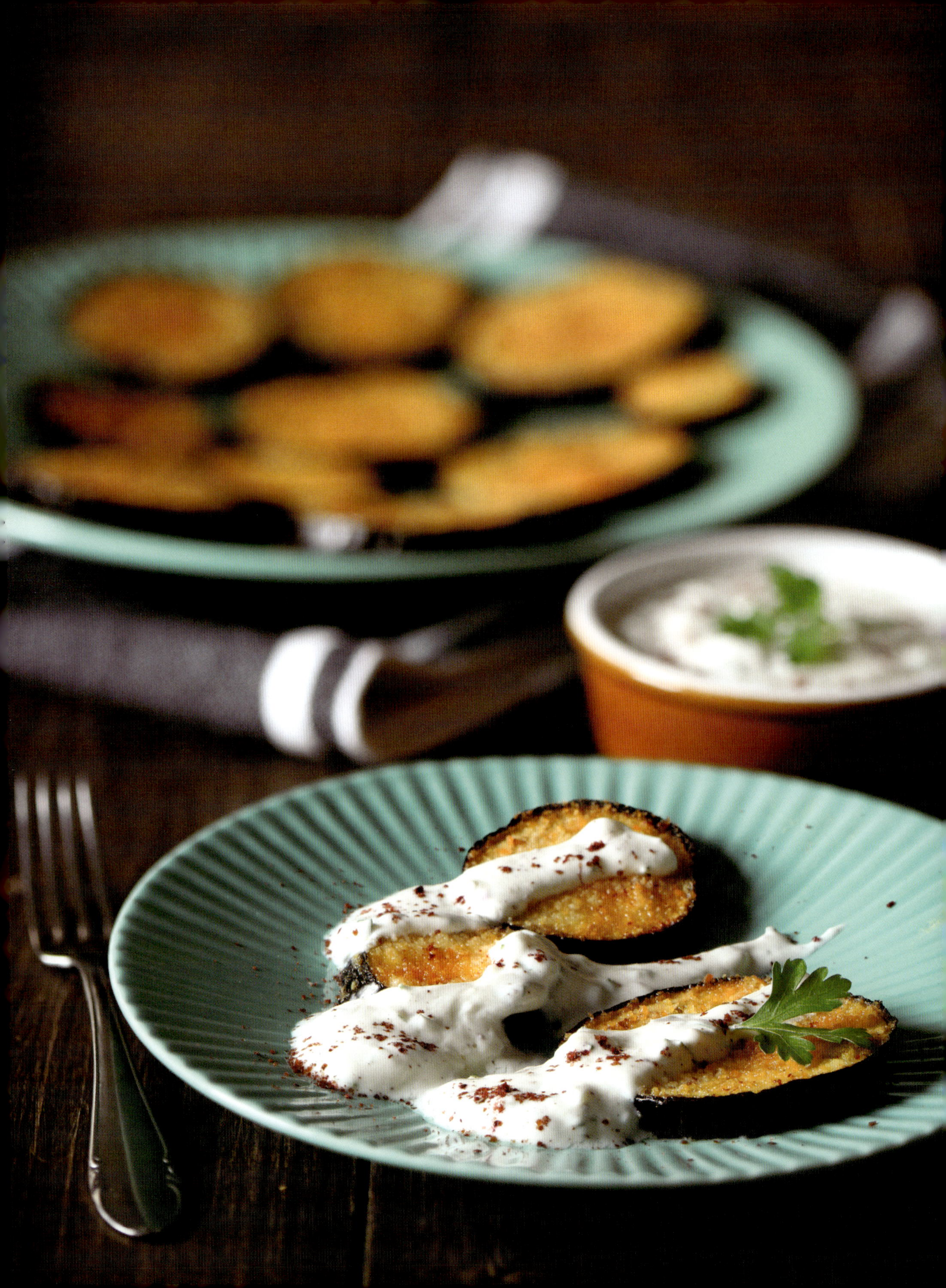

Eggplant and Tahini Yogurt

2 small eggplants (aubergines)
2 tablespoons of vegetarian oil
2 cloves of garlic, crushed
1 tablespoons tahini
250 g (9 oz) low fat yogurt
Juice of 1 lime
Pinch of salt
2 tablespoons parsley, chopped
1 tablespoon extra virgin olive oil
1 tablespoon sumac

Preheat the oven to 220°C (425°F). Slice the eggplants in 5 millimeter slices, oil them with vegetarian oil and place into a medium bowl. Next arrange them over a roaster tray grill rack and bake for 20 minutes. Meanwhile in a medium bowl mix together the crushed garlic, tahini, yogurt, lime juice, a pinch of salt and chopped parsley. Arrange the eggplant slices on a large plate and pour the yogurt mixture over. Serve with a sprinkle of sumac on top.

Serves 8

Per serving
107 kcal, 8.8 g fat (1.4 g saturated), 3.4 g protein, 3.8 g carbs (3.5 g sugar), 2.2 g fibre, 0.4 g salt

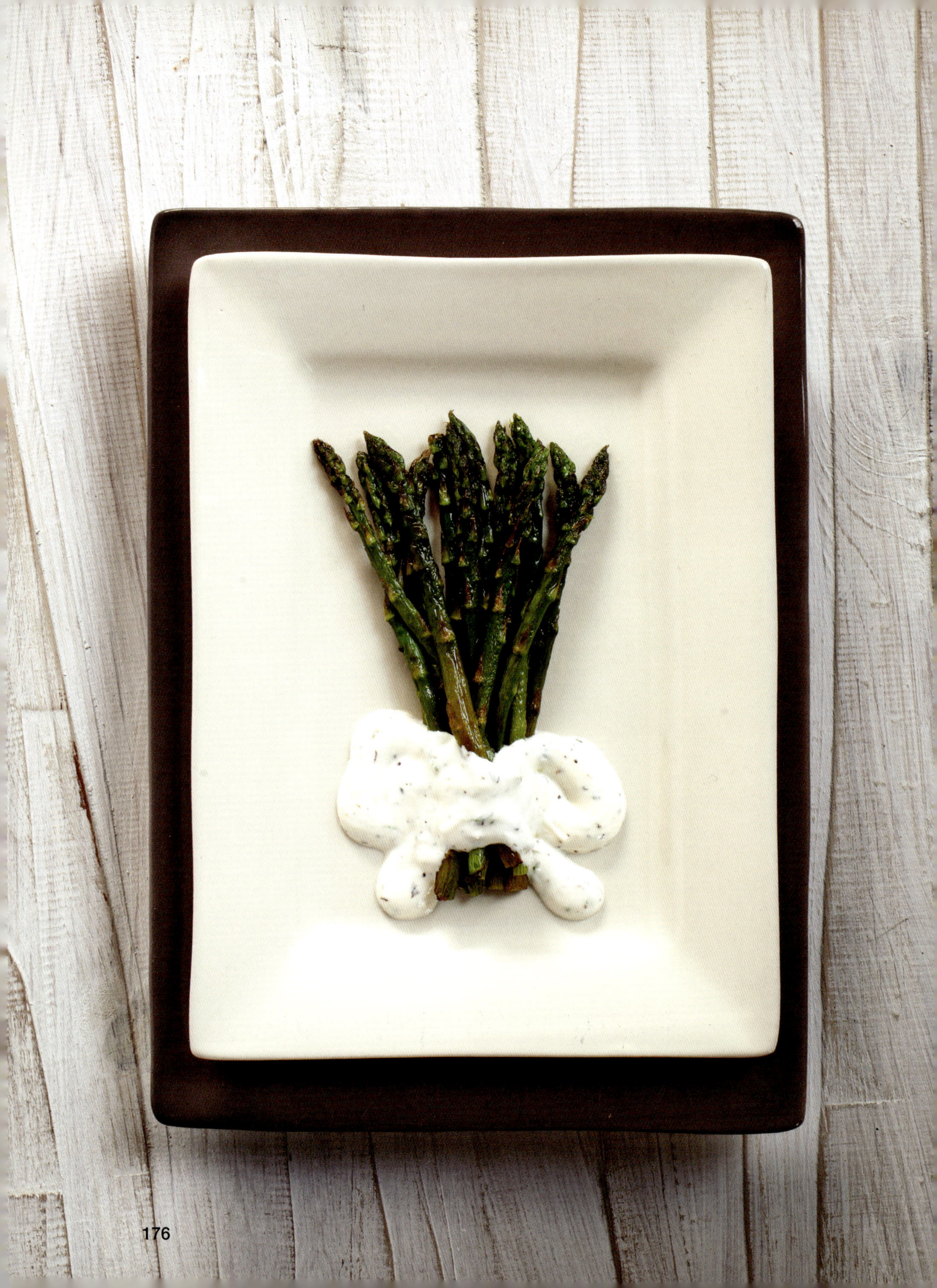

Pan Roasted Asparagus and Yogurt Dip

200 g (7 oz) low fat yogurt
1 clove garlic, finely chopped
1 tablespoon tahini paste
2 tablespoons fresh thyme, chopped
1 tablespoon dry marjoram
2 tablespoons extra virgin olive oil
2 bunches fresh asparagus, washed and bottoms trimmed
2 tbsp olive oil
a pinch of salt

Combine the yogurt, chopped garlic, tahini paste, chopped fresh thyme, dry marjoram, olive oil, a pinch of salt in a medium bowl and mix well then set aside. Meanwhile throw the asparagus into a large frying pan, gently oil each and every one of them, cover the frying pan with a lid and cook over high heat for about 2 minutes. Shake the asparagus and cook for another 2 minutes, lid on, repeat until the asparagus are crisp but still tender. Remove from the heat and serve warm with the yogurt dip.

Serves 4

Per serving
240 kcal, 20.5 g fat (3.2 g saturated), 7.6 g protein, 6.6 g carbs (5.3 g sugar), 3.3 g fibre, 0.8 g salt

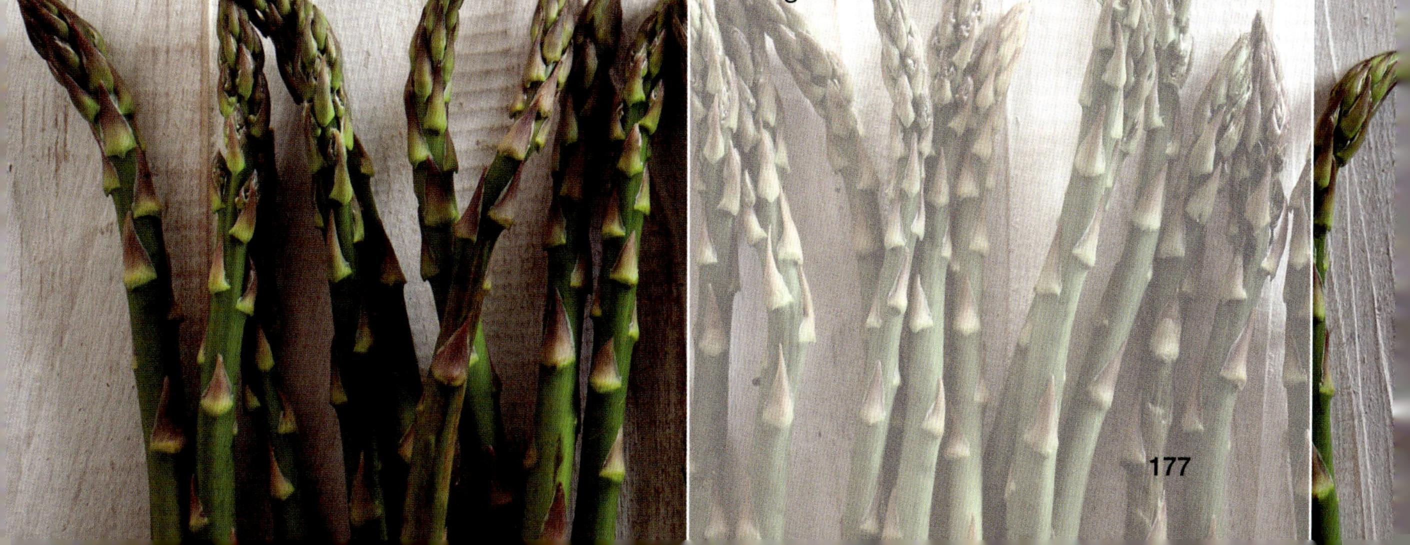

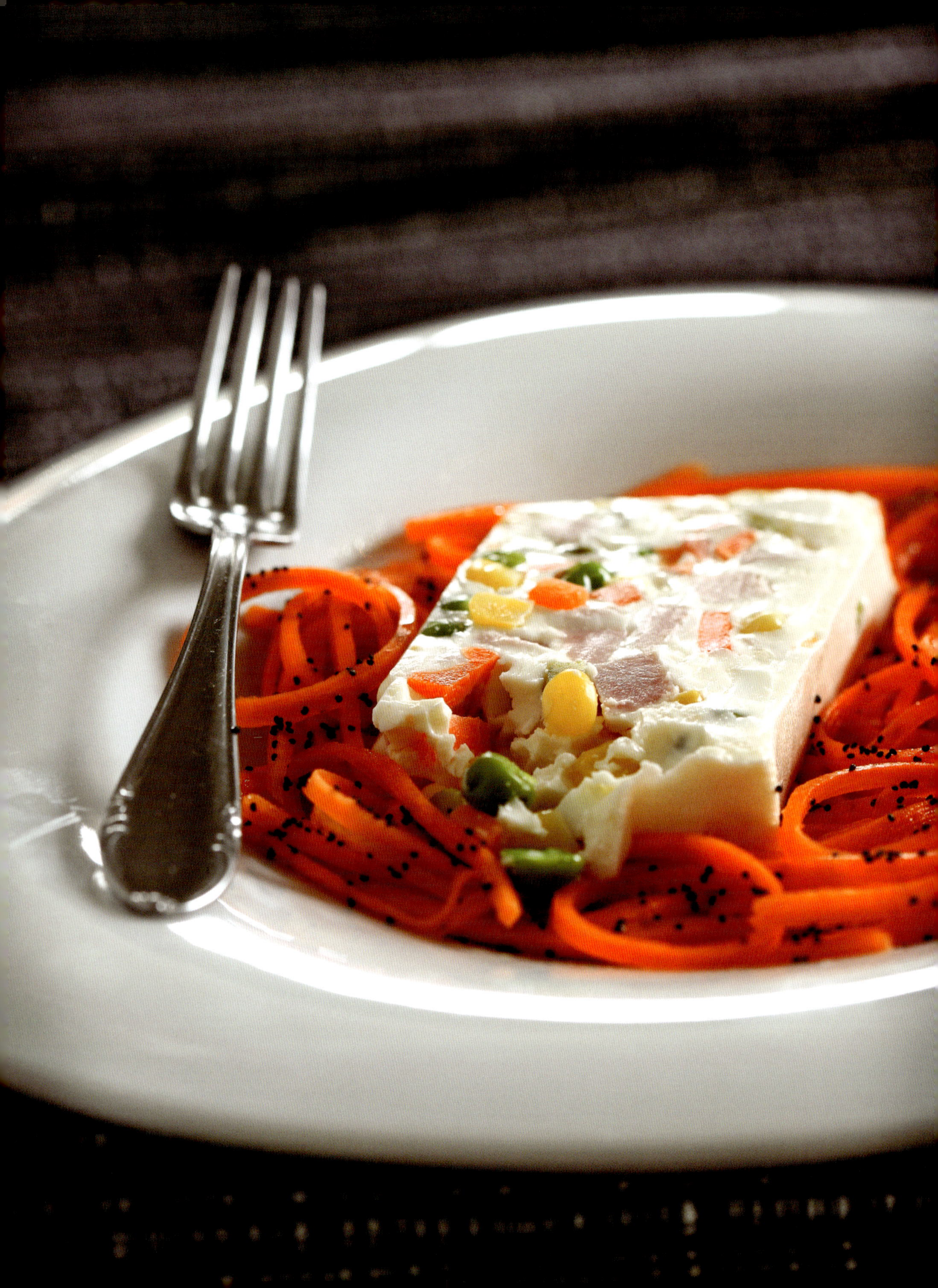

Yogurt Terrine

500 g (17½ oz) low fat yogurt
24 g (¾ oz) gelatin
200 g (7 oz) mayonnaise
2 boiled eggs, diced
200 g (7 oz) ham, diced
70 g (3 oz) pickled gherkins, diced
100 g (3½ oz) garden peas, frozen
50 g (2 oz) sweetcorn, frozen
1 carrot peeled, diced
a pinch of salt

carrot and poppy seed salad:
2 carrots, peeled and grated
1 lime juice, freshly squeezed
1 tablespoon extra virgin oil
a pinch of poppy seeds
a pinch of salt

Boil the eggs for about 10 minutes, peel and dice and set aside. Peel, dice and throw the carrot into a small pot, add the garden peas, sweetcorn and add boiling water and boil for about 5 minutes, then drain. In a large bowl combine the diced pickled gherkins, boiled carrot, boiled garden peas, boiled sweetcorn mix and set aside. Then in a medium bowl combine the yogurt and mayonnaise, mix well. Next dissolve the gelatin, following the instructions on the packet. In a small bowl, put 120 ml (4 fl oz) boiling water and sprinkle in the gelatin while stirring briskly until thoroughly dissolved. Leave it to cool for a few minutes. Afterwards, add the gelatin to the yogurt mixture and stir well. Add the mixture to the chopped products and mix well again. Finally pour it into a bread-baking silicone mould around 10 x 26 cm (4 x 10 inches) and 6 cm (2½ inches) deep and leave in the refrigerator for 4 hours or overnight. Then transfer the terrine to a chopping board and put in the freezer for no more than 30 minutes to cool and become easy to slice. Remove from the freezer, slice and serve cold over carrot and poppy seeds salad or any green leaves salad.

Serves 8

Per serving
286 kcal, 22.0 g fat (4.0 g saturated), 13.2 g protein, 9.4 g carbs (7.0 g sugar), 1.3 g fibre, 1.6 g salt

Devilled Eggs

4 tablespoons low fat yogurt, strained
8 hard boiled eggs, peeled
2 teaspoons wholegrain mustard
1 tablespoon extra virgin olive oil
pinch of chili pepper, ground
pinch of salt
pinch of sumac for garnish
8 pickled gherkins, halved lengthwise

Boil the eggs for about 10 minutes in a small pot with cold water. Then rinse the eggs with cold water to cool down for a couple of minutes. Next gently crack the eggshells, peel the eggs and halve lengthwise. Carefully separate the yolks from the boiled egg halves and put in a small bowl while placing the whites on a serving plate. To make the filling, add the strained yogurt, wholegrain mustard, extra virgin olive oil, a pinch of ground chili pepper and a pinch of salt to the bowl with yolks. Using a fork mash it all together. Finally spoon the mixture back into the empty egg whites and garnish with sprinkled sumac and half pickled gherkins.

Serves 8

Per serving
222 kcal, 16.9 g fat (4.2 g saturated), 14.6 g protein, 3.1 g carbs (3.1 g sugar), 0.2 g fibre, 1.3 g salt

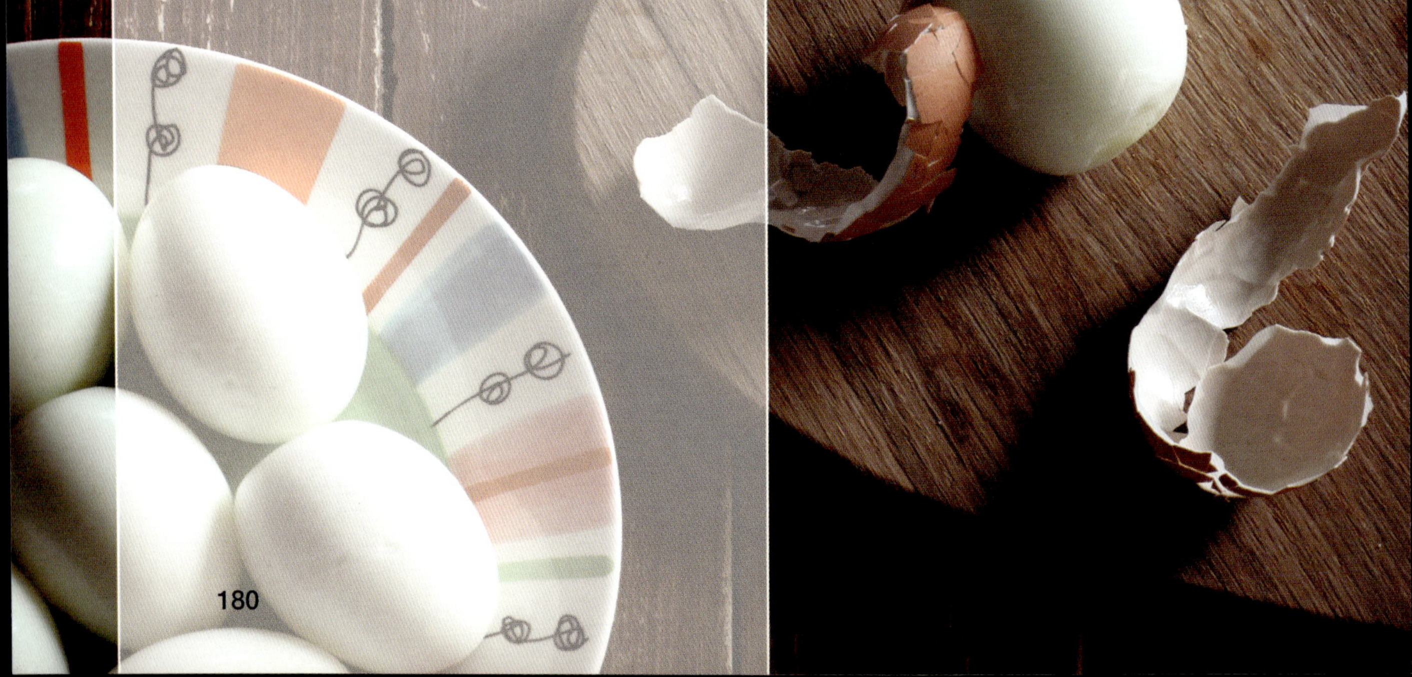

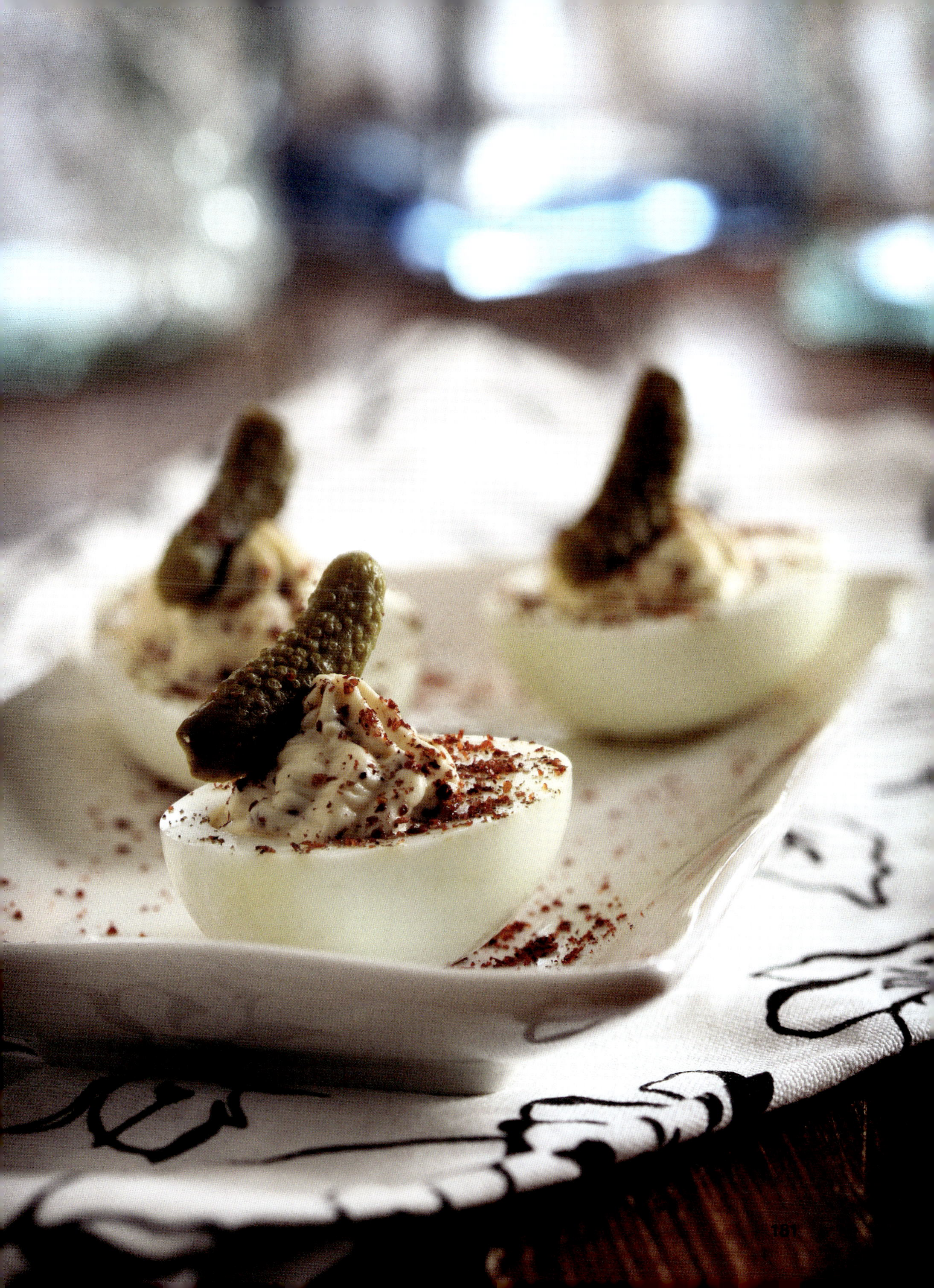

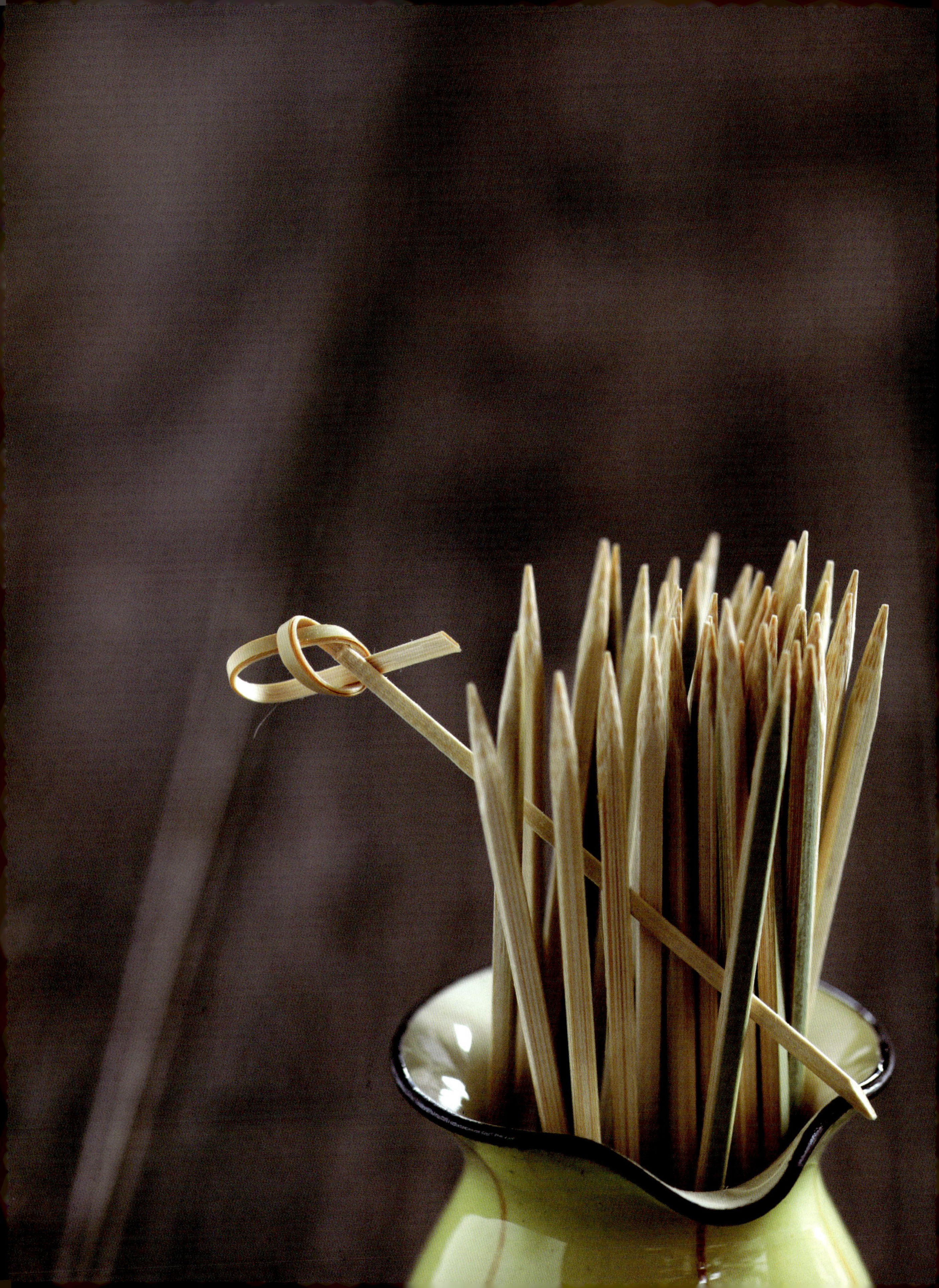

Nibbles

Fried Yogurt Fritters

500 g (17½ oz) strained yogurt
30 g (1 oz) walnuts, finely chopped
2 garlic cloves, crushed
2 tablespoons finely chopped fresh mint leaves
1 teaspoon freshly ground black pepper
50 g (2 oz) plain white flour
50 g (2 oz) golden breadcrumbs
1 teaspoon bicarbonate of soda
pinch of salt
2 eggs
200 ml (6¾ fl oz) sunflower oil, for frying
sweet chili sauce, to serve

Combine the strained yogurt, walnuts, garlic, mint and black pepper in a medium bowl and set aside. Combine the flour, breadcrumbs, bicarbonate of soda and a pinch of salt on a large plate. Beat the eggs in a small bowl. Using two tablespoons, give the fritters shape and then roll into the breadcrumb mixture. Heat the oil in a small frying pan. Dip the fritters into the beaten eggs and then dip fry in the oil for about 2 minutes or until golden. Remember to turn them over in the pan to cook both sides. Once ready, remove from the oil and leave to drain on kitchen paper. Serve warm with sweet chili sauce.

Serves 6

Per serving
184 kcal, 10 g fat (2 g saturated), 8 g protein,
17 g carbs (7 g sugar), 0.8 g fibre, 1.2 g salt

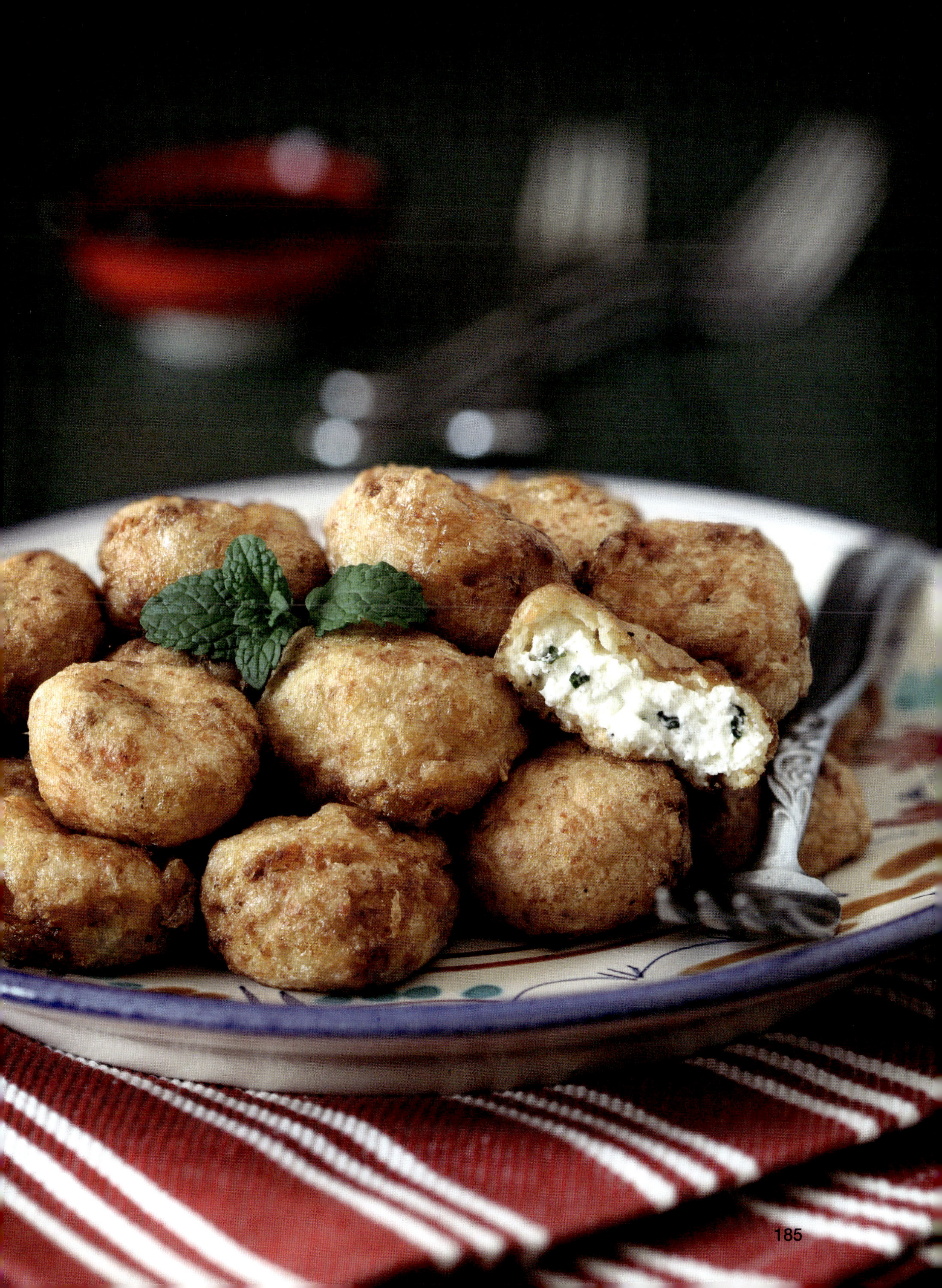

Vegetable Wraps

100 g (3½ oz) shredded cheddar cheese
2 roasted red or yellow bell pepper, peeled, seeded and thinly sliced
100 g (3½ oz) strained yogurt
50 g (2 oz) celeriac, peeled and grated
1 handful fresh parsley, finely chopped
1 teaspoon horseradish sauce
1 teaspoon poppy seeds
4 tortilla wrap breads
a pinch of salt

Cut up the celaric so you are only using 50 g (2 oz), peel and grate it and place in a medium bowl, sprinkle over a pinch of salt and mix well. Leave to rest for 1–2 hours. Meanwhile in a large bowl mix together the strained yogurt and horseradish sauce and add the sliced roasted peppers.
Next lay the tortilla wrap breads over a wooden chopping board. Spread a quarter of the yogurt and pepper mixture over the first bread. Sprinkle over a quarter of the grated celeriac, quarter of the parsley, quarter of the shredded cheddar cheese and a pinch of poppy seeds. Roll and serve, repeat with the rest of the wraps.
Ideal for lunch box.

Serves 4

Per serving
350 kcal, 11.2 g fat (6.2 g saturated), 14.5 g protein, 52.9 g carbs (5.9 g sugar), 4.2 g fibre, 1.8 g salt

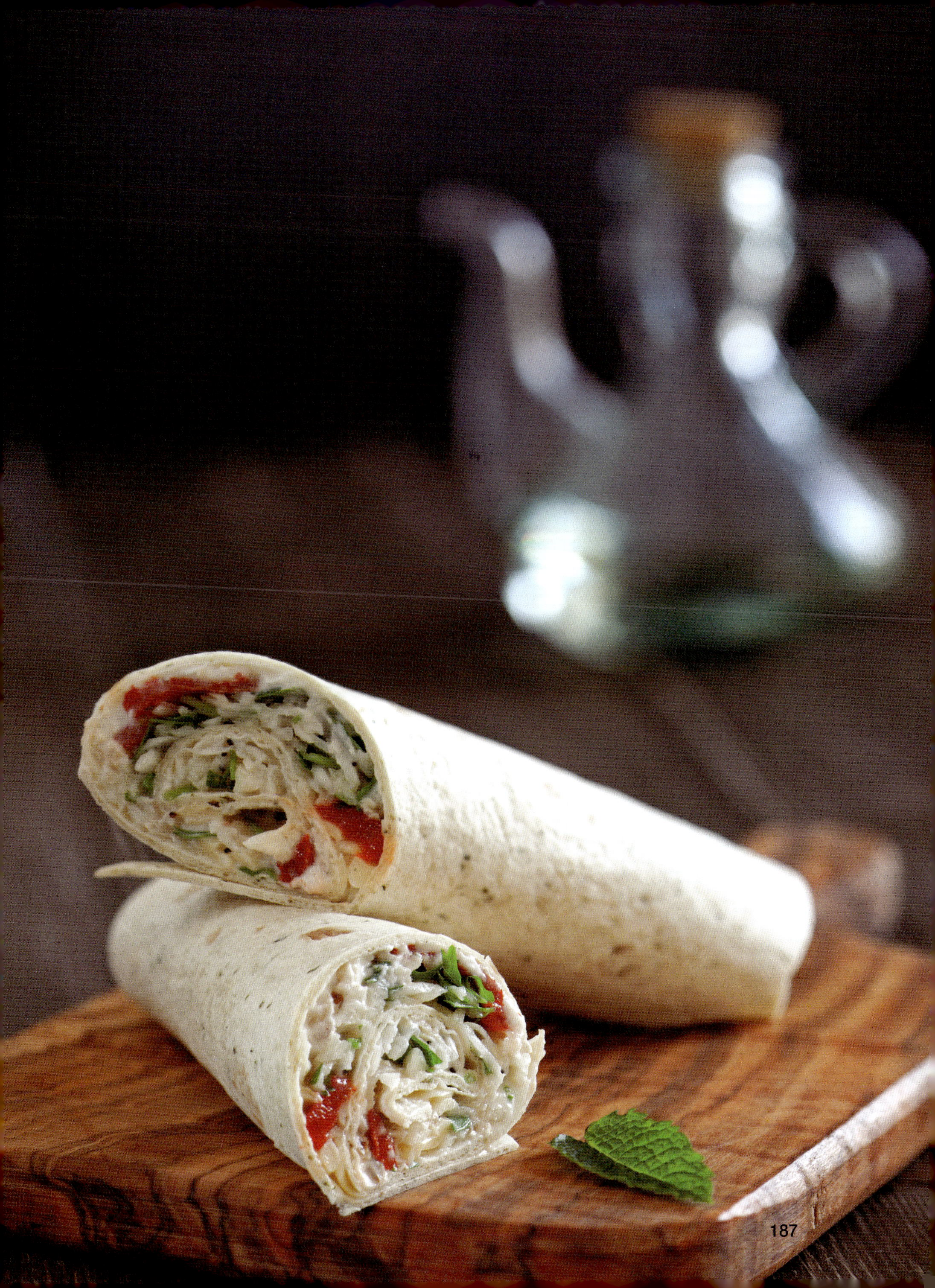

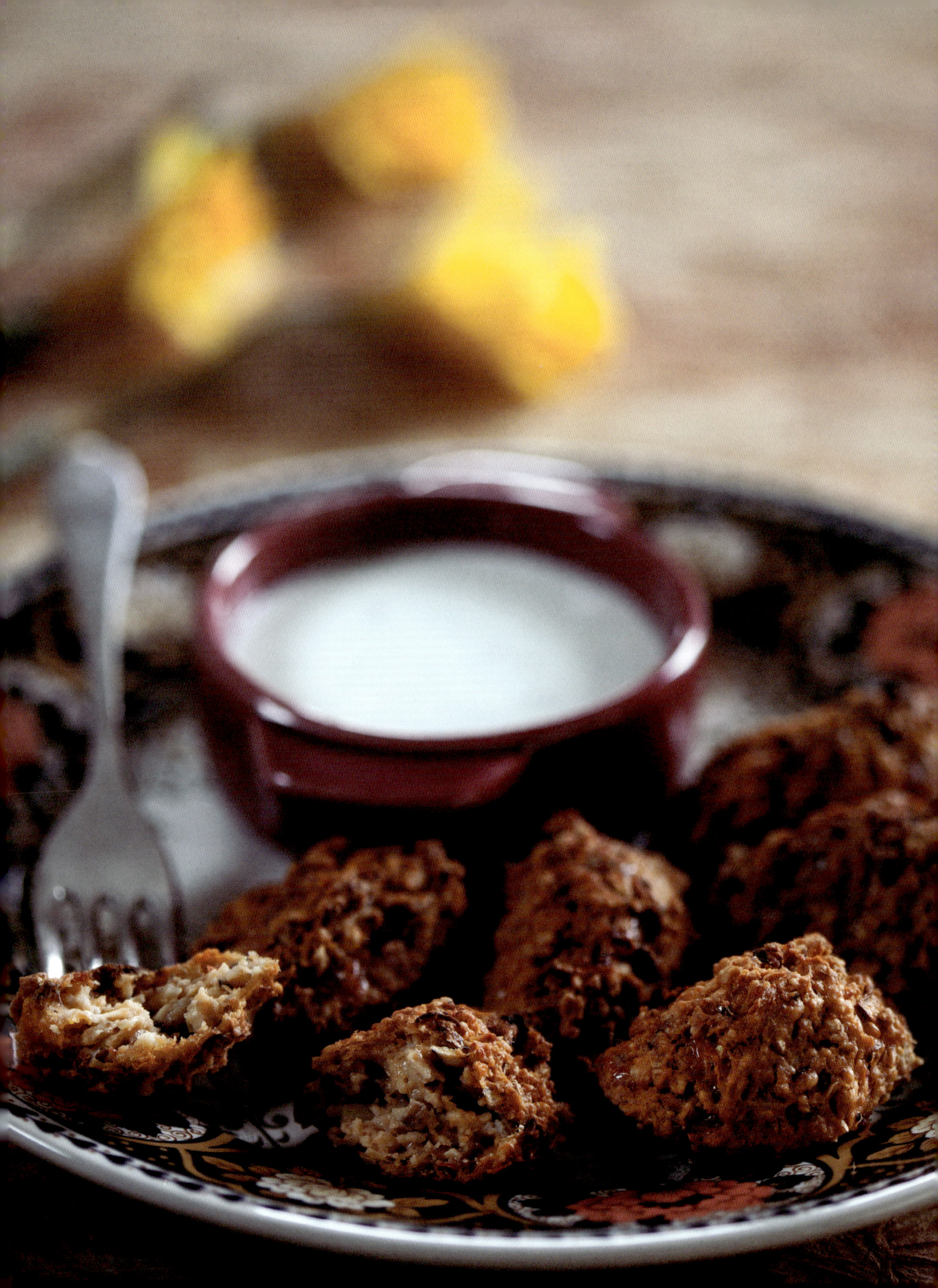

Oat Fritters

250 g (9 oz) oatmeal
50 g (2 oz) cheddar cheese, shredded
2 tablespoons olive oil
1 medium leek, finely chopped
1 large free-range egg
1 tablespoon tomato puree
1 teaspoon paprika
1 teaspoon dry thyme
1 teaspoon cumin powder
1 teaspoon grounded black pepper
pinch of salt

In a large bowl soak the oatmeal in 200 ml (6¾ fl oz) boiling water. Add more water if needed. After 5 minutes add the egg, shredded cheddar cheese, olive oil, finely chopped leek, tomato puree, paprika, dry thyme, cumin powder, grounded black pepper and a pinch of salt. Mix well until it becomes a sticky mess. Using two tablespoons make small balls and arrange on a parchment lined baking sheet. Bake in the oven at 200°C (400°F) for 30 minutes. Leave the fritters to cool for about 30 minutes and serve together with yogurt topping.

Yogurt topping:
250 g (9 oz) low fat yogurt
1 clove garlic, crushed
pinch of salt

in a small bowl mix together the low fat yogurt, crushed garlic, season with salt and serve.

Serves 4

Per serving
418 kcal, 17.8 g fat (4.4 g saturated), 16.5 g protein, 51.3 g carbohydrates (5.5 g sugar), 6.4 g fibre, 1.9 g salt

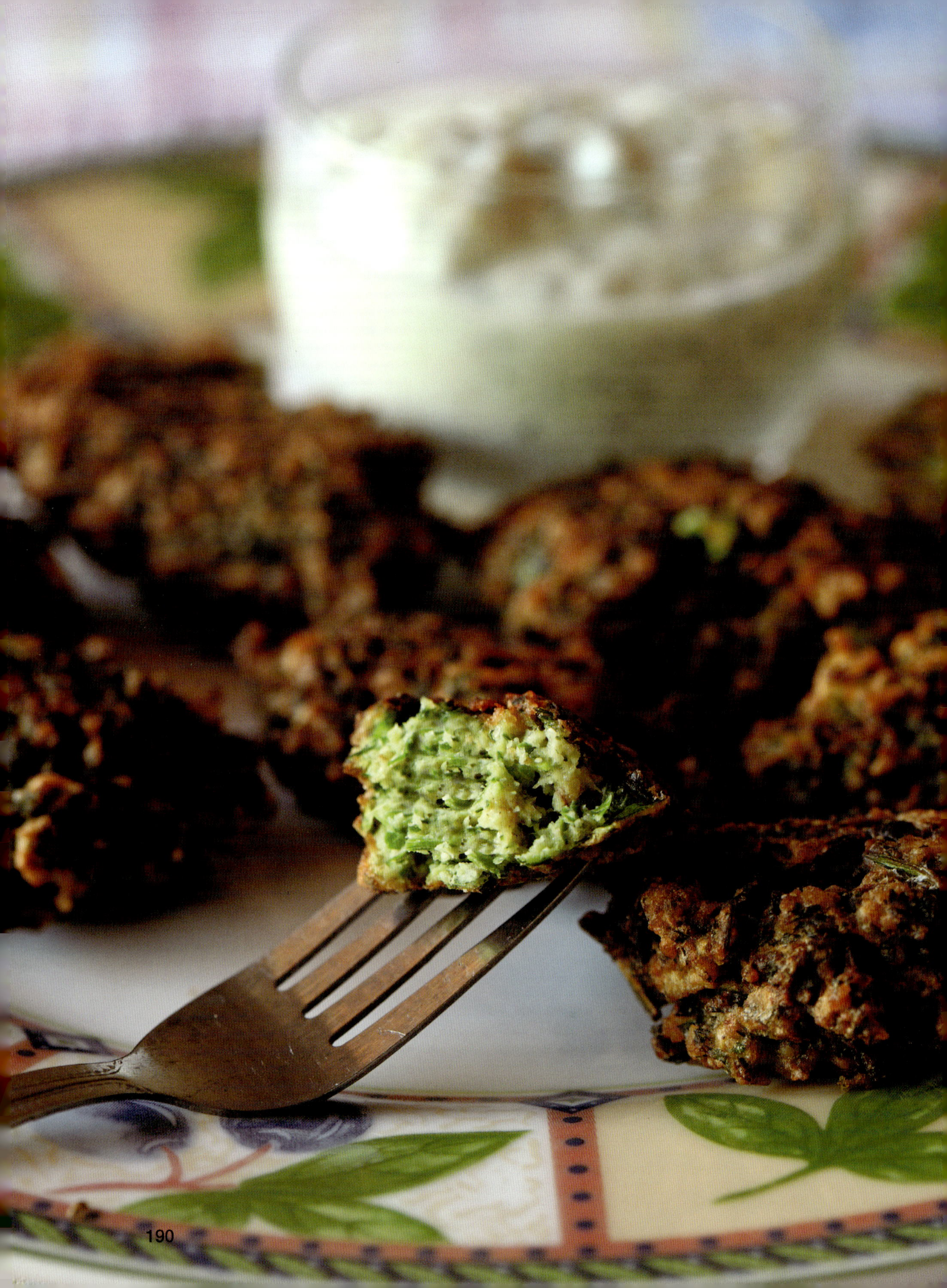

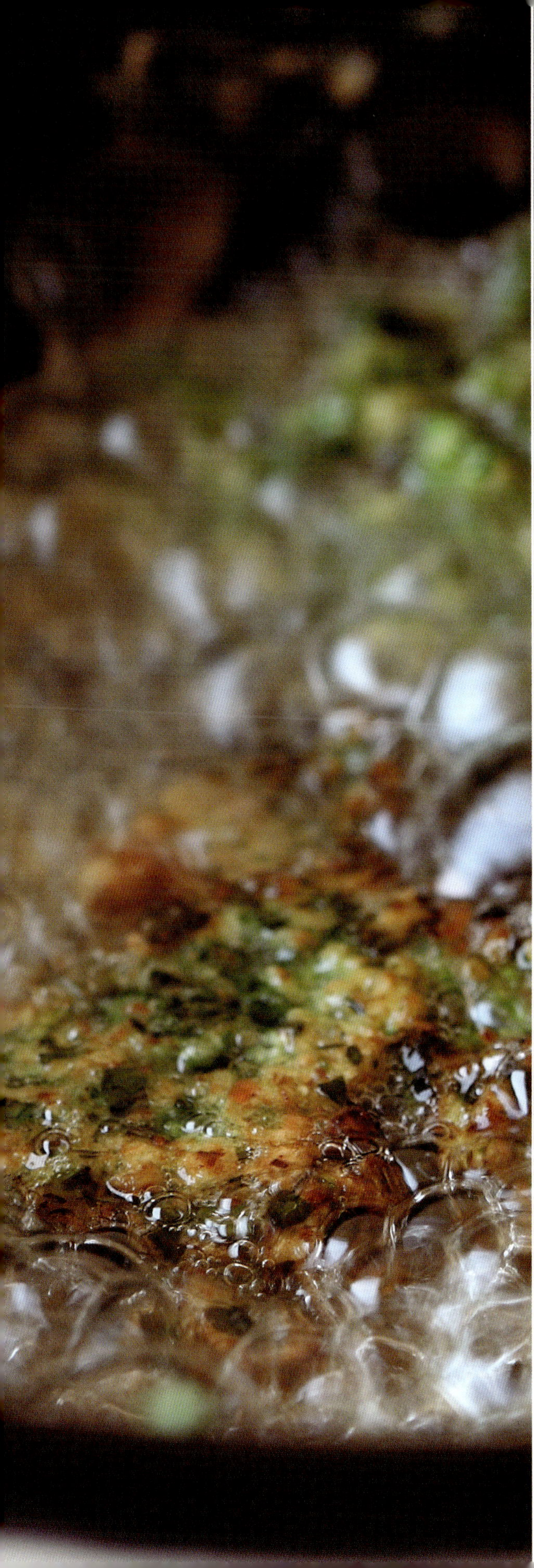

Vegetarian Fritters

100 g (3½ oz) chopped parsley
3 spring onions
2 small zucchini (courgettes)
4 eggs
3 tablespoons white wheat plain flour
180 g (6 oz) oatbran
1 teaspoon ground black pepper
1 teaspoon salt
200 ml (6¾ fl oz) sunflower oil for dip fry

Throw the parsley, spring onions and zucchini into a blender and blend for a couple of minutes until smooth. Transfer the mixture to a large bowl and add the eggs, flour, oat bran, black pepper and salt. Mix well to make a dense grain mash. Add more oat bran if you need to make it thicker.
Leave to rest for about 10 minutes. Preheat 200 ml (6¾ fl oz) sunflower oil in a small saucepan and using 2 spoons prepare small balls from the mixture and deep fry on both sides for about 2 minutes until brown. Quickly remove from the pan and strain off the oil.

Topping:
500 g (17½ oz) yogurt
1 clove of garlic
20 g (¾ oz) chopped fresh dill
pinch of salt and black pepper
1 tablespoon mustard mayo.

Serve warm with some yogurt topping.

Serves 6

Per serving
437 kcal, 28.5 g fat (8.8 g saturated), 15.6 g protein, 28.7 g carbs (5.6 g sugars), 1.6 g salt, 7.7 g fibre

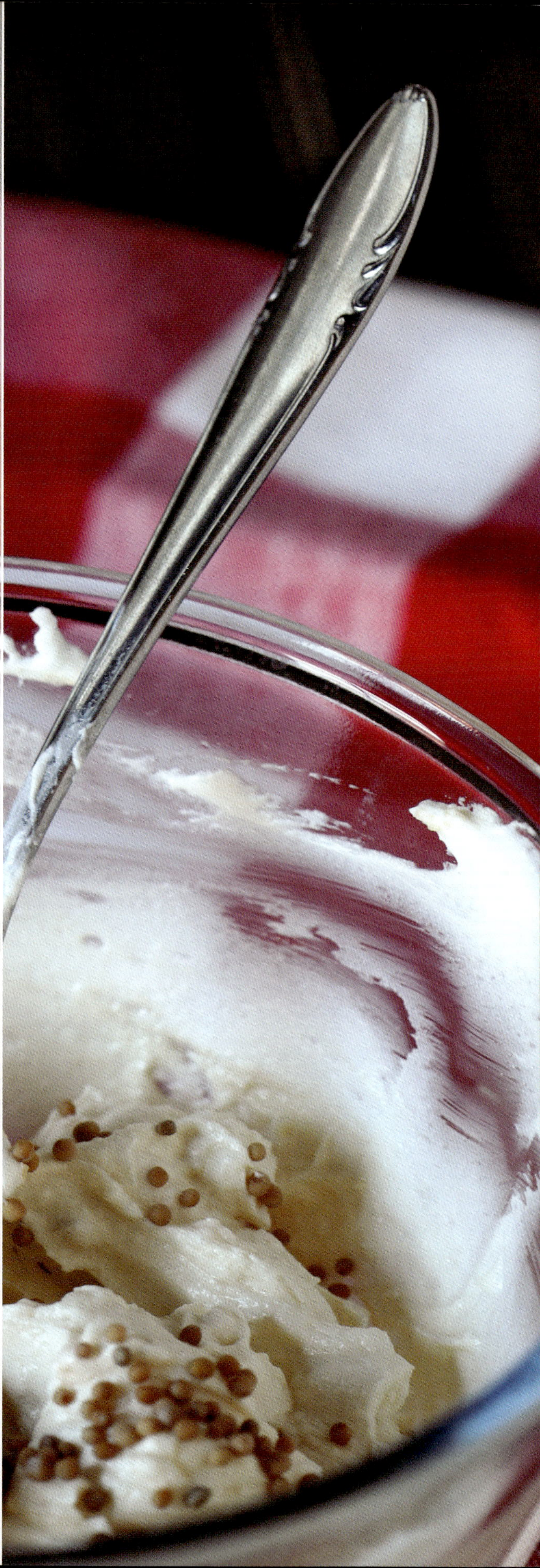

Mustard Seed Ham Rolls

300 g (10½ oz) Ham, sliced
1 teaspoon mustard seeds
1 tablespoon extra virgin olive oil
1 Egg yolk, boiled
3 medium pickled gherkins cut on stripes
200 g (7 oz) yogurt, strained
pinch of salt

Boil one large egg for about 10 minutes, peel and separate the yolk into a medium bowl. Squash the yolk with a fork and add the strained yogurt and oil. Season with pinch of salt and mix well. Finally add a teaspoon of mustard seeds and mix well. Leave it to rest for a moment. Meanwhile cut the pickled gherkins into strips. Lay out the ham slices on a chopping board and spread a tablespoon of the yogurt mixture over. Add a pickled gherkin and roll up.

This is an excellent starter, you can garnish with some arugula (rocket) salad and kalamata olives.

Serves 6/2 rolls per serving.

Per serving
120 kcal, 6.4 g fat (2.0 g saturated), 13.2 g protein, 3.1 g carbs (3.1 g sugar), 0.1 g fibre, 1.5 g salt

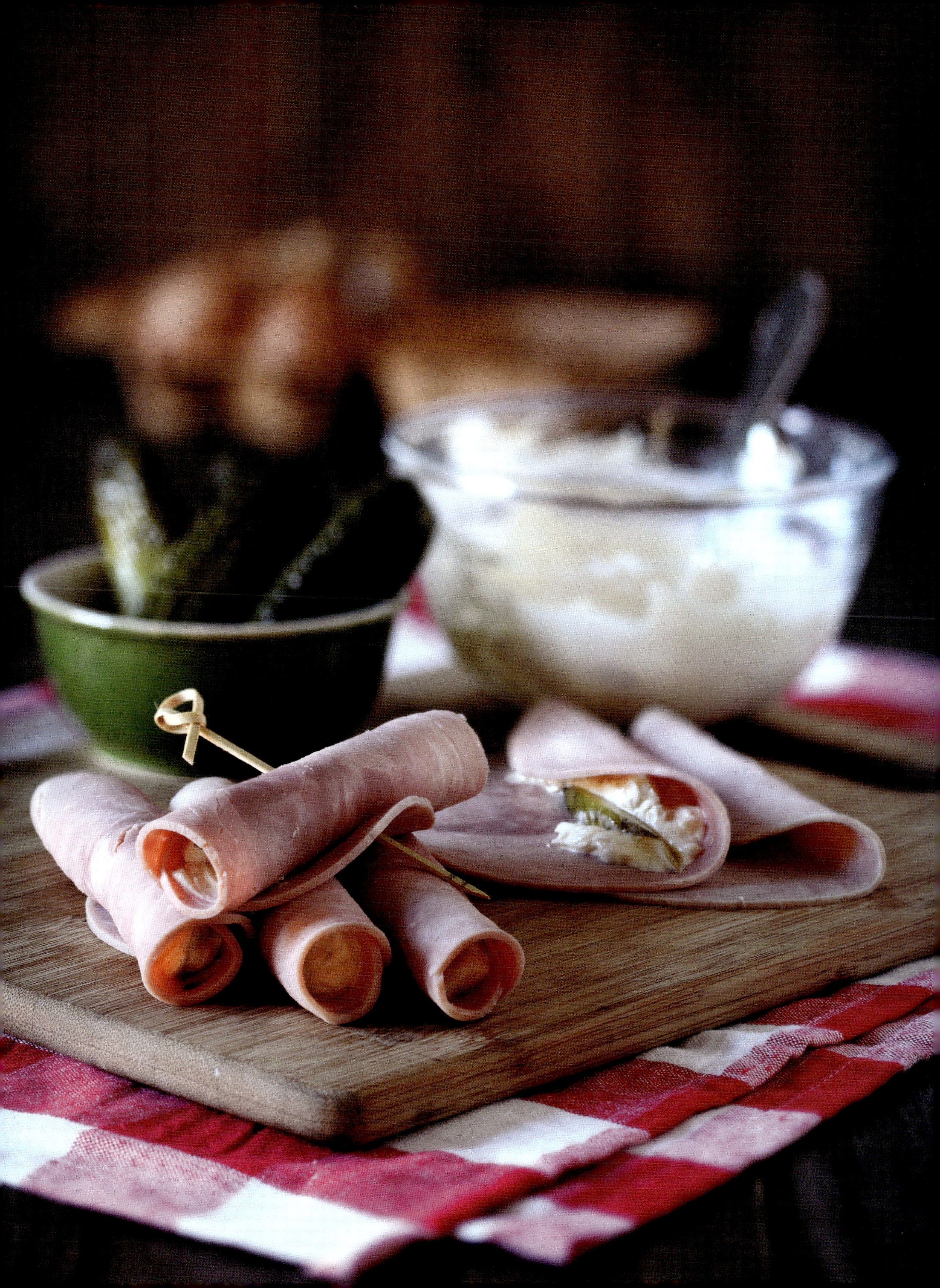

Pastrami Sandwiches

100 g (3½ oz) Pastrami
2 teaspoons horseradish
200 g (7 oz) yogurt, strained
1 clove garlic, crushed
1 handful chopped chives
pinch of salt
pinch of black pepper, freshly ground
bread, toast

Combine the strained yogurt, garlic, horseradish, salt and black pepper in a medium bowl and mix well. Spread a tablespoon of the yogurt mixture over toasted bread, place a slice of pastrami on top and sprinkle over some chopped chives.

Serves 6/2 sandwiches per person

Per serving
193 kcal, 3.3 g fat (1.3 g saturated), 11.1 g protein, 31.8 g carbs (4.9 g sugar), 3.3 g fibre, 1.8 g salt

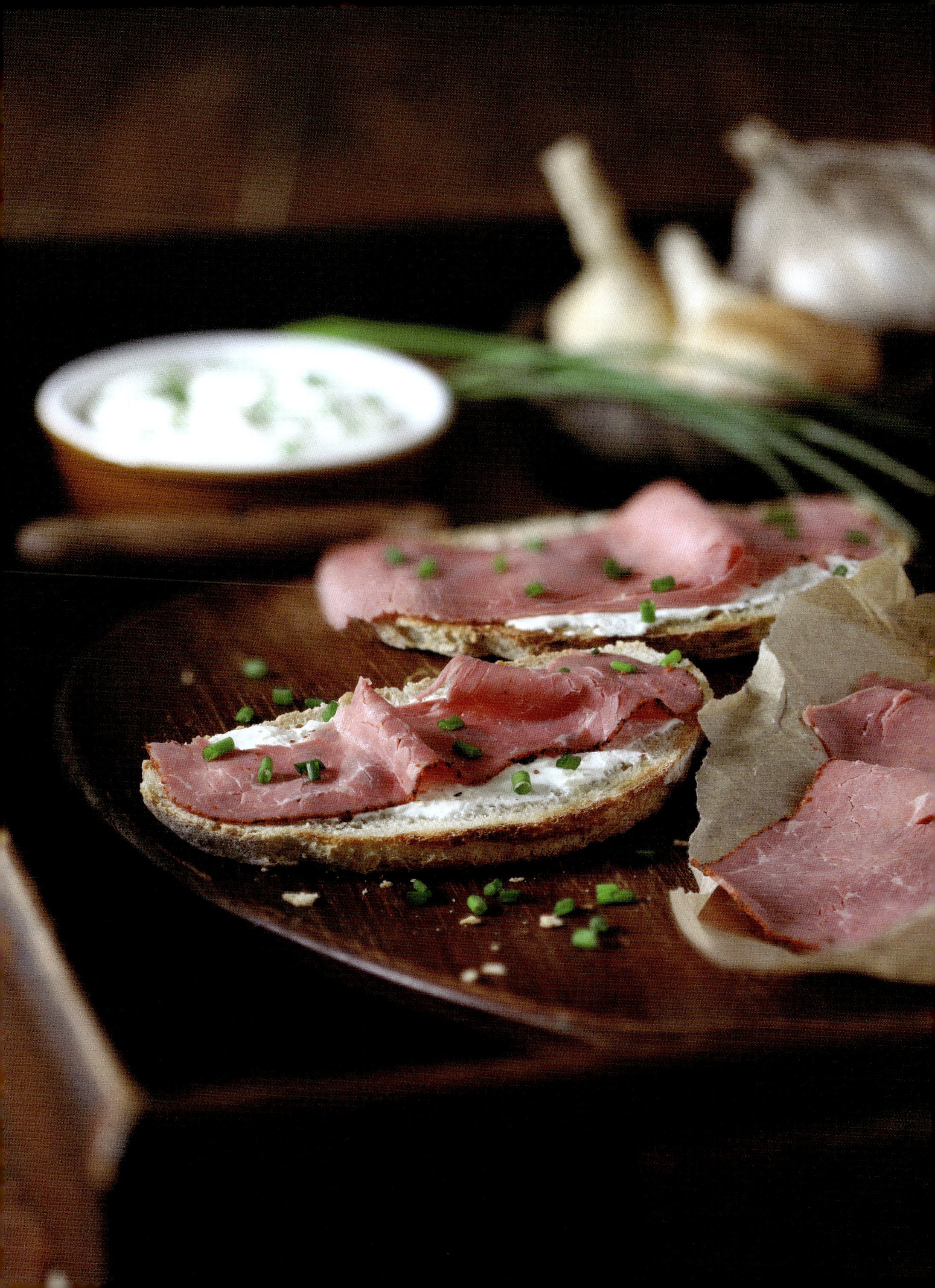

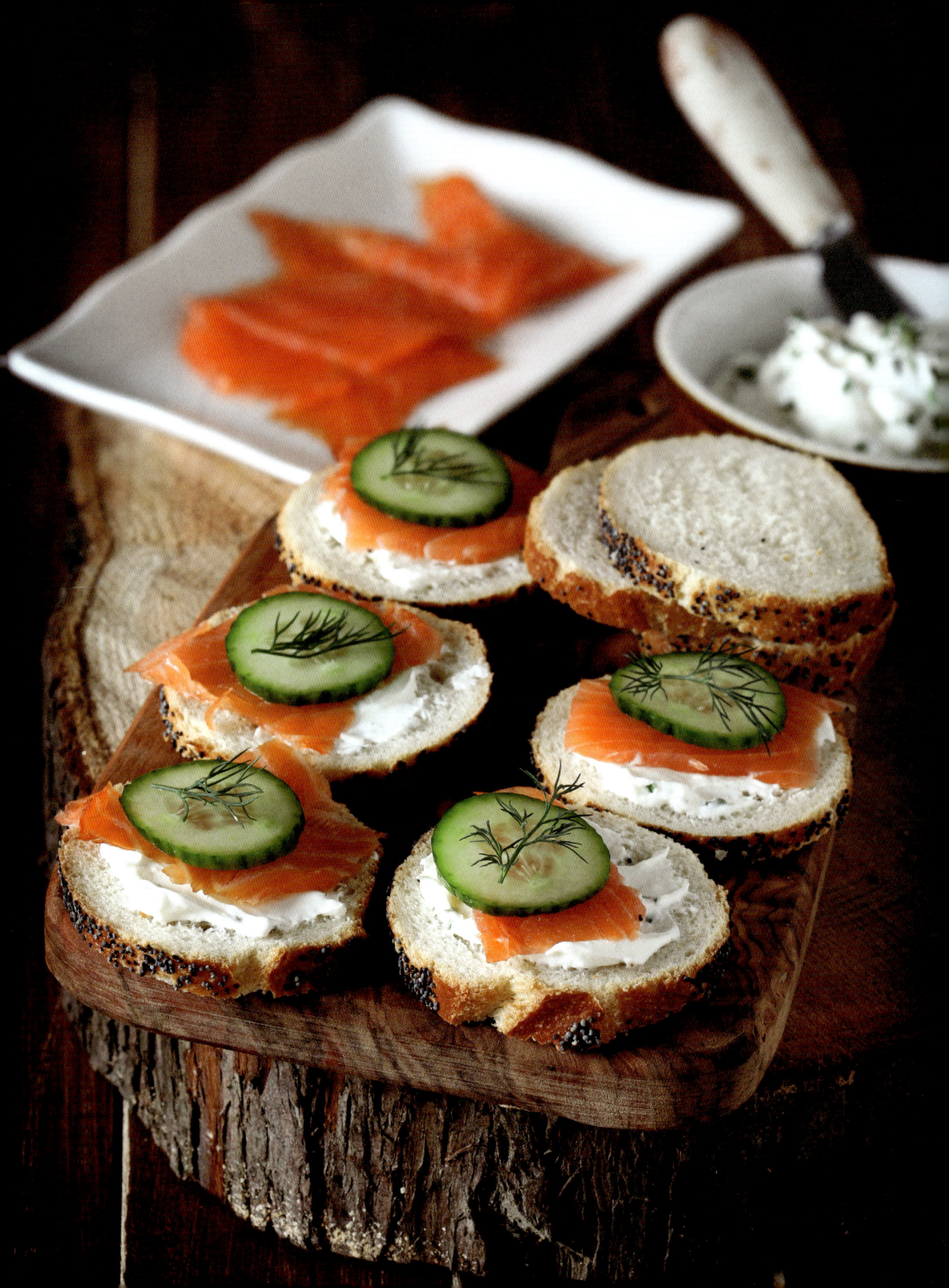

Salmon Sandwiches

120 g (4½ oz) smoked salmon, sliced
200 g (7 oz) yogurt, strained
1 clove garlic, crushed
1 teaspoon dry tarragon
100 g (3½ oz) cucumber, sliced
1 shallot, peeled and finely chopped
½ lime fresh juice
pinch of salt
1 baguette
fresh dill to garnish

In a small bowl combine the strained yogurt, crushed garlic, tarragon, finely chopped shallot, lime juice and salt, mix well. Cut the baguette into ring slices, spread a tablespoon of yogurt mixture over each ring, lay on a slice of salmon and slice of cucumber and garnish with fresh dill.

Serves 6

Per serving
217 kcal, 3.2 g fat (1.1 g saturated), 13 g protein, 36.2 g carbs (4.7 g sugar, 1.6 g fibre, 2.4 g salt

Zucchini Pancakes

500 g (17½ oz) small zucchini (courgette), grated
a pinch of salt
100 g (3½ oz) feta cheese, finely crushed with a fork
2 tablespoons grapeseed oil
3 large eggs, beaten
ground black pepper
3 spring onions, finely chopped
1 garlic clove, crushed
2 tablespoons spelt flour
a pinch of ground nutmeg
½ teaspoon baking powder
50 ml (1½ fl oz) sunflower oil, for frying

For the yogurt sauce:
300 g (10½ oz) low fat yogurt
1 garlic clove, crushed
2 tablespoons finely chopped fresh dill
pinch of salt (optional)
juice of ½ lime

First make the yogurt sauce by putting all the ingredients in a bowl and mixing together.
To make the pancakes, grate the zucchini and throw into a large bowl. Sprinkle over a pinch of salt, mix well and transfer to a colander to drain for about 45 minutes. Return the drained zucchini to the bowl and add the feta cheese, grapeseed oil, beaten eggs, black pepper, spring onions, garlic, spelt flour, nutmeg and baking powder and mix well. Preheat a frying pan over a medium heat, add 1 tablespoon of sunflower oil and, using a tablespoon, gently spoon in the pancake mixture and fry for about 2 minutes until golden brown. Carefully turn over and fry the other side for about 2 minutes until golden. When cooked, remove from the pan and leave to drain on kitchen paper. Clean the frying pan with kitchen paper and repeat with the rest of the pancake mixture. Serve with the yogurt sauce.

Serves 6

Per serving
250 kcal, 19 g fat (4.7 g saturated), 10 g protein, 12 g carbs (6 g sugar), 2.7 g fibre, 1.8 g salt

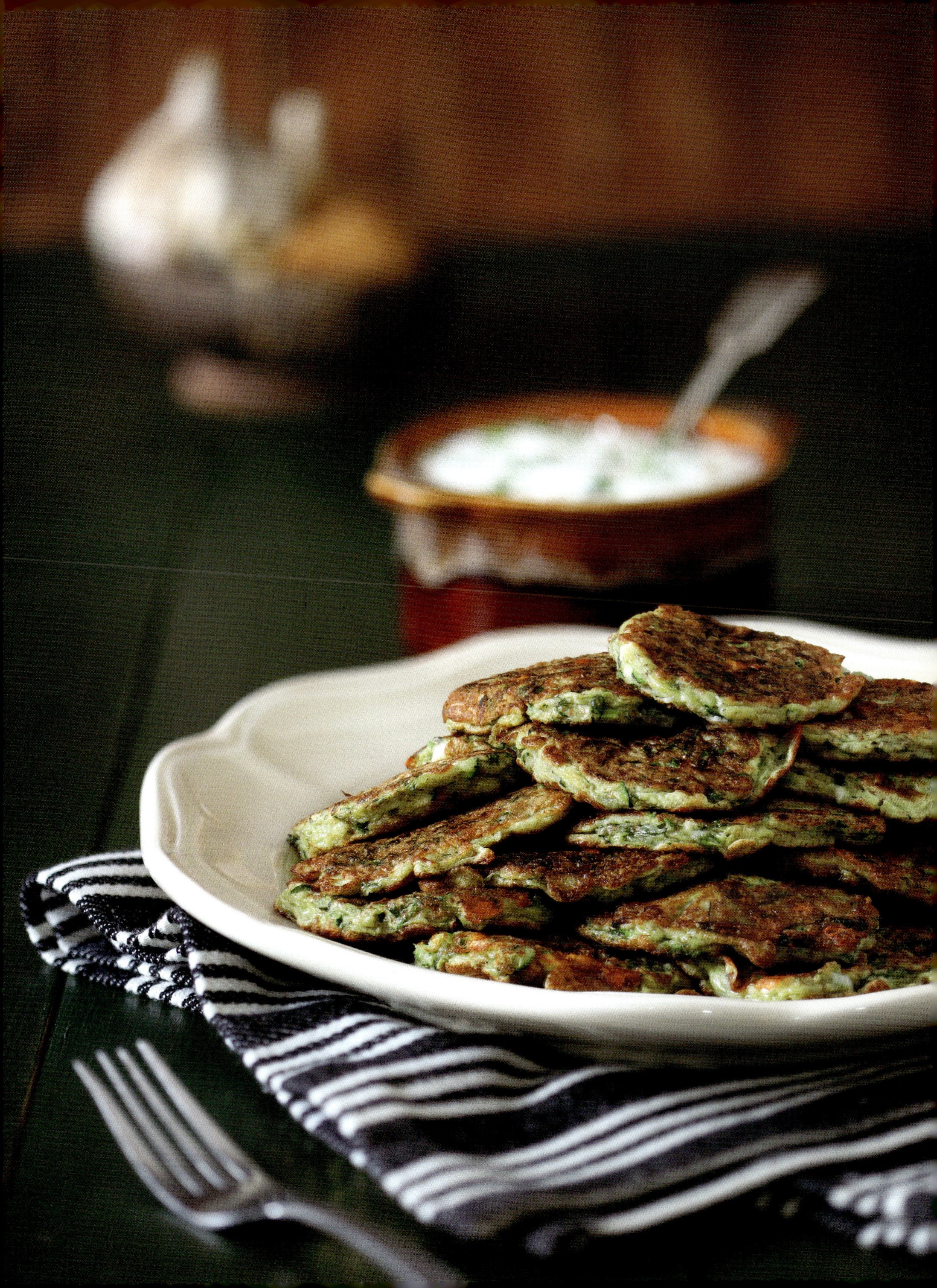

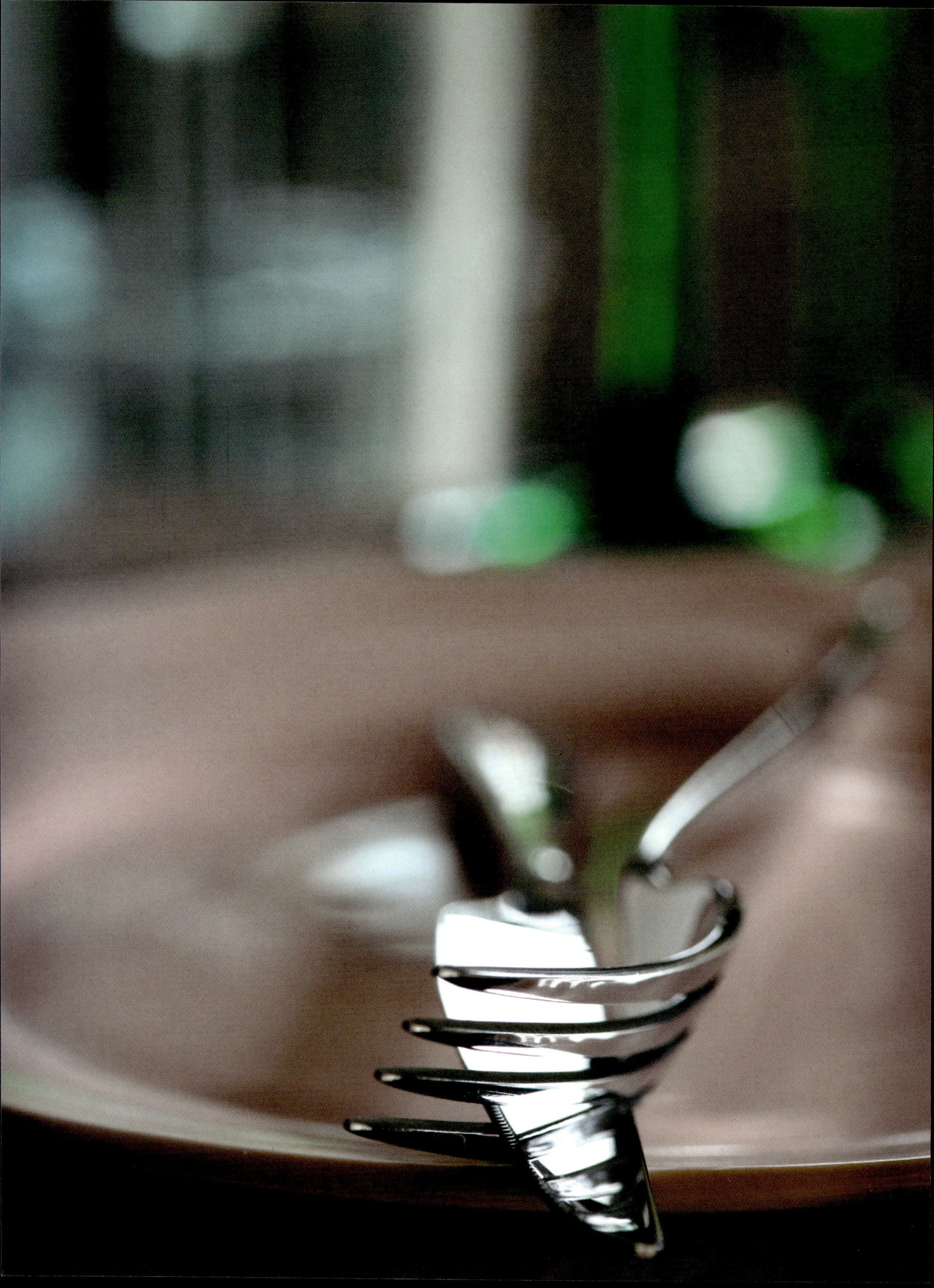

Main Meals

Conchiglie

300 g (10½ oz) conchiglie pasta, boiled
1 medium eggplant (aubergine), diced
2 tablespoons fresh mint leaves, chopped
100 g (3½ oz) light mayonnaise
100 g (3½ oz) low fat yogurt
100 g (3½ oz) radishes, sliced
30 ml (1 fl oz) vegetarian oil
pinch of salt

Throw the conchiglie into a medium pot, add boiling water to cover and boil for about 12 minutes then drain. Meanwhile in a large frying pan throw the diced eggplant, vegetarian oil and cook for about 10 minutes on high heat. Remove from the heat and add the boiled conchiglie, chopped fresh mint leaves, sliced fresh radishes, yogurt, mayonnaise and mix well, serve warm. You will be surprised!

Serves 4

Per serving
372 kcal, 17 g fat (2 g saturated), 11 g protein, 48 g carbs (6 g sugar), 1.7 g fibre, 1.4 g salt

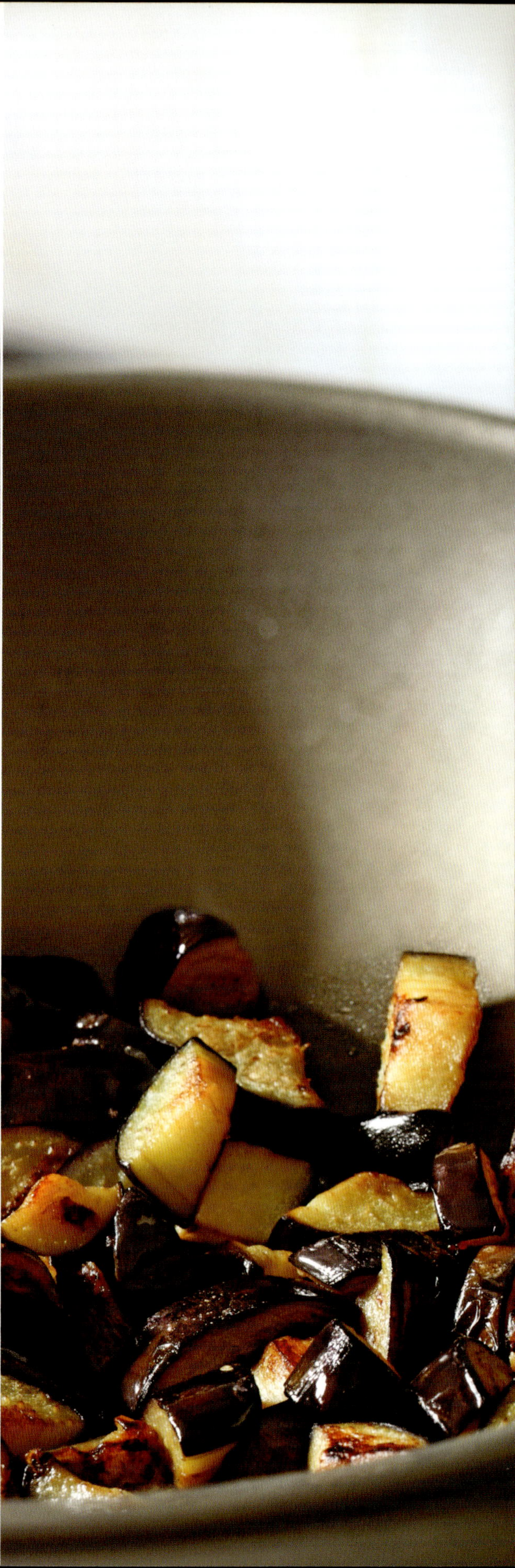

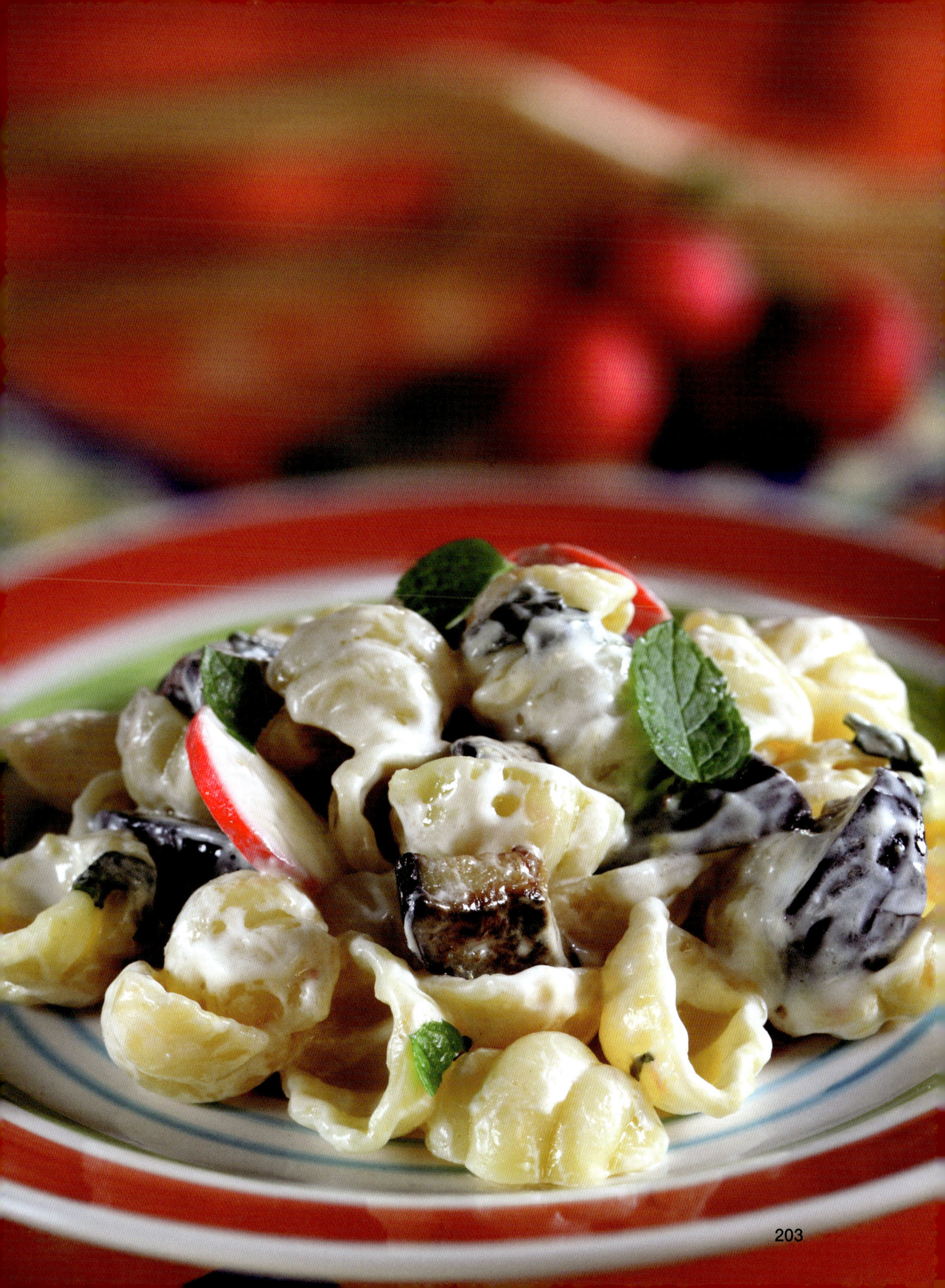

Zucchini Tart

3 medium zucchinis (courgettes)
4 eggs
100 g (3½ oz) white wheat plain flour
1 teaspoon baking soda
150 ml (5 fl oz) semi-skimmed milk
1 red salad onion
2 cloves garlic
100 g (3½ oz) prosciutto
100 g (3½ oz) mozzarella
30 g (1 oz) butter
1 tablespoon olive oil
50 g (2 oz) Parmesan cheese - grated
10 g (½ oz) fresh thyme leaves

Combine the eggs, flour, baking soda, milk, chopped mozzarella and butter in a large bowl and mix well with a wooden spoon. Cut the zucchini into long thin slices, oil them and toss half of them gently onto a parchment - lined baking try. Pour the mixture over the zucchinis and sprinkle chopped onions then and add the rest of the zucchinis. Arrange the prosciutto pieces on top. Bake for about 25 minutes at 200°C (400°F), then sprinkle over some grated Parmesan cheese and bake for few more minutes. Garnish the top with some fresh thyme leaves.

Serve warm with mixed yogurt with chopped garlic and black pepper.

200 g (7 oz) yogurt
1 clove garlic
black pepper

Serves 6

Per serving 339 kcal, 21.5 g fat (10.9 g saturated), 20 g protein, 17.4 g carbs (3.8 g sugar), 1.5 g salt, 1.9 g fibre

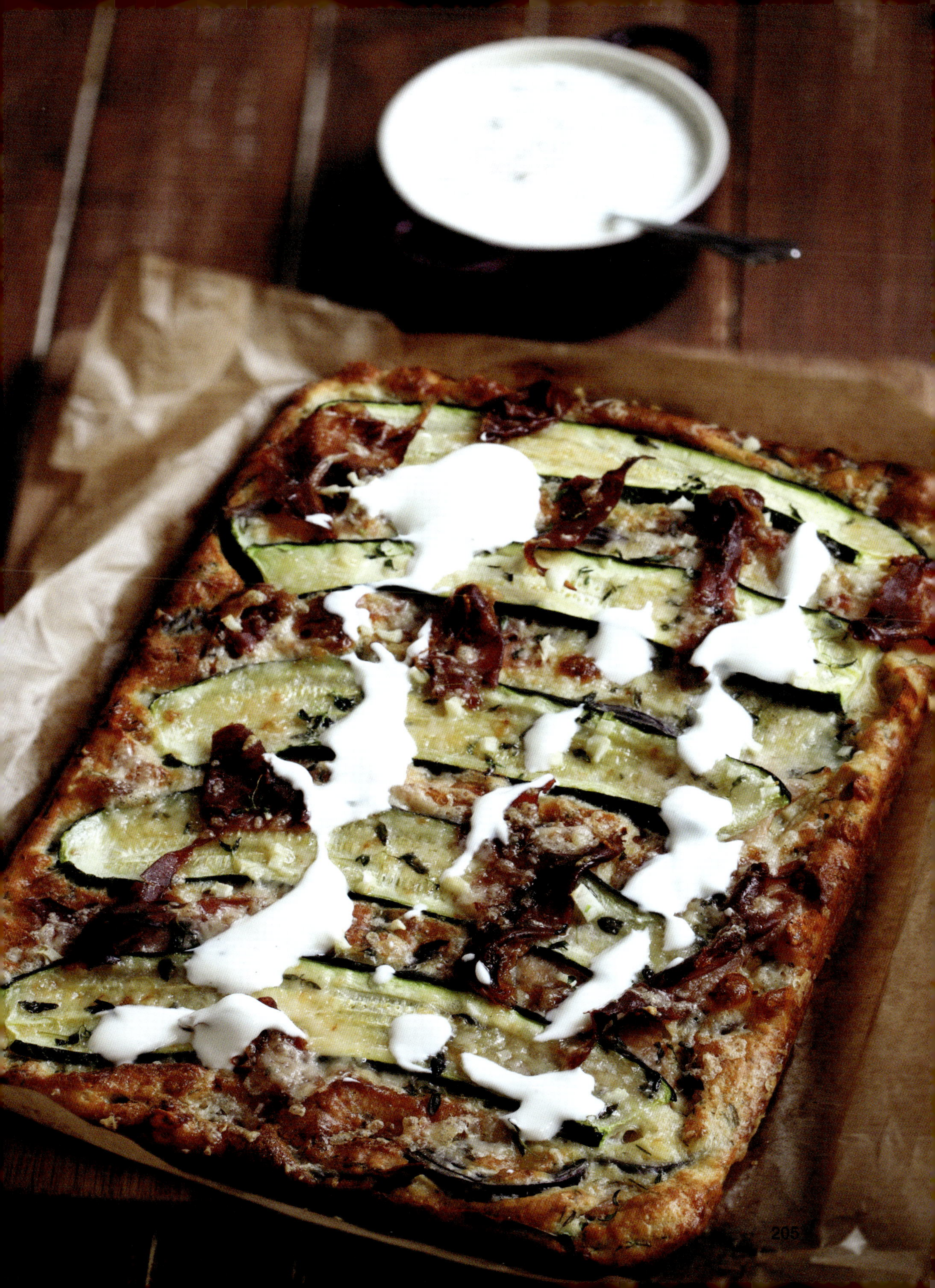

Chicken Fricassee

1 middle size chicken – 1 kg (2.2 lb)
200 ml (6¾ fl oz) chicken broth
200 g (7 oz) yogurt
3 eggs
8 tablespoon white wheat plain flour
30 g (1 oz) butter
1 lemon - juice
20 g (¾ oz) toasted flaked almonds
pinch of salt
pinch of black pepper ground

Boil the chicken in a large saucepan in 2 litres (4¼ pints) of water for 25 minutes. Once cooled, debone the chicken and separate 200ml (6¾ fl oz) of the chicken broth for later. Add the flour and butter to the remaining broth in a deep saucepan and simmer over a low heat for about 2 minutes.

Mix together the yogurt, eggs, lemon juice and chicken broth you set aside earlier and stir well. Combine the yogurt mixture with the flour, butter and broth, then add the chicken chopped into large pieces and cook for 10 more minutes, stiring constantly. Serve warm with some sprinkled almonds flakes and black pepper.

Serves 6

Per serving
372 kcal, 18.1 g fat (7.4 g saturated), 30.9 g protein, 22.8 g carbs (2.2 g sugars), 0.9 g salt, 1.6 g fibre

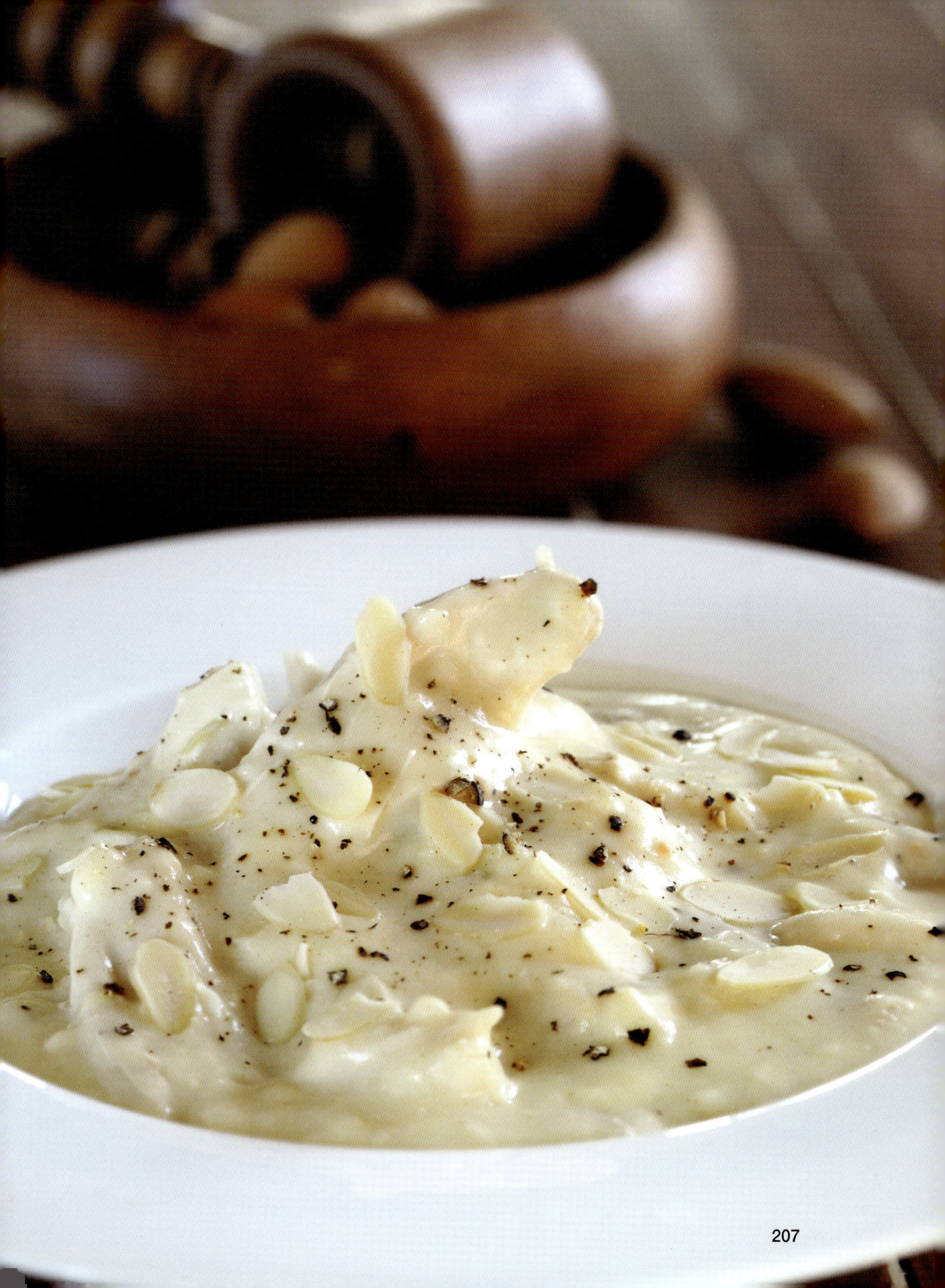

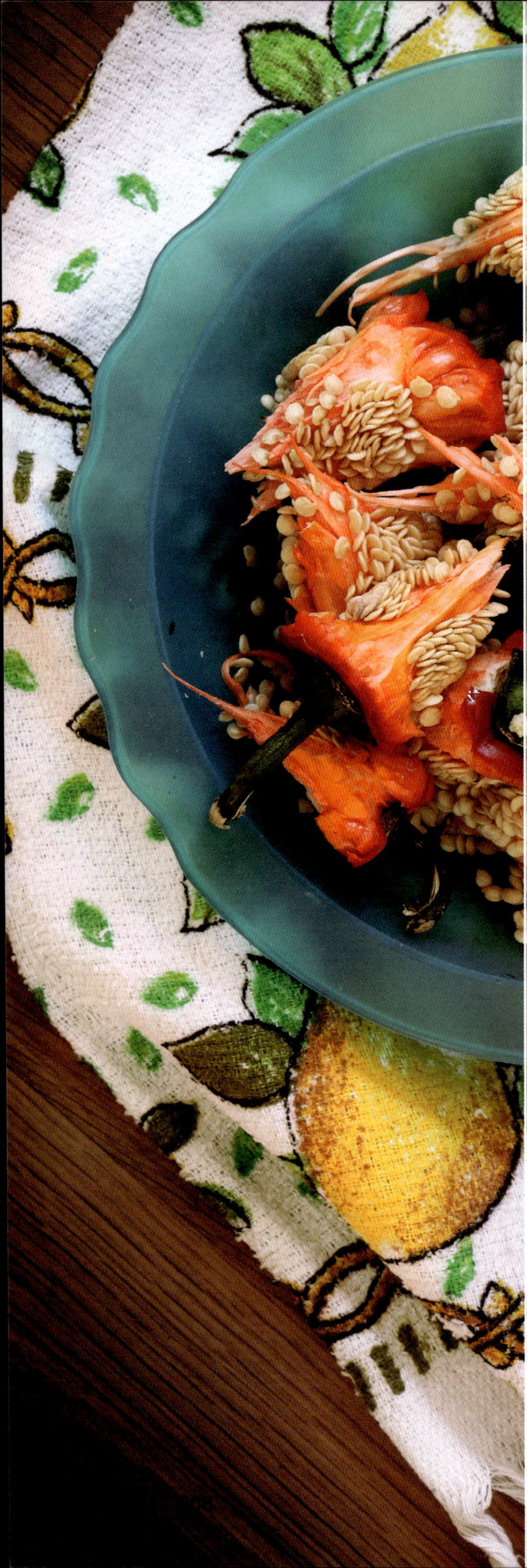

Stuffed Peppers

6 sweet pointed peppers
1 leek chopped
200 g (7 oz) basmati rice
500 g (17½ oz) beef mince
1 teaspoon of thyme
pinch of salt
1 carrot – chopped
1 litre (1¾ pints) water
1 vine tomato, sliced

Preheat oven to 220°C (425°F).

To make the stuffing:
Put the mince in a large saucepan, add 100 ml (3½ fl oz) water and stir with a fork until the mince gets a loose texture and brown color. Next add the chopped leek and carrot. Meanwhile boil the basmati rice in 500 ml (17 fl oz) of cold water in a small pot for no more than 7 minutes so that it is almost but not completely cooked. Drain the water and add to the mince and vegetables. Mix well and set aside.

To prepare the peppers:
Wash the peppers, cut the stems, remove the seeds and stuff the empty peppers with the rice and mince mixture. Close each pepper with a slice of vine tomato, to keep the stuffing in. Arrange the peppers in a baking tray. Add 200 ml (6¾ fl oz) of boiling water to cover the bottom of the tray and bake in the oven for about 30 minutes. Serve warm with a good tablespoon of yogurt on top of each pepper.

Serves 8

Per serving pepper
374 kcal, 14.4 g fat (6 g saturated), 21 g protein, 40 g carbs (8.8 g sugar), 0.7 g salt, 3.8 g fibre

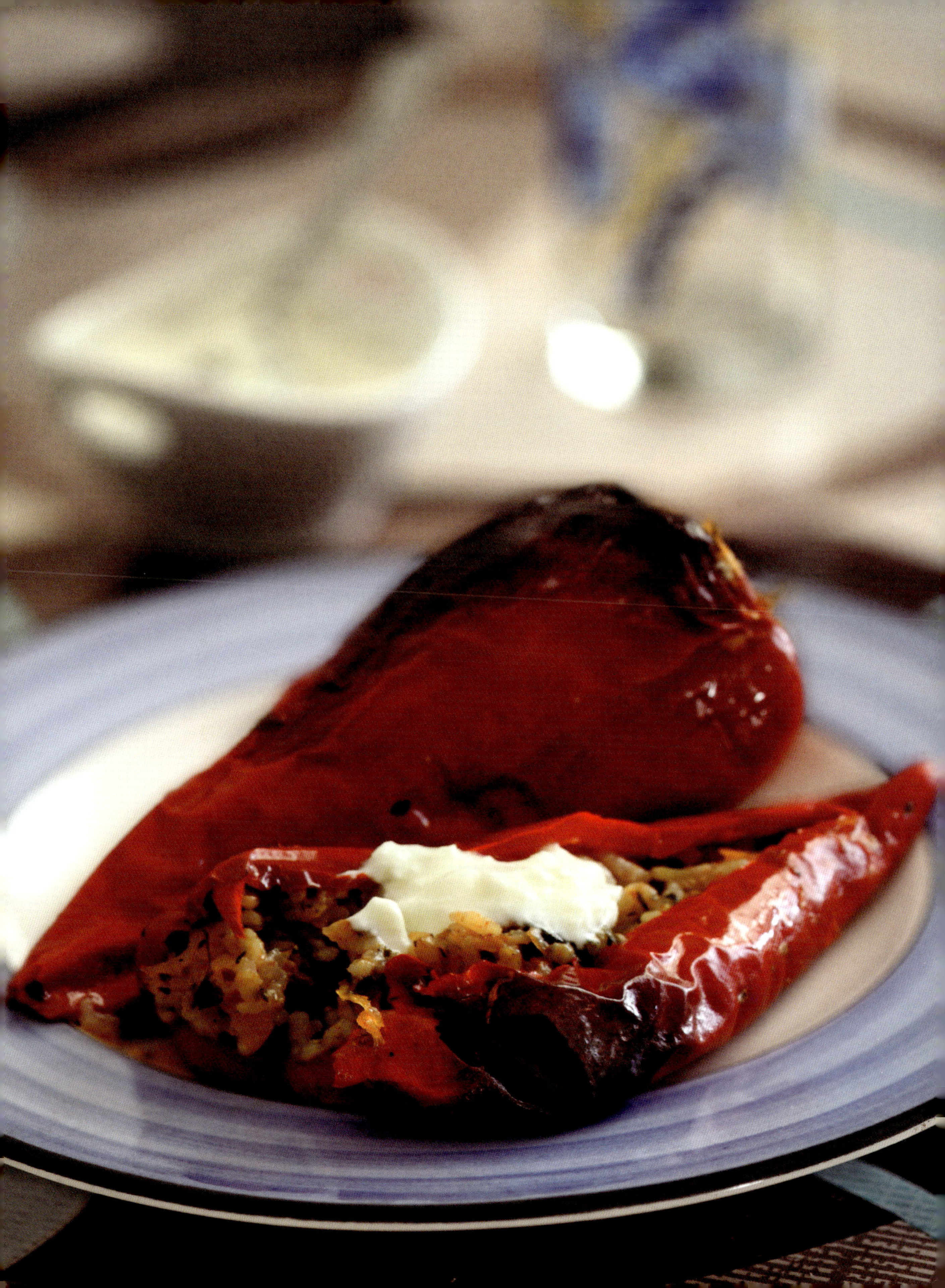

Roasted Greens with Pancetta and Yogurt Dressing

150 g (5 oz) yogurt
1 tablespoon extra-virgin olive oil
1 lemon, freshly squeezed juice

Mix the yogurt, oil, lemon juice and pinch of salt in a small bowl and set aside.

200 g (7 oz) diced bacon
a pinch of caraway seeds
1 onion, sliced
a handful of fresh dill coarsely chopped
50 g (2 oz) pine kernels
350 g (12 oz) mange tout – mix, tender stem and fine beans, trimmed
a pinch of salt

Boil the mange tout, tender stem and fine beans in 1 litre (2 pints) of water for no more than 4 minutes in a large saucepan.

Meanwhile, heat a frying pan over a high heat. Add the pancetta and cook for about 3 minutes. Then add the caraway seeds, onion and pine kernels and cook for about 3 more minutes stirring constantly. Remove from the heat and sprinkle over the chopped dill.

Combine the greens with the pancetta mixture and serve warm with a spoonful of yogurt mixture on top.

Serves 4

Per serving
303 kcal, 23.8 g fat (6.6 g saturated), 15.8 g protein, 7.3 g carbs (6.1 g sugar), 3.4 g fibre, 2.7 g salt

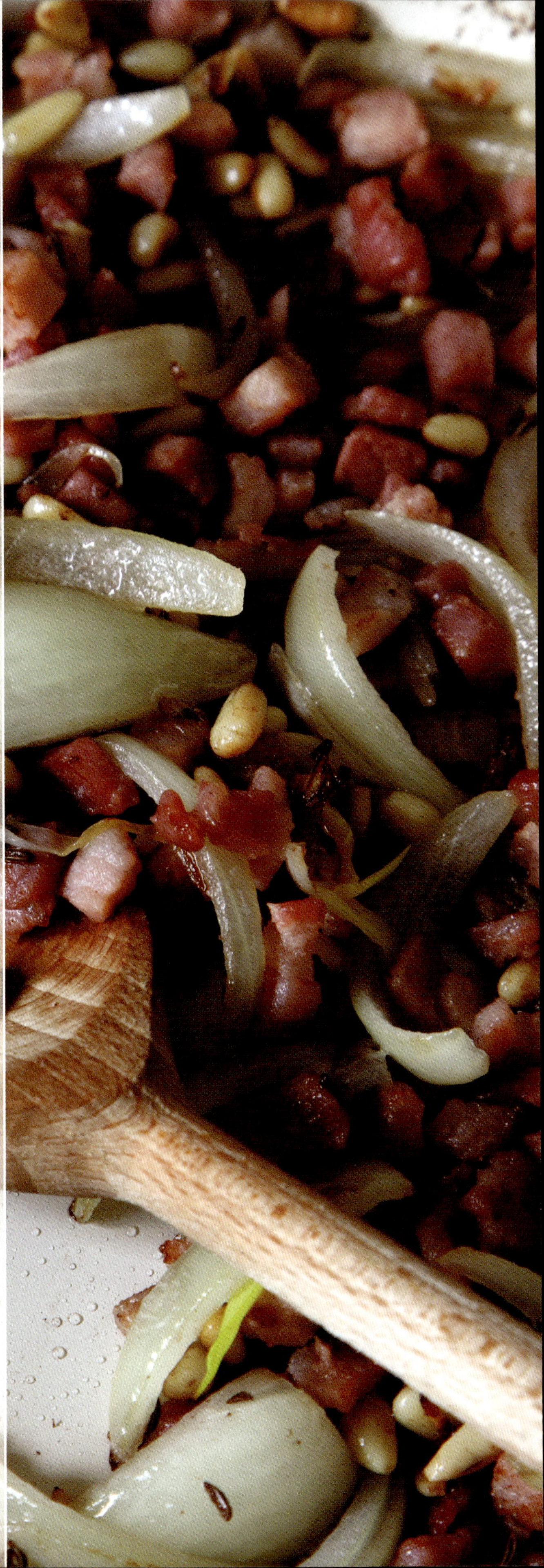

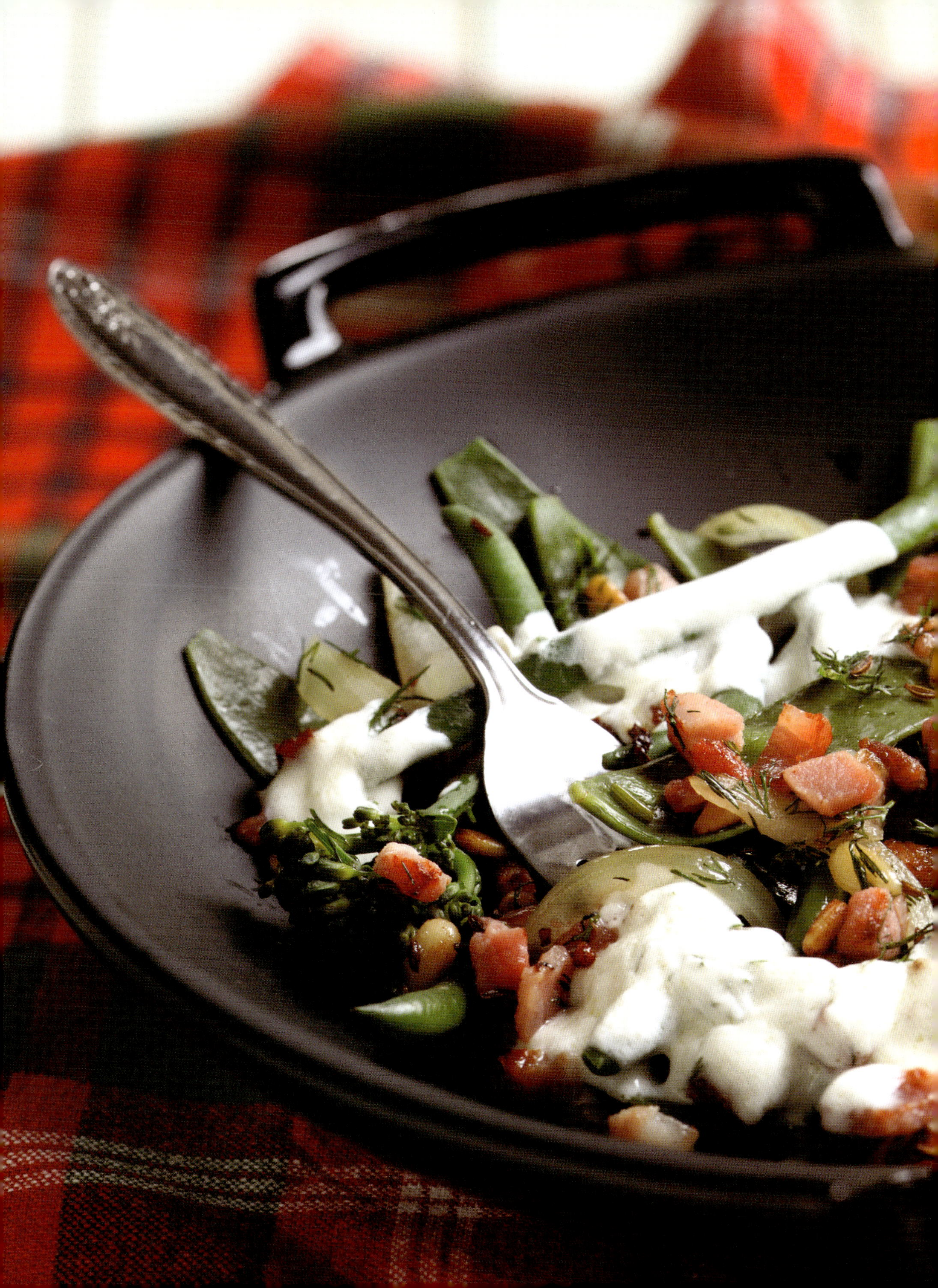

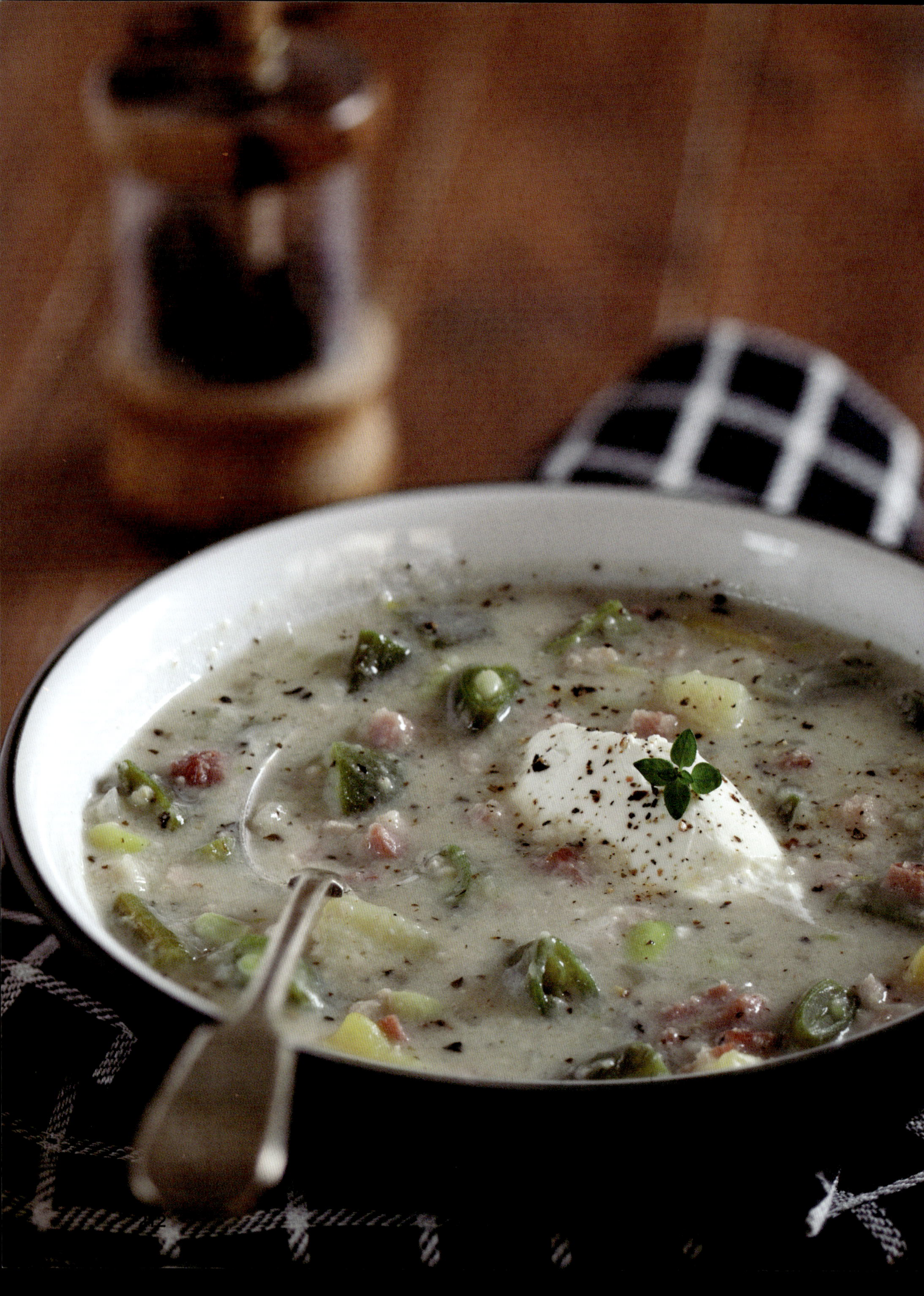

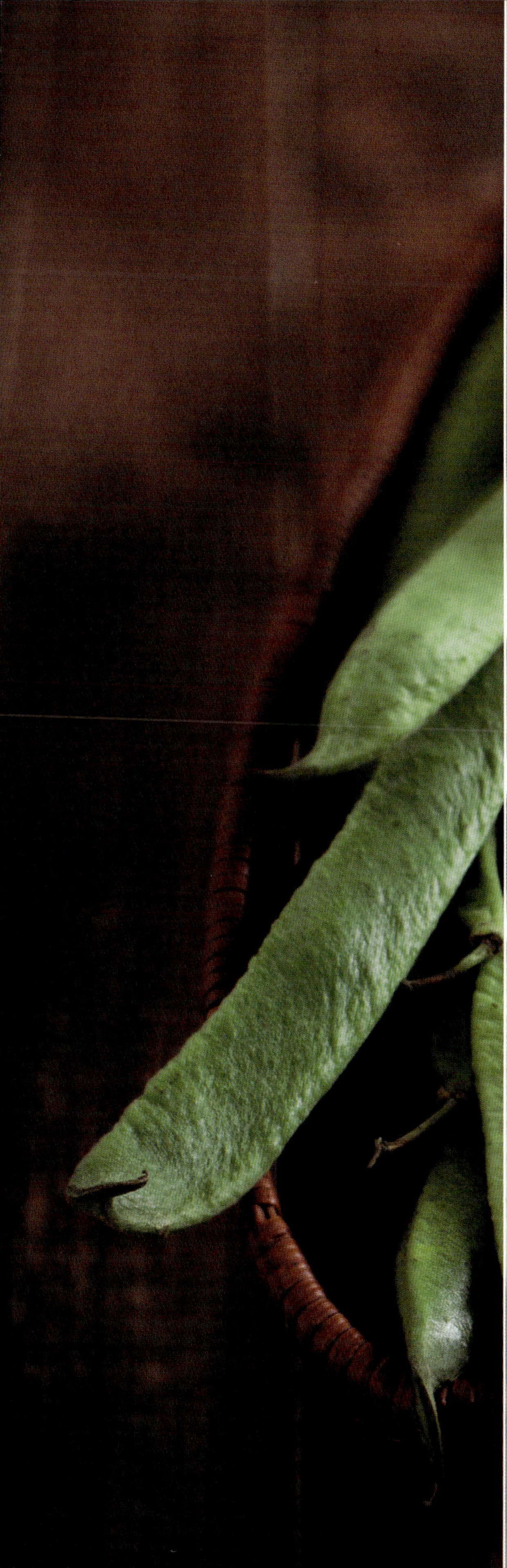

Runner Bean Stew

400 g (14 oz) runner beans
400 g (14 oz) potatoes
50 g (2 oz) butter
2 tablespoons oatbran
1 large chopped onion
200 g (7 oz) diced bacon
1 teaspoon Marjoram
pinch of black pepper
200 ml ($6\frac{3}{4}$ fl oz) milk
600 ml (20 fl oz) mineral water
pinch of salt
6 tablespoons strained yogurt
some fresh thyme leaves

Boil the potatoes in a medium saucepan for 20 minutes, until soft but not too soft. Cool and cut into small cubes.
Next cut the runner beans into small chunks. Boil 1 litre ($1\frac{3}{4}$ pints) of water in a medium saucepan and throw the beans in. Boil for 15 minutes until just barely tender and immediately transfer to a large bowl with cold water. The cold water will preserve the nice green color.
Meanwhile, heat a large saucepan over a high heat. Add the diced bacon and cook for about 3 minutes, then add the butter, chopped onion, marjoram and 100 ml ($3\frac{1}{2}$ oz) water. Cook, until the onion is translucent for about 3 more minutes stirring constantly. Add the oatbran, milk and 500 ml (17 fl oz) mineral water and bring to a simmer and thicken for no more than 10 minutes.
Turn the heat off for a minute, add the potato and beans and stir. Season with black pepper and salt. Serve hot on a plate with a tablespoon of strained yogurt and garnish with some fresh thyme leaves.

Serves 6

Per serving
298 kcal, 18.5 g fat (10 g saturated), 12.7 g protein, 20.1 g carbs (6.7 g sugar), 4.0 g fibre, 2.0 g salt

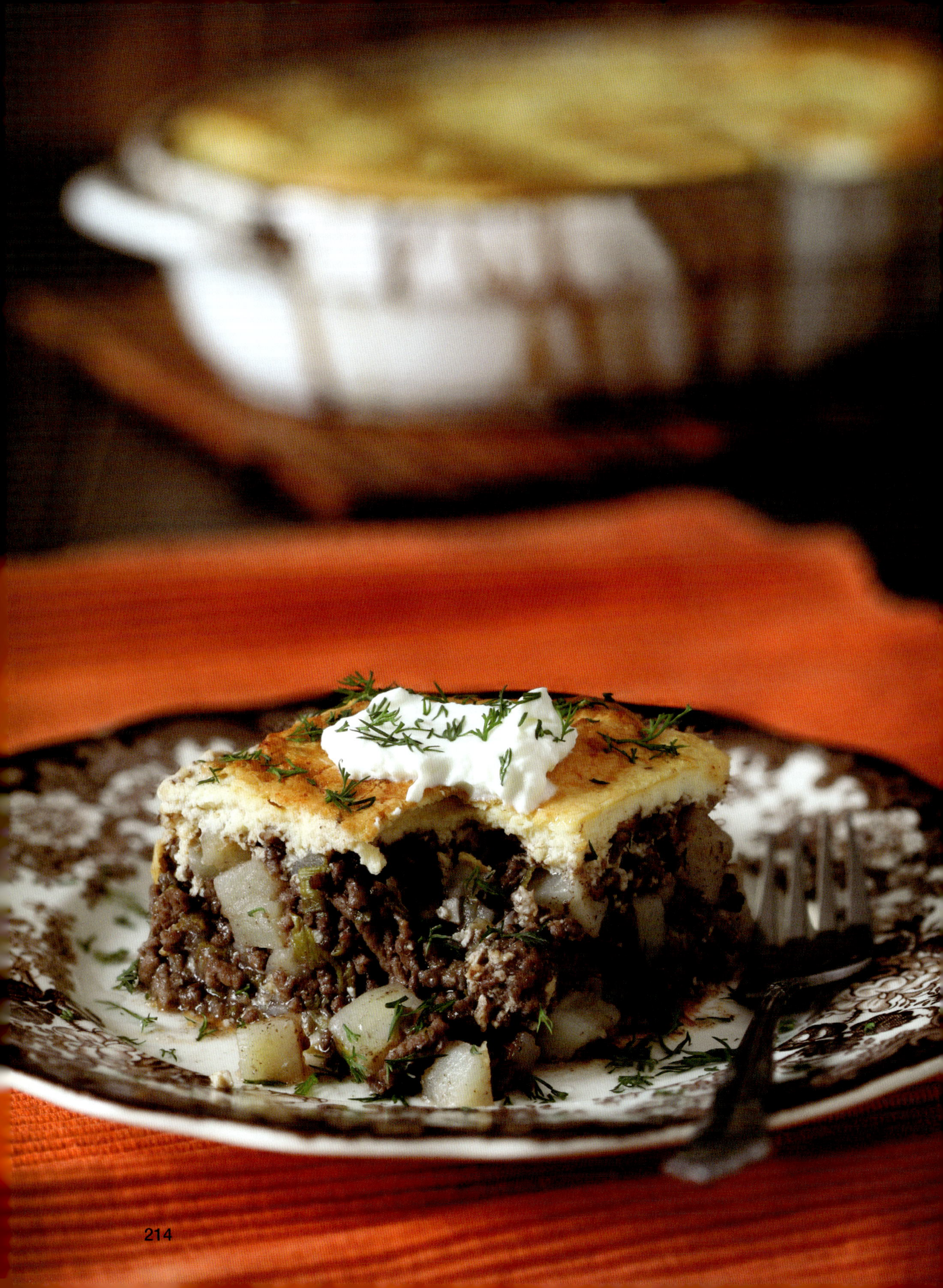

Northern Moussaka

75 ml (3 fl oz) olive oil
1 large onion, finely chopped
500 g (17½ oz) beef mince
3 garlic cloves, chopped
500 g (17½ oz) potatoes, cut into small cubes
1 cinnamon stick
1 teaspoon allspice
150 g (5 oz) vine tomatoes, chopped
200 ml (6¾ fl oz) red wine
250 ml (8½ fl oz) boiling water
Salt and freshly ground black pepper

topping:
50 ml (1½ fl oz) milk
100 g (3½ oz) low fat yogurt
2 tablespoons plain white flour
3 free-range eggs, beaten
1 teaspoon carom seeds

For serving:
400 g (14 oz) low fat yogurt

Preheat the oven to 200°C (400°F). Heat 2 tablespoons of olive oil and 50 ml (1½ fl oz) water in a large pot. Add the onion and cook gently for 2 minutes or until the onion becomes transparent, but not colored. Add the beef mince and the garlic and break up the mince with a fork until it has a loose texture and continue cooking until the mince browns. Next add the chopped potatoes, mix well, take off the heat and set aside.
In another medium saucepan stir together the cinnamon stick, allspice, tomato purée and the wine, bring to the boil and then take out the cinnamon stick. Transfer the mince mixture and the cinnamon sauce to a flameproof casserole. Add 250 ml (8½ fl oz) boiling water or just to cover it. Bake in the oven for 40 minutes.
Meanwhile, make the topping. In a medium bowl beat the eggs then add the milk and yogurt and mix well. Last add the white flour, mix again and set aside.
Pour the topping over the meat and bake, uncovered, for a further 10 minutes or until the topping sauce gets a nice golden brown color. Allow to cool for about 20 minutes before serving. For best results serve each portion with some tablespoons of yogurt.

Serves 8

Per serving
533 kcal, 34.7 g fat (14.7 g saturated), 25.7 g protein, 27.0 g carbs (10.9 g sugar), 2.7 g fibre, 1.0 g salt.

Bulgur and Mushrooms Stuffed Zucchinis

6 medium zucchinis (courgettes)
2 tablespoons olive oil
1 finely chopped leek
200 ml (6¾ fl oz) bulgur, macerated
100 g (3½ oz) Walnuts finely chopped
200 g (7 oz) chestnut mushrooms finely chopped
2 tablespoons fresh thyme leaves
30 g (1 oz) red cheddar cheese, shredded

Preheat oven to 200°C (400°F). In a small bowl with 200 ml (6¾ fl oz) cold water macerate the bulgur for about 20 minutes. Using a long teaspoon make a tube carving the inside of the zucchini. To make the stuffing, in a large saucepan throw in the chopped mushrooms and olive oil and cook for no more than 10 minutes then add the chopped leek. Cook for another 2 minutes. Take off the heat and add the chopped walnuts, bulgur and thyme. Mix well and stuff the zucchinis. Arrange the stuffed zucchinis in a deep porcelain dish or glass baking tray and add boiling water to cover almost to the middle of the zucchinis. Bake in the oven for about 30 minutes. Then sprinkle shredded cheddar cheese over the zucchinis and bake for 3 more minutes. Leave to cool for a couple of minutes while you prepare the topping. Serve on a plate with a few tablespoons of yogurt.

Topping:
500 g (17½ oz) low fat yogurt
2 garlic cloves crushed
1 tablespoon chopped fresh dill
pinch of salt

In a medium bowl pour the yogurt, crushed garlic, chopped dill and some salt. Mix well and serve.

Serves 6

Per serving
373 kcal, 19.1 g fat (3.6 g saturated), 14.9 g protein, 36.3 g carbs (9.9 g sugar), 3.9 g fibre, 0.7 g salt

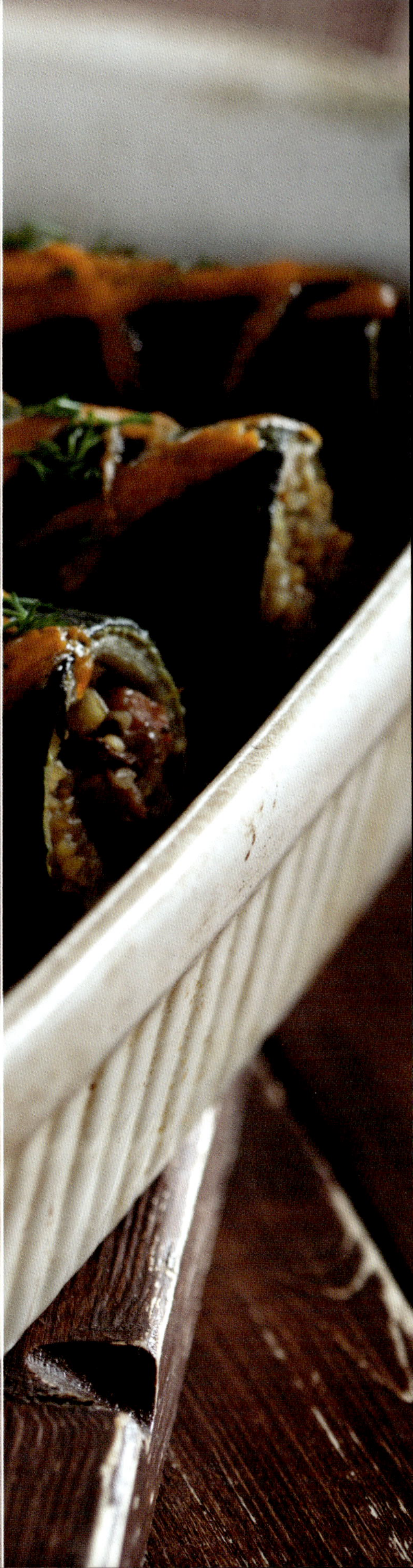

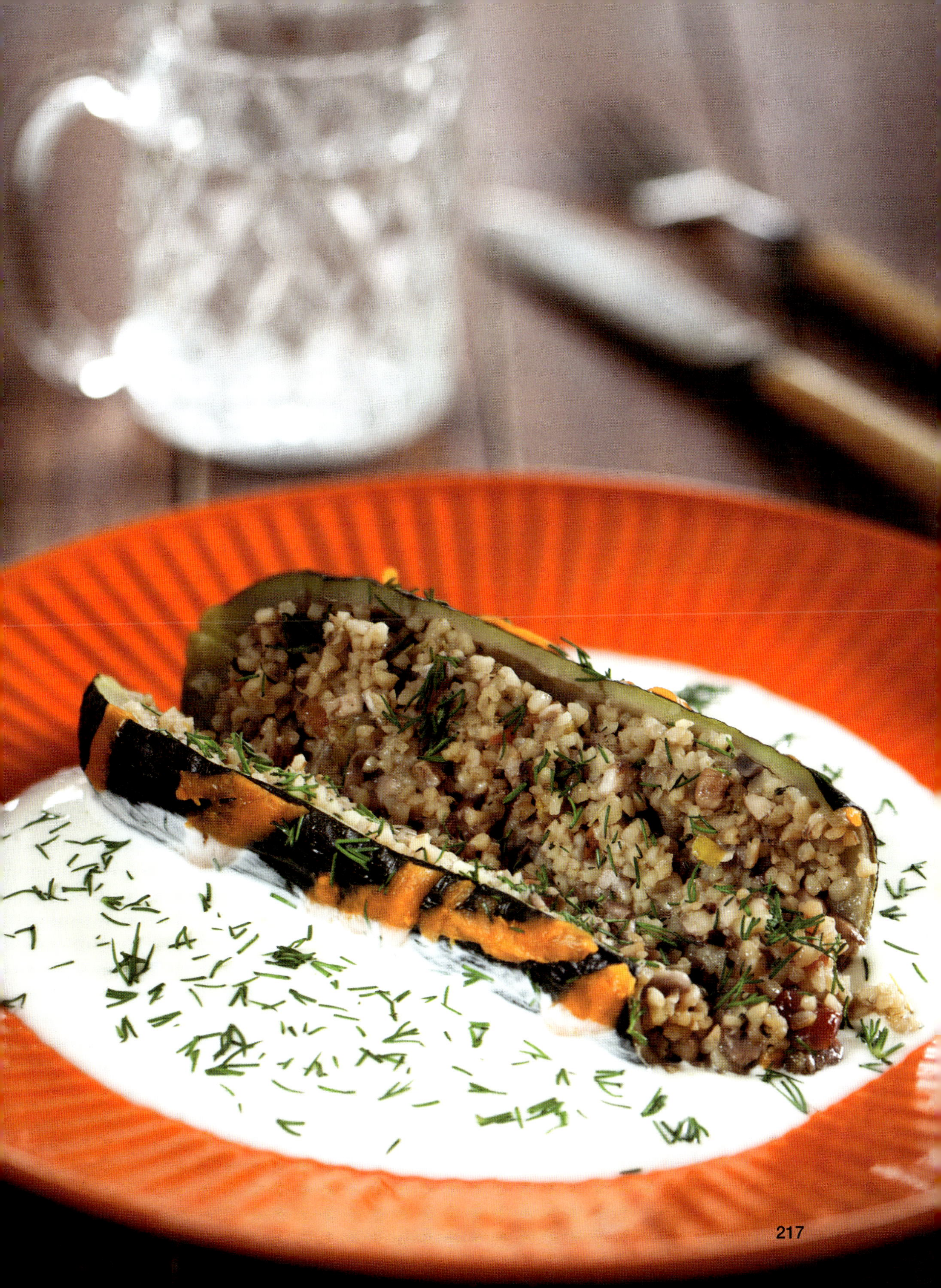

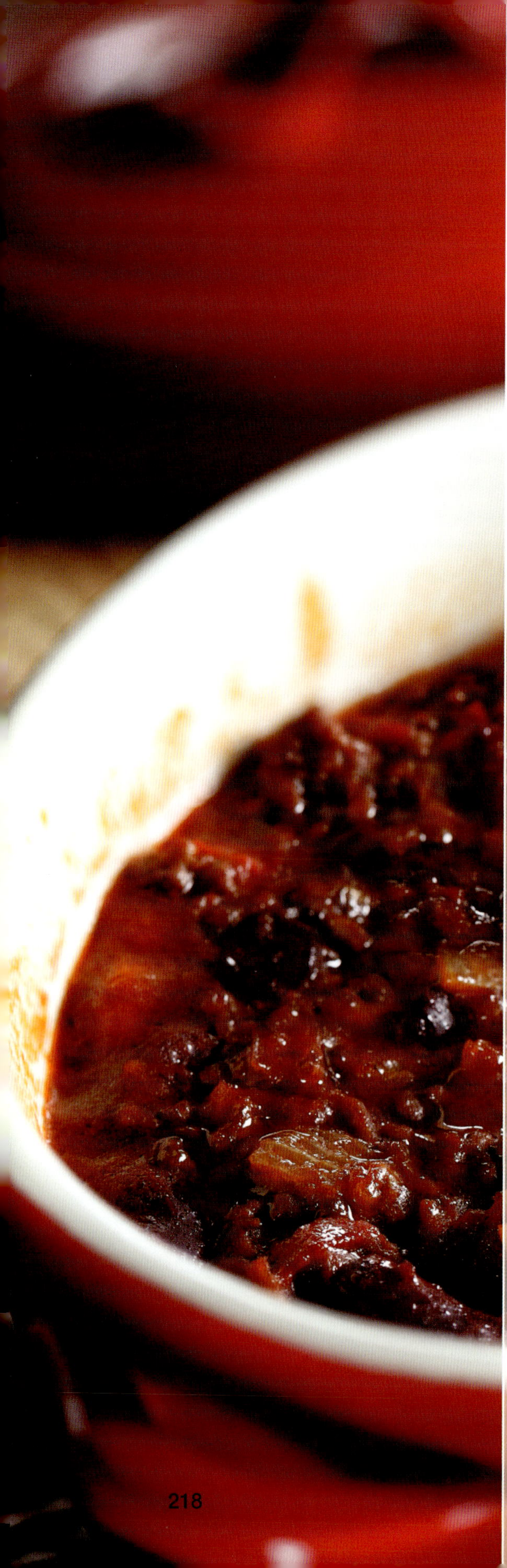

Chili Con Carne Potatoes

2 tablespoon olive oil
1 medium onion, finely chopped
3 garlic cloves, crushed
1 tablespoon ground cumin
1 red pepper, finely chopped
600 g (21 oz) beef mince
1 can 400 g (14 oz) peeled plum tomatoes
1 can 400 g (14 oz) kidney beans, drained and rinsed
1 tablespoon tomato paste
1 small chili pepper/optional
100 g (3½ oz) sweetcorn, frozen
pinch of salt and black pepper

Throw the chopped onion, red pepper, sweetcorn, crushed garlic, ground cumin, olive oil and 50 ml (1½ fl oz) water in a large saucepan. Cook over a medium heat for about 5 minutes while stirring constantly with a wooden spoon. Next add the mince and cook for another 5 minutes. Keep stirring and try to break up any lumps. When the mince browns, add the tomatoes, tomato paste and kidney beans and stir well. Simmer for another 10 minutes occasionally stirring.

6 large potatoes
2 tablespoons of olive oil
60 g wild arugula (rocket)
250 g (9 oz) low fat yogurt

Meanwhile preheat the oven to 200°C (400°F). Wash the potatoes well, dry and prick several times with a fork. Bake for about 45 minutes in the oven. Once cooked, transfer a potato to a serving plate, halve it and pour over some of the chill and one tablespoon of yogurt. Arrange around some wild arugula or any green salad and serve.

Serves 6

Per serving
468 kcal, 24.9 g fat (8.4 g saturated), 28.1 g protein, 34.8 g carbohydrates (9 g sugar), 6.8 g fibre, 1.2 g salt

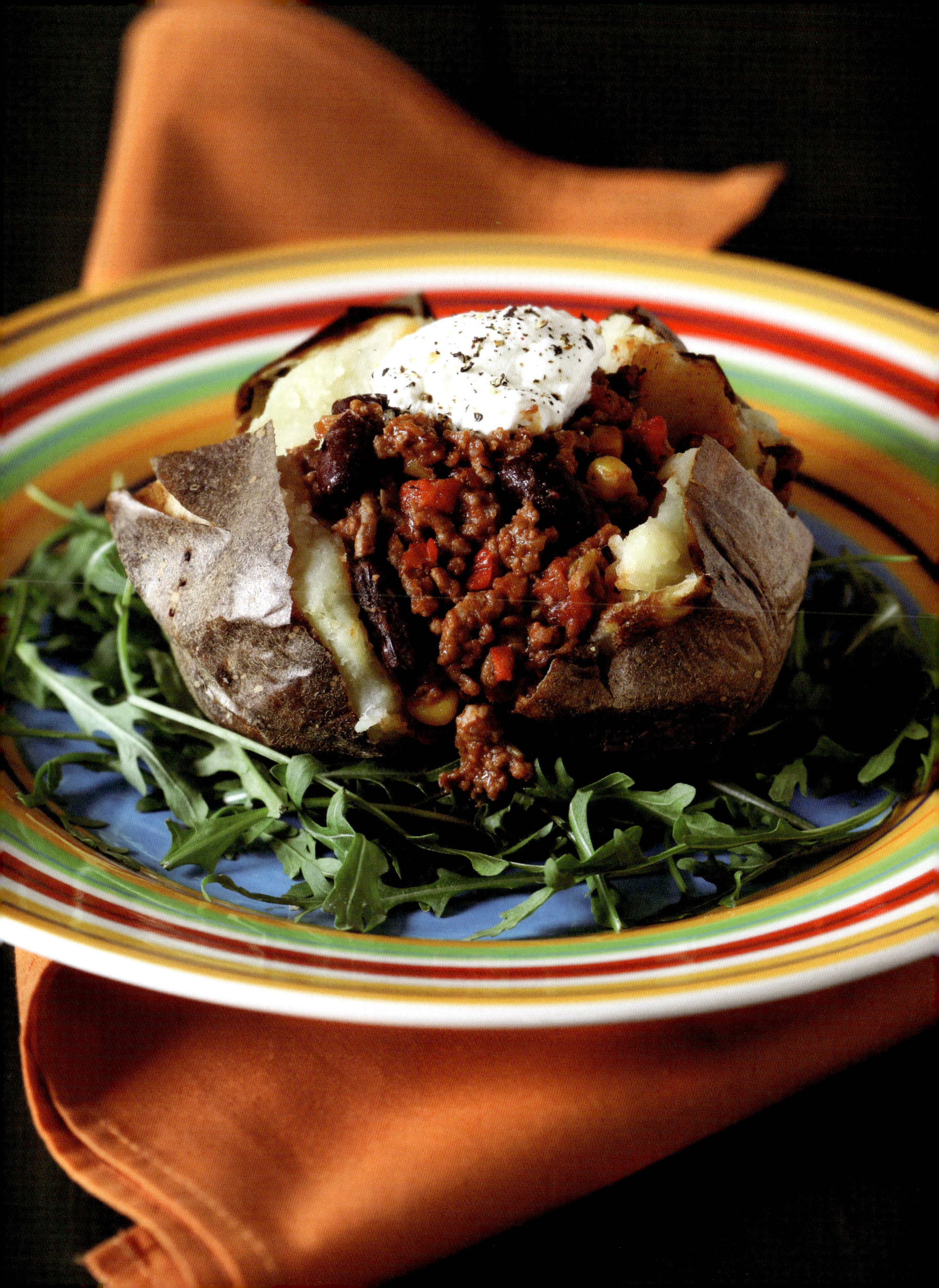

Poached Eggs in Yogurt Sauce

4 large free range eggs
250 g (9 oz) low fat yogurt
100 g ($3\frac{1}{2}$ oz) feta cheese, diced
2 tablespoons wine vinegar
1 clove garlic, crushed
pinch of paprika
pinch of salt
2 tablespoon olive oil

Pour the wine vinegar in 1 litre ($1\frac{3}{4}$ pints) of boiling water in a medium pot and add a pinch of salt. Separately, in a small bowl break one egg and gently pour into the boiling water. Boil the egg for about 5 minutes. The shorter the time, the runnier the egg will be. Repeat the procedure with the rest of the eggs. Meanwhile in another medium bowl mix the yogurt and garlic and add the diced feta cheese. Finally, warm the olive oil and paprika in a small saucepan until it starts sizzling but not burning.
To serve, cover the bottom of a plate with a couple of spoons of the yogurt mixture, two eggs and drizzle over some sizzling oil and paprika. Sprinkle with a pinch of salt.

Serves 2

Per serving
496 kcal, 36.8 g fat (13.4 g saturated), 30.8 g protein, 10.6 g carbohydrates (10.2 g sugar), 0.1 g fibre, 3.9 g salt

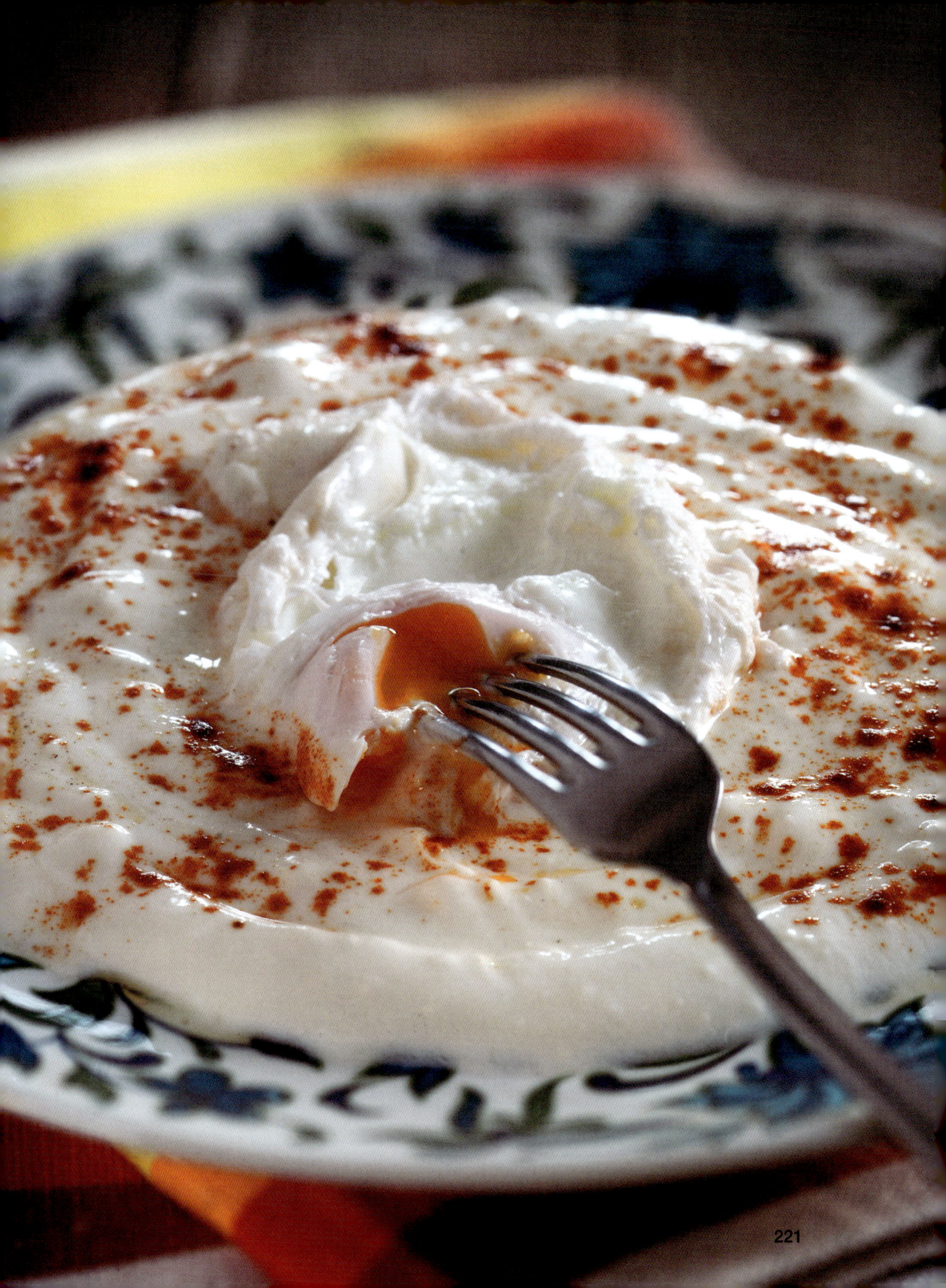

Meatballs with Yogurt Sauce

600 g (21 oz) low fat beef mince
1 egg
1 red onion, finely chopped
handful fresh parsley, finely chopped
1 teaspoon ground cinnamon
1 teaspoon ground cumin
pinch of salt and black pepper
1 tablespoon brown sugar

Preheat oven to 200°C (400°F). In a large bowl combine the mince, egg, chopped onion, chopped parsley, cinnamon, cumin and season with salt and pepper. Mix well and the form the mixture into small balls. Place the meatballs onto a baking tray and bake in the oven for about 40 minutes. Sprinkle some brown sugar over each meatball and cook for 2 more minutes. Serve warm with yogurt sauce.

Yogurt sauce:
250 g (9 oz) low fat yogurt
2 minced garlic cloves
1 tablespoon extra virgin olive oil
1 handful fresh mint, finely chopped
1 teaspoon sesame seeds

Put all the ingredients in a blender and blend together till smooth.

Serves 6

Per serving
250 kcal, 13.4 g fat (5.1 g saturated), 25.6 g protein, 8 g carbs (7.1 g sugar), 0.7 g fibre, 0.8 g salt

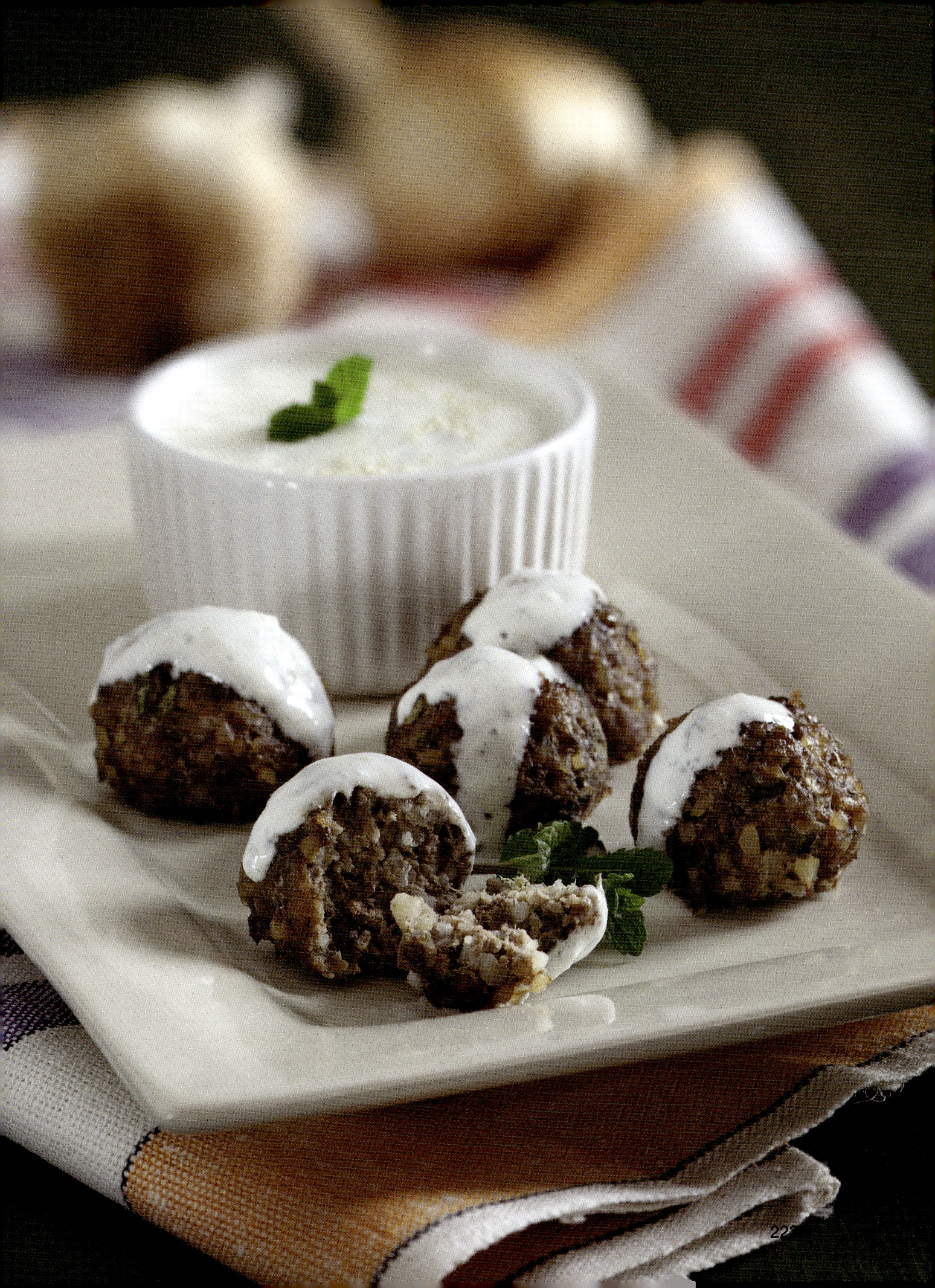

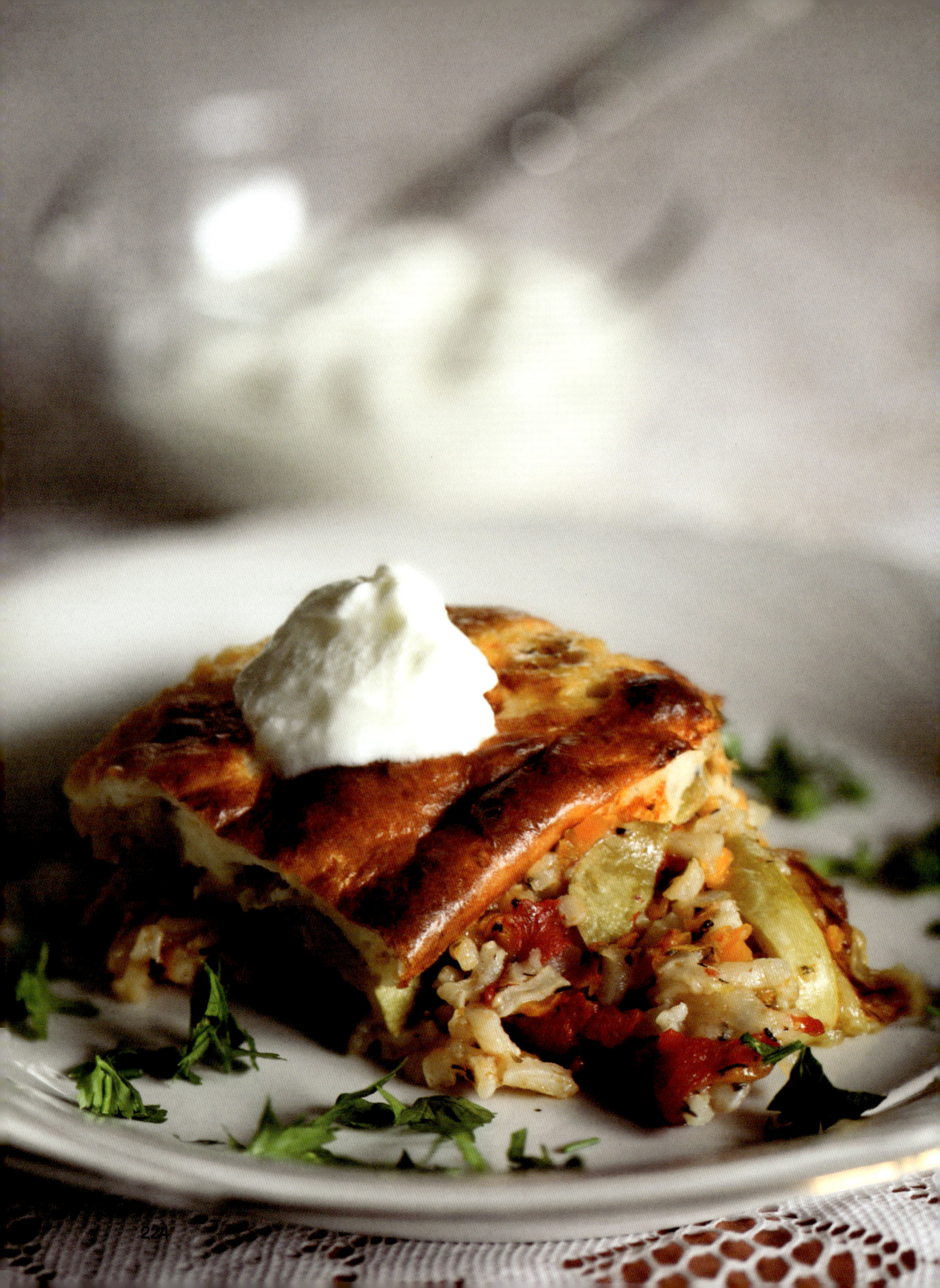

Zucchini Moussaka

3 middle size zucchinis (courgettes)
2 sweet pointed peppers, chopped
1 large carrot, grated
75 ml (3 fl oz) vegetarian oil
100 g (3½ oz) white flour
100 g (3½ oz) corn flour
500 g (17½ oz) yogurt + 200 g (7 oz) extra for serving
2 eggs
3 garlic cloves, crushed
100 g (3½ oz) feta cheese, diced
1 tablespoon dry oregano
1 handful fresh dill, chopped
1 handful fresh parsley, chopped
pinch of salt

Preheat oven to 200°C (400°F). Wash and trim off the ends of the zucchinis and cut into 5mm thick slices. Sprinkle with a pinch of salt and leave to drain for 20 minutes in a colander. Meanwhile, in a small baking tray mix together the dry oregano, white flour and corn flour. In another large bowl place the sliced zucchinis and chopped peppers and oil each piece. Next, one by one wallow each piece in the flour mixture and arrange in layers on a pre-greased large baking tray and sprinkle from time to time with some grated carrot and chopped fresh dill. Bake in the oven for about 20 minutes until the zucchini are golden. Finally in a large bowl mix together the yogurt, the eggs, crushed garlic and 3 tablespoons of the flour mixture. Arrange the diced feta cheese over the cooked zucchini and pour over the yogurt mixture and bake for another 10 minutes or until golden. Serve cold with a spoonful of yogurt and sprinkle with some parsley.

Serves 6

Per serving
531 kcal, 21.6 g fat (6.6 g saturated), 16.8 g protein, 71.8 g carbs (14.4 g sugar), 3.8 g fibre, 1.4 g salt

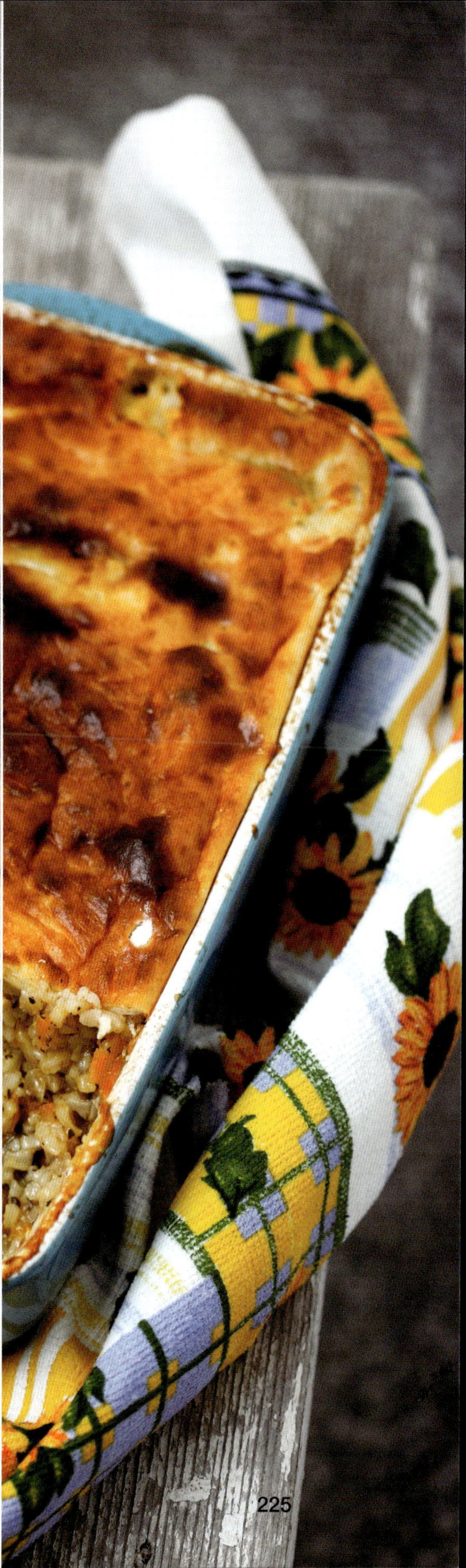

Salmon Topped with Yogurt and Ricotta

750 g (26½ oz) Salmon fillet
100 g (3½ oz) ricotta
100 g (3½ oz) low fat yogurt, strained
1 red bell pepper, chopped
1 tablespoon sunflower oil
2 shallots
1 teaspoon black pepper
1 tablespoon dry tarragon
1 teaspoon salt
300 g (10½ oz) broccoli
1 tablespoon olive oil
2 tablespoons chives, chopped

Preheat the oven to 200°C (400°F).
Cut the salmon fillet into 6 portions. Rub the skin with salt and put the fillets on a baking tray. Bake in the oven for about 20 minutes until the edges are golden. Meanwhile preheat the oil in a small saucepan and throw in the chopped red pepper and a pinch of salt, cook for about 2 minutes until tender. Cover and leave aside to rest.
Then in a medium bowl combine the ricotta, strained yogurt, chopped shallots, dry tarragon and black pepper, mix well.
Next, cook the broccoli in boiling water for no more than 3 minutes. Drain, drizzle with some olive oil and season with a pinch of salt.
After the salmon is cooked, place on serving dishes and spread a big tablespoon of the yogurt mixture over each fillet and arrange on top some of the cooked red pepper pieces. Sprinkle with chopped chives over and serve with the broccoli to garnish.

Serves 6

Per serving
348 kcal, 21.3 g fat (4.8 g saturated), 35.3 g protein, 4.0 g carbs (3.4 g sugar), 2.2 g fibre, 1.1 g salt

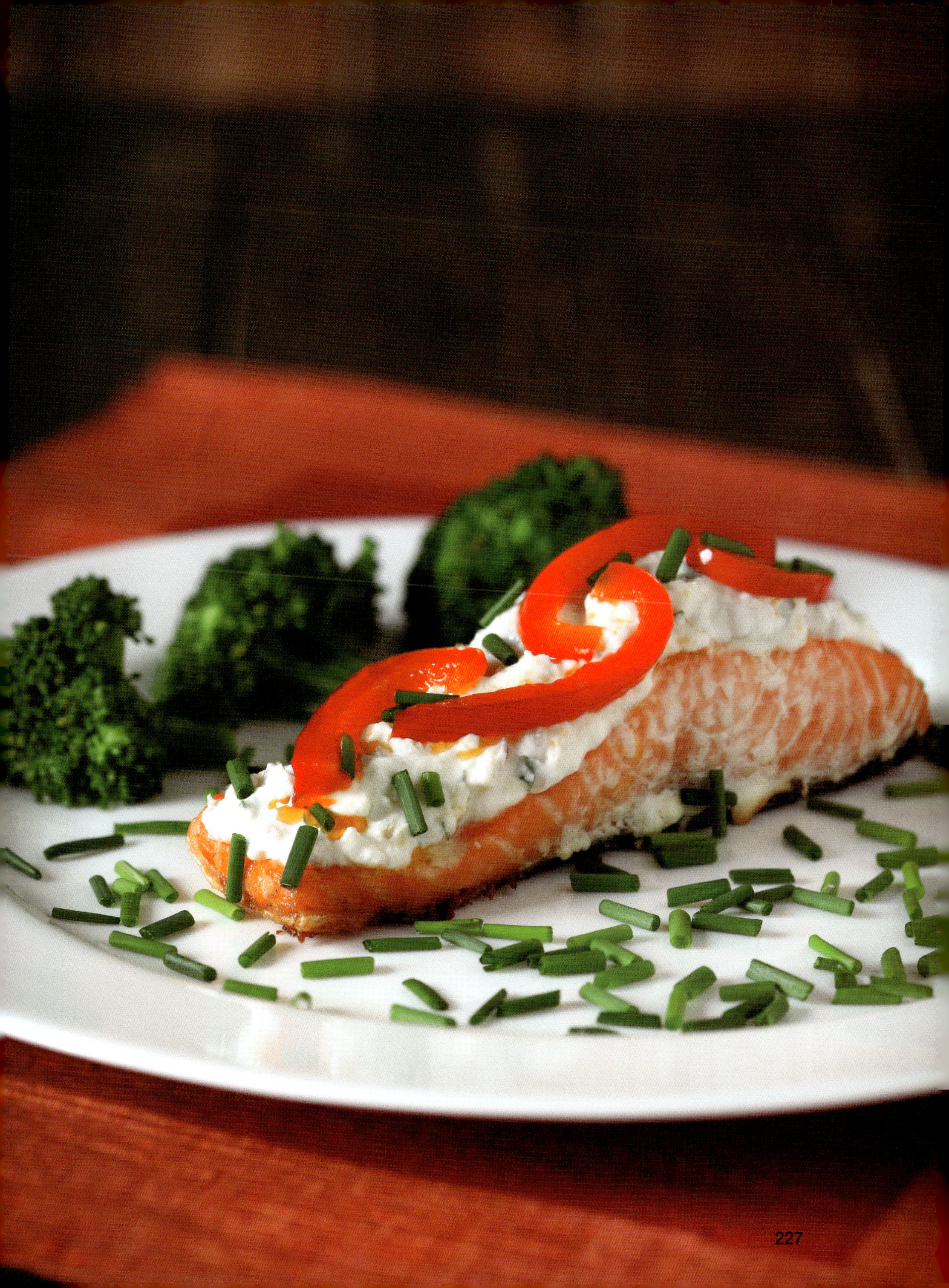

Meatballs in White Sauce

Meatballs:
600 g (21 oz) beef mince
100 g (3½ oz) bulgur
1 onion finely chopped
1 handful fresh parsley, finely chopped
1 egg
1 teaspoon cumin
pinch of salt
pinch of black pepper
some spoonsfuls of flour to coat the meatballs

Soak 100 g (3½ oz) bulgur in 200 ml (6¾ fl oz) cold water for 15 minutes. Mix the mince, soaked bulgur, finely chopped onion, fresh parsley, egg, cumin, salt and black pepper. Make small meatballs and coat them in flour. Put the meatballs into a large saucepan in 2 litres (4½ pints) boiling water and a pinch of salt and boil for 30 minutes.

White sauce:
500 g (17½ oz) yogurt
3 tablespoons flour
2 eggs
3 tablespoons olive oil
pinch of salt
pinch of dried thyme
250 g (9 oz) chestnut mushrooms coarsely chopped
1 teaspoon mustard seeds
fresh thyme to serve

Combine the oil and mushrooms in a large saucepan and cook for 5 minutes. Meanwhile in a medium bowl, mix together the yogurt, eggs, mustard seeds and flour. Add the yogurt mixture to the cooked mushrooms and simmer until thickened. Next add 2-3 ladles of the bullion from the meatballs, season with salt and dried thyme, mix well and cook for another 2 minutes. Finally add the boiled meatballs and serve warm. Sprinkle some fresh thyme on top of each plate.

Serves 6

Per serving
541 kcal, 33.8 g fat (14.2 g saturated), 31.7 g protein, 29.3 g carbs (5.4 g sugar) 1.7 g fibre, 1.4 g salt

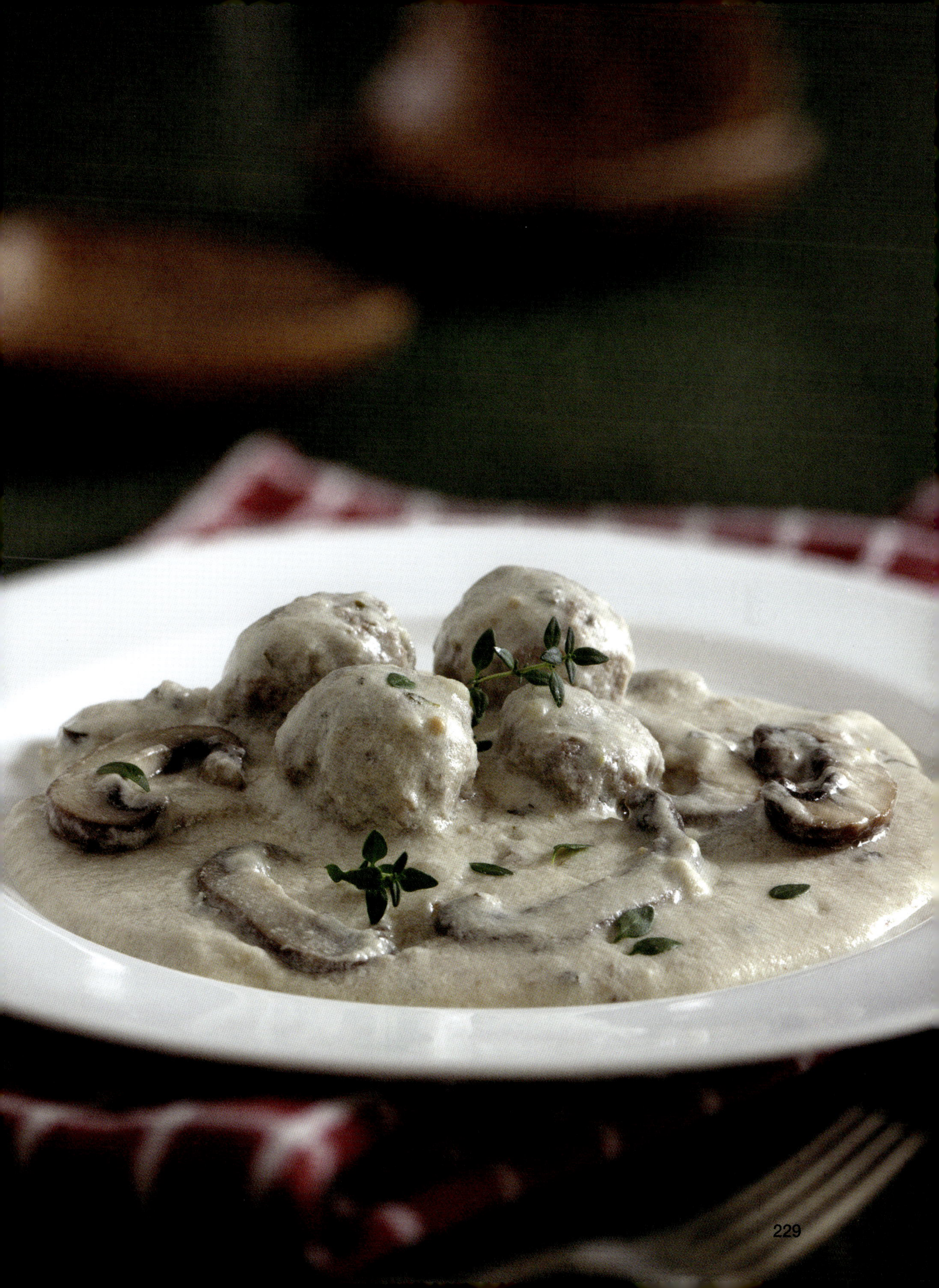

Yogurt Chicken

600 g (21 oz) chicken thighs fillets, boneless, skinless
250 g (9 oz) low fat yogurt
3 tablespoons Parmesan cheese, grated
2 tablespoons fresh thyme, finely chopped
1 large garlic clove, crushed
juice of 1 lime
pinch of black pepper
pinch of salt
1 teaspoon chili powder, optional
4 tablespoons golden bread crumbs

Preheat the oven to 200°C (400°F). Combine the yogurt, parmesan cheese, thyme, garlic, lime juice, black pepper and salt in a large bowl and mix well. Then add the chicken thighs and mix well again. Leave in a refrigerator for about 30 minutes. Place the chicken on a foiled baking sheet, sprinkle over the golden bread crumbs and bake for about 40 minutes.

Serves 4

Per serving
453 kcal, 27.2 g fat (9.9 g saturated), 38.7 g protein, 14.3 g carbs (5.7 g sugar), 0.6 g fibre, 1.7 g salt

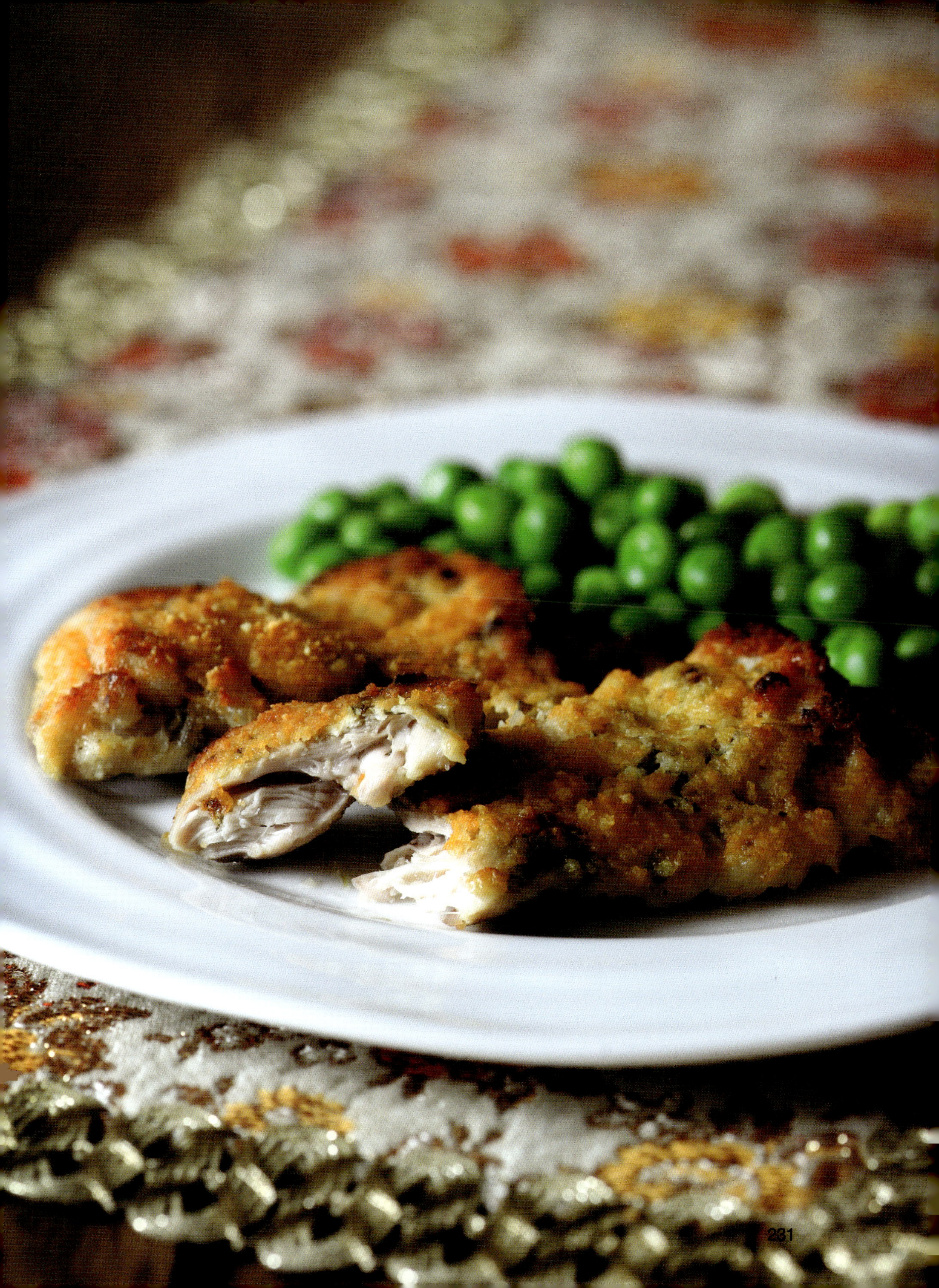

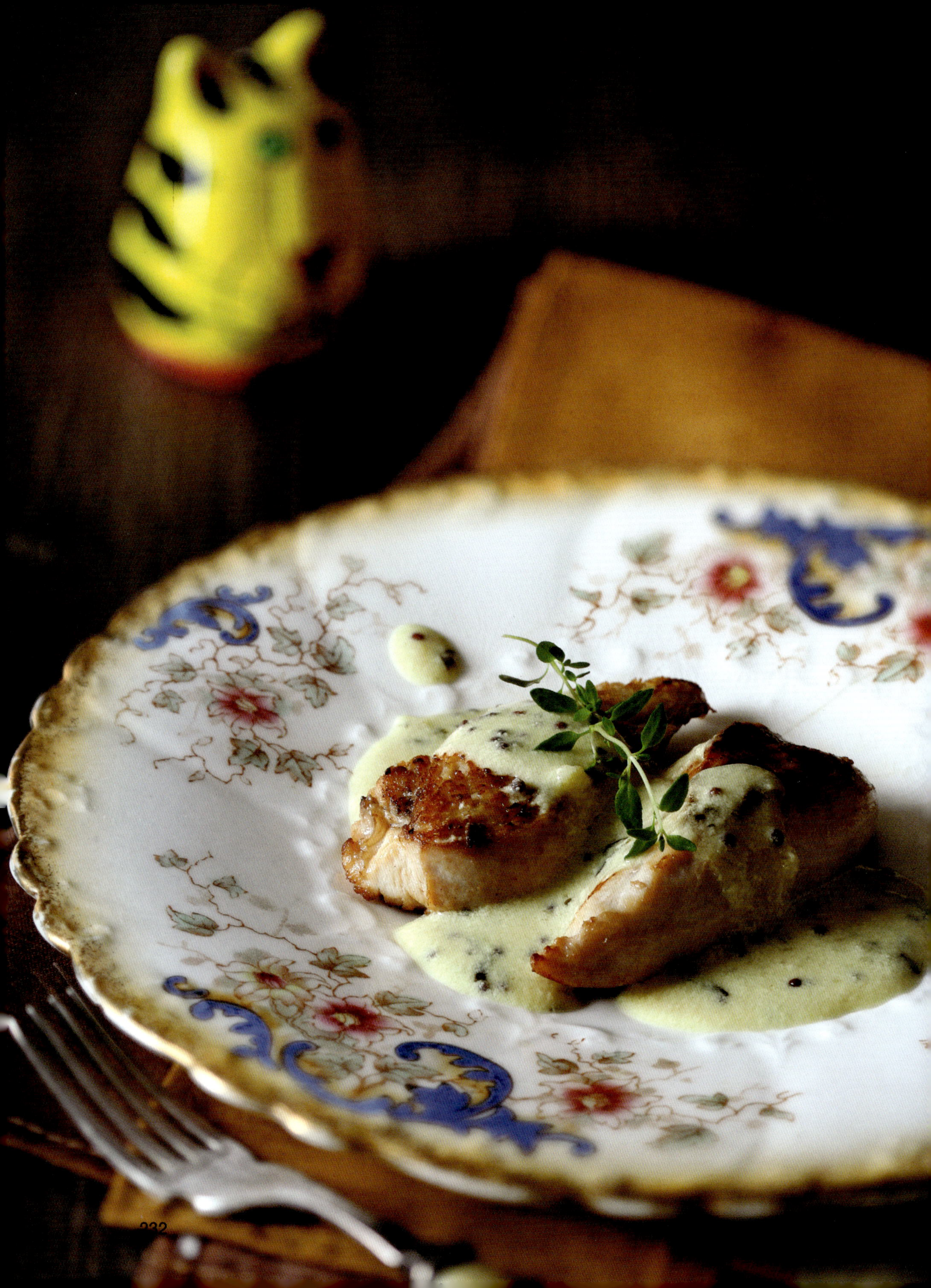

Chicken with Mustard Yogurt Sauce

150 g (5 oz) low fat yogurt
1 tablespoon wholegrain mustard
1 tablespoon chopped fresh thyme
2 tablespoons grapeseed oil
1 tablespoon teriyaki sauce
a pinch of salt
400 g (14 oz) chicken breast fillets, cut for chunks
75 ml (3 fl oz) chicken stock
1 tablespoon plain white flour

Combine the yogurt, mustard seeds and thyme in a small bowl and leave aside for later. To make the marinate, pour the grapeseed oil, teriyaki sauce and salt into a medium bowl and mix together. Add the chicken pieces and leave to marinate for about 15 minutes. To cook the chicken, sauté in a frying pan for 2-3 minutes on all sides, until cooked. Take the pan off the heat and transfer the chicken filets into another pot and keep warm with a lid on top. Then pour the chicken stock into the pan and cook for about 1 minute, remove from the heat, add the yogurt mixture and mix well. Serve the chicken with the sauce poured over the top.

Serves 4

Per serving
263 kcal, 13.2 g fat (1.8 g saturated), 31.9 g protein, 7.1 g carbs (2.9 g sugar), 0.2 g fibre, 1.2 g salt

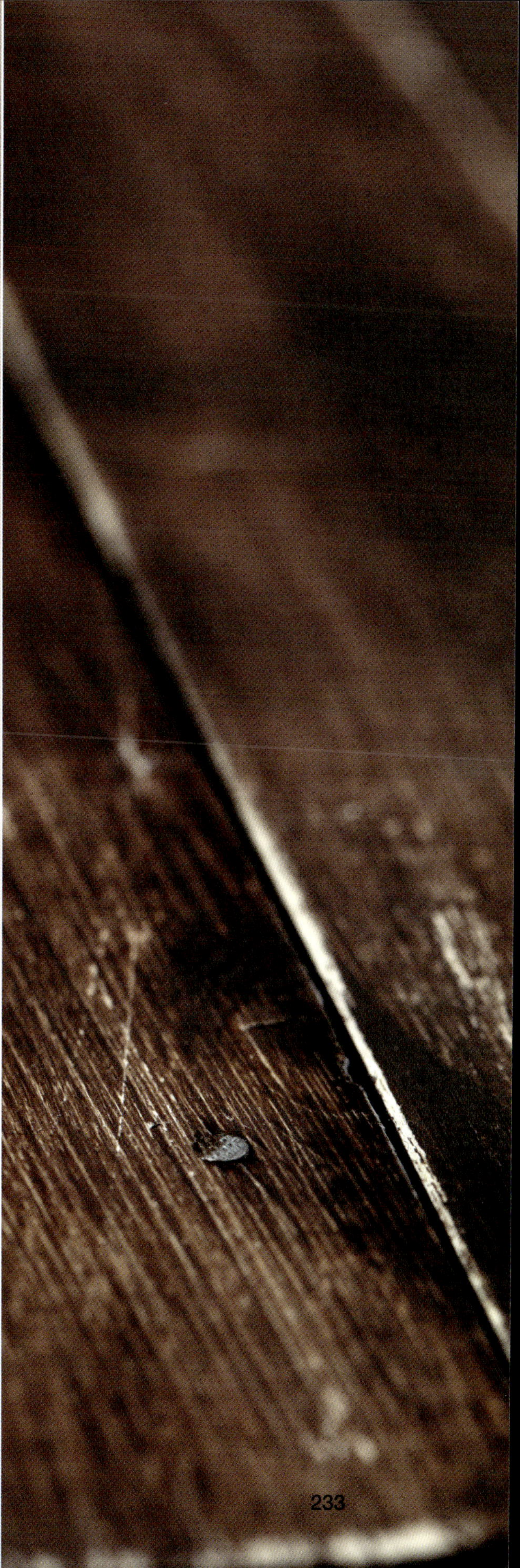

Grilled Vegetables and Yogurt Dip

1 small eggplant (aubergine)
2 small zucchinis (courgettes)
1 red pepper
1 yellow pepper
200 g (7 oz) mushrooms
1 large red salad onion

Marinade:
1 teaspoon fresh rosemary, chopped
75 ml (3 fl oz) vegetarian oil
1 clove garlic, crushed
1 tablespoon of balsamic vinegar
pinch black pepper, freshly ground
pinch salt

Yogurt Dip:
200 g (7 oz) yogurt
1 teaspoon tahini
1 handful basil, freshly chopped
1 clove garlic, crushed
juice of 1 lemon
1 teaspoon extra virgin oil
pinch of salt
pinch of sugar

To prepare the marinade, combine the vegetable oil, rosemary, garlic, balsamic vintgar, a pinch of salt and pepper into a small bowl and mix well. Next, cut the onion in rings 5mm thick. Cut peppers in four pieces lengthwise. Cut the mushrooms in halves. Slice the eggplant and zucchinis. Place all the vegetables in a large bowl and pour the marinate over and mix gently. Leave it for about 15 minutes to rest. Meanwhile in a small bowl combine the yogurt, tahini, fresh chopped basil, one crushed clove of garlic, lemon juice, extra virgin oil, a pinch of salt and sugar and mix well. Grill the vegetables for about 7 to 8 minutes until lightly charred and tender and arrange on a platter. Serve with the yogurt dip.

Serves 6

Per serving
193 kcal, 15.6 g fat (2.4 g saturated), 4.5 g protein, 9.4 g carbs (8.0 g sugar), 2.8 g fibre, 1.1 g salt

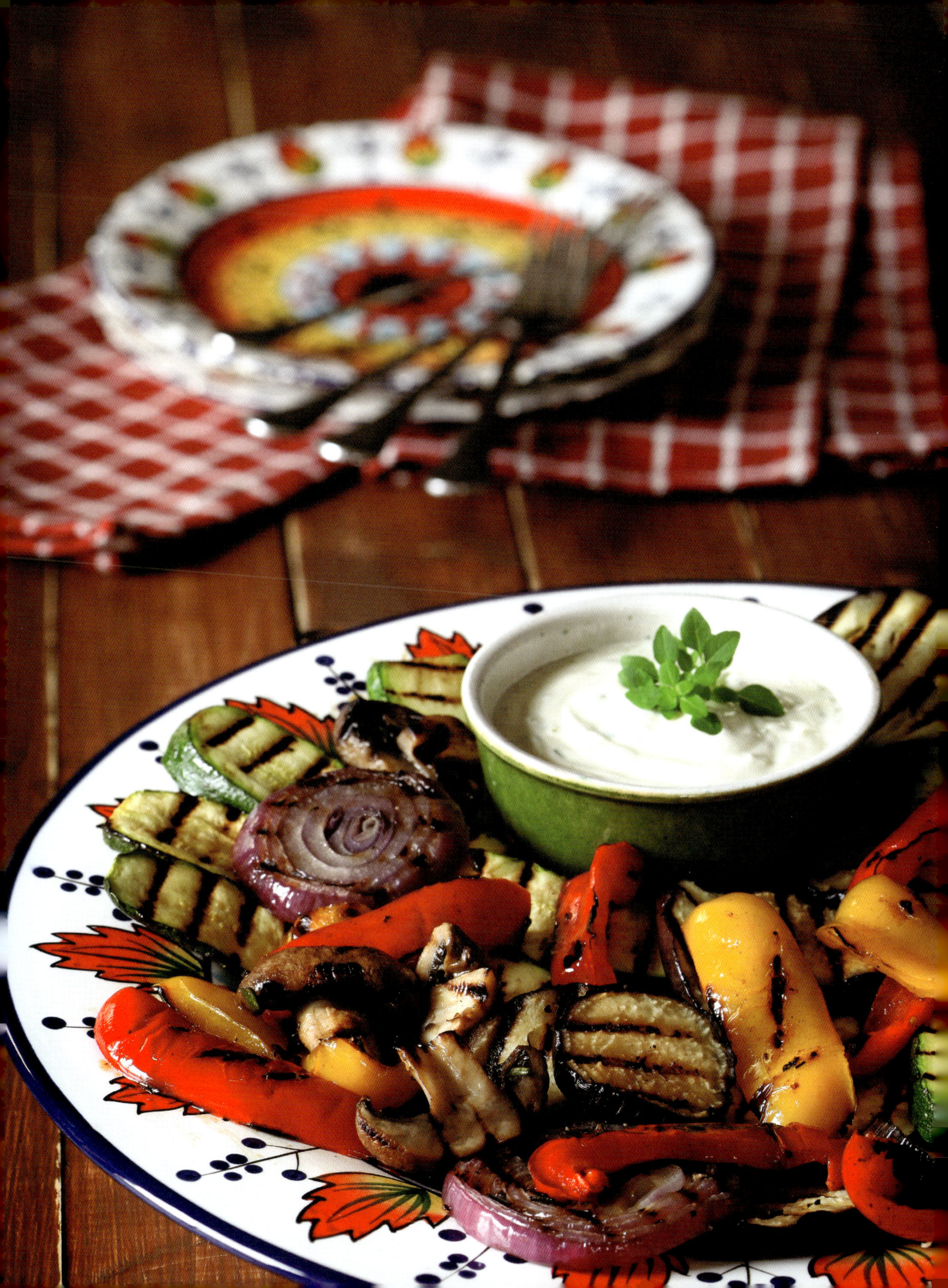

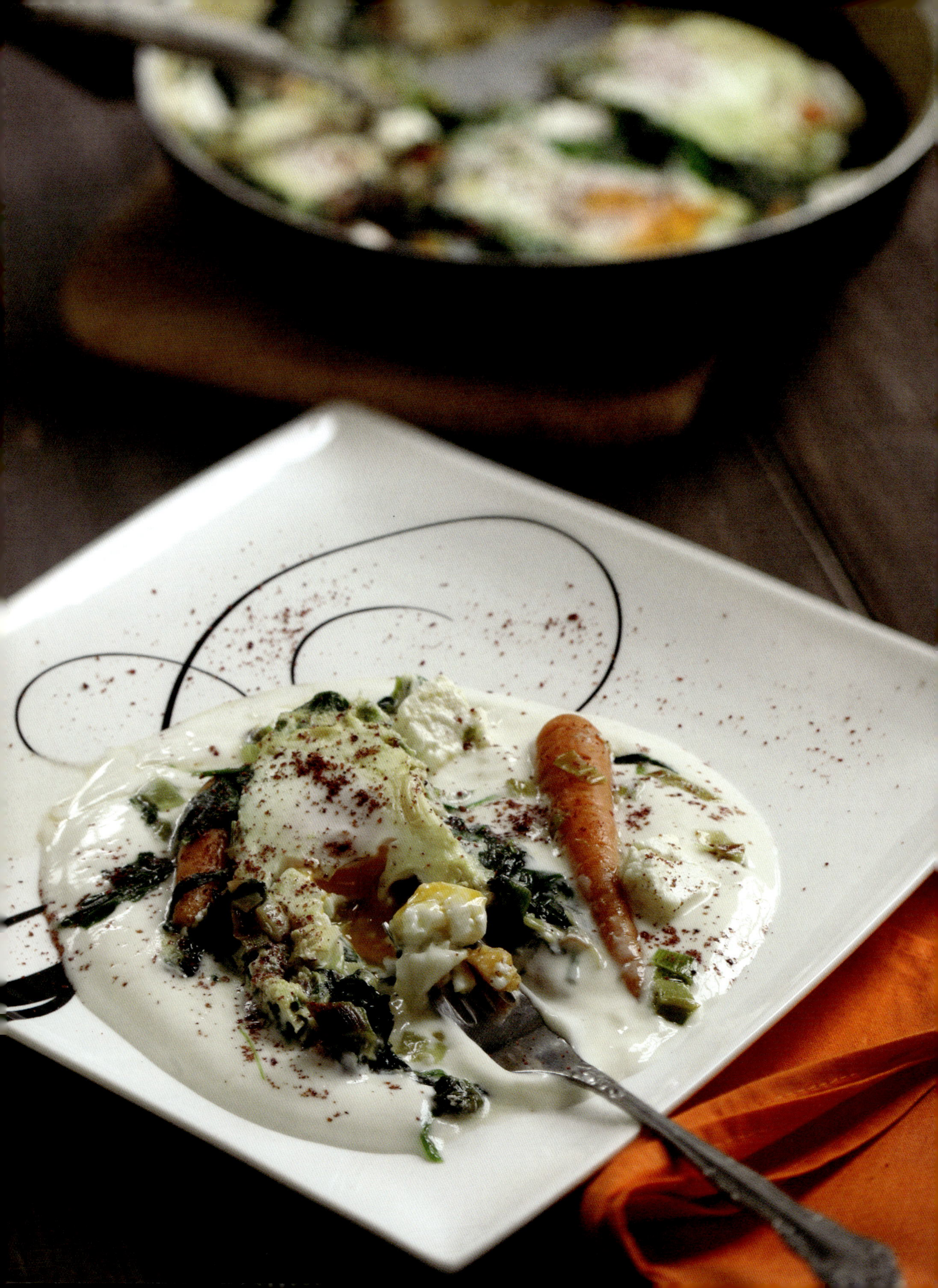

Spinach and Carrots Baked Eggs

2 tablespoons sunflower oil
50 ml (1½ fl oz) boiling water
1 medium leek, roughly chopped
6 small carrots
250 g (9 oz) baby spinach
4 large eggs
100 g (3½ oz) feta cheese, diced
a pinch of salt
250 g (9 oz) low fat yogurt
1 teaspoon sumac

Heat the oil and water In a medium frying pan over a medium heat for a few minutes. Throw in the chopped leek and carrots and sauté for about 5 minutes. Meanwhile, wash the spinach in a colander, transfer to a large bowl, pour over boiling water and scald for about 2 minutes, then return in the colander to drain. Throw the spinach into the frying pan, stir together with the leek and carrots and simmer for about 3 minutes. Using a spoon, make an indentation in the spinach and crack one egg into each indentation. Cover the frying pan and cook for about 5 minutes and then add the feta cheese and cook for 2 more minutes. Put 2 tablespoons of yogurt on each plate. Serve the spinach on top and sprinkle over the sumac and salt if needed.

Serves 4

Per serving
200 kcal, 12.1 g fat (4.7 g saturated), 9.6 g protein, 13.9 g carbs (13.2 g sugar), 5.4 g fibre, 2.0 g salt

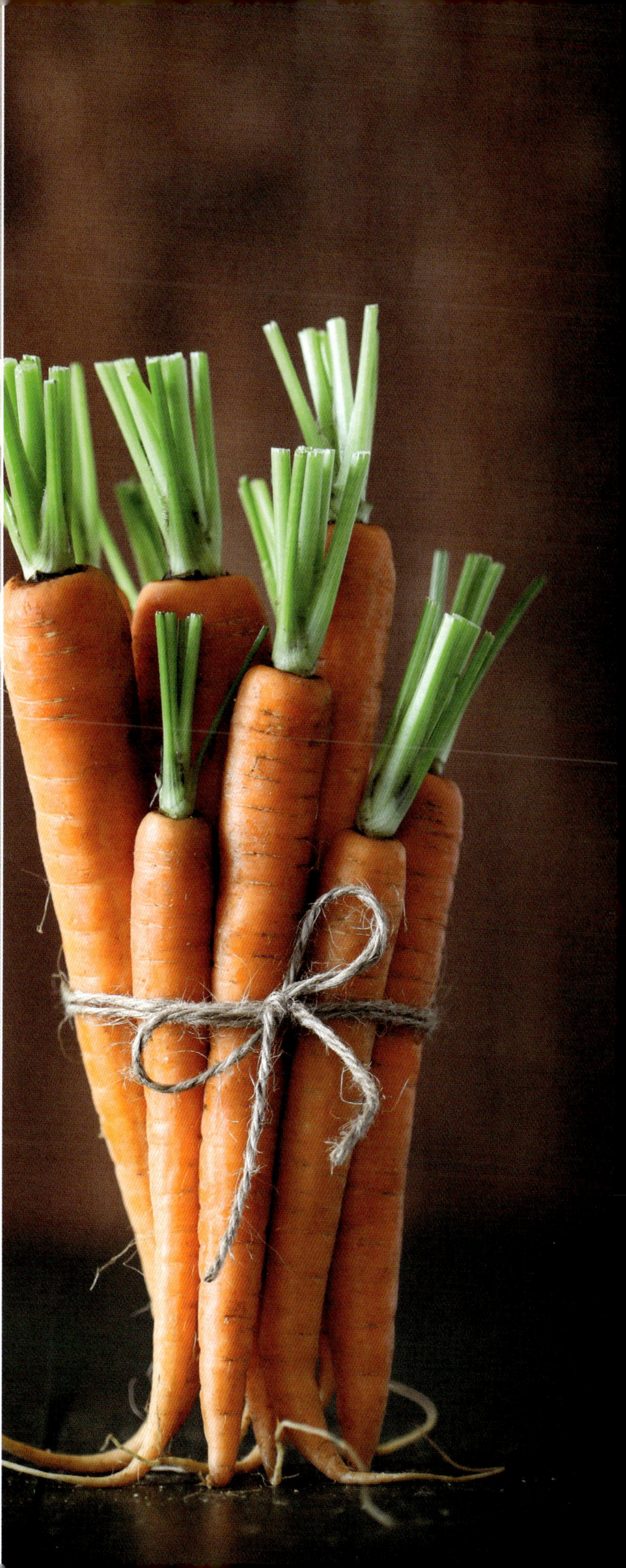

Cod Fillets with Creamy Yogurt Sauce

500 g (17½ oz) skinned and boneless cod fillets
6 tablespoons sunflower oil
200 g (7 oz) spring onions, finely chopped
1 garlic clove, crushed
1 tablespoon dried tarragon
1 teaspoon black pepper
a pinch of salt
150 ml (5 fl oz) double cream
25 ml (¾ fl oz) brandy
200 g (7 oz) low fat yogurt

Wash the fish and cut in 4 chunks. Heat the oil in a medium frying pan and fry the fish in batches over a medium heat for about 2 minutes on each side, until lightly browned. When cooked, take out of the pan and lay on cooking paper to drain the oil. Meanwhile, in a preheated pan with oil and 50ml (1½ fl oz) boiling water, throw in the spring onions, garlic, tarragon, black pepper and salt to season and cook, stirring all the time, for about 3 minutes. Add the cream and cook for another 2 minutes. Just before taking off the heat, add the brandy and stir well. Remove from the heat, add the yogurt and stir well again. Serve the yogurt sauce warm dividing on to 4 plates with a chunk of fish on top. Offer a glass of chardonnay white wine as optional.

Serves 4

Per serving
484 kcal, 37.3 g fat (14.4 g saturated), 27.3 g protein, 8.7 g carbs (7.9 g sugar), 1.1 g fibre, 1.0 g salt

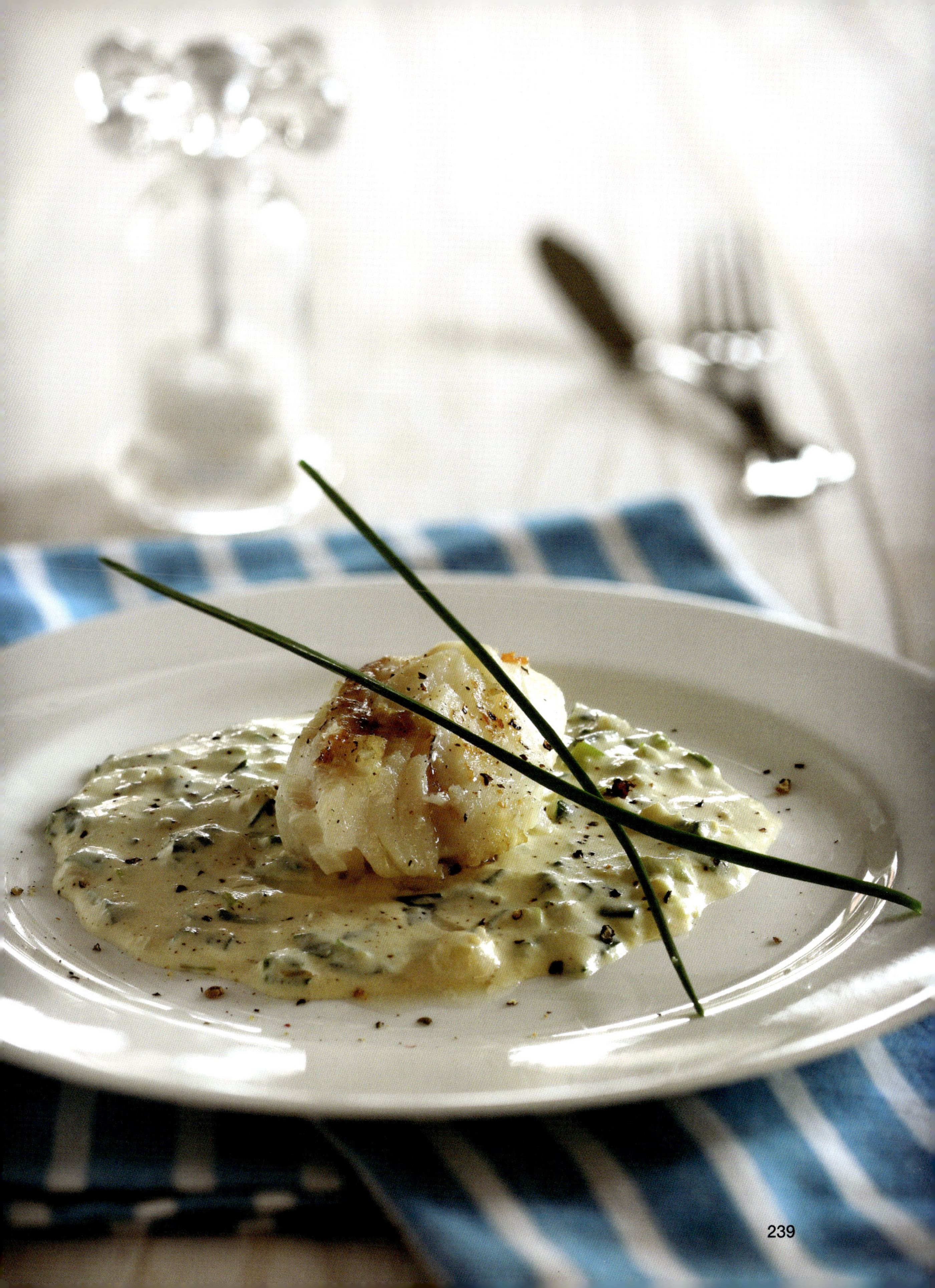

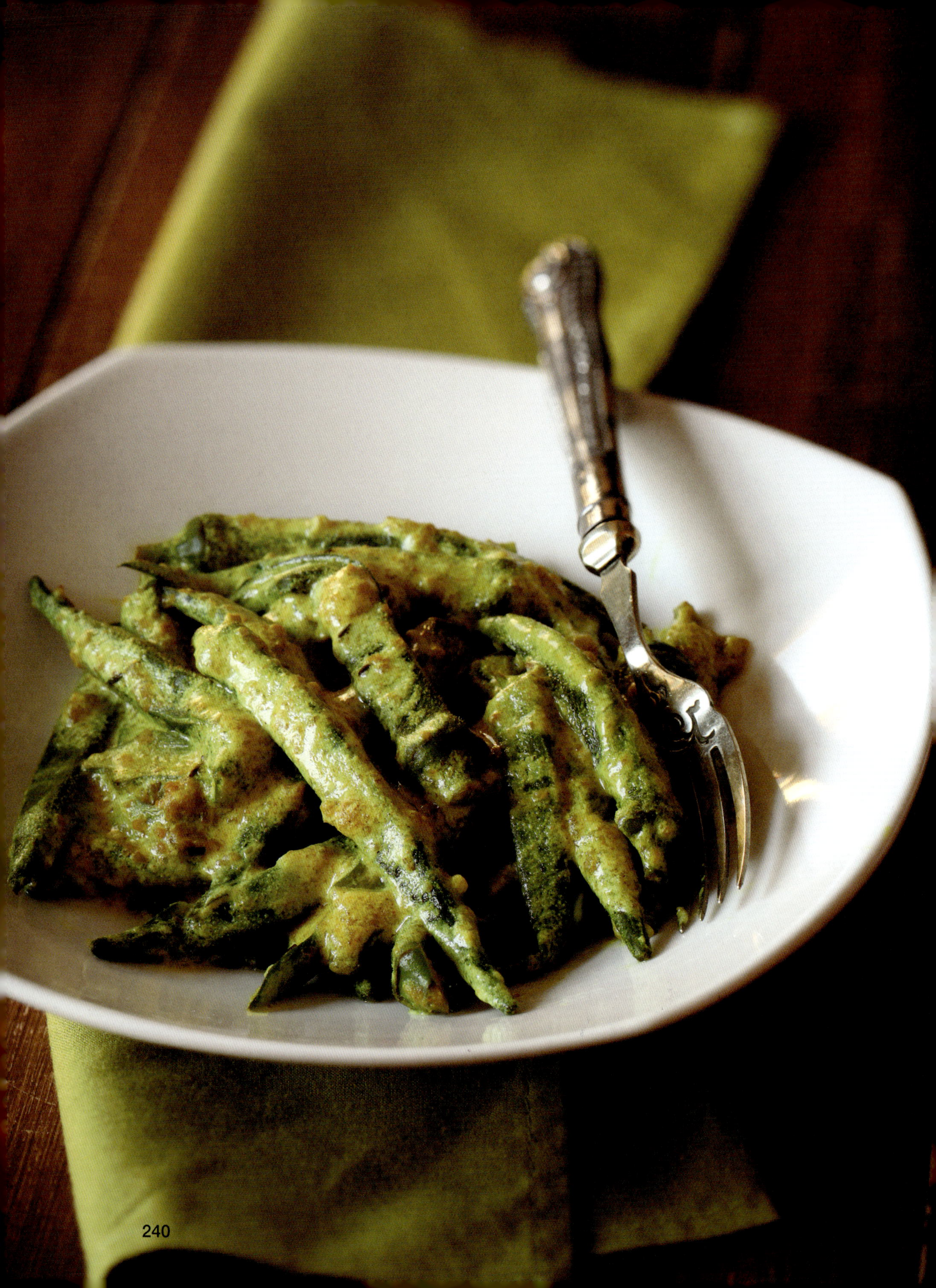

Okra in Yogurt

1 tablespoon caraway seeds
4 tablespoons vegetable oil
4 garlic cloves, chopped
1 tablespoon paprika
1 tablespoon brown sugar
a pinch of salt
2 tablespoons ground turmeric
600 g (21 oz) okra pods, halved
500 ml (17 fl oz) boiling water
3 tablespoons rye flour
200 g (7 oz) low fat yogurt

Toss the caraway seeds in a large dry frying pan and heat over high heat for about 1 minute until fragrant. Add the oil, garlic, paprika, sugar, salt and turmeric and cook for about 2 minutes until the garlic is soft. Add the halved okra and cook for about 1 minute before adding the boiling water. Bring to a simmer and cook for about 5 minutes until the okra is tender. Finally add the rye flour and cook for another 2 minutes, stirring all the time, until thickened. Once ready, remove from the heat and let it cool for 5 minutes. Pour the yogurt over the okra and mix well. Serve warm.

Serves 4

Per serving
240 kcal, 14.1 g fat (2.2 g saturated), 9.0 g protein, 22.7 g carbs (11.4 g sugar), 10.0 g fibre, 0.9 g salt

Russian Pelmeny

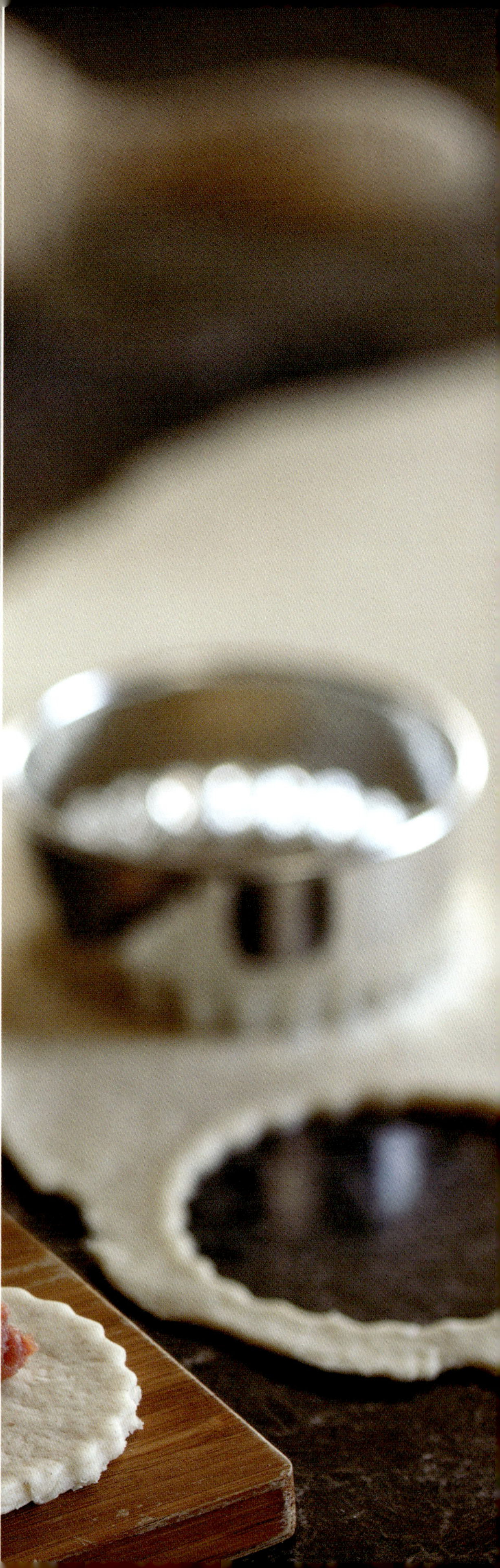

Dough:
3 egg
150 ml (5 fl oz) water
800 g (28 oz) flour
1 teaspoon vinegar
pinch of salt

Stuffing:
400 g (14 oz) beef mince
1 onion, finely chopped
1 carrot, finely chopped
1 handful fresh dill, finely chopped
1 teaspoon black pepper, freshly ground
pinch of salt

Yogurt dip:
200 g (7 oz) low fat yogurt to serve
1 tablespoon fresh dill, chopped
1 teaspoon black pepper, freshly ground

Mix thoroughly the beef mince with onion, chopped carrots, chopped dill, salt and pepper. Leave it to rest in the refrigerator.

Meanwhile make a pastry dough: combine the self raising flour, eggs, water, vinegar into a large bowl and knead to make a dough. Roll the dough with a rolling pin to a 2 mm thin base. Cut it into 50 mm circles with a biscuit cutter or if you haven't got one, use a large wine glass to cut the circles. Next add a tablespoon of the mince mixture on top of each circle and fold in half to close. You can choose to cook now or freeze for later. To cook, drop the pelmeny into a large pot with boiling salted water or broth. The pelmeny are ready when they emerge on the top in about 3 minutes or until meat is fully cooked. Drain them and serve in deep dishes, with a tablespoon of yogurt dip and garnish with dill.

Serves 8

Per serving
507 kcal, 12.1 g fat (4.5 g saturated), 23.5 g protein, 81 g carbs (4.5 g sugar), 4.6 g fibre, 1.0 g salt

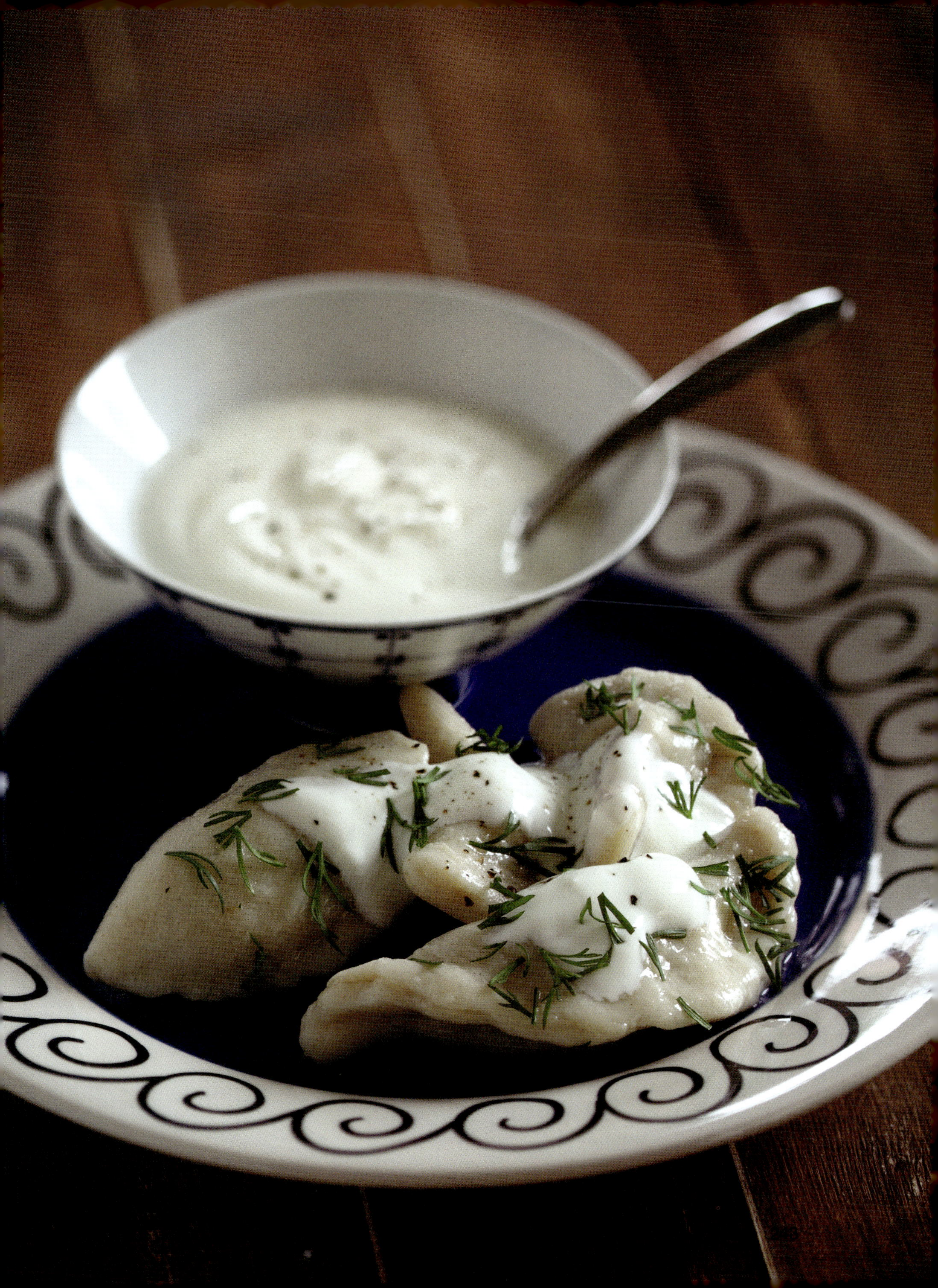

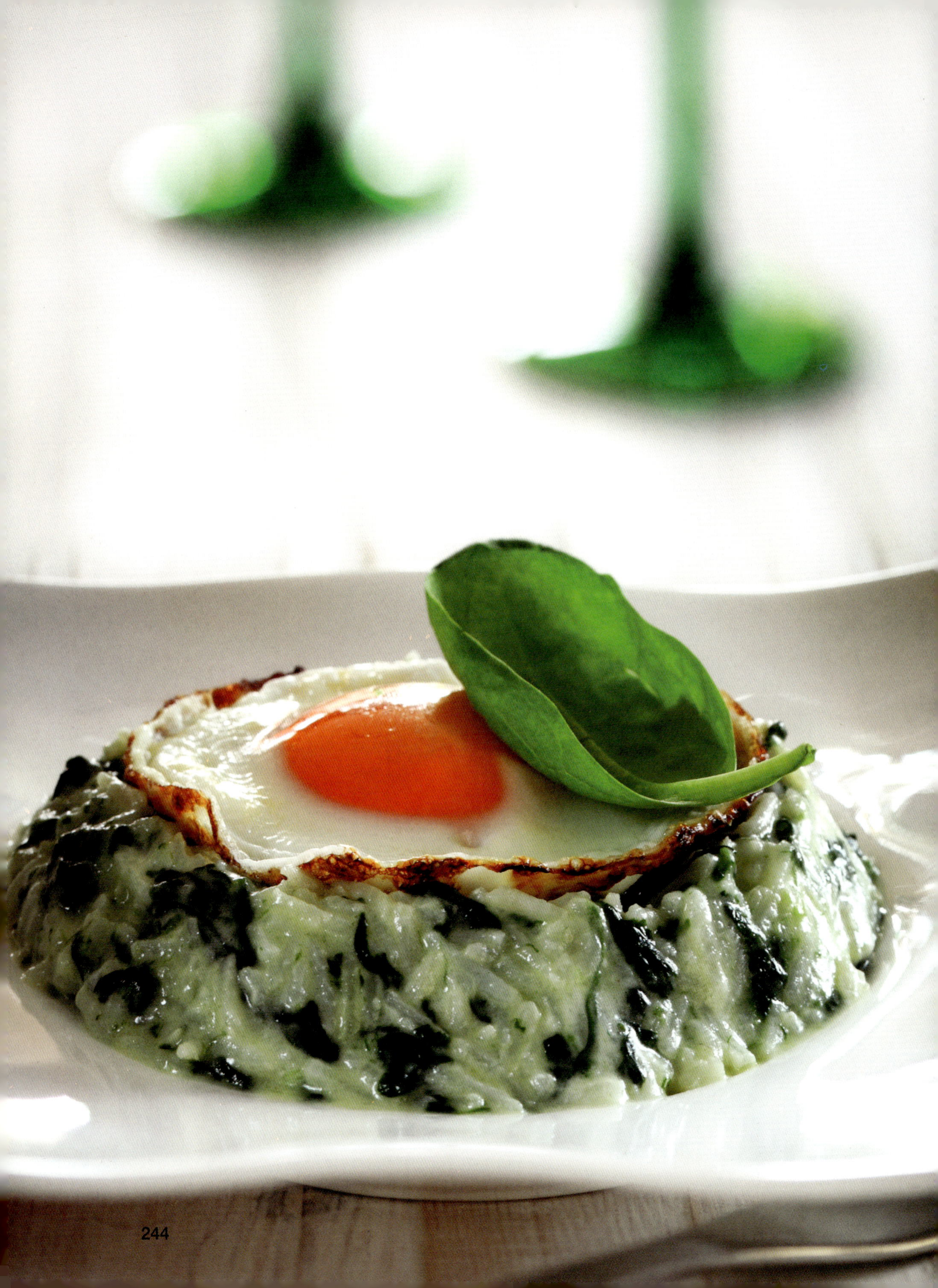

Spinach and Rice

200 g (7 oz) basmati rice, washed and boiled
450 g (16 oz) spinach, washed and roughly chopped
200 ml ($6\frac{3}{4}$ fl oz) semi-skimmed milk
70 g (3 oz) butter
200 g (7 oz) low fat yogurt
4 eggs
4 tablespoons vegetable oil

Wash the basmati rice a put into small pan with 500 ml (17 fl oz) boiling water and boil for about 10 minutes on medium heat while stirring constantly. Drain the rice and set aside. Meanwhile wash the spinach in a colander, roughly chop and throw in a large pan. Place the pan over a medium heat, add the butter, a cup of cold milk, and cook for about 5 minutes until the spinach softens. Add the boiled rice, mix well and cook for one more minute. Remove the pot from the heat. Meanwhile, preheat a frying pan with vegetable oil and fry the eggs in batches over a medium heat until lightly browned and crispy. Serve dividing the spinach and rice onto four plates, add 2-3 tablespoons of yogurt to each plate and on the top arrange a fried egg.

Serves 4

Per serving
557 kcal, 33.0 g fat (12.8 g saturated), 16.9 g protein, 47.9 g carbs (7.9 g sugar), 3.2 g fibre, 1.7 g salt

Stuffed Peppers in White Sauce

500 g (17½ oz) beef mince
100 g (3½ oz) basmati rice
1 tablespoons olive oil
6 bell peppers
1 medium leek, finely chopped
1 vine tomato, shredded
2 tablespoons fresh thyme, finely chopped
1 teaspoon ground black pepper
a pinch of salt

Sauce:
3 large free-range eggs
2 tablespoons white flour
150 g (5 oz) low fat yogurt
50 g (2 oz) butter

To prepare the stuffing, wash the basmati rice and boil in 500 ml (17 fl oz) of cold water in a small pan on medium heat for no more than 7 minutes so that it is almost but not completely cooked. Drain the water and set aside. Meanwhile throw the beef mince into a large saucepan and add 100 ml (3½ oz) cold water, 1 tablespoon olive oil and cook at high heat. Break up the mince with a wooden spoon until it has a loose texture. Keep cooking and stirring for about 15 minutes until the mince browns. Next add the finely chopped leek, chopped vine tomato, chopped fresh thyme, pinch of ground black pepper and salt. Cook for another 3 minutes, then add the boiled basmati rice, mix well and remove from the heat. Set aside the mixture for couple of minutes to cool.

Preheat the oven to 200°C (400°F). To prepare the stuffed peppers, wash and cut the stems of the peppers, remove the seeds and stuff the empty peppers with the mixture above. Arrange the peppers on a baking tray. Put the stems back on top of the peppers, add 300ml (10 fl oz) of boiling water to cover the bottom of the tray and bake in the oven for about 40 minutes.

To prepare the white sauce, whisk 3 eggs in a small pan, add melted butter and gradually add the flour while whisking constantly to break any lumps. Finally add one ladle of about 100ml (3½ oz) or more, if needed, of the sauce from the baking tray with the cooked peppers. Bring over high heat for about 5 minutes until the sauce becomes creamy. Remove from the heat and add the yogurt while stirring constantly. Serve the stuffed peppers warm over some white sauce and sprinkle some freshly grounded black pepper.

Serves 8

Per serving
325 kcal, 20 g fat (8.8 g saturated), 18.4 g protein, 18.0 g carbs (5.7 g sugar), 1.8 g fibre, 0.7 g salt

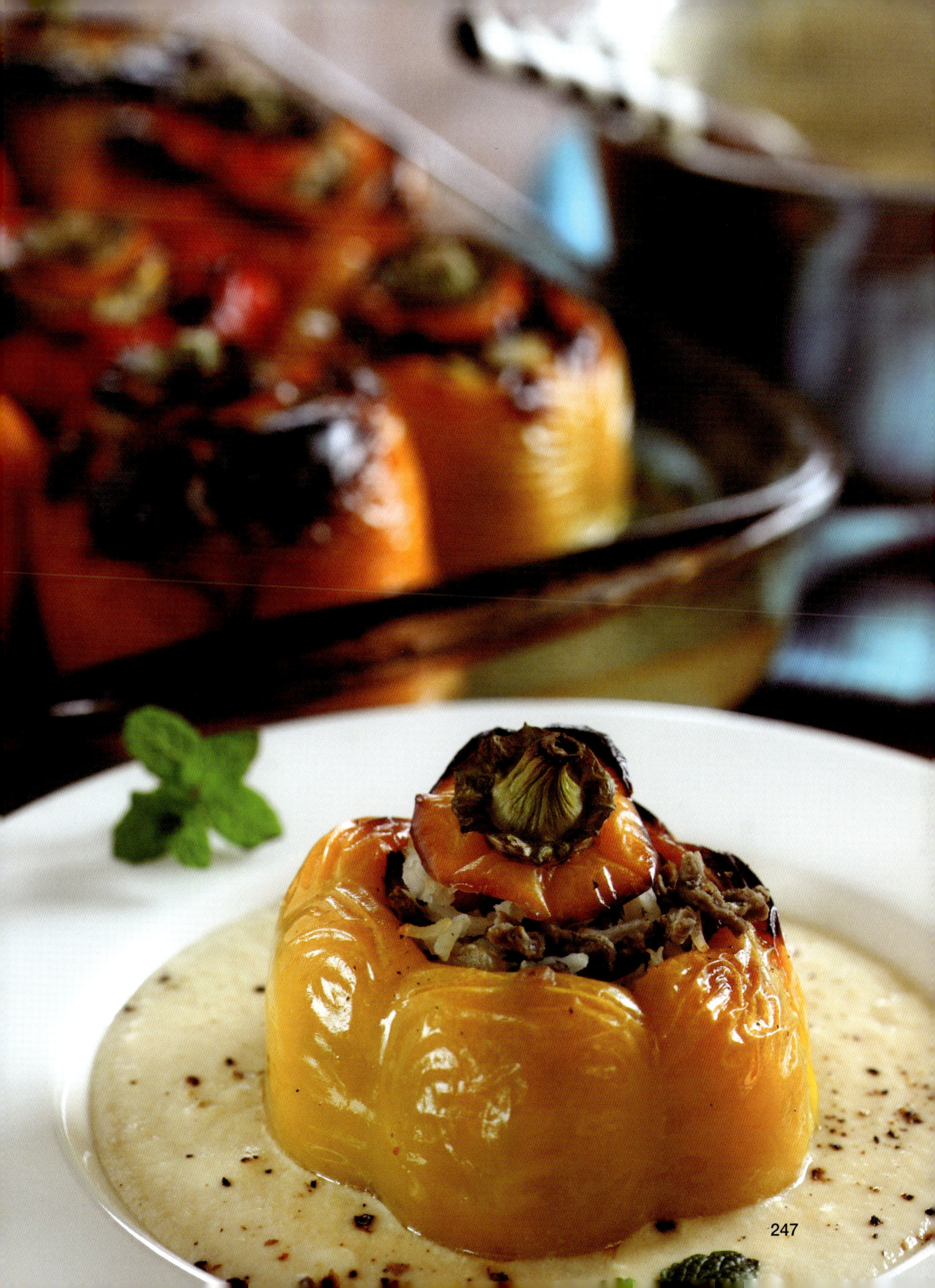

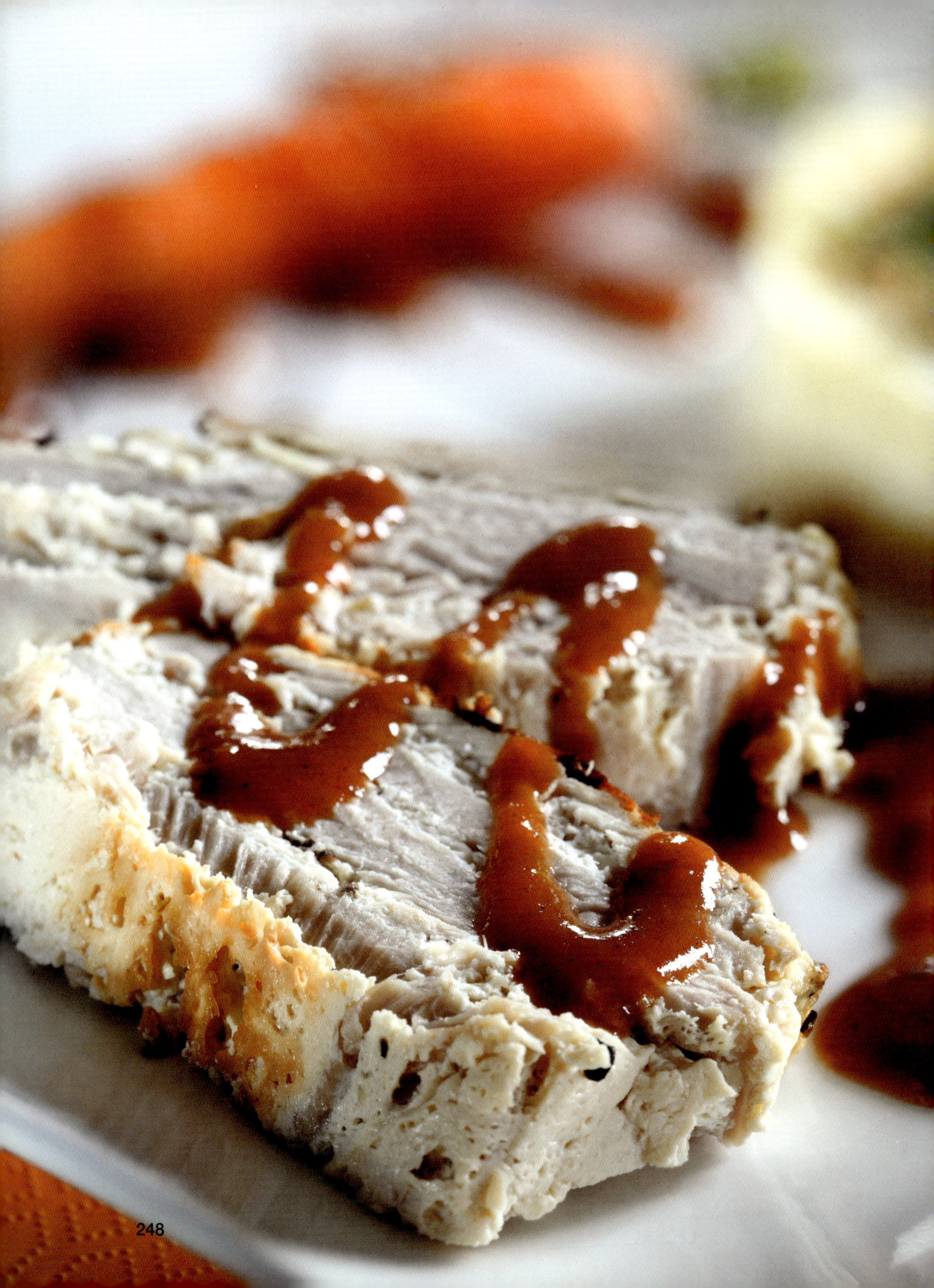

Turkey Yogurt Fillets

400 g (14 oz) turkey fillets
500 g (17½ oz) low fat yogurt
½ lime freshly squeezed juice
2 tablespoons sunflower oil
1 tablespoon mustard seeds
pinch black paper, grounded
pinch of salt

Preheat the oven to 200°C (400°F). Combine the yogurt, lime juice, sunflower oil, mustard seeds, freshly grounded black pepper, a pinch of salt and mix well. Arrange the turkey fillets in a small casserole pot with a lid, making alternate layers with the yogurt mixture. Cover the casserole pot with a lid and cook in the oven for about 50 minutes. Remove the lid and cook for another 5 minutes until the top becomes golden. Remove from the oven, gently take the yogurt fillets out of the casserole pot and place on a chopping board. Cut into 1 cm (½ inch) thick slices across the meat to reveal the different the layers. Serve warm together with mash potato and some boiled green peas and carrots.

Serves 4

Per serving
225 kcal, 9.2 g fat (2.0 g saturated), 29.4 g protein, 9.5 g carbs (9.5 g sugar), 0.0 g fibre, 1.1 g salt

Yellow Split Peas Casserole

250 g (9 oz) low fat yogurt, strained
250 g (9 oz) yellow split peas
2 medium carrots, chopped
2 medium parsnips, chopped
1 medium leek, finely chopped
4 whole cloves garlic, peeled
2 tablespoons vegetable oil
1 tablespoon mint, dry
1 teaspoon paprika
1 teaspoon thyme, dry
some freshly grounded black pepper
a pinch of salt

Put the yellow split peas in a small pan, add water and bring to boil for about 5 minutes over high heat. Remove from the heat, drain the water and transfer into a large pan. Add the chopped carrots, parsnip, leek, peeled whole cloves garlic, vegetable oil, dry mint, paprika, dry thyme, a pinch of salt and 2 litres (4¼ pints) of cold water and bring to boil. Cook on the stove over medium heat for about 45 minutes. Serve warm with a tablespoon of strained yogurt and sprinkle with freshly grounded black pepper.

Serves 6

Per serving
227 kcal, 5.6 g fat (1.0 g saturated), 12.5 g protein, 33.8 g carbs (7.7 g sugar), 6.6 g fibre, 0.6 g salt

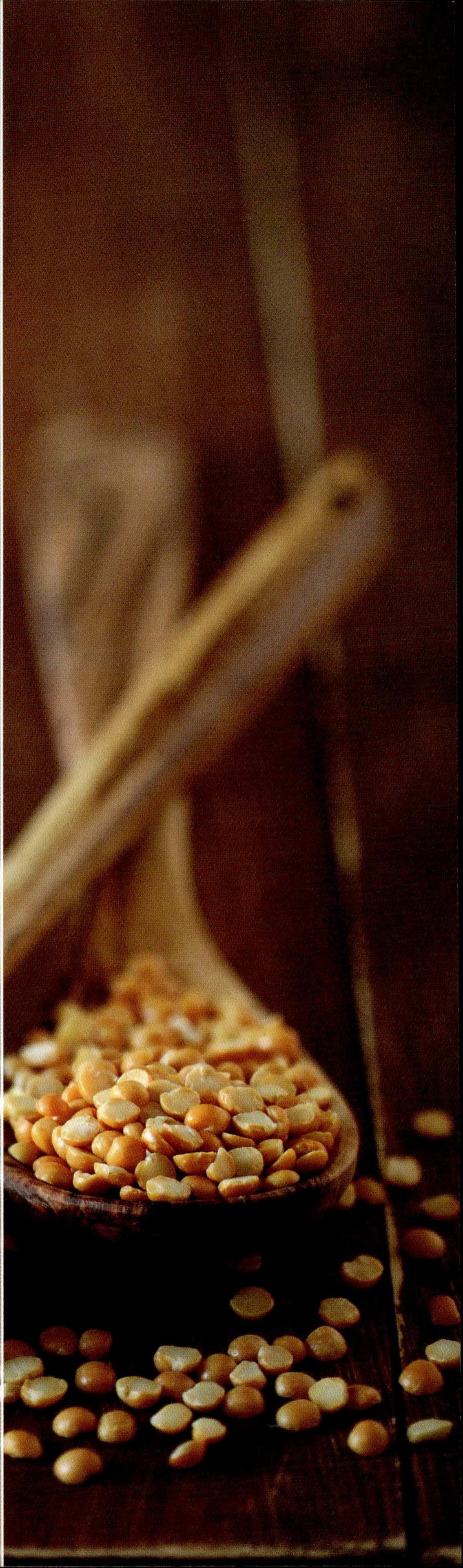

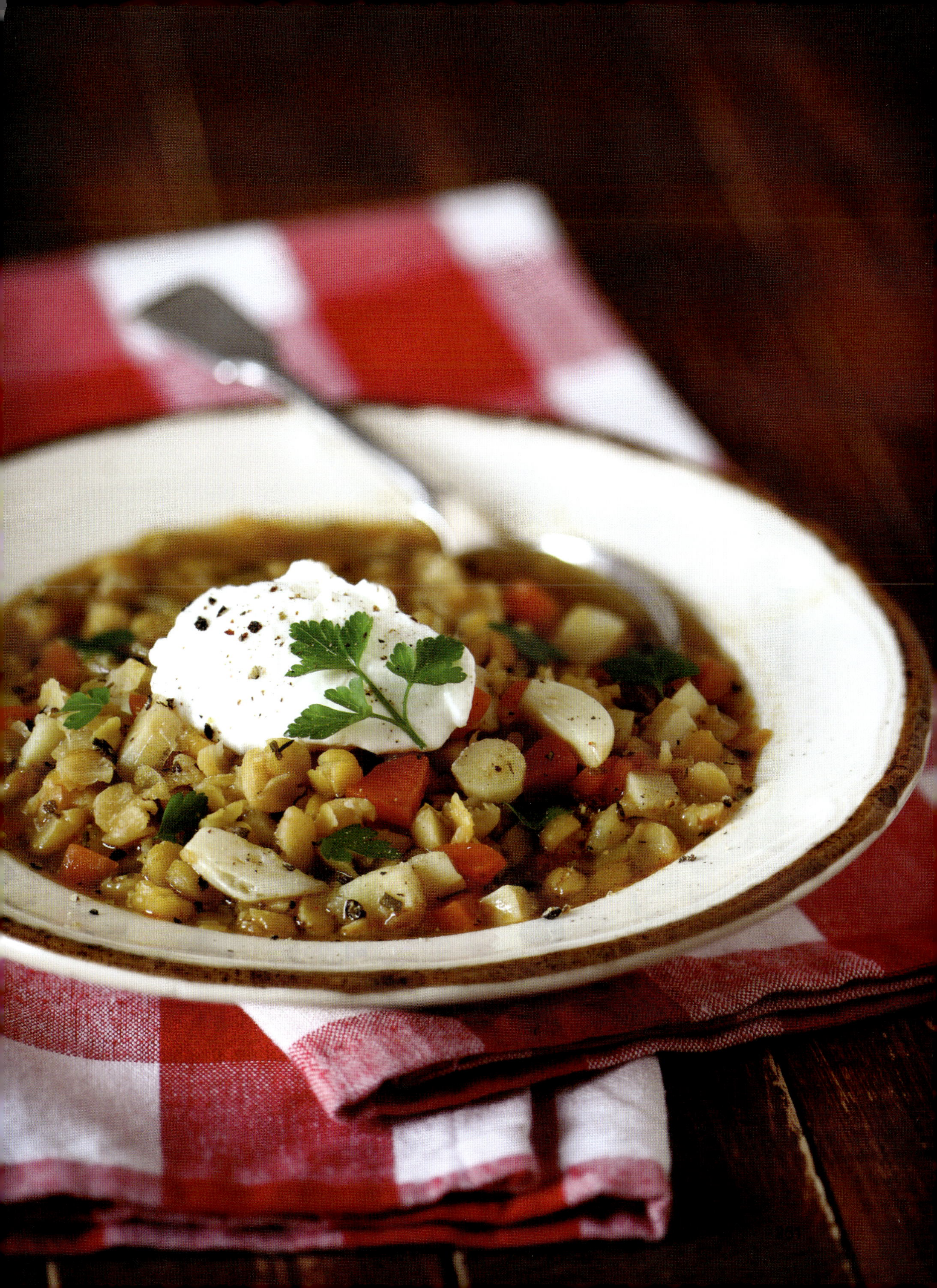

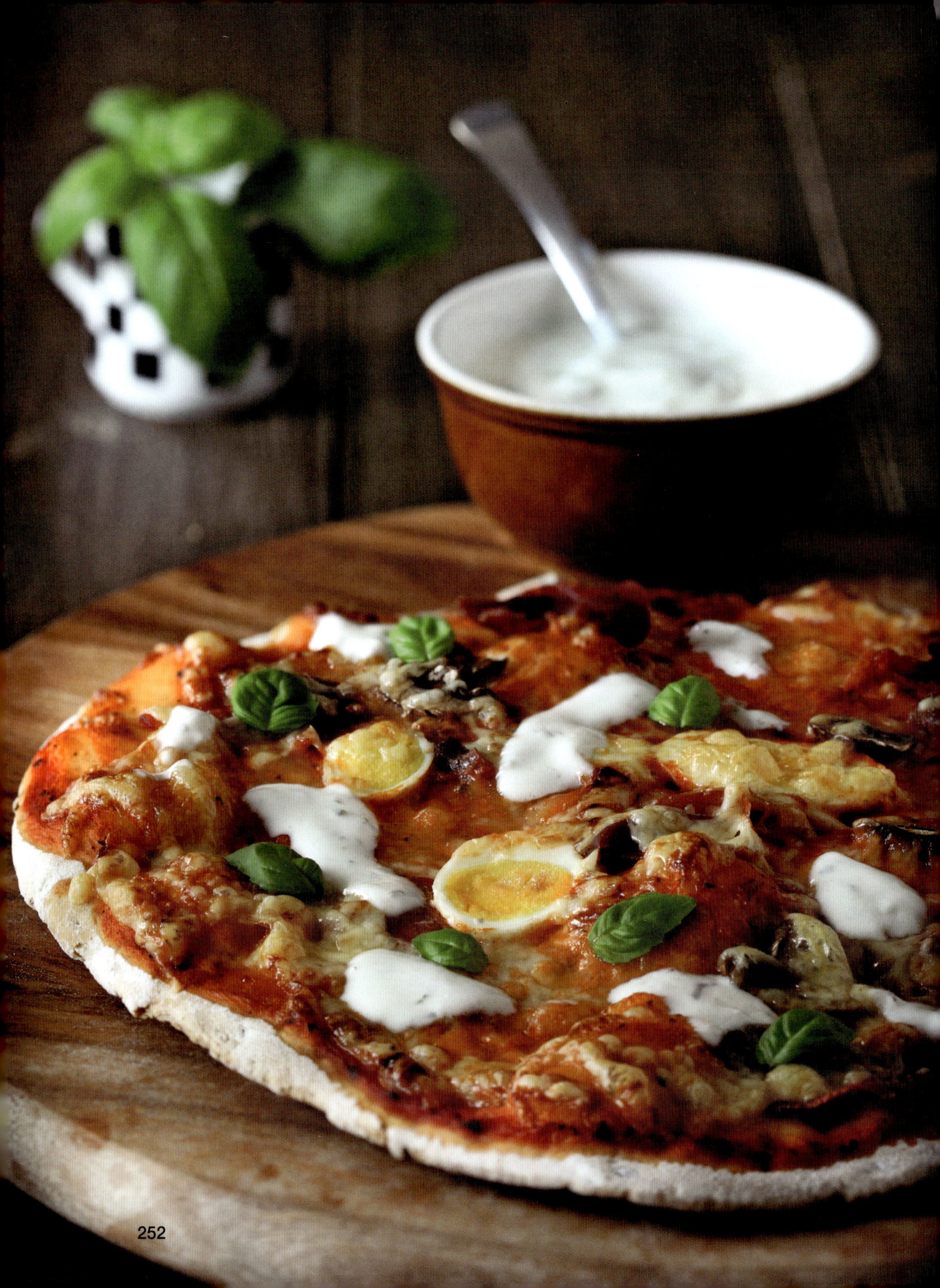

Homemade Pizza and Garlic Yogurt Sauce

300 ml (10 fl oz) warm but not boiling water, about 40°C/104°F
2 teaspoons active dry yeast
500 g (17½ oz) plain white flour
a pinch of sugar
2 pinches of salt
1 tablespoon linseeds
3 tablespoons sunflower oil, plus extra to glaze

For the topping:
150 g (5 oz) tomato and basil sauce
150 g (5 oz) mozzarella cheese, ripped by hand
3 mushrooms, sliced
80 g (3 oz) Serrano ham
2 eggs, hard-boiled and sliced
150 g (5 oz) Cheddar cheese, grated
15 fresh basil leaves

For the garlic yogurt sauce:
200 g (7 oz) low fat yogurt
2 garlic cloves, crushed
2 tablespoons extra virgin olive oil
1 tablespoon dried oregano
a pinch of salt

To make the yogurt sauce, in a small bowl, combine the yogurt, garlic, olive oil, oregano and salt and mix well. Leave to rest in the refrigerator for 15 minutes or longer.

To make the pizza base, pour the warm water into a small bowl and add the yeast. Stir gently to allow the yeast to dissolve completely. Meanwhile, in a large bowl add the flour, sugar, salt and linseeds. Then add the olive oil and the dissolved yeast, mix well and knead to make a smooth and elastic dough. If needed, add more flour or water. Brush over some oil to cover and glaze the dough, cover with kitchen towel and leave in a warm place for about 1 hour or longer until it doubles In size.

Preheat the oven to 200°C (400°F). Knead the dough a little and then divide into three balls. Take the first dough ball, flatten using a rolling pin or your hands to make a round base about 5mm thick. The thinner the base, the crispier the pizza will be when baked. Oil the surface and spoon over a third of the tomato sauce. Arrange a third of the mozzarella cheese, mushrooms, ham and sliced boiled eggs on top and sprinkle over the grated Cheddar cheese. Repeat with the remaining dough and ingredients. Put the pizza on a pizza stone or a baking tray and bake for about 15 minutes. Serve the pizza warm with the garlic yogurt sauce and fresh basil leaves over the top.

Serves 3

Per serving
623 kcal, 32.9 g fat (12.1 g saturated), 31.2 g protein, 53.9 g carbs (8.4 g sugar), 3.9 g fibre, 4.1 g salt

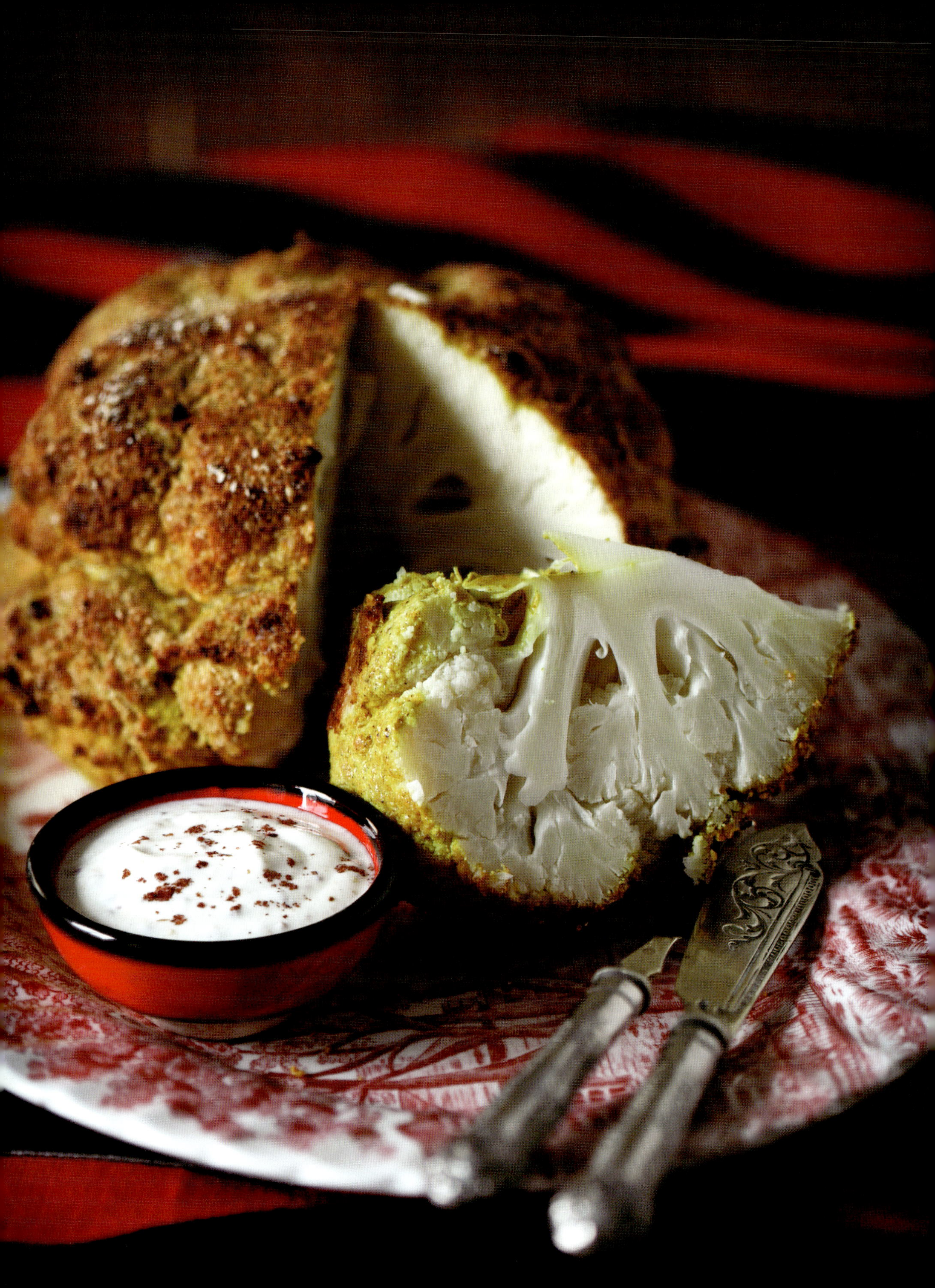

Roasted Cauliflower

1 cauliflower head
250 g (9 oz) low fat yogurt
2 tablespoons grape seed oil
2 cloves garlic, crushed
1 teaspoon allspice, ground
1 teaspoon turmeric, ground
2 tablespoons oatbran
generous pinch of salt

Yogurt dip:
100 g (3½ oz) low fat yogurt
1 tablespoon extra virgin olive oil
1 teaspoon wholegrain mustard
1 teaspoon sumac, ground

Prehea the oven to 200°C (400°F). Gently remove the green leaves and cut the woody stem of the cauliflower head. Trim off the base and wash and set aside. Meanwhile into a large bowl combine the low fat yogurt, the grape seed oil, crushed garlic, ground allspice, ground turmeric and a generous pinch of salt and mix well. Then steep the cauliflower head into the bowl and by hand spread the mixture all over the cauliflour. Then remove the cauliflower head to a slightly oiled baking sheet and roast it in the oven for about 30 minutes until the cauliflower surface is dry and slightly brown. Remove from the oven and leave it to rest and cool a bit before cutting and serving. Meanwhile prepare the dressing, in a small bowl combine the low fat yogurt, extra virgin olive oil, coarse mustard, grounded sumac and mix well. Serve a piece of roasted cauliflower over some green salad and pour over the yogurt dressing.

Serves 6

Per serving
105 kcal, 6.8 g fat (1.2 g saturated), 4.9 g protein, 6.4 g carbs (5.5 g sugar), 1.5 g fibre, 1.0 g salt

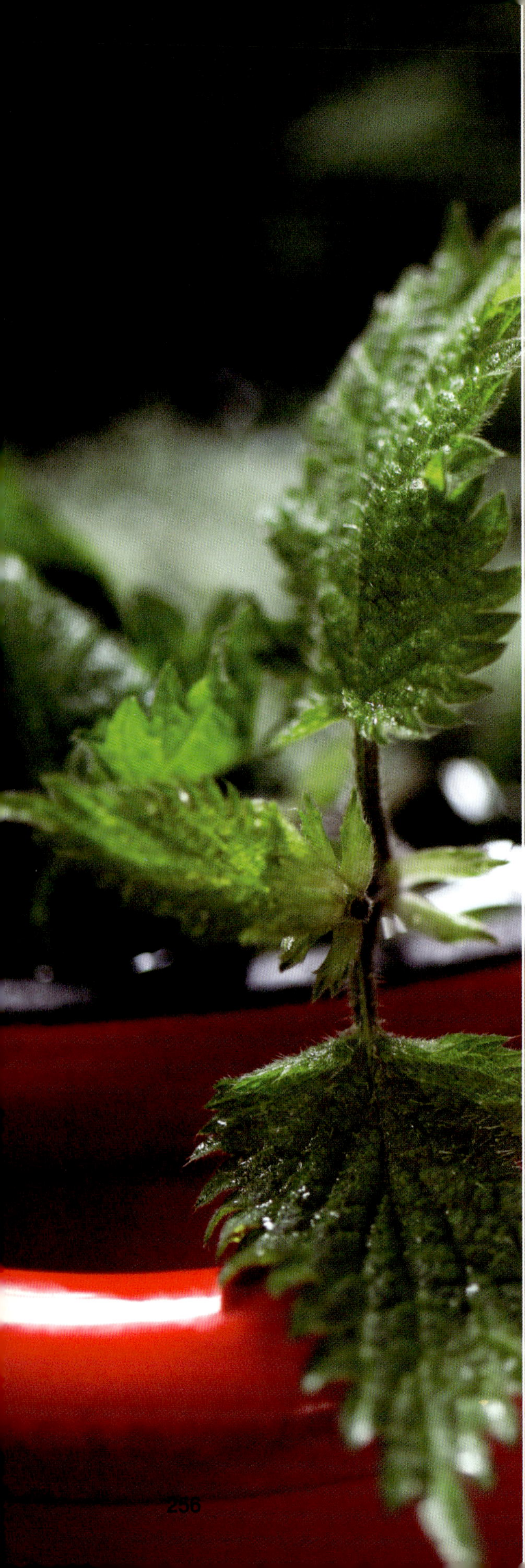

Spring Nettles and Eggs

150 g (5 oz) young nettle tips
2 litres (4½ pints) boiling water
50 g (2 oz) butter
12 spring onions, finely chopped
a pinch of salt
8 large eggs
100 g (3½ oz) feta cheese, diced
250 g (9 oz) low fat yogurt
a pinch of sumac
handful flat leaf parsley, chopped
1 dried sweet red pointed peppers, chopped (optional)

Personally, I pick young nettle tips from the local park or wood, which is great in spring time! Remember to use silicone gloves to pick them and wash the nettles thoroughly in a colander. Throw into a large pan, add the boiling water and boil over a high heat for about 5 minutes until tender. Drain into a colander and keep pressing to make a green ball. Transfer to a chopping board, chop finely and set aside. Meanwhile, melt the butter in a large frying pan and throw in the spring onions and a pinch of salt. Cook over a high heat for about 2 minutes until tender. Add the chopped nettles and cook for another 2 minutes. Crack In the eggs, mix well and cook for another 2 minutes. Remove from the heat, add the feta cheese, pour over a spoonful of yogurt and mix well. Serve garnished with a pinch of sumac and chopped parsley.

Serves 4

Per serving
353 kcal, 27.3 g fat (13.5 g saturated), 21.0 g protein, 6.5 g carbs (6.4 g sugar), 2.0 g fibre, 2.5 g salt, Nettles are also rich in vitamin C and iron.

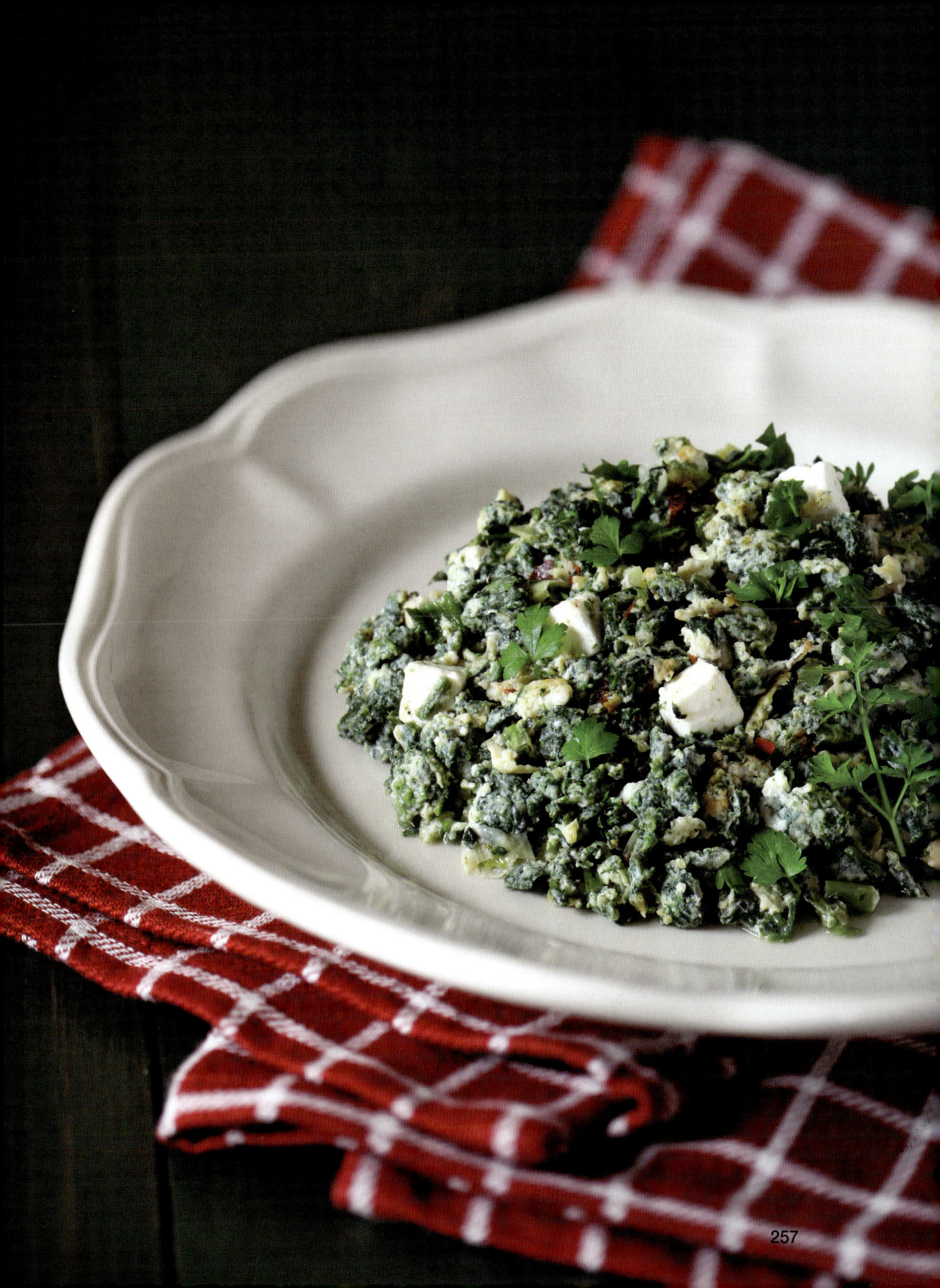

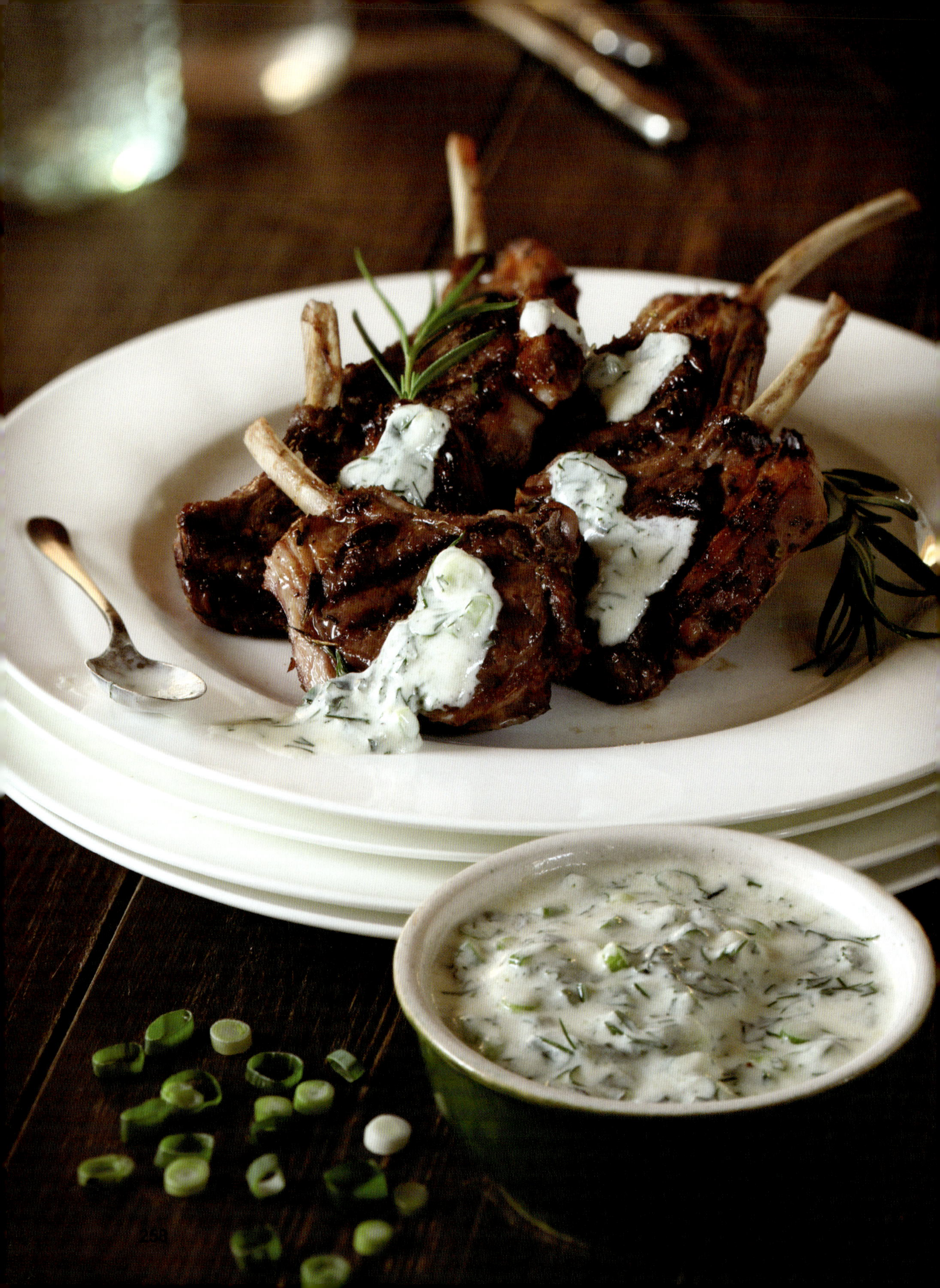

Lamb with Yogurt Minty Sauce

Lamb:
2 tablespoons fresh rosemary, chopped
4 cloves garlic
1 tablespoon oregano, dried
a pinch of salt
100 ml (3½ oz) grape seed oil
100 ml (3½ oz) red wine
freshly squeezed juice of ½ lime
1 rack of lamb, cut on chops, 600 g (21 oz)

Sauce:
250 g (9 oz) low fat yogurt
1 tablespoon extra virgin olive oil
freshly squeezed juice of ½ lime
100 g (3½ oz) spring onions, finely chopped
4 tablespoons fresh mint, finely chopped
2 tablespoons fresh dill, finely chopped
pinch of freshly ground black pepper
pinch of salt

To make the marinade, place the garlic, rosemary, oregano and a pinch of salt into the bowl of a food processor and blend until the herbs are finely minced. Add the lime juice, olive oil, and red wine and blend again.
Place the lamb chops in a ceramic dish just large enough to hold them in a single layer. Pour the marinade over the chops. Cover with plastic wrap and refrigerate for about 3 hours or overnight.
To cook the lamb, preheat a grill pan on high heat and grill the lamb chops for about 5 minutes on each side. Remove from the pan to a pan with a lid to keep them warm and leave to rest for about 5 minutes.
To make the yogurt minty sauce, combine the yogurt, olive oil, lime juice, chopped spring onions, chopped mint, chopped dill, freshly ground black pepper and a pinch of salt in a medium bowl and mix well. Serve the lamb chops warm with some Yogurt Minty Sauce on top.

Serves 6

Per serving
576 kcal, 49.2 g fat (17.2 g saturated), 25.8 g protein, 4.8 g carbs (3.8 g sugar), 0.6 g fibre, 1.2 g salt

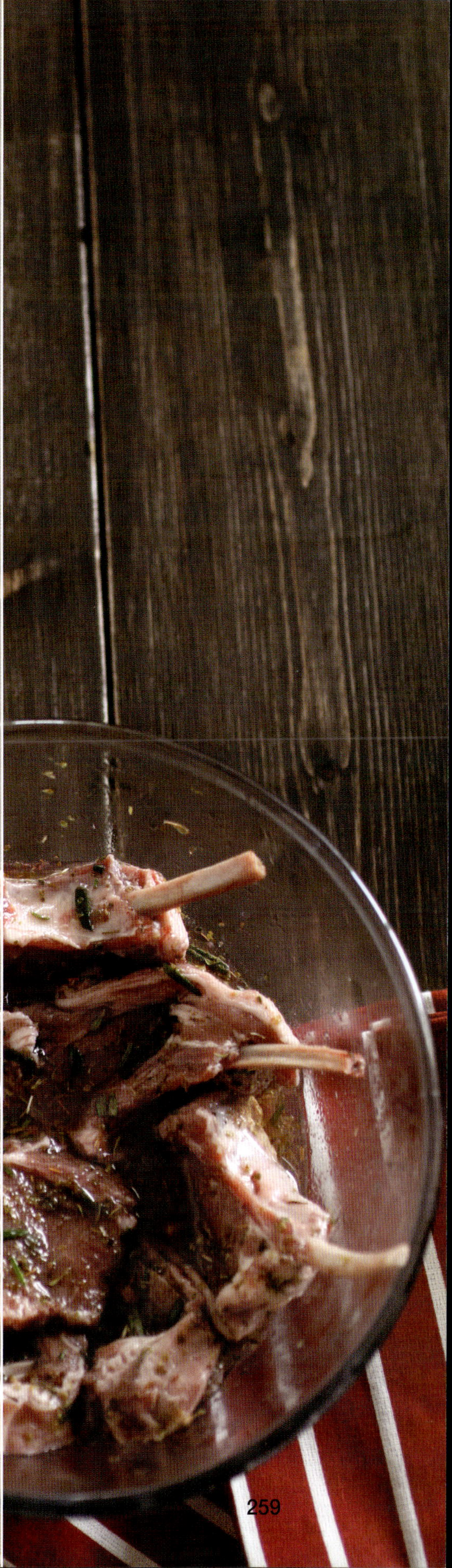

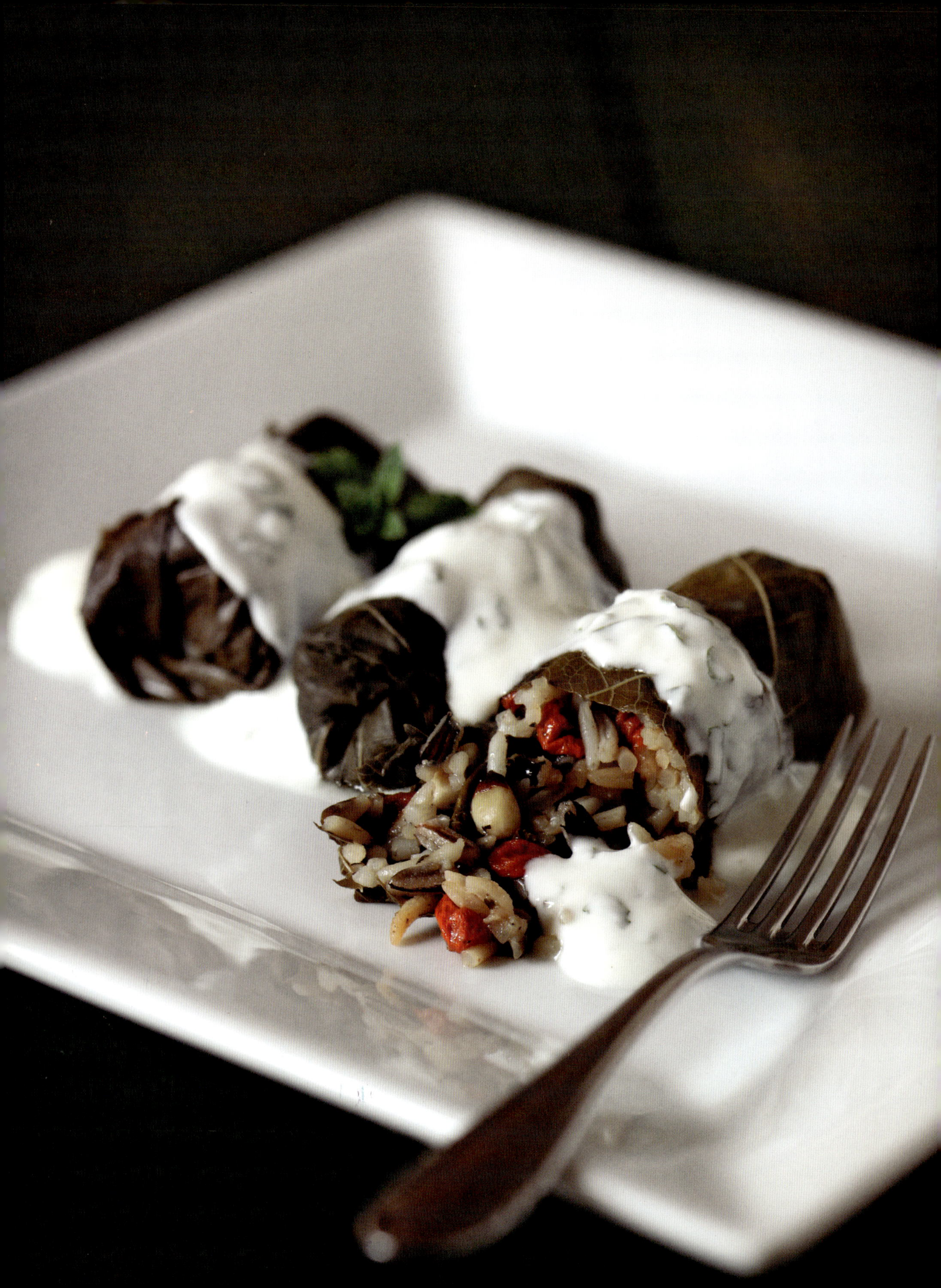

Stuffed Vine Leaves (Sarmy)

100 g (3½ oz) basmati and wild rice
50 ml (1½ fl oz) sunflower oil
3 large shallots, chopped
20 g (¾ oz) dried goji berries
20 g (¾ oz) pine nuts, toasted
1 teaspoon asafoetida
1 teaspoon nutmeg
1 tablespoon dried mint
a pinch of salt
200 g (7 oz) vine leaves preserved in brine
sliced carrots, for cooking if necessary

For the yogurt topping:
250 g (9 oz) low fat yogurt
freshly squeezed juice of ½ lime
2 tablespoons chopped fresh mint leaves
a pinch of salt

To make the stuffing, boil the basmati and wild rice in a small saucepan in 500 ml (17 fl oz) water for no more than 7 minutes so that it is almost but not completely cooked. Drain the water and set aside. Heat the sunflower oil and 50 ml (1½ fl oz) boiling water in a large saucepan, add the shallots and cook over a high heat for about 5 minutes until tender. Remove from the heat, add the goji berries, pine nuts, turmeric, nutmeg, dried mint and salt and mix well. Add the cooked rice, mix well.

Place a vine leave on a chopping board and spoon one tablespoon of stuffing on top. Fold in the edges of the leaf and roll up. Repeat with the rest of the leaves and stuffing.

Cover the bottom of a large saucepan with the leftover leaves or slice some carrots to prevent the wraps sticking to the bottom of the pan. Arrange the stuffed vine leaves on top, in compact layers to prevent breaking. Cover the wraps with a small porcelain plate to press them, and prevent them from moving, and pour over boiling water just to cover the plate. Put the lid on the top and cook over medium heat for about 25 minutes.

Meanwhile, in a small bowl combine the yogurt, lime juice, chopped mint, pinch of salt and mix well. Serve the stuffed vine leaves warm with some yogurt mixture on top.

Serves 6

Per serving
192 kcal, 11 g fat (1 g saturated), 5 g protein, 18 g carbs (4 g sugar), 0.5 g fibre, 2.4 g salt

Lamb Casserole with Yogurt Topping

600 g (21 oz) lamb, boned and diced
1 tablespoon paprika
2 tablespoon corn flour
2 leeks, finely chopped
1 carrot, peeled and sliced
200 g (7 oz) baby button mushrooms, halved
3 tablespoons olive oil
100 g (3½ oz) red wine
200 g (7 oz) vine tomatoes, chopped
50 g (2 oz) prunes
1 teaspoon cinnamon, ground
3 small bay leaves
pinch of black pepper, ground
pinch of sugar
pinch of salt

Preheat the oven to 180°C (350°F). In a large bowl mix the diced lamb with the corn flour, ground black pepper, sugar and salt, make sure each piece of lamb is coated. Leave to rest for a few minutes to allow the meat to absorb the flavor. Heat the oil mixed with 200 ml (6¾ fl oz) boiling water in a large pan. Add the chopped leek, carrot and the lamb and cook for about 10 minutes until the lamb becomes brown. Next transfer to flameproof casserole dish and add the red wine, chopped tomatoes, prunes, ground cinnamon, bay leaves, halved mushrooms and stir well and cook in the oven for about 50 minutes. Serve warm with a spoonful of yogurt topping over the top.

Yogurt topping:
200 g (7 oz) low fat yogurt
2 cloves garlic, crushed
1 tablespoon fresh mint leaves, chopped

In a small bowl combine the low fat yogurt, crushed garlic, chopped mint leaves and mix well.

Serves 4
Per serving
282 kcal, 16 g fat (6 g saturated), 23 g protein, 10 g carbs (9 g sugar), 3.1 g fibre, 0.8 g salt

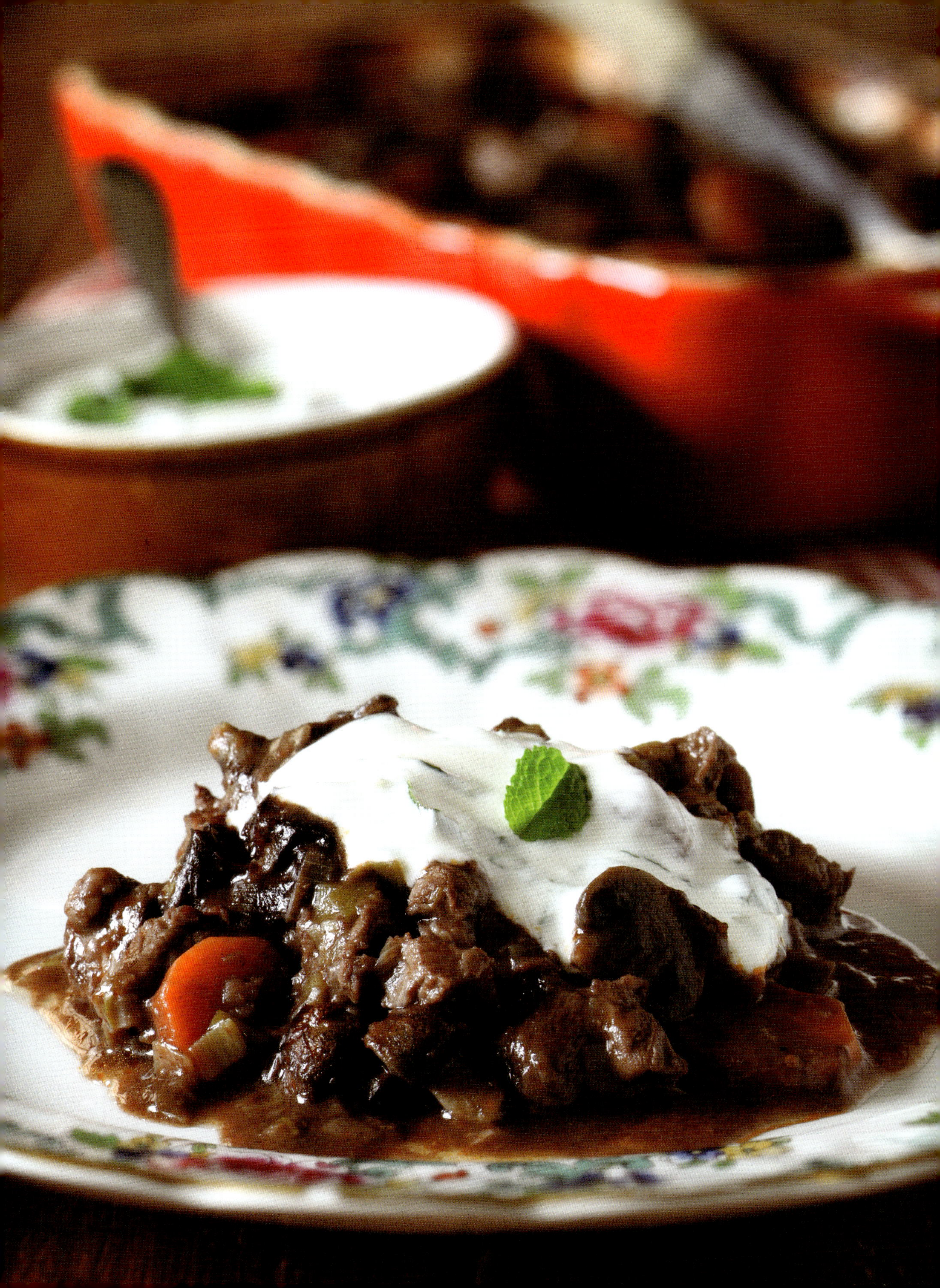

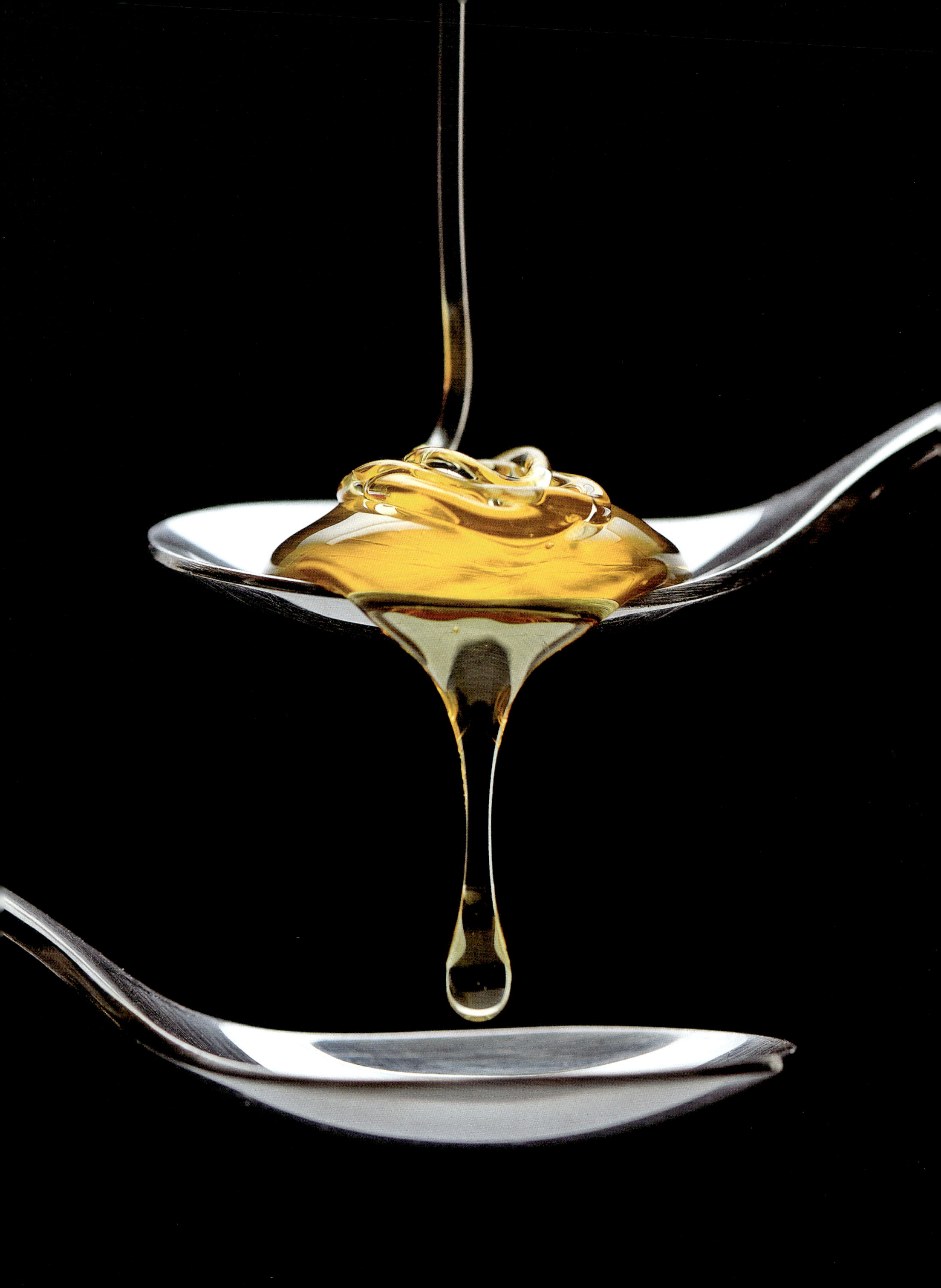

Desserts

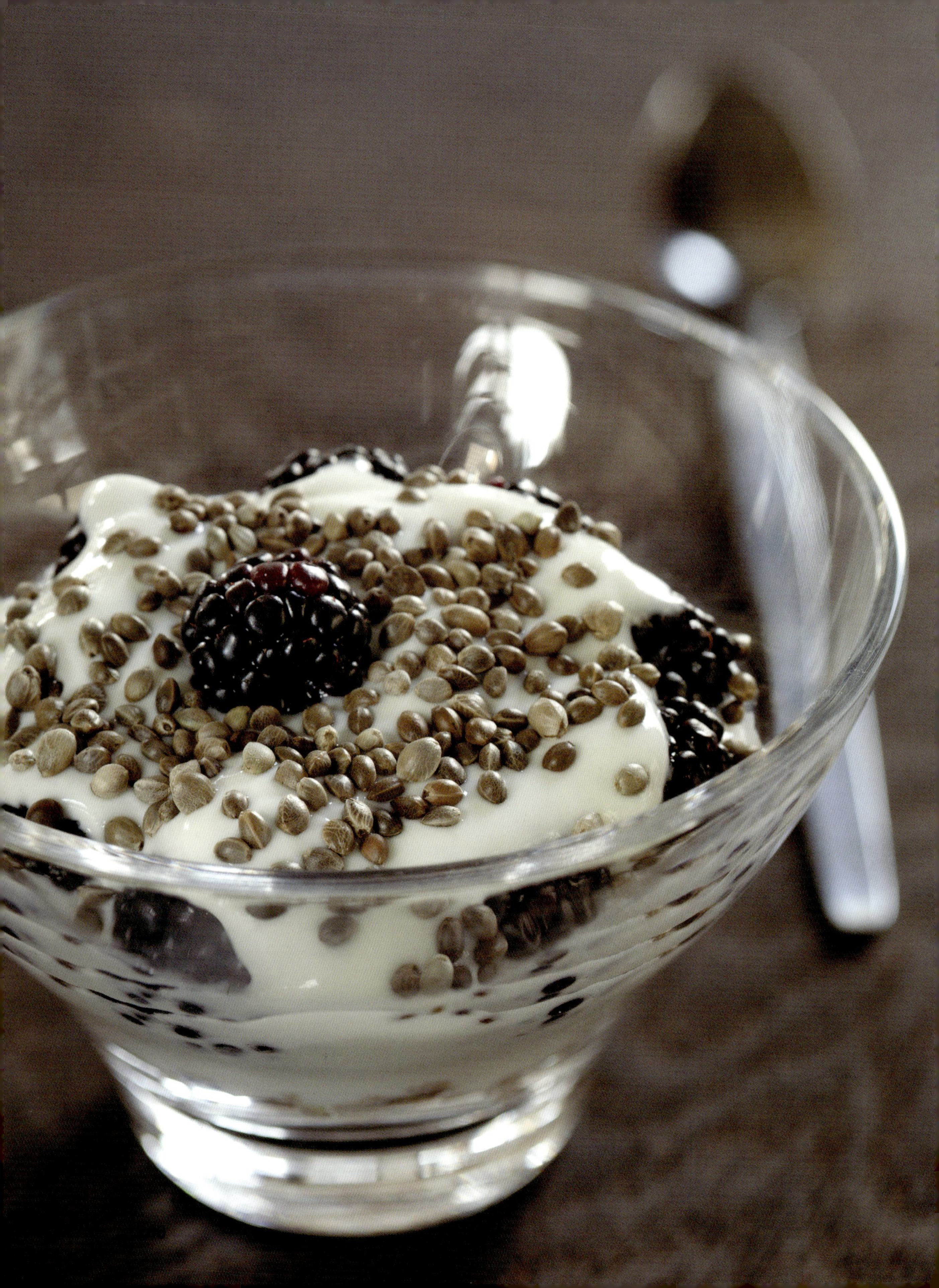

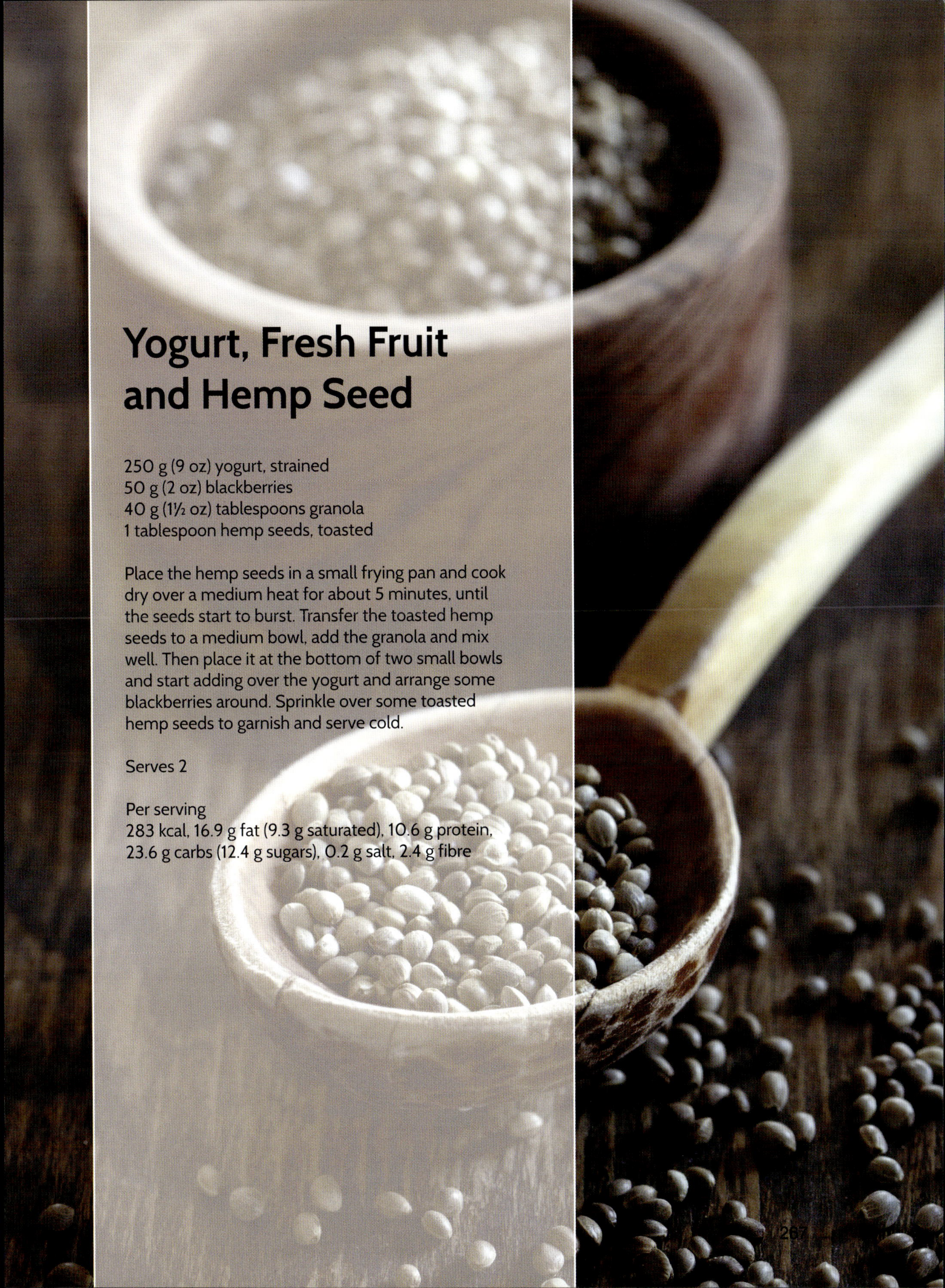

Yogurt, Fresh Fruit and Hemp Seed

250 g (9 oz) yogurt, strained
50 g (2 oz) blackberries
40 g (1½ oz) tablespoons granola
1 tablespoon hemp seeds, toasted

Place the hemp seeds in a small frying pan and cook dry over a medium heat for about 5 minutes, until the seeds start to burst. Transfer the toasted hemp seeds to a medium bowl, add the granola and mix well. Then place it at the bottom of two small bowls and start adding over the yogurt and arrange some blackberries around. Sprinkle over some toasted hemp seeds to garnish and serve cold.

Serves 2

Per serving
283 kcal, 16.9 g fat (9.3 g saturated), 10.6 g protein, 23.6 g carbs (12.4 g sugars), 0.2 g salt, 2.4 g fibre

Chia Yogurt Dessert

2 tablespoons Chia
500 g (17½ oz) yogurt - strained
50 g (2 oz) raspberries
5 drops rum flavoring
pinch of ground cinnamon
flaked almonds to garnish

In a medium bowl pour the yogurt, chia, rum flavoring, cinnamon and mix well. Transfer to large glasses or bowls, sprinkle with the flaked almonds and garnish with some raspberries. Leave it to rest for about 1 hour in the refrigerator before you serve.

Serves 2

Per serving
402 kcal, 31.5 g fat (17.5 g saturated), 17.3 g protein, 18.2 g carbs (12.6 g sugar), 0.4 g salt, 4.4 g fibre

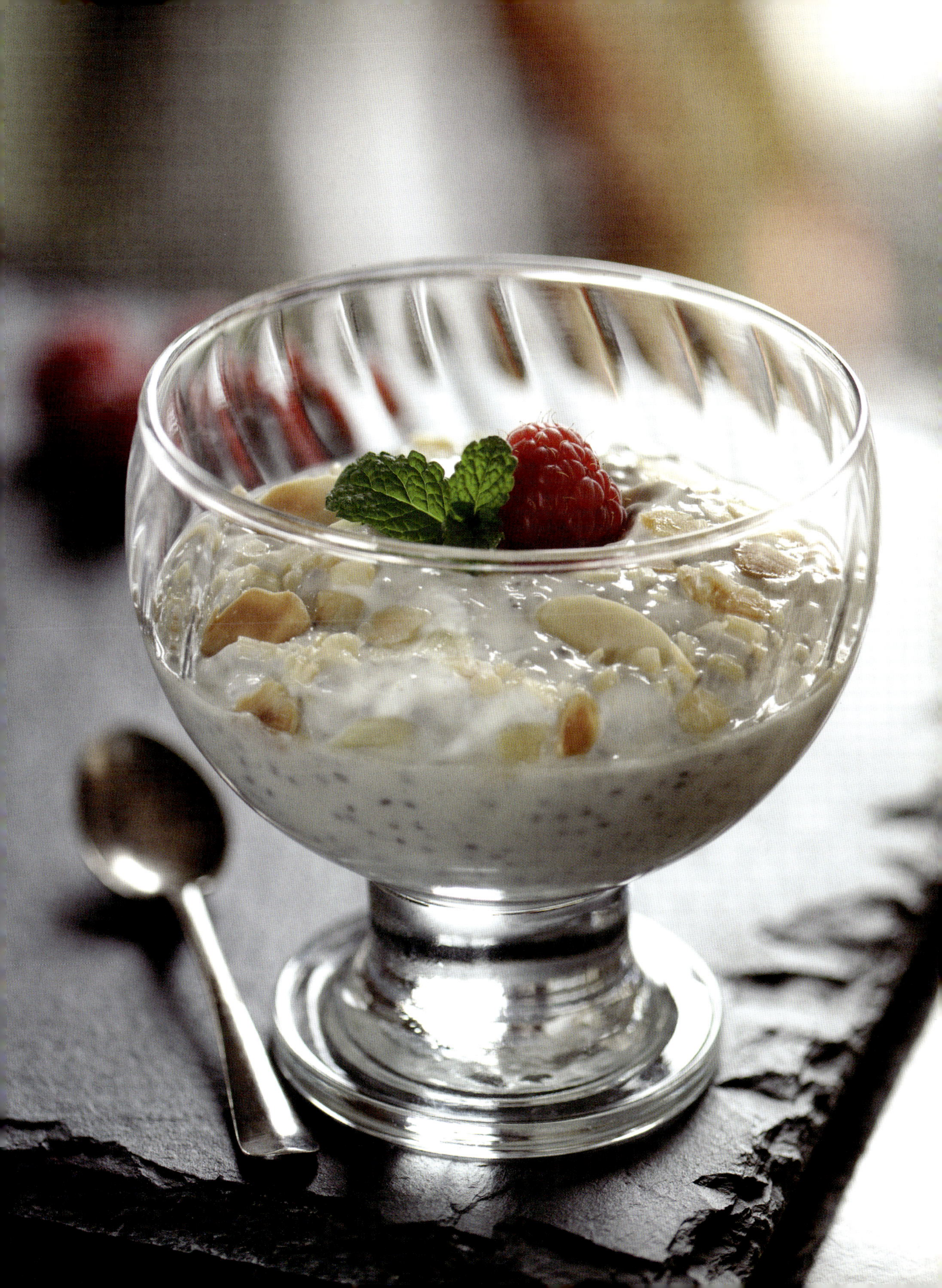

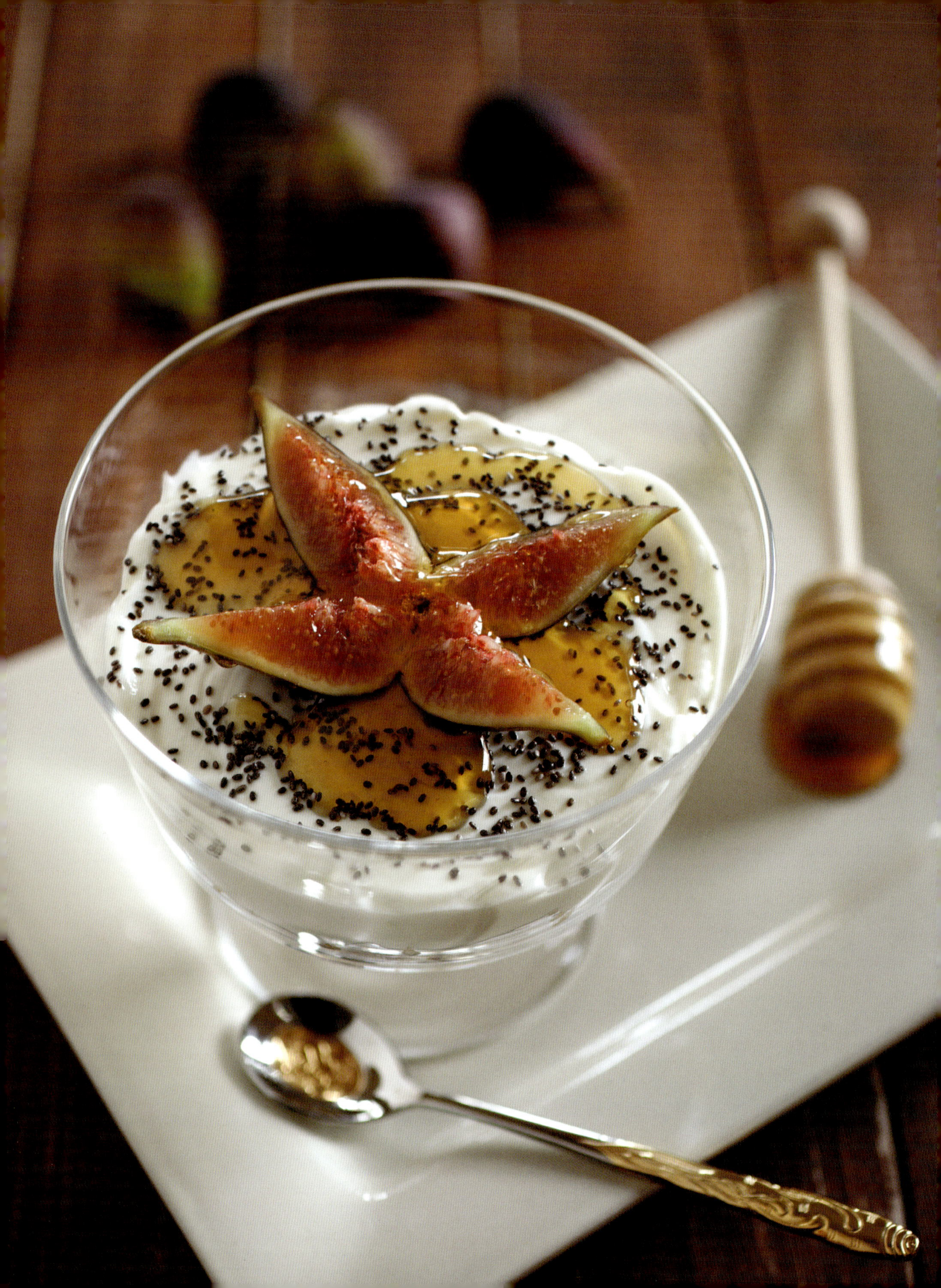

Figs and Chia

300 g (10½ oz) strained yogurt
100 g (3½ oz) ricotta
6 small figs
1 tablespoon chia seeds
3 teaspoons running honey

In a medium bowl combine the yogurt, ricotta and chia. Wash and chop each the figs into four pieces. Pour two tablespoons of the mixture into three serving glasses or small bowls. Then arrange the fig pieces, you can save some for final decoration and then add the rest of the mixture. Arrange the rest of the figs, sprinkle some chia seeds and pour one teaspoon of honey over. Leave in the refrigerator for a couple of minutes and serve cold.

Serves 3

Per serving
228 kcal, 15 g fat (9.2 g saturated), 9.8 g protein, 15.9 g carbs (14.1 g sugar), 0.3 g salt, 1.8 g fibre

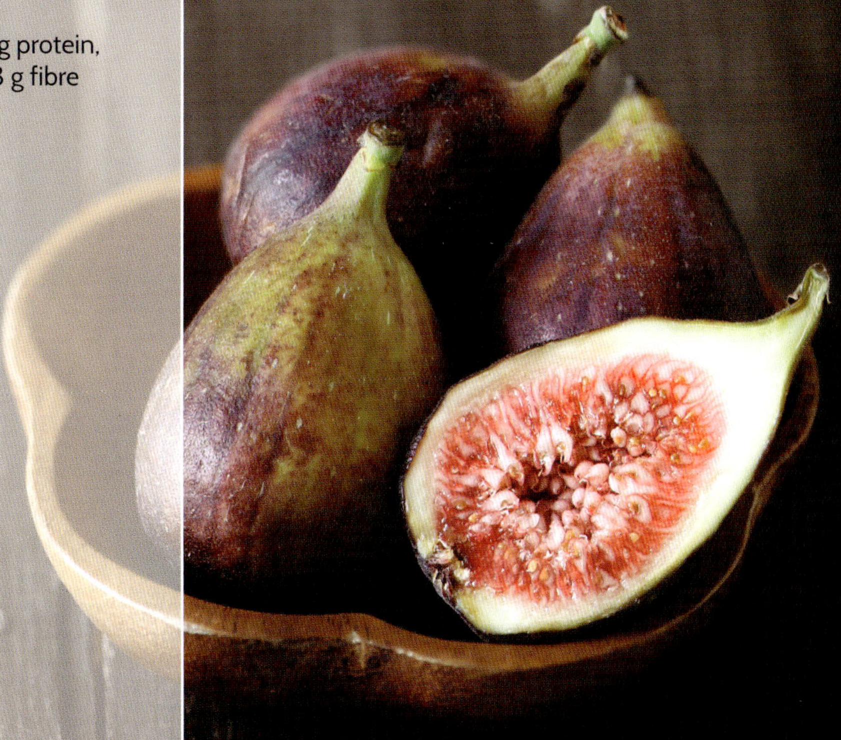

Dried Dates and Egg Cream

100 · dried chopped dates
250 g (9 oz) yogurt
3 egg yolks
2 tablespoons sugar

In a small bowl pour 200 g (7 oz) warm water and soak the dried dates for 10 min, then dice them in small pieces. Arrange the pieces at the bottom of four small fireproof soufflé bowls. In another small bowl mix the eggs yolk, yogurt and sugar. Then pour the mixture over the dates in the four bowls. Bake it in a water bath for about 30 minutes until slightly golden. Leave for some time to cool at room temperature, than move to the refrigerator for one hour or more and serve cold.

Serves 4

Per serving
236 kcal, 10.5 g fat (5.4 g saturated), 6.6 g protein, 30.5 g carbs (30.3 g sugar), 0.1 g salt, 1.3 g fibre

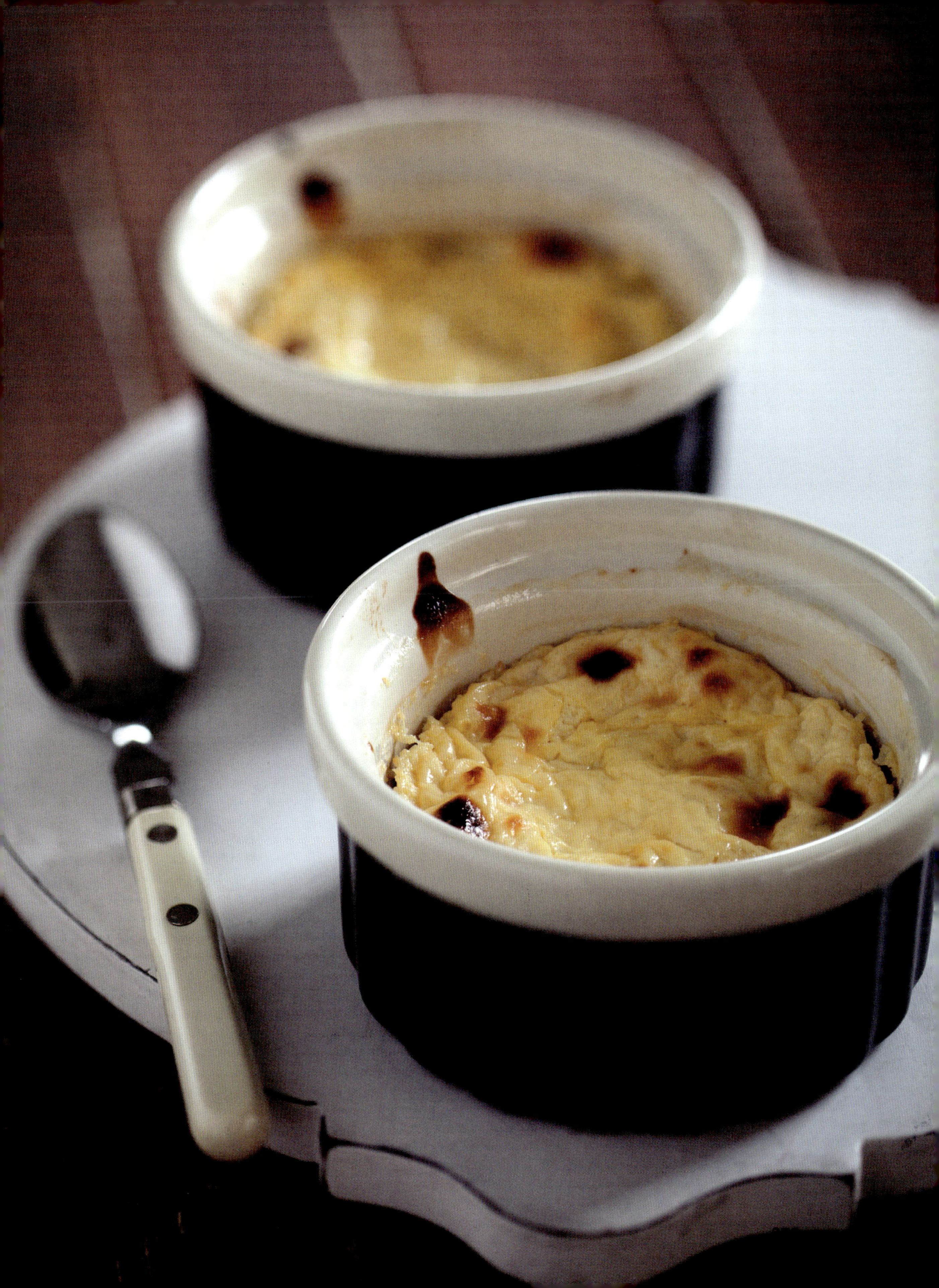

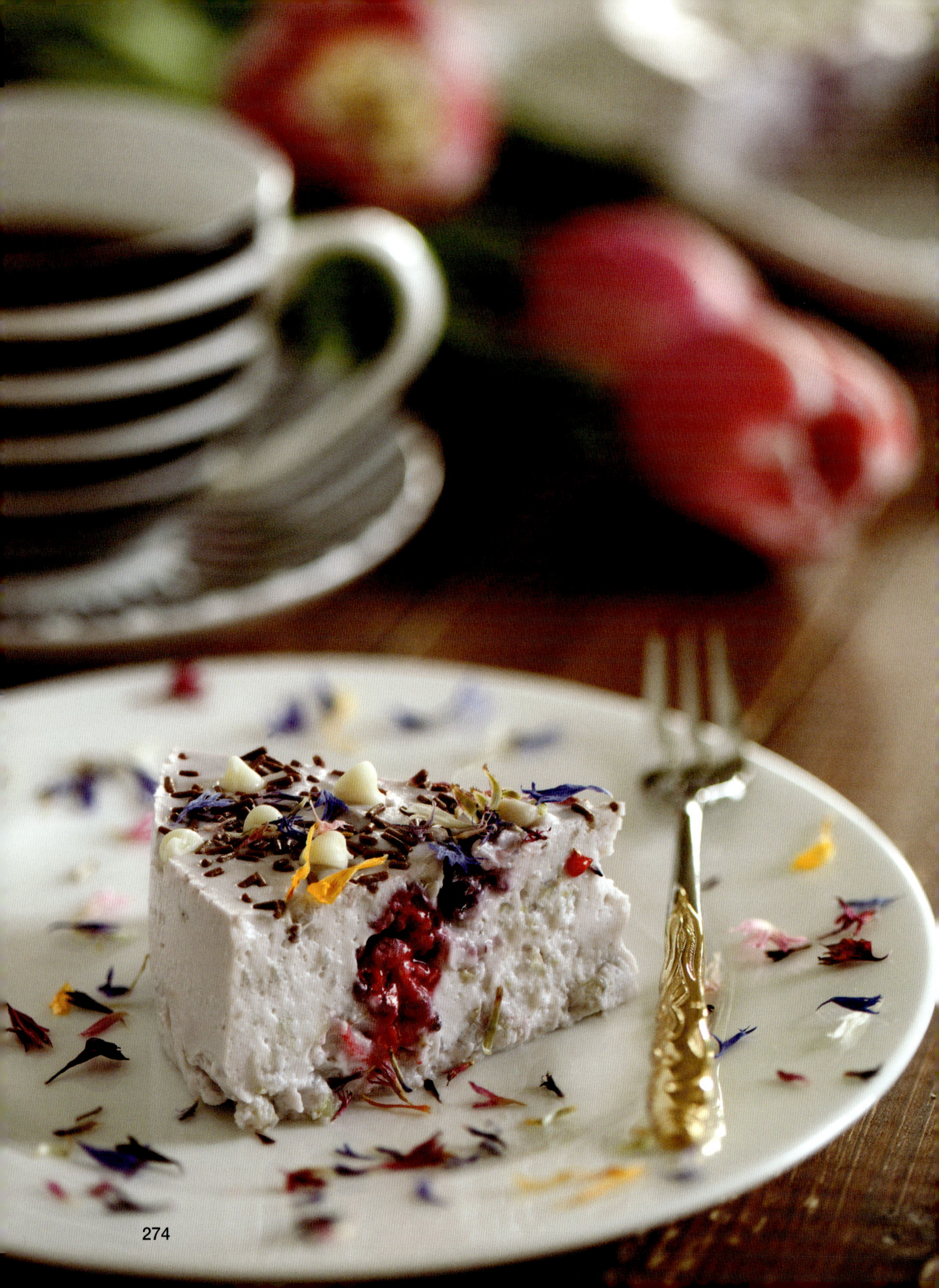

Blackcurrant Parfait

200 g (7 oz) strained yogurt
200 g (7 oz) ricotta
70 g (3 oz) blackcurrant jam
12 g (½ oz) gelatin
30 g (1 oz) sugar
50 g (2 oz) buckwheat
5 g (1/4 oz) vanilla

For decoration:
pinch of dried edible flower petals
white chocolate drops
sugar strands

Boil the buckwheat in 2 litres (4½ pints) water for about 20 minutes in a medium saucepan. Once ready, set aside.
Throw into a blender the yogurt, ricotta, blackcurrant jam, sugar, vanilla and blend until smooth. Transfer to a medium bowl, add the cooked buckwheat and mix well. Dissolve the gelatin, following the instructions on the packet. In a small bowl, put 120 ml (4 fl oz) boiling water and sprinkle the gelatin while stirring briskly until thoroughly dissolved. Leave it to cool for a few minutes. Add the gelatin to the yogurt mixture prepared earlier and stir with a whisk until well mixed. Pour the ready mixture into a small round springform cake tin and leave it to cool overnight in the refrigerator. Next release from the cake tin and transfer to a reasonable sized serving plate. To decorate sprinkle with the chocolate drops, sugar strands and the dried edible flower petals. Serve cold!

Serves 6

Per serving
182 kcal, 7.3 g fat (4.6 g Saturated), 5.8 g protein, 24.9 carbs (17.6 g sugar), 0.2 g fibre, 0.2 g salt.

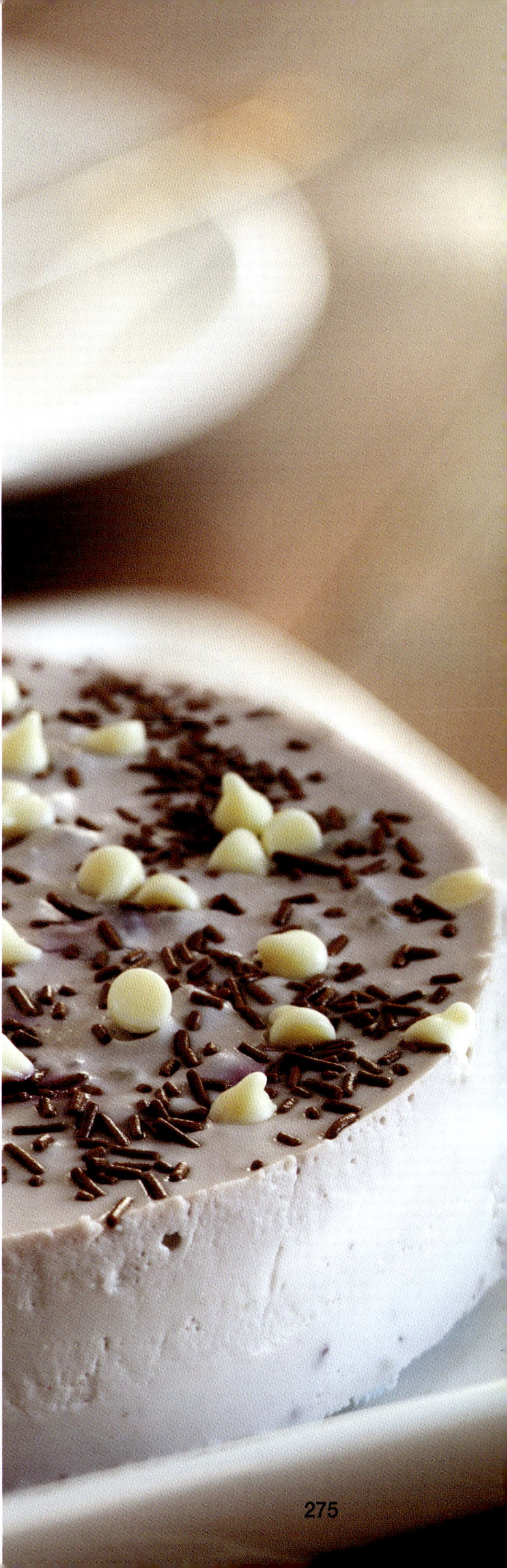

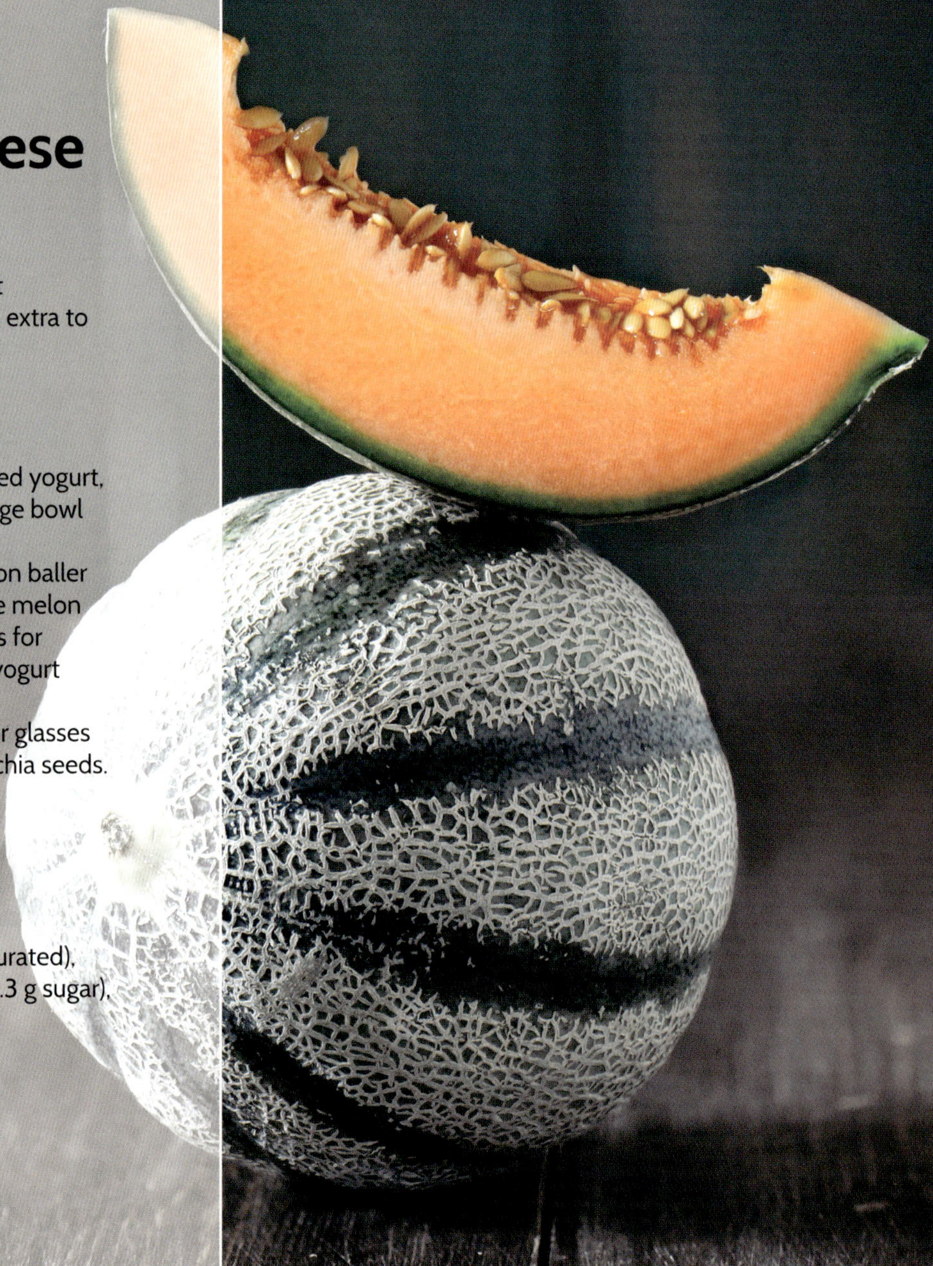

Melon and Ricotta Cheese

100 g (3½ oz) ricotta cheese
400 g (14 oz) strained yogurt
1 tablespoon chia seeds, plus extra to decorate
1 tablespoon honey
200 g (7 oz) melon

Put the ricotta cheese, strained yogurt, chia seeds and honey in a large bowl and mix together.
Dice the melon or use a melon baller to make melon balls. Add the melon pieces, reserving a few pieces for decoration If wished, to the yogurt mixture and stir.
Divide between four bowls or glasses and sprinkle over a pinch of chia seeds. Serve cold.

Serves 4

Per serving
207 kcal, 13.8 g fat (8.6 g saturated), 8.8 g protein, 13.7 g carbs (12.3 g sugar), 1.4 g fibre, 0.3 g salt

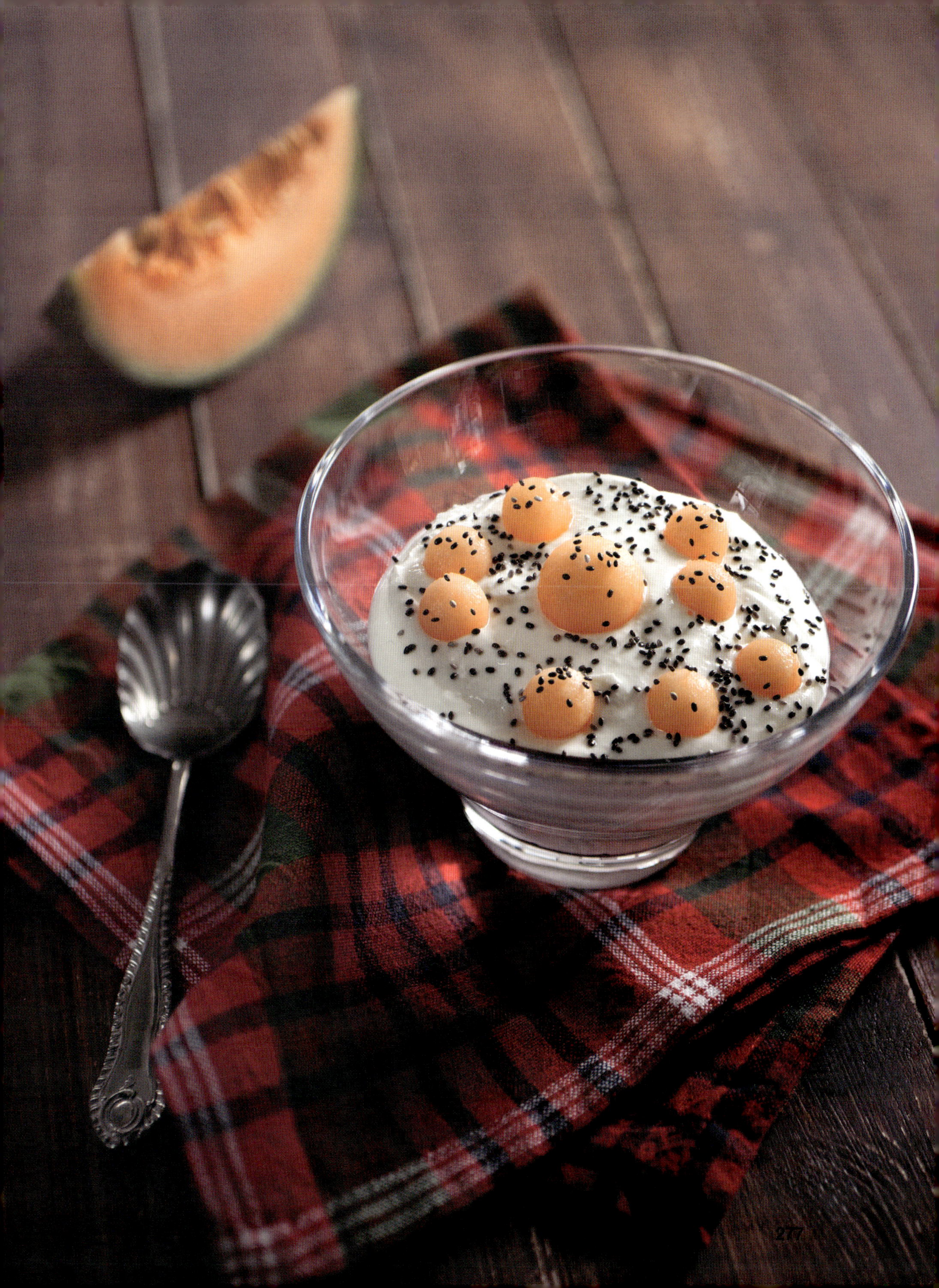

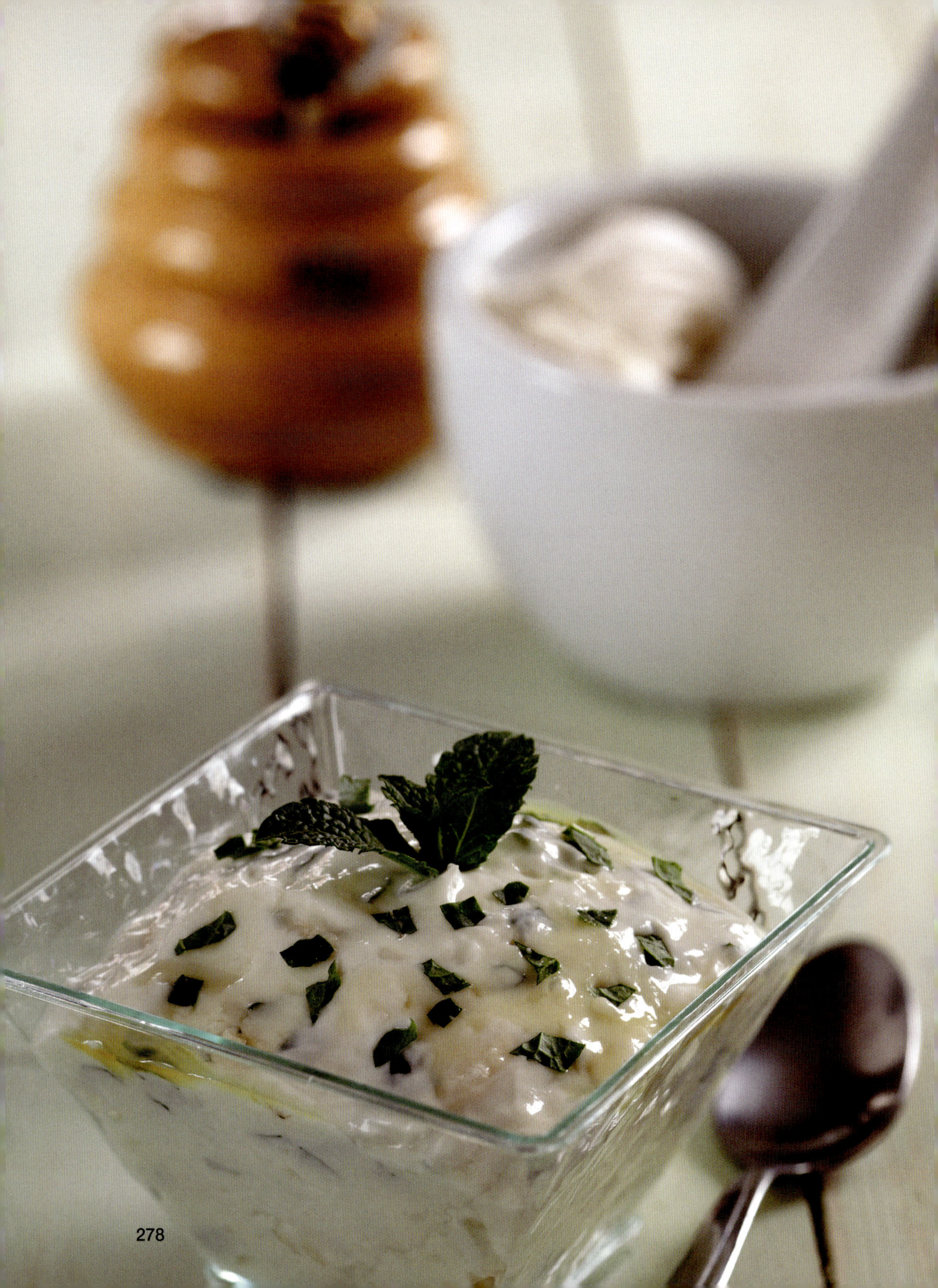

Yogurt and Meringues

300 g (10½ oz) strained yogurt
1 teaspoon honey
150 g (5 oz) meringues
2 tablespoons chopped fresh mint leaves

Break the meringues into small pieces in a large mortar. Next in a medium bowl mix the yogurt, honey, meringue pieces and finely chopped fresh mint leaves. Finally divide into four bowls or glasses and leave to rest for no more than 15 minutes in the refrigerator. Serve cool!

Serves 4

Per serving
249 kcal, 7.7 g fat (5.1 g saturated), 6.4 g protein, 41.3 g carbs (40.9 g sugar), 0 g fibre, 0.2 g salt

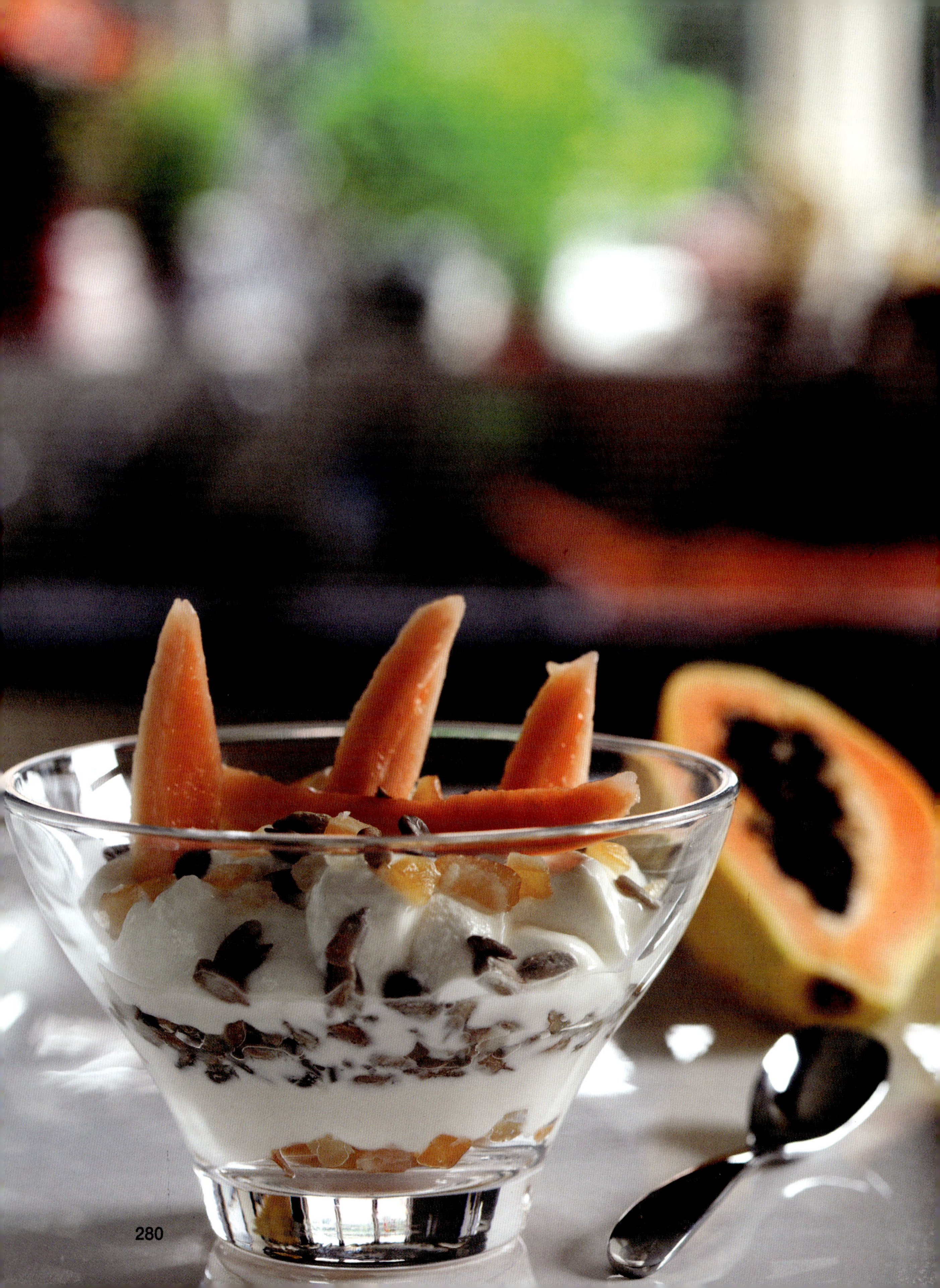

Papaya and Yogurt

300 g (10½ oz) strained yogurt
1 small papaya, seeded and sliced
50 g (2 oz) citrus mixed peel
30 g (1 oz) sunflower seeds, roasted

Place the sunflower seeds in a small frying pan and toast dry over a medium heat for about 3 minutes, until the seeds start to burst. Once ready, set aside. Next, arrange layers in four bowls, starting with yogurt then some citrus mixed peel and some papaya slices. Garnish with the toasted sunflower seeds. Cover the glasses with kitchen foil and leave it to rest for no more than 30 minutes in the refrigerator. Serve cold!

Serves 4

Per serving
201 kcal, 11.6 g fat (5.6 g saturated), 6.8 g protein, 17.9 g carbs (10.9 g sugar), 3.4 g fibre, 0.3 g salt

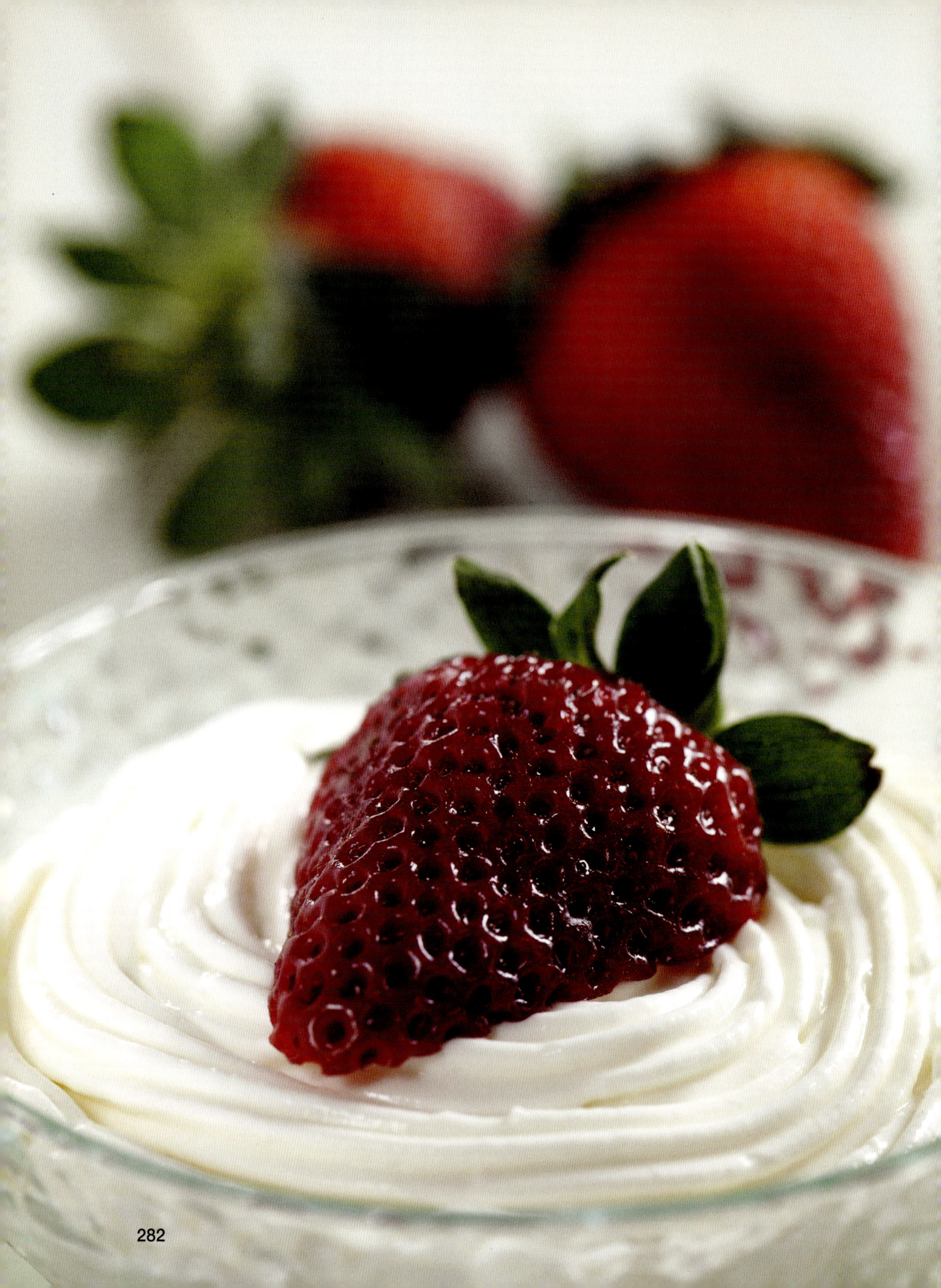

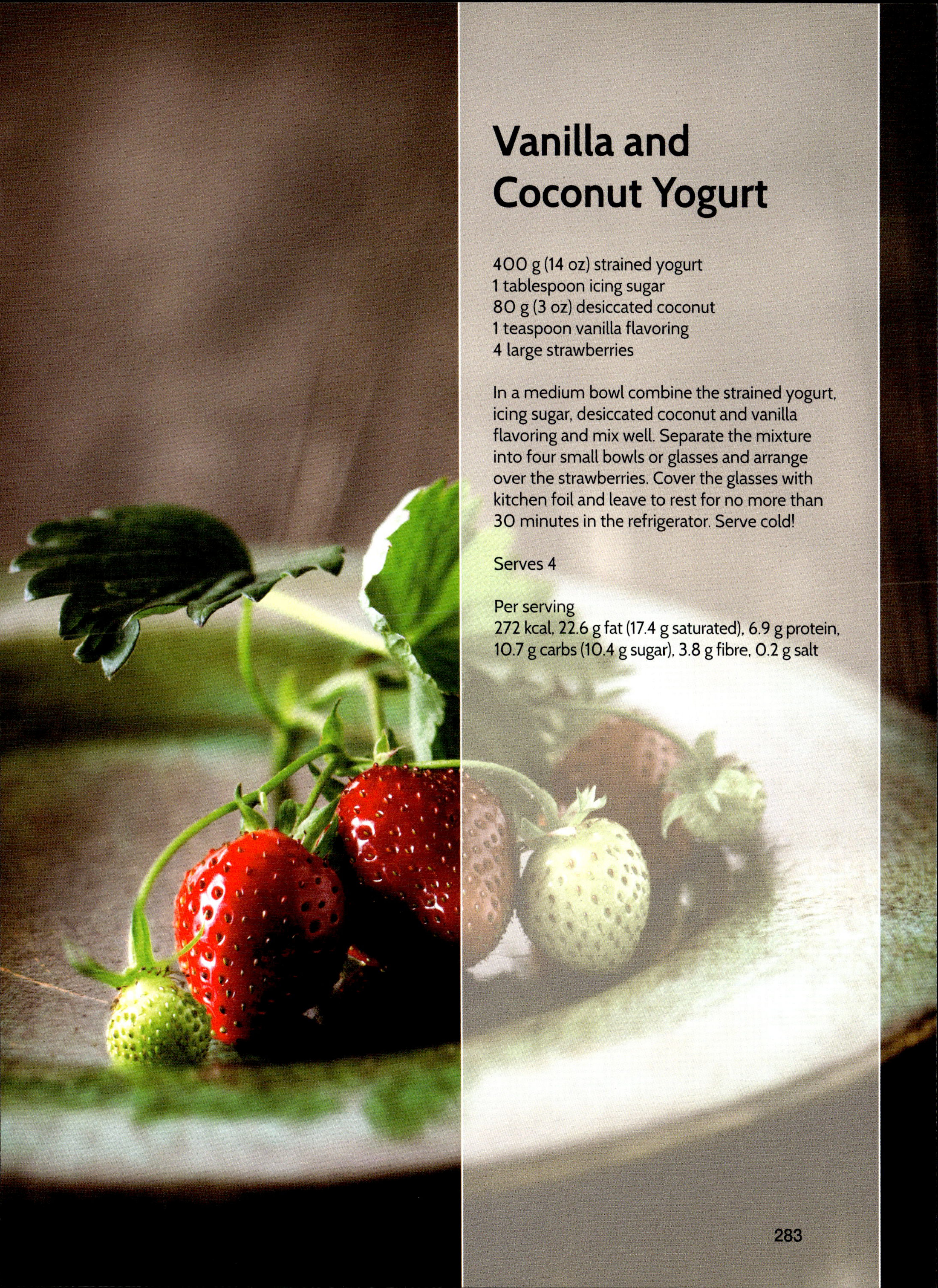

Vanilla and Coconut Yogurt

400 g (14 oz) strained yogurt
1 tablespoon icing sugar
80 g (3 oz) desiccated coconut
1 teaspoon vanilla flavoring
4 large strawberries

In a medium bowl combine the strained yogurt, icing sugar, desiccated coconut and vanilla flavoring and mix well. Separate the mixture into four small bowls or glasses and arrange over the strawberries. Cover the glasses with kitchen foil and leave to rest for no more than 30 minutes in the refrigerator. Serve cold!

Serves 4

Per serving
272 kcal, 22.6 g fat (17.4 g saturated), 6.9 g protein, 10.7 g carbs (10.4 g sugar), 3.8 g fibre, 0.2 g salt

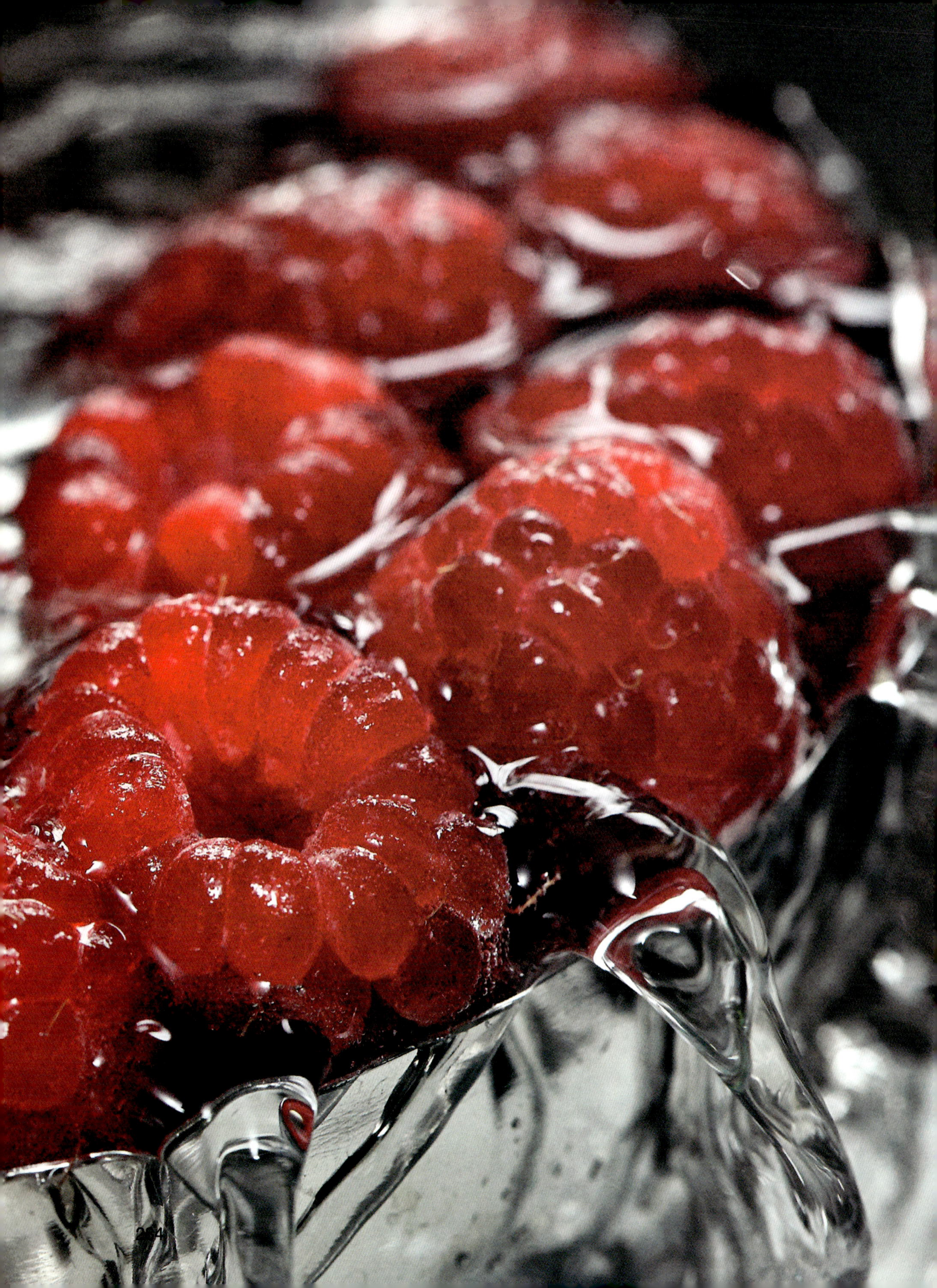

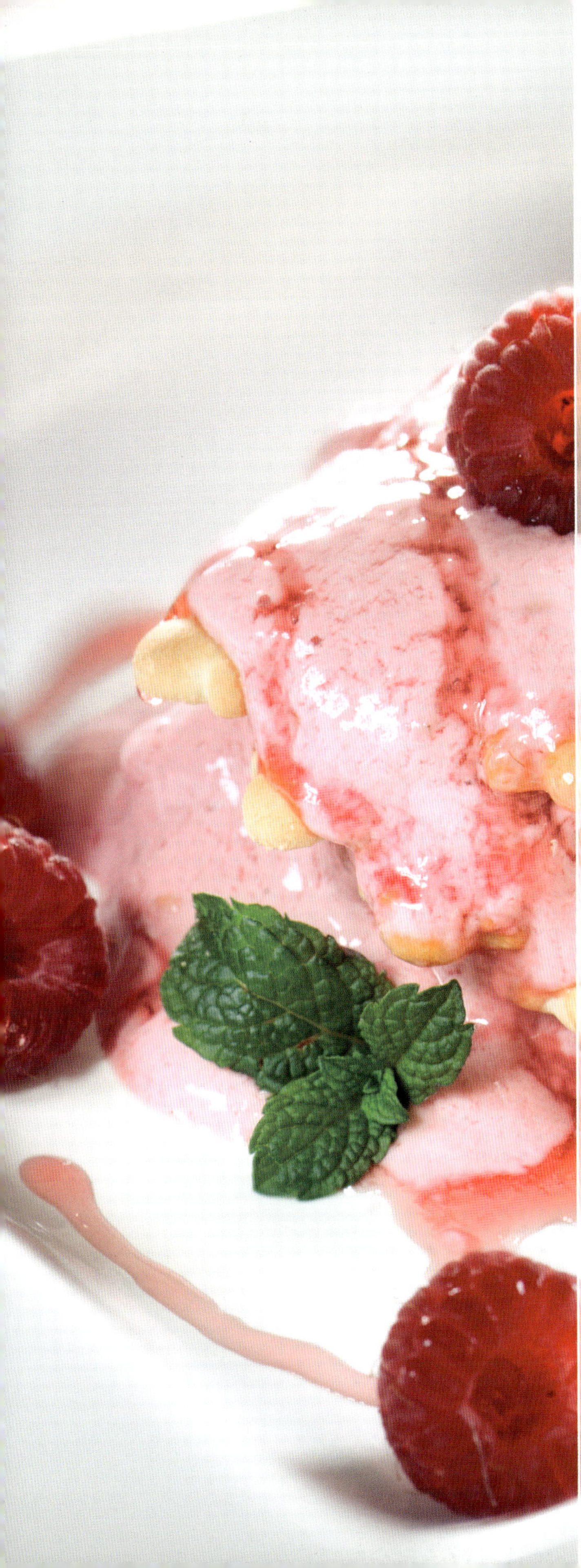

Raspberry Biscuit Dessert

1 teaspoon raspberry or strawberry syrup
6 tablespoons strained yogurt
100 g (3½ oz) fresh raspberries (leave some for decoration)
20 tea biscuits
some fresh mint leaves for garnish
drizzle of raspberry or strawberry syrup for garnish

Combine the yogurt, syrup and the fresh raspberries in a food processor and whiz until it turns into a paste. Then arrange layers of flavor, repeating one biscuit and one tablespoon of the paste. Prepare just before you serve, garnish with some fresh mint leaves, some fresh raspberries and drizzle some raspberry or strawberry syrup over.

Serves 4

Per serving
254 kcal, 11.2 g fat (6.7 g saturated), 6 g protein, 32.7 g carbs (11 g sugar), 0.8 g fibre, 0.1 g salt

Strawberry yogurt

400 g (14 oz) strained yogurt
100 g (3½ oz) strawberries
30 g (1 oz) sunflower seeds, roasted
1 tablespoon strawberry syrup
some fresh mint leave to garnish

Place the sunflower seeds in a small frying pan and toast dry over a medium heat for about 3 minutes, until the seeds start to burst, then set aside. Dividine into four small bowls or glasses, place the strained yogurt at the bottom of each. Next cut and arrange the strawberries. Sprinkle the roasted sunflower seeds and drizzle strawberry syrup. Decorate with fresh mint leaves. Cover the glasses with kitchen foil and leave it to rest for no more than 30 minutes in the refrigerator. Serve cold!

Serves 4

Per serving
266 kcal, 20.1 g fat (8.1 g saturated), 10 g protein, 11.6 g carbs (7.7 g sugar), 2.0 g fibre, 0.2 g salt

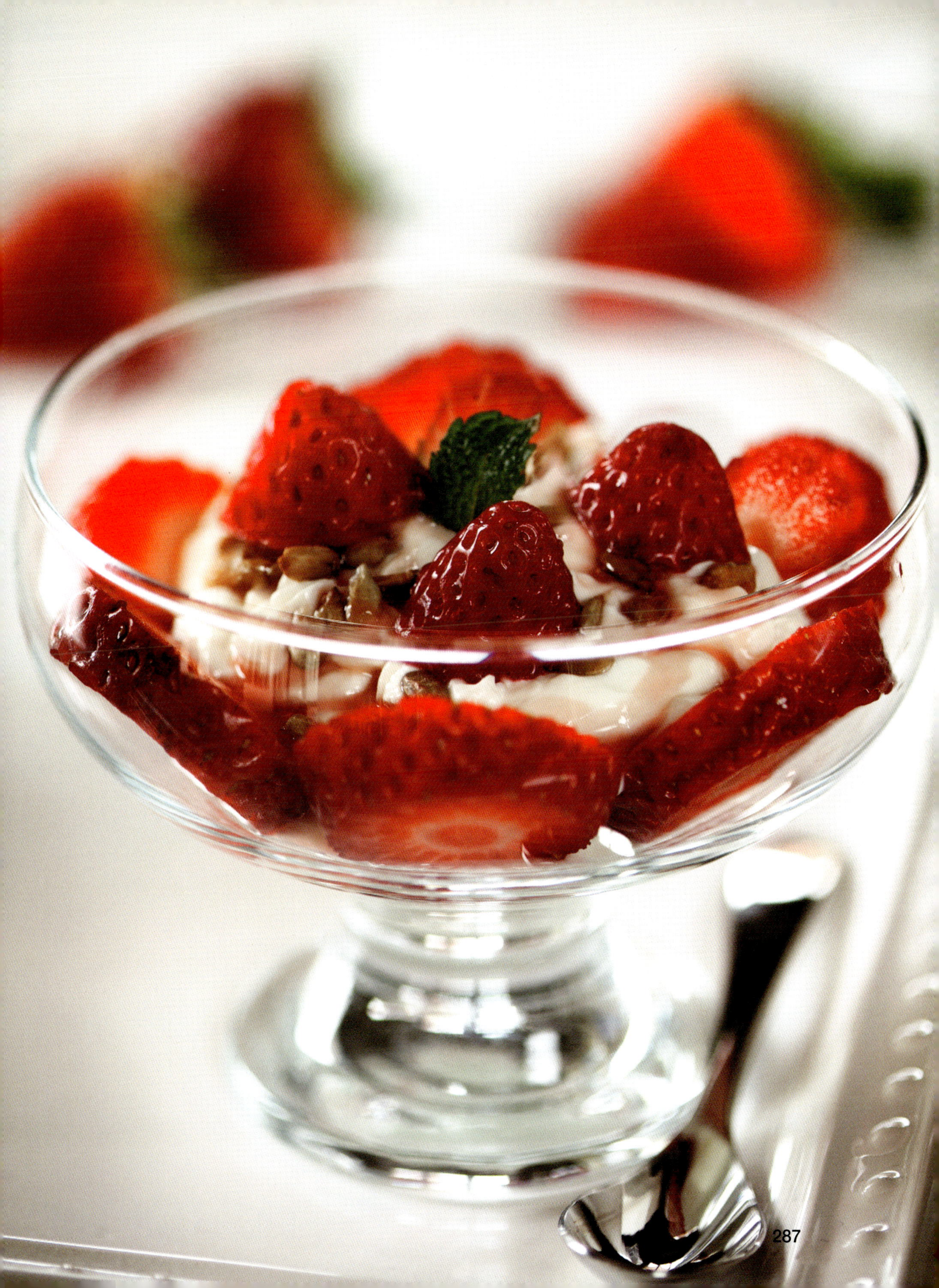

Kiwi Mousse

3 egg whites
50 g (2 oz) caster sugar
2 middle kiwis
200 ml (6¾ fl oz) low fat yogurt, strained

Separate the whites from the yolks of 3 large eggs. The eggs must be fresh as this makes them easier to separate. Place the whites into the whisking bowl and using a hand mixer beat them on slow speed until the mixture resembles a fluffy cloud and stands up in stiff peaks when the blades are lifted. After that, switch to a medium speed and start adding the sugar slowly, beat it for about 5 minutes, until the meringue mixture is cool, and holds its shape. Make sure you don't over-beat and set aside. Peel the kiwis and blend in the blender until you have green kiwi puree. In a medium bowl combine the kiwi puree and the strained yogurt and mix well. Than add the meringue mixture and mix it again and serve it as quick as possible.

Serves 2

Per serving
278 kcal, 10.5 g fat (6.8 g saturated),
10.7 g protein, 37.4 g carbs (36.9 g sugar),
1.5 g fibre, 0.4 g salt

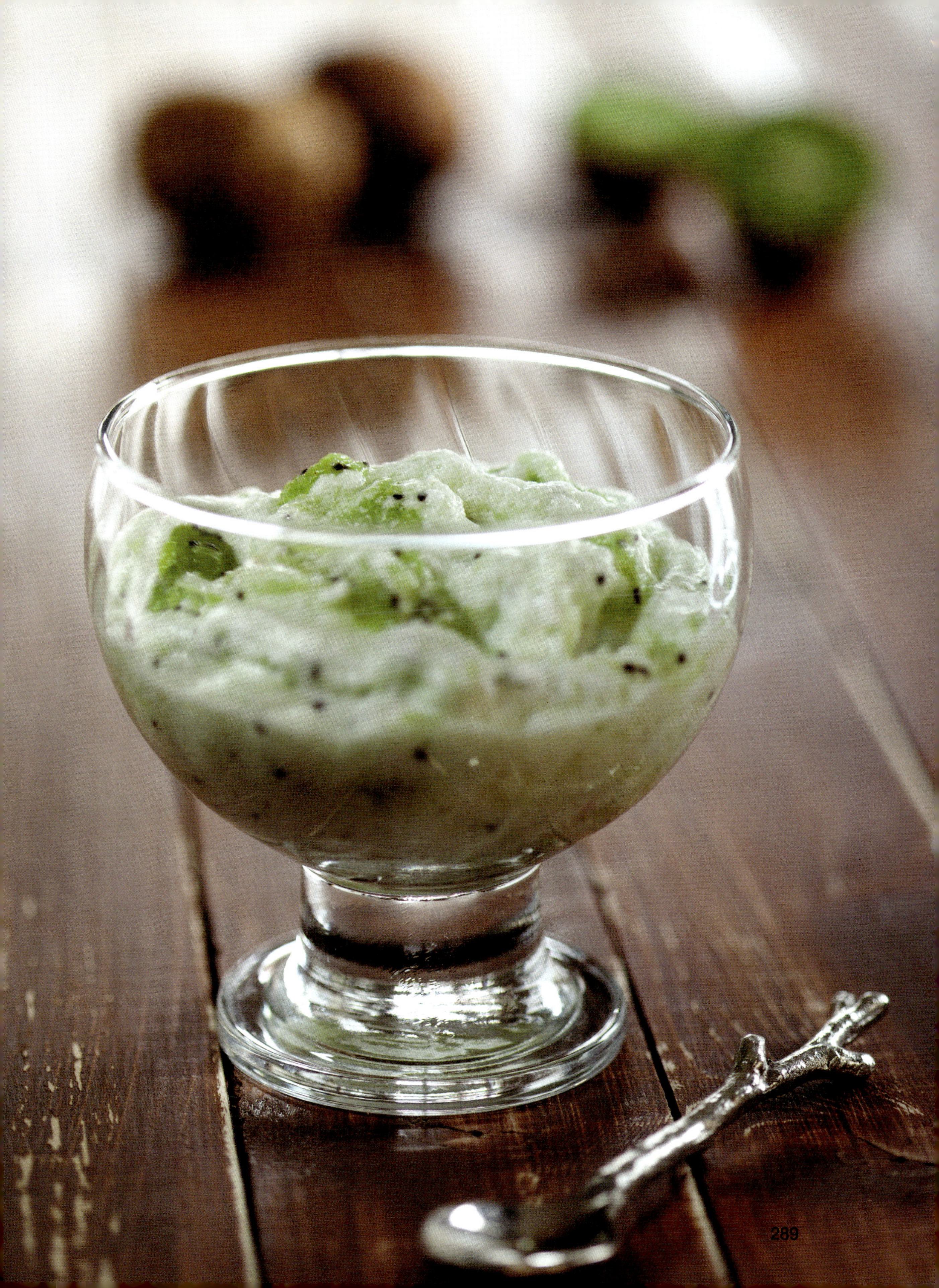

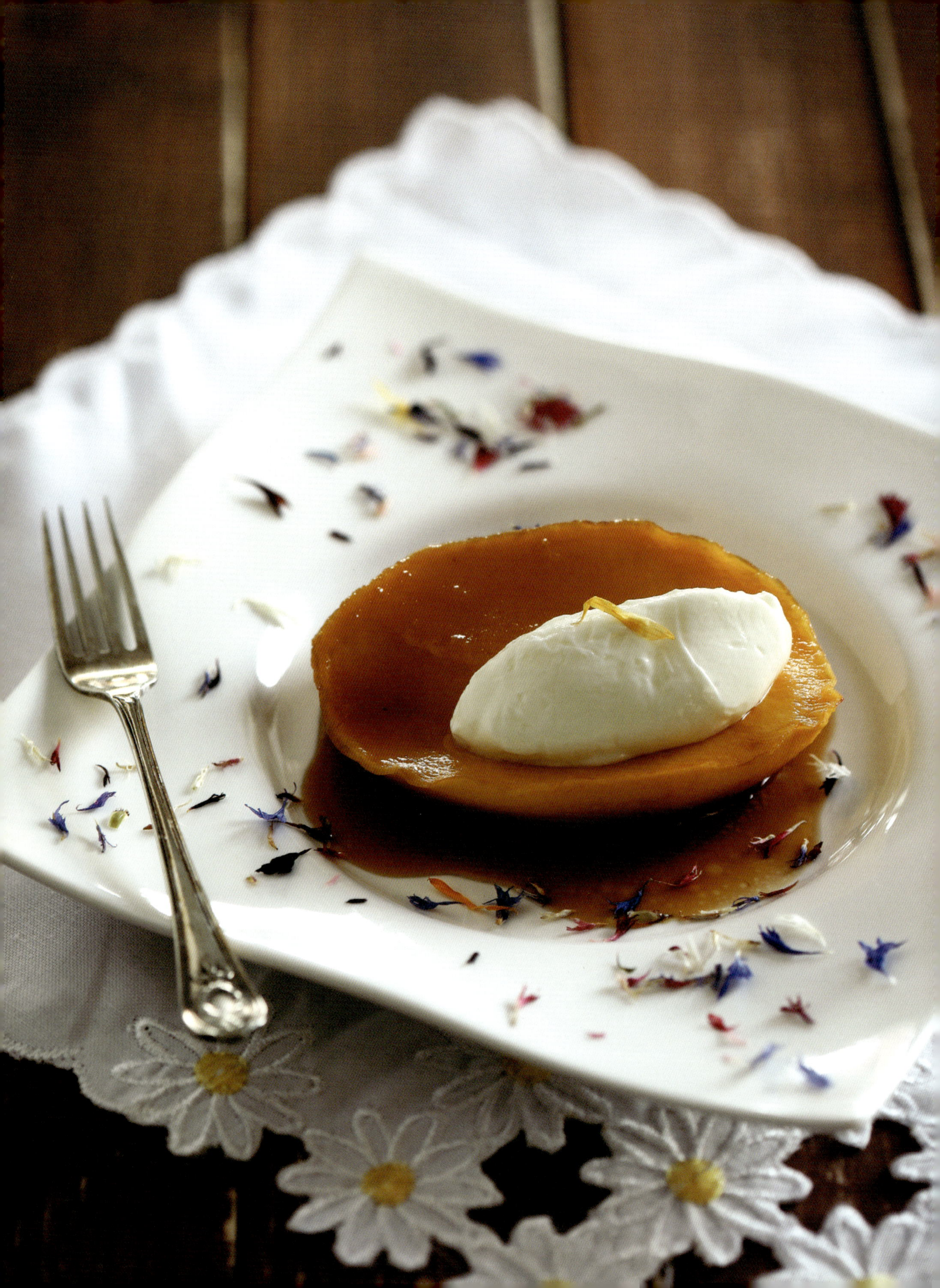

Liqueur Glazed Mango with Yogurt

2 large mangoes sliced in half, skin off
1 teaspoon vanilla extract
6 tablespoons dark brown sugar
150 g (5 oz) yogurt, strained
pinch of salt
50 ml (1½ fl oz) Tia Maria dark Liqueur or Kahlua Coffee Liqueur

Preheat oven to 200°C (400°F). Mix the yogurt, vanilla extract and a pinch of salt in a medium bowl. Let it rest for 1 hour in the refrigerator. In a large bowl combine Liqueur, sugar, pinch of salt and stir with a whisk. Next gently toss the mango pieces in the sugar mixture and soak for about 10 minutes. Then arrange the mango pieces, on a small baking tray and pour over the remaining sugar mixture. Bake in the ovem for about 15 minutes or until just tender. Serve it with tablespoon of the yogurt mixture on the top.

Serves 4

Per serving
244 kcal, 4 g fat (2.6 g saturated), 2.7 g protein, 46.4 g carbs (40.7 g sugar), 3.9 g fibre, 0.9 g salt.

Pecans and Honey Yogurt

200 g (7 oz) strained yogurt
4 tablespoons runny honey
80 g (3 oz) pecans
100 g (3½ oz) granola

Arrange layers of granola and yogurt into four bowls or glasses. Decorate with pecans on the top and drizzle over a spoonful of honey. Leave it to rest for no more than 15 minutes in the refrigerator. Serve cold!

Serves 4

Per serving
381 kcal, 22.5 g fat (4.5 g saturated), 7.3 g protein, 39 g carbs (26.2 g sugar), 3.0 g fibre, 0.1 g salt

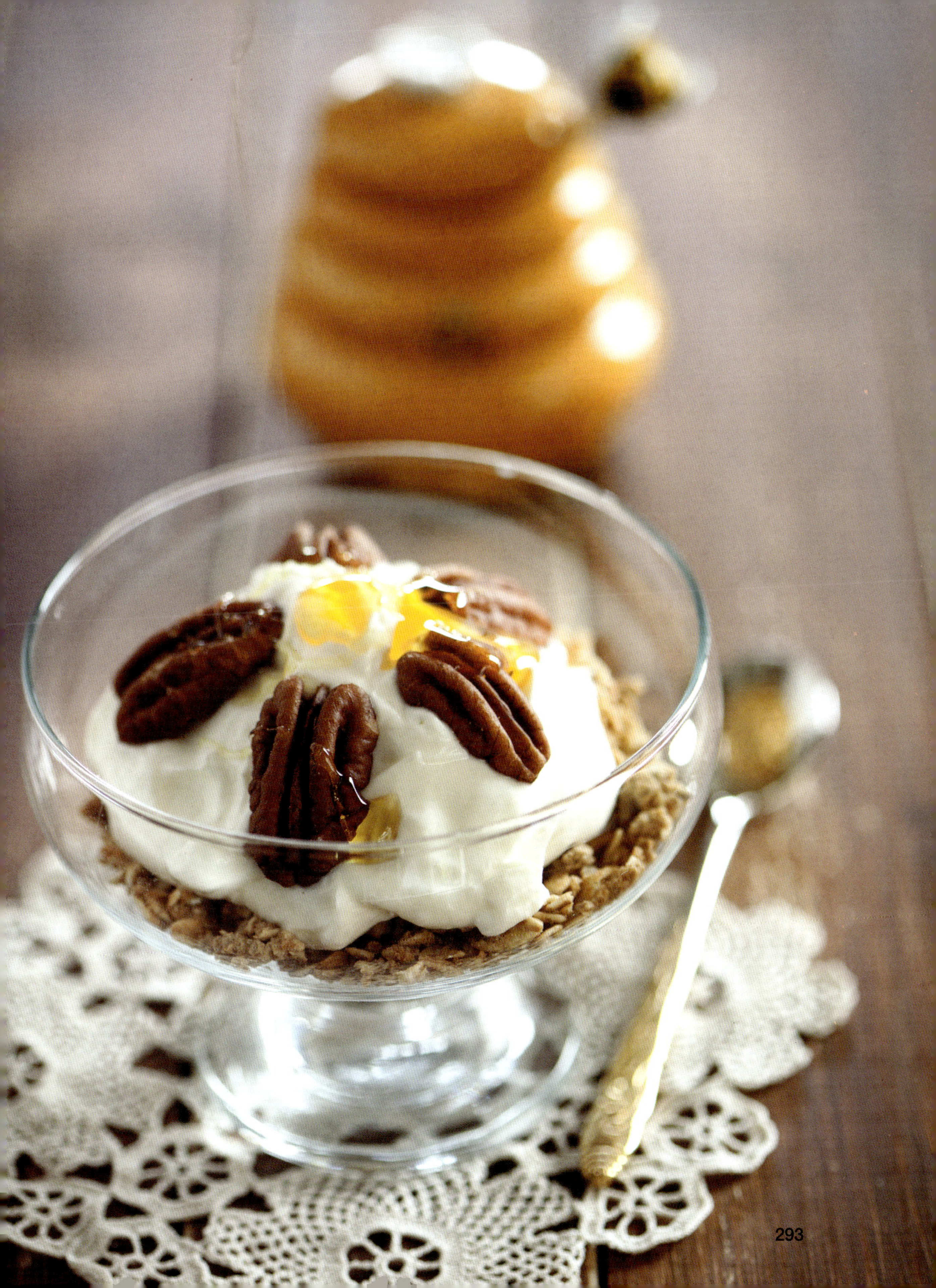

Pomegranate Granola and Pumpkin Seeds

200 g (7 oz) low fat yogurt, strained
80 g (3 oz) pomegranate seeds
40 g (1½ oz) pumpkin seeds, roasted
8 drops vanilla flavoring
100 g (3½ oz) granola

Mix the strained yogurt and vanilla flavoring into a medium bowl. Separating into four bowls or glasses arrange layers of the granola and then vanilla yogurt. Sprinkle over some pomegranate and some pumpkin seeds. Leave it to rest for no more than 15 minutes in the refrigerator. Serve cold!

Serves 4

Per serving
241 kcal, 13 g fat (4.1 g saturated),
8 g protein, 23.4 g carbs (9.5 g sugar),
3.4 g fibre, 0.1 g salt

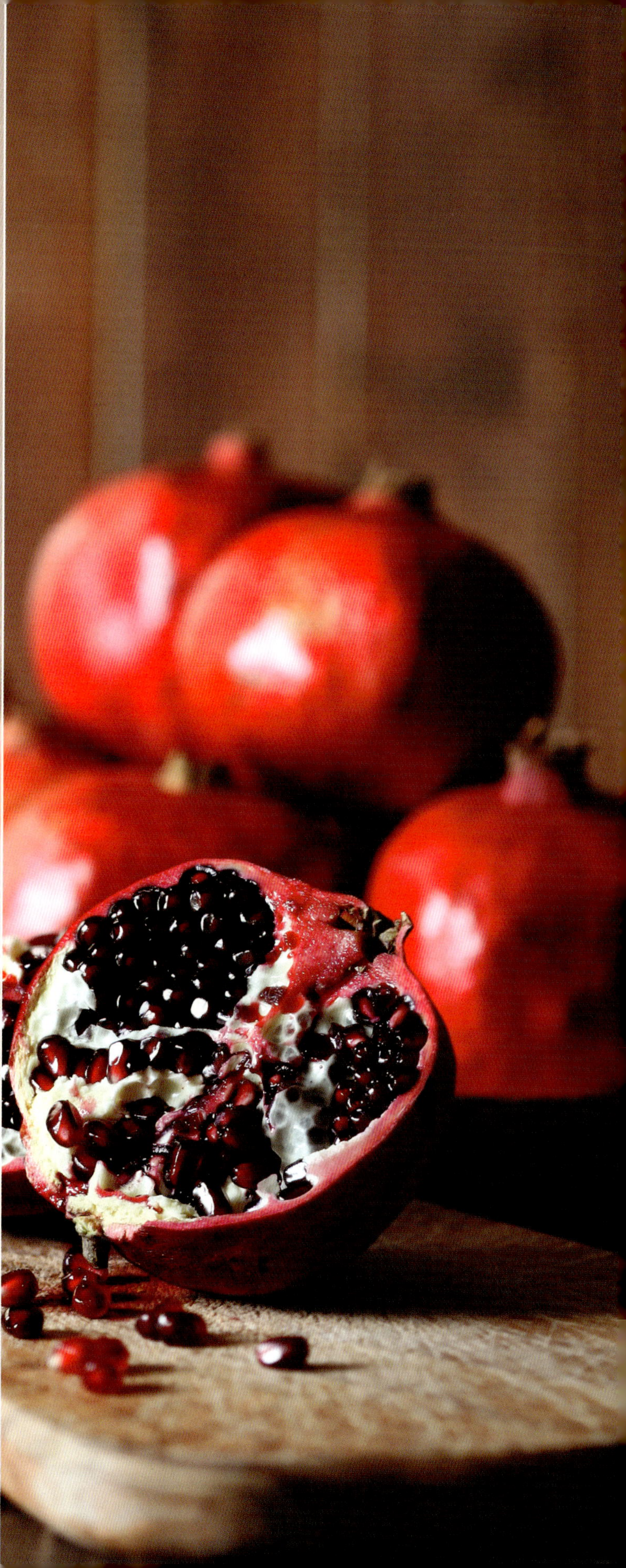

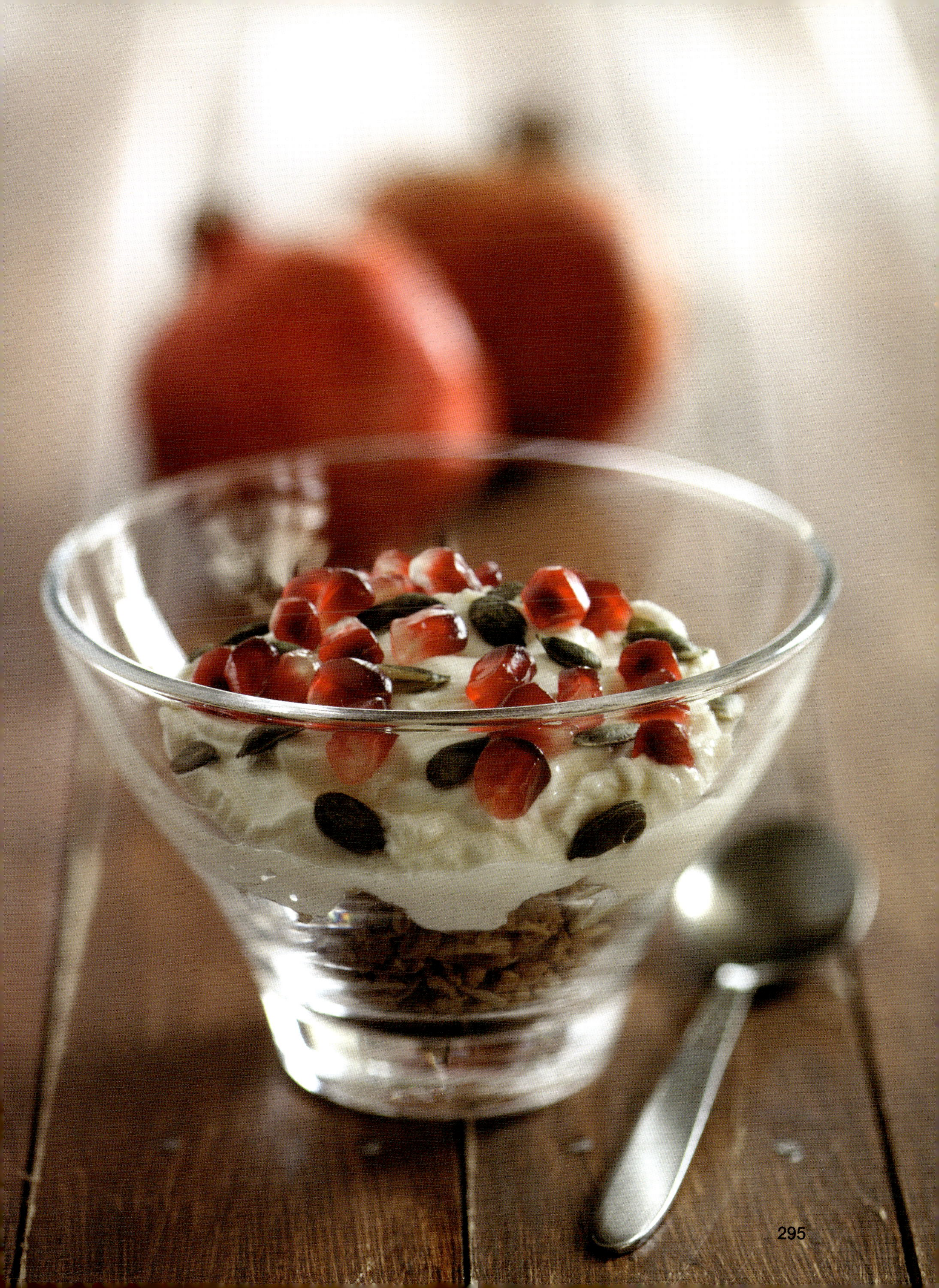

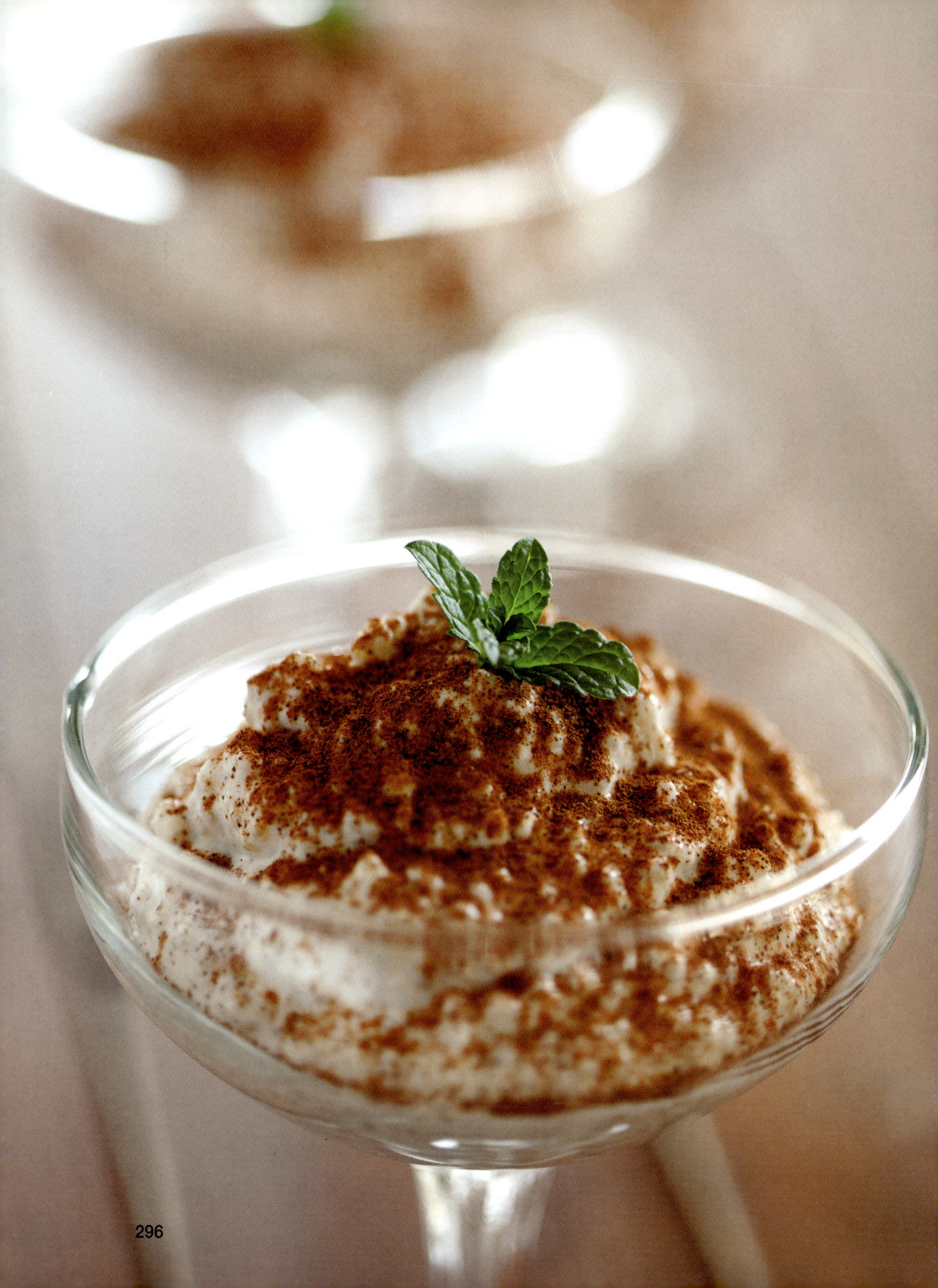

Quinoa and Rum Flavored Yogurt

50 g (2 oz) Quinoa, boiled
350 g (12 oz) yogurt, strained
1 tablespoon runny honey
5 drops of rum flavoring
1 teaspoon ground cinnamon

In a medium saucepan boil the Quinoa for about 10 minutes in 2 litres (4½ pints) water. Then transfer into a cooking strainer and drain for 5 minutes. Combine the drained quinoa and the strained yogurt, add the rum flavoring and mix well. Finally pour into large serving glasses or bowls, sprinkle over a pinch of cinnamon and decorate with mint leaves.

Serves 4

Per serving
172 kcal, 9.6 g fat (6 g saturated), 6.8 g protein, 15.7 g carbs (9.3 g sugar), fibre – nil, 0.2 g salt

Raspberry and Banana Cream

200 g (7 oz) yogurt
1 banana
100 g (3½ oz) strawberry
80 g (3 oz) muesli with dry fruits and nuts

Peel the banana and throw into the blender bowl, add the strawberries and yogurt and blend well until smooth. Separate the mixture into four small bowls or glasses and sprinkle over muesli with dry fruits and nuts.

Serves 2

Per serving
343 kcal, 12.9 g fat (6.8 g saturated),
10.8 g protein, 48.8 g carbs (26.9 g sugar),
1.5 g fibre, 0.3 g salt

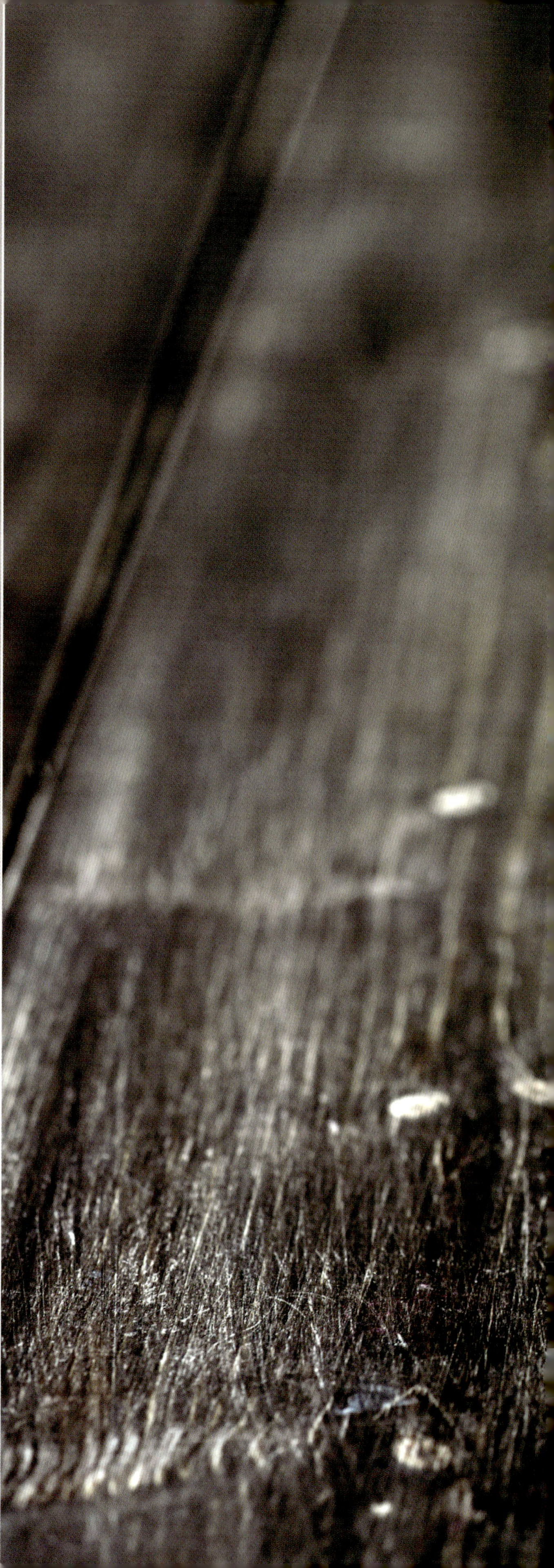

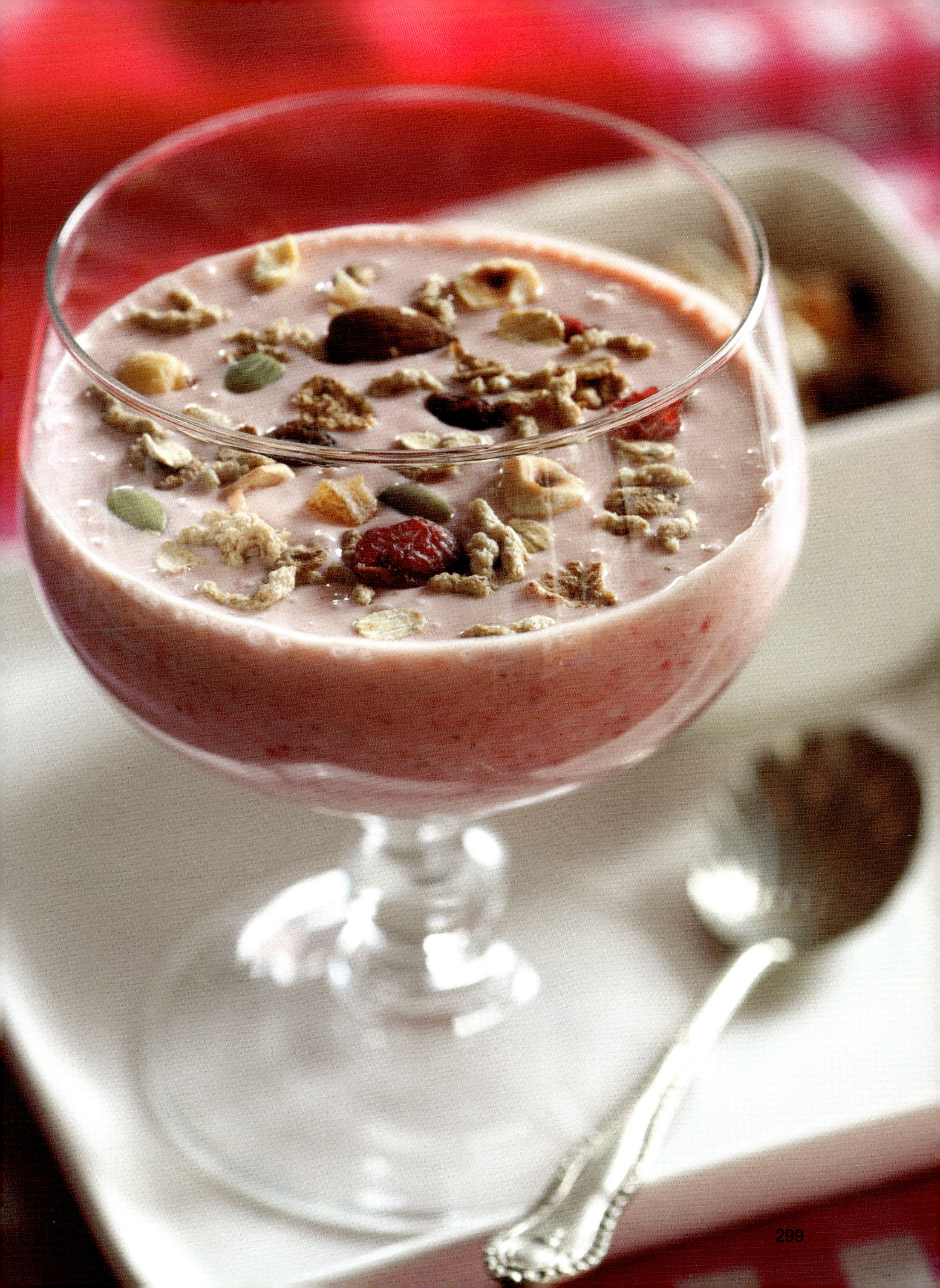

Raspberry and Pistachio Honey Yogurt

200 g (7 oz) yogurt
100 g (3½ oz) ricotta cheese
50 g (2 oz) raspberry
30 g (1 oz) pistachios
2 teaspoons honey

Combine the yogurt and ricotta cheese in the blender bowl and blend well until smooth. Separate the mixture into two small bowls or glasses. Arrange on the top some raspberries, pistachios and drizzle over some runny honey.

Serves 2

Per serving
385 kcal, 29.6 g fat (12.1 g saturated), 15.3 g protein, 15.1 g carbs (14.2 g sugar), 2.9 g fibre, 0.6 g salt

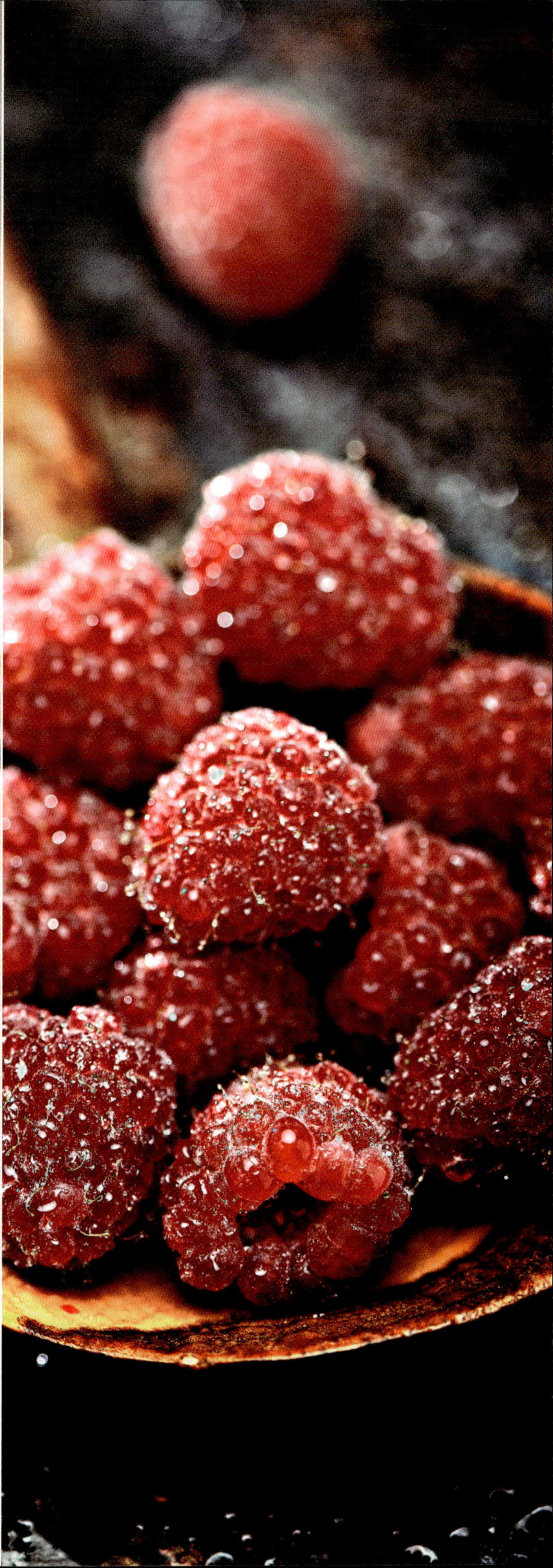

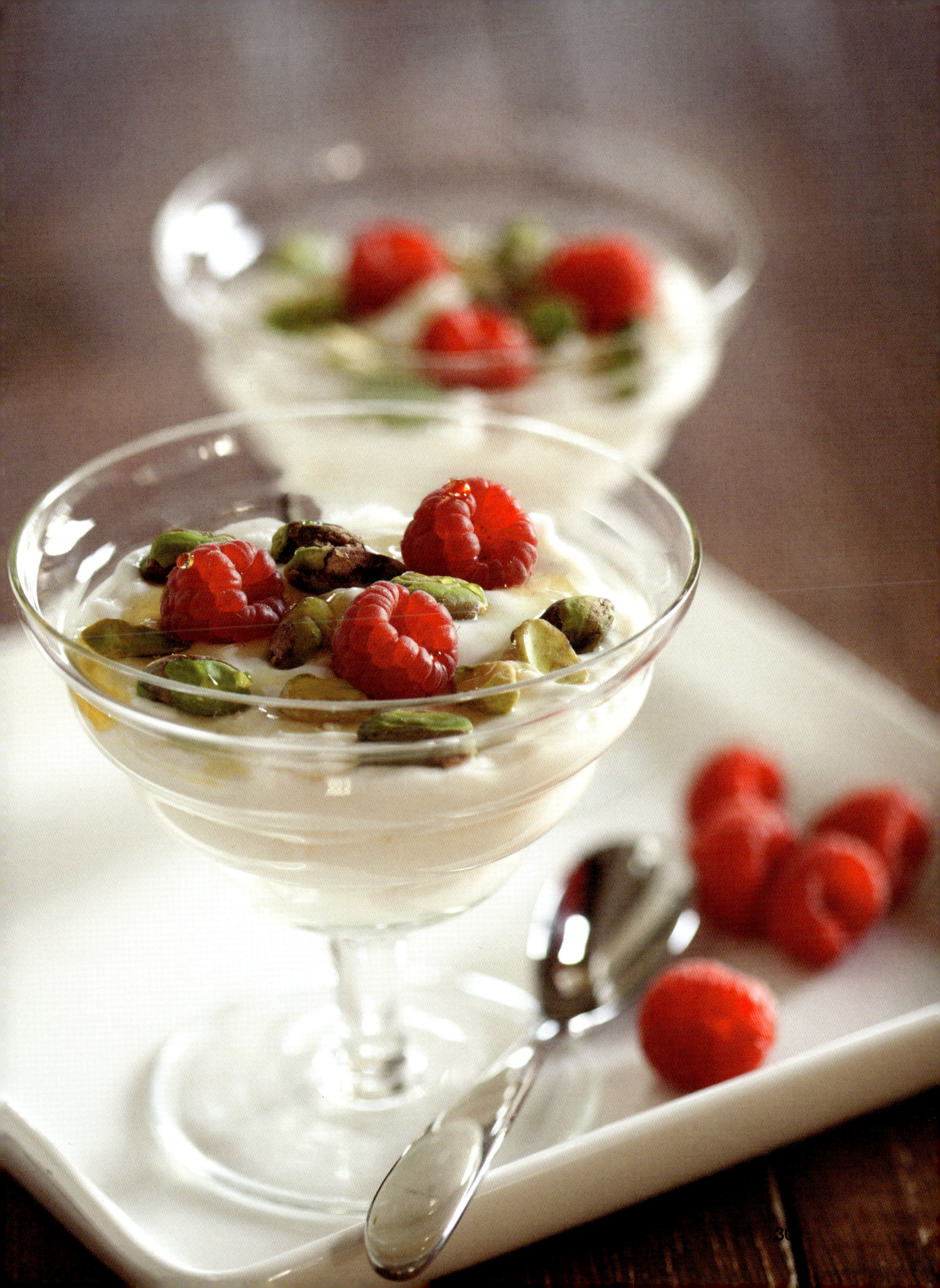

Tiramisu

600 g (21 oz) strained yogurt
300 g (10½ oz) mascarpone cheese
3 tablespoons icing sugar
50 ml (1½ fl oz) Tia Maria dark Liqueur or Kahlua Coffee Liqueur
250 g (9 oz) biscotti
2 tablespoons cocoa powder
fresh mint leaves, to decorate

Put the strained yogurt, mascarpone cheese, icing sugar and the liqueur, into a large bowl and mix well until you make a cream. Put layers of biscotti and cream onto a large plate or tray as shown in the picture. Finally sprinkle over sifted cocoa powder to decorate. Leave the tiramisu to rest in the refrigerator for about 2 hours before serving, decorated with fresh mint leaves.

Serves 10

Per serving
321 kcal, 20.8 g fat (10.9 g saturated), 8.5 g protein, 24.2 g carbs (22.4 g sugar), 1.6 g fibre, 0.2 g salt

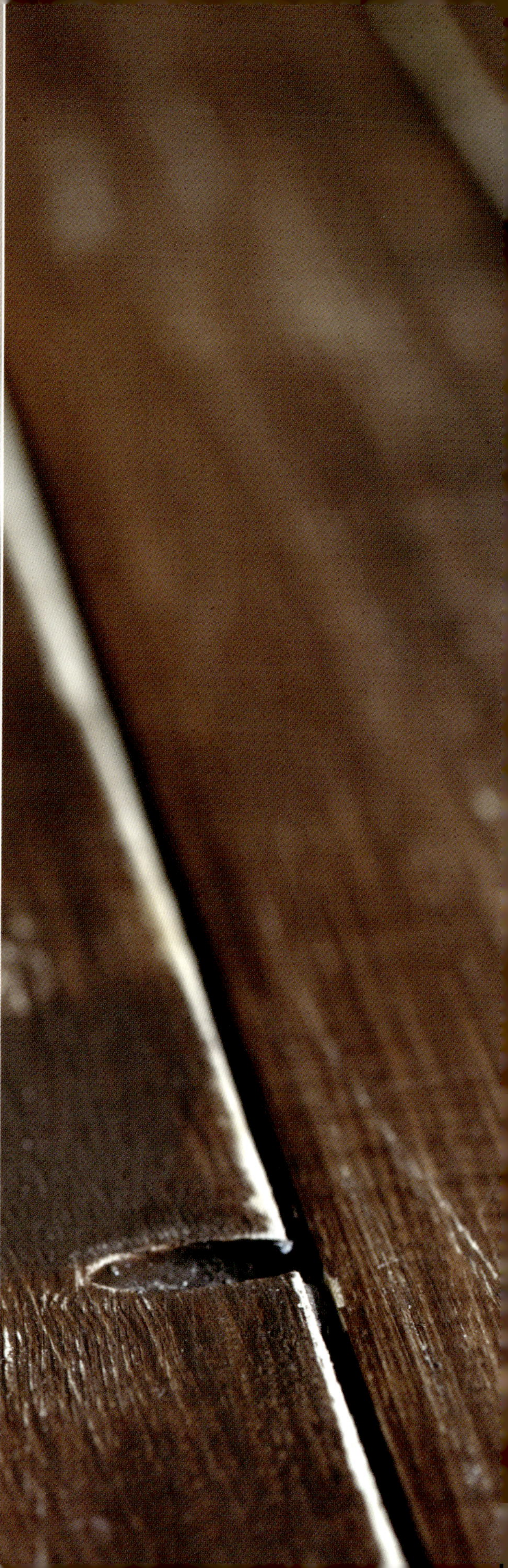

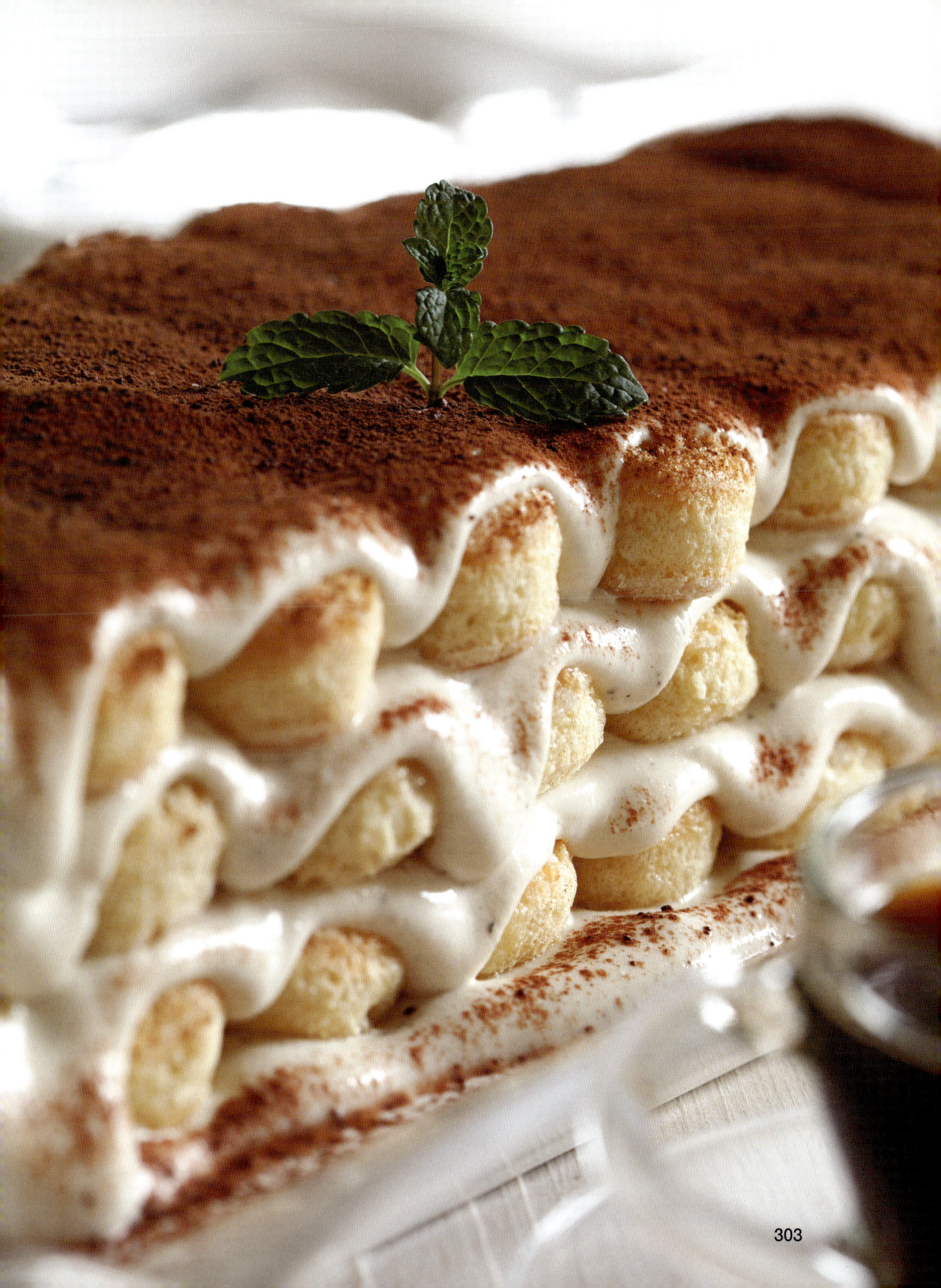

Goji Berries Yogurt Dessert

500 g (17½ oz) strained yogurt
50 g (2 oz) dried goji berries
50 g (2 oz) dried blackcurrants
50 g (2 oz) almond flakes
40 g (1½ oz) dark chocolate, broken into smaller pieces
1 banana

Add the banana and strained yogurt to a blender and blend until smooth. Next add the almond flakes, dried black currants, goji berries and pieces of dark chocolate, mix well with spoon. Divide the mixture into six serving glasses and leave in the refrigerator to rest for 30 minutes.

Serves 6

Per serving
242 kcal, 16.4 g fat (8.0 g saturated), 7.4 g protein, 16.6 g carbs (15.5 g sugar), 1.8 g fibre, 0.1 g salt

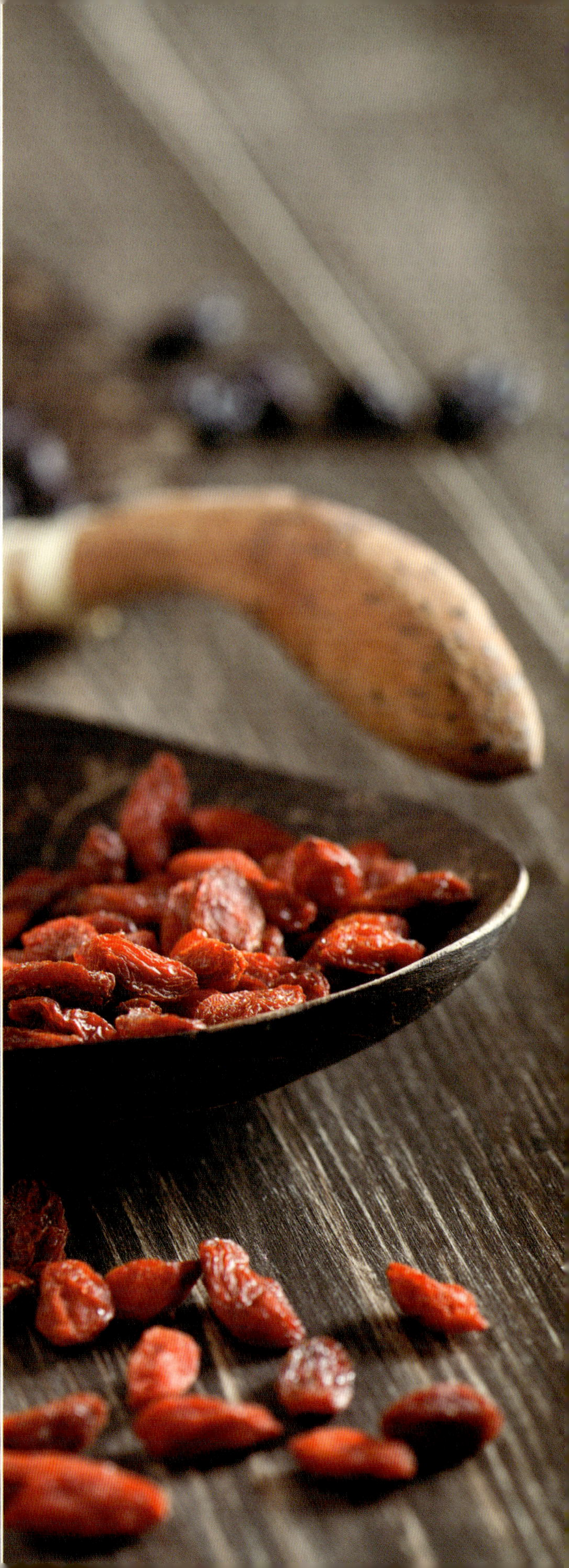

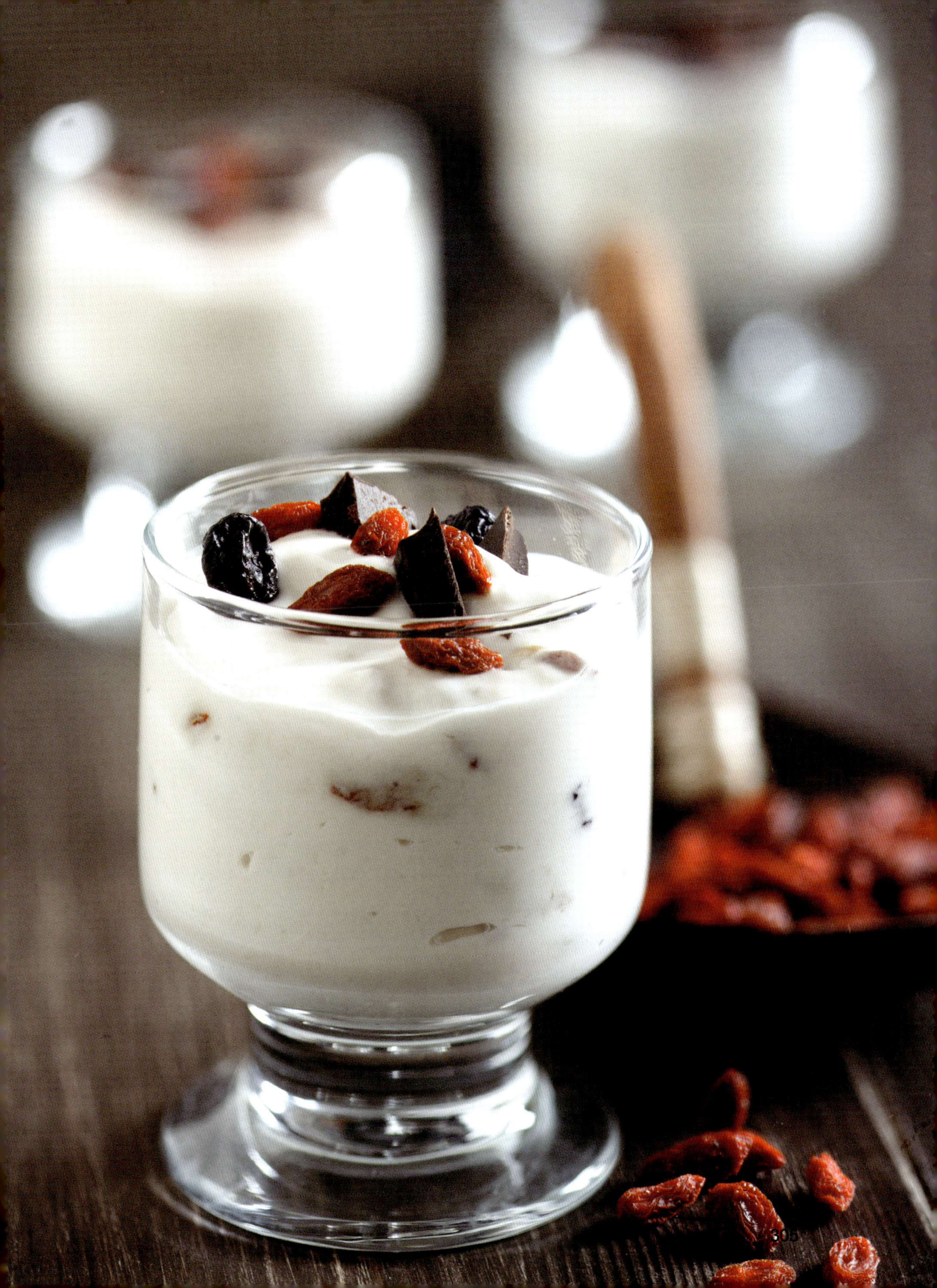

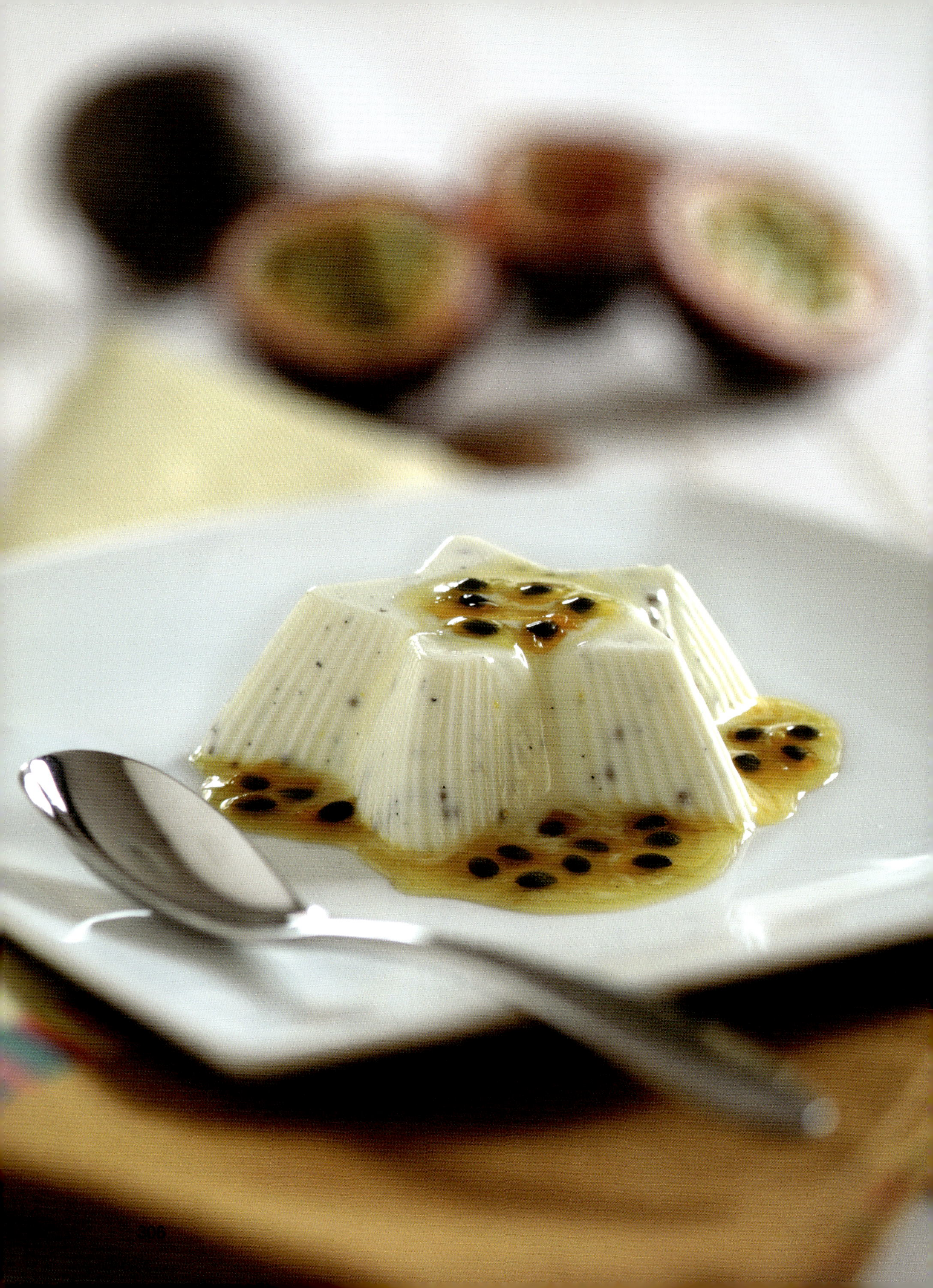

Yogurt Panna Cotta with Passion Fruit Syrup

vegetable oil, for greasing
100 ml (3½ oz) single cream
500 g (17½ oz) low fat yogurt
1 tablespoon chia seeds
4 teaspoons of vegetarian gelatine
200 ml (6¾ fl oz) cold water
4 tablespoons honey
seeds from 1 vanilla pod

For the passion fruit syrup:
50 ml (1½ fl oz) mineral water
50 g (2 oz) caster sugar
4 passion fruit
freshly squeezed juice of ½ lime

Lightly grease 8 panna cotta moulds with a little vegetable oil. In a medium bowl, combine the cream, yogurt and chia seeds, whisk together until smooth and set aside. Soften the gelatine in the cold water. In a small saucepan, bring the honey and vanilla seeds to simmering point and then add the gelatine and stir to dissolve. Pour the honey mixture over the yogurt mixture. Fill the prepared moulds with the mixture and leave them in the refrigerator for about 5 hours to set.

To make the passion fruit syrup, in a small saucepan bring the mineral water to simmering point. Add the sugar and stir well for about 3-5 minutes. Add the pulp from the passion fruit and lime juice and simmer over a medium heat for about 5 minutes or until the liquid becomes syrupy. Set aside to cool.

Before serving, dip the bases of the panna cotta moulds in warm water for a few seconds, and then turn out onto serving plates. Spoon over some of the passion fruit syrup and serve quickly.

Serves 8

Per serving
193 kcal, 7.9 g fat (4.7 g saturated), 4.8 g protein, 28.0 g carbs (27.2 g sugar), 1.0 g fibre, 0.1 g salt

Mascarpone Yogurt

300 g (10½ oz) strained yogurt
3 tablespoons mascarpone
3 tablespoons icing sugar
50 g (2 oz) biscotti
8 medium strawberries
Some fresh mint leaves for decoration

In a blender grind the biscotti into crumbs then add the strained yogurt, mascarpone and icing sugar. Mix well until smooth.
Slice the strawberries and arrange layers of flavor, strawberries and mixture and decorate with fresh mint leaves. Let the desert rest for no more than 30 minutes in the refrigerator and serve.

Serves 4

Per serving
284 kcal, 14.6 g fat (6.4 g saturated), 8.8 g protein, 30.8 g carbs (29.0 g sugar), 1.7 g fibre 0.16 g salt

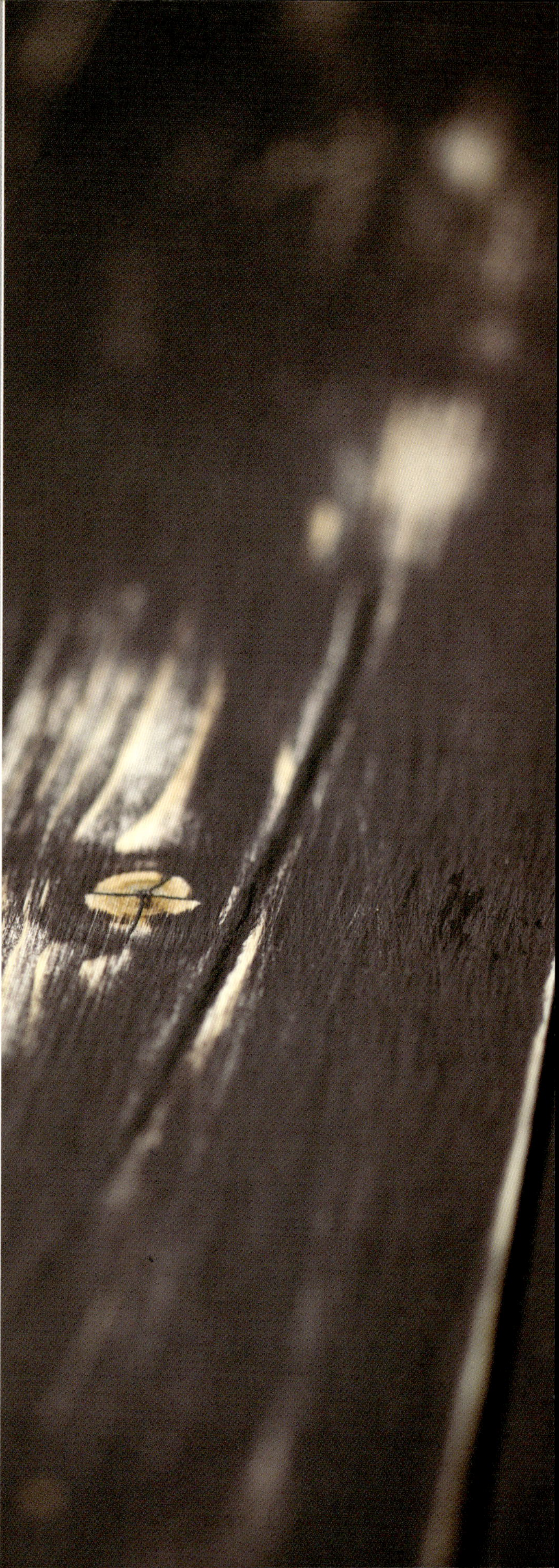

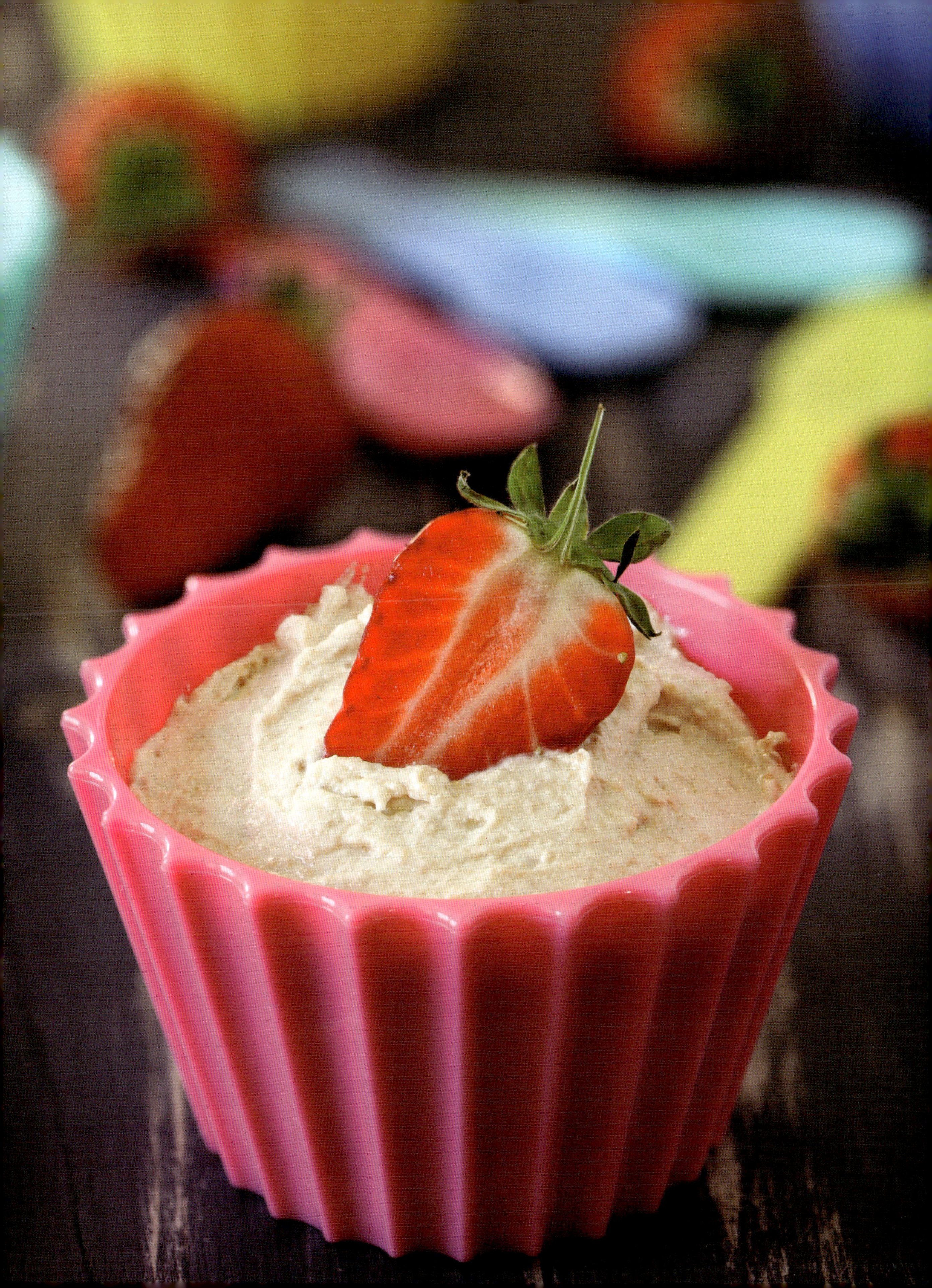

Strawberry Panna Cotta

500 g (17½ oz) low fat yogurt
10 tablespoons icing sugar
600 g (21 oz) strawberry, washed and halved
12 g (½ oz) vegetarian gelatine, softened in 200 ml (6¾ fl oz) cold water
1 teaspoon vanilla flavoring

For decoration:
pinch of dried edible flower petals
50 g (2 oz) toasted almonds, slices

Arrange the washed and halved strawberries at the bottom of a 25.5 cm (10 inch) round crispy tart pan. Combine the yogurt, the icing sugar and vanilla flavoring in a large bowl and mix well. Add the softened vegetarian gelatin and stir with a whisk. Carefully pour the yogurt mixture over the strawberries and cover up with kitchen cling film and leave overnight in the refrigerator. Remove the film and dip the base of the tart pan in a large tray filled with hot water for a few seconds. Transfer the panna cotta gently to a large plate upside down and sprinkle over some dried edible flower petals and toasted almonds slices.

Serves 8

Per serving
134 kcal, 4.2 g fat (0.7 g saturated), 6.2 g protein, 18.8 g carbs (18.5 g sugar), 1.7 g fibre, 0.1 g salt

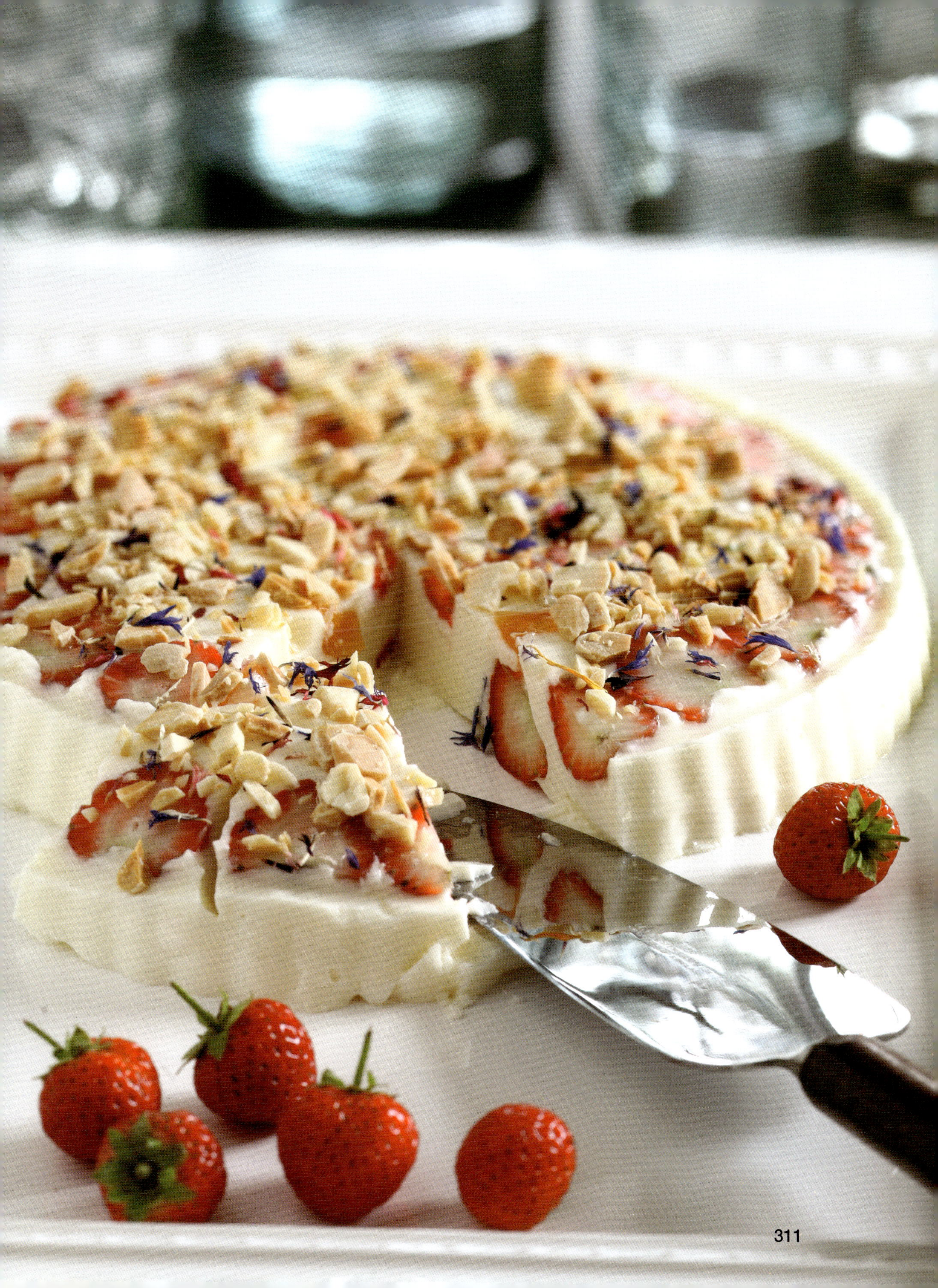

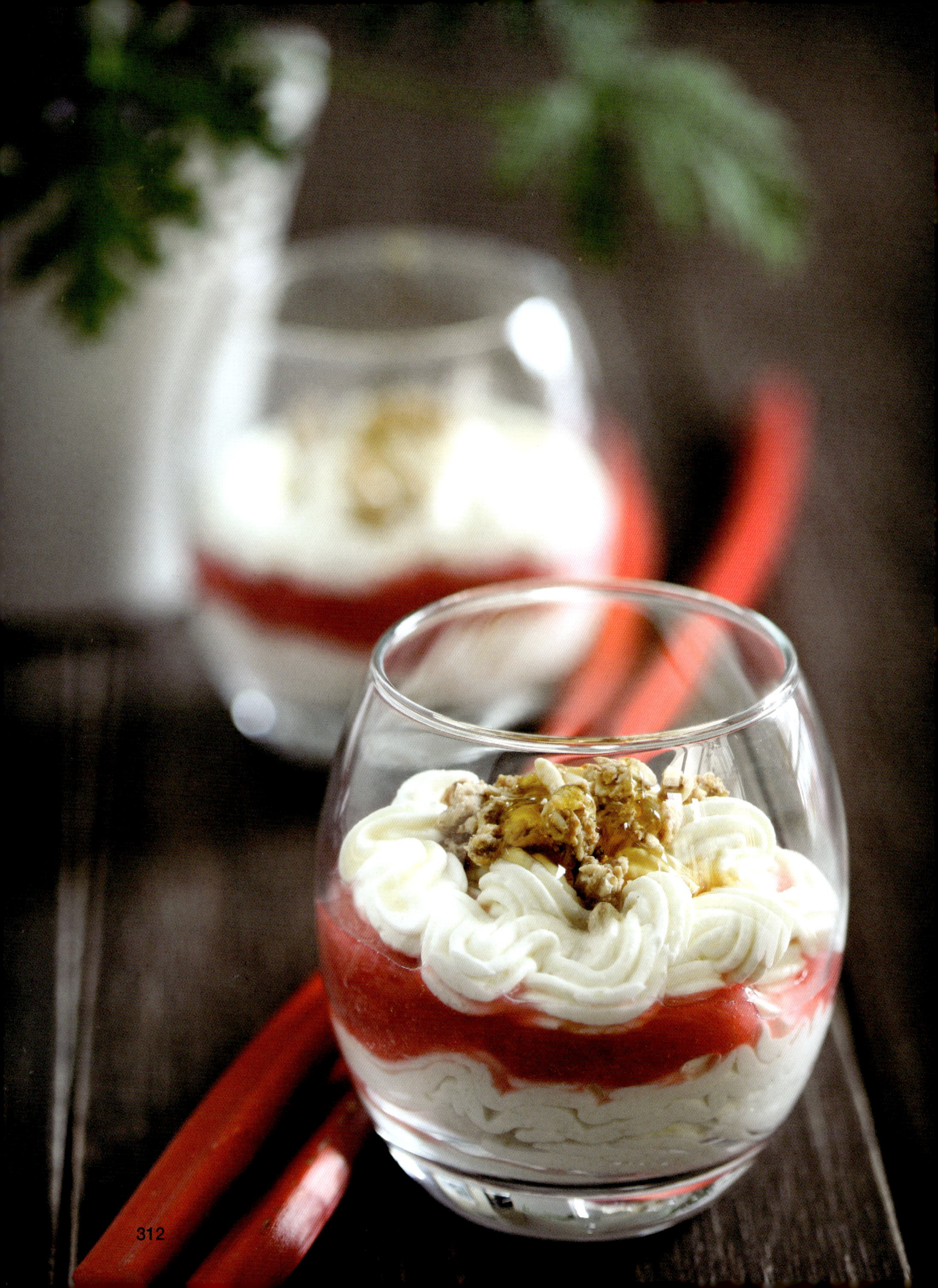

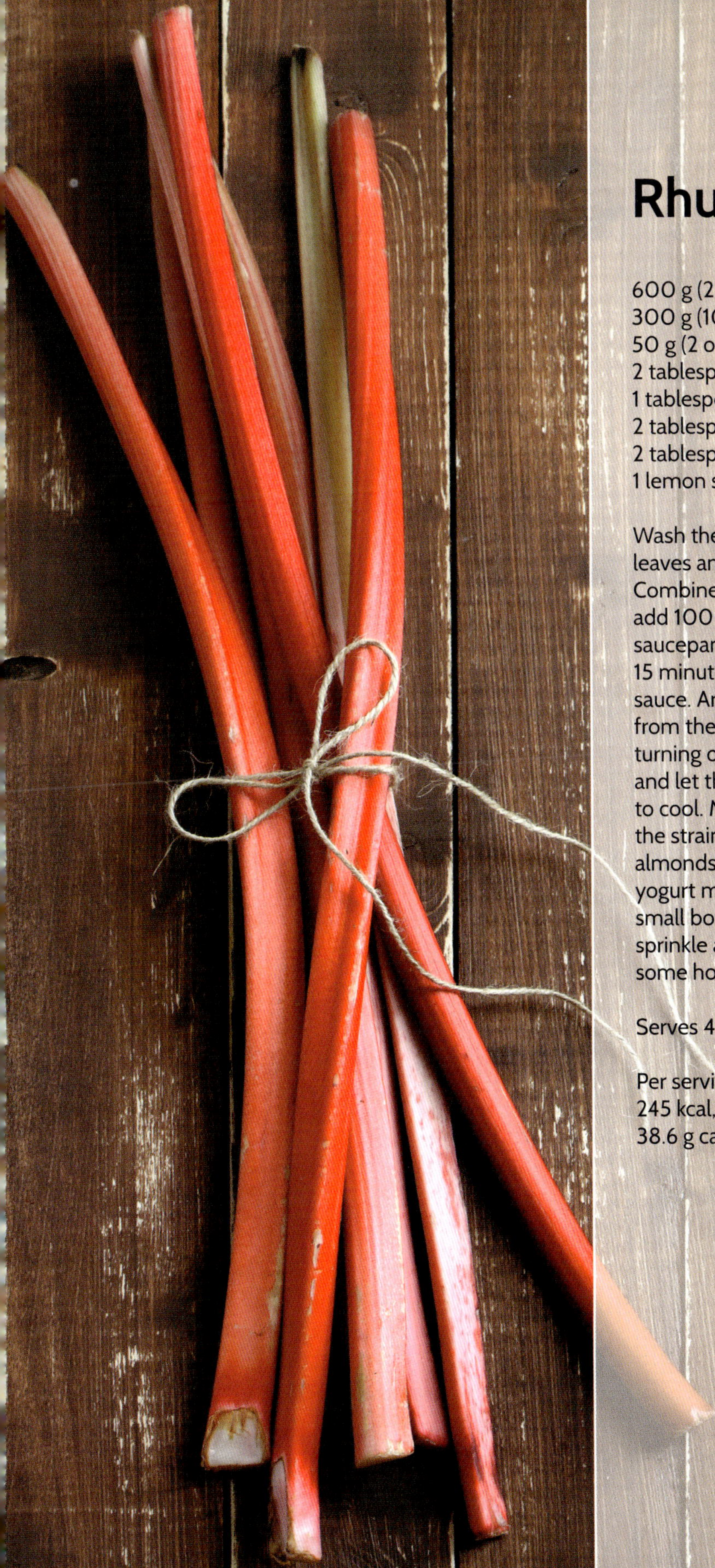

Rhubarb Parfaits

600 g (21 oz) yogurt, strained
300 g (10½ oz) rhubarb
50 g (2 oz) brown sugar
2 tablespoons icing sugar
1 tablespoon honey
2 tablespoons granola
2 tablespoon almonds, grounded
1 lemon scented geranium leaf

Wash the rhubarb and trim off any remaining leaves and chop it into 2.5 cm (1-inch) pieces. Combine the rhubarb pieces with sugar and add 100 ml (3½ oz) cold water Into a medium saucepan and cook on a low heat for about 15 minutes until the rhubarbs become a chunky sauce. Around 3 minutes before removing it from the heat, add the geranium leaf. After turning off the heat remove the geranium leaf and let the mixture rest for another 20 minutes to cool. Meanwhile in a medium bowl combine the strained yogurt, icing sugar and grounded almonds and mix it well. To serve divide the yogurt mixture and cooked rhubarb into four small bowls or glasses making layers then sprinkle a pinch of granola on the top and pour some honey over. Serve immediately.

Serves 4

Per serving
245 kcal, 6.8 g fat (1.3 g saturated), 10.2 g protein, 38.6 g carbs (34.7 g sugar), 1.9 g fibre, 0.3 g salt

Yogurt and White Chocolate Dessert

150 g (5 oz) sour cream
250 g (9 oz) white chocolate, melted
225 g (8 oz) low fat yogurt
1 teaspoon cardamom seeds, crushed
7 g (1/4 oz) gelatin
handful fresh berries
some pistachio sugar syrup for decoration
30 g (1 oz) hazelnuts, chopped

Dissolve the gelatin following the instructions on the packet. Then in a large bowl pour the yogurt and the melted chocolate and mix well. Next add the gelatin to the yogurt mixture and stir again. Finally add to the mixture the sour cream, cardamom seeds, chopped hazelnuts and mix well again. Pour the ready mixture into a large silicone chocolate mould. Leave it to cool overnight in the refrigerator. Serve cold decorated with fresh berries and pistachio sugar syrup.

Serves 12

Per serving
164 kcal, 10.6 g fat (5.5 g saturated), 3.7 g protein, 14.5 g carbs (14.4 g sugar), 0.3 g fibre, 0.1 g salt

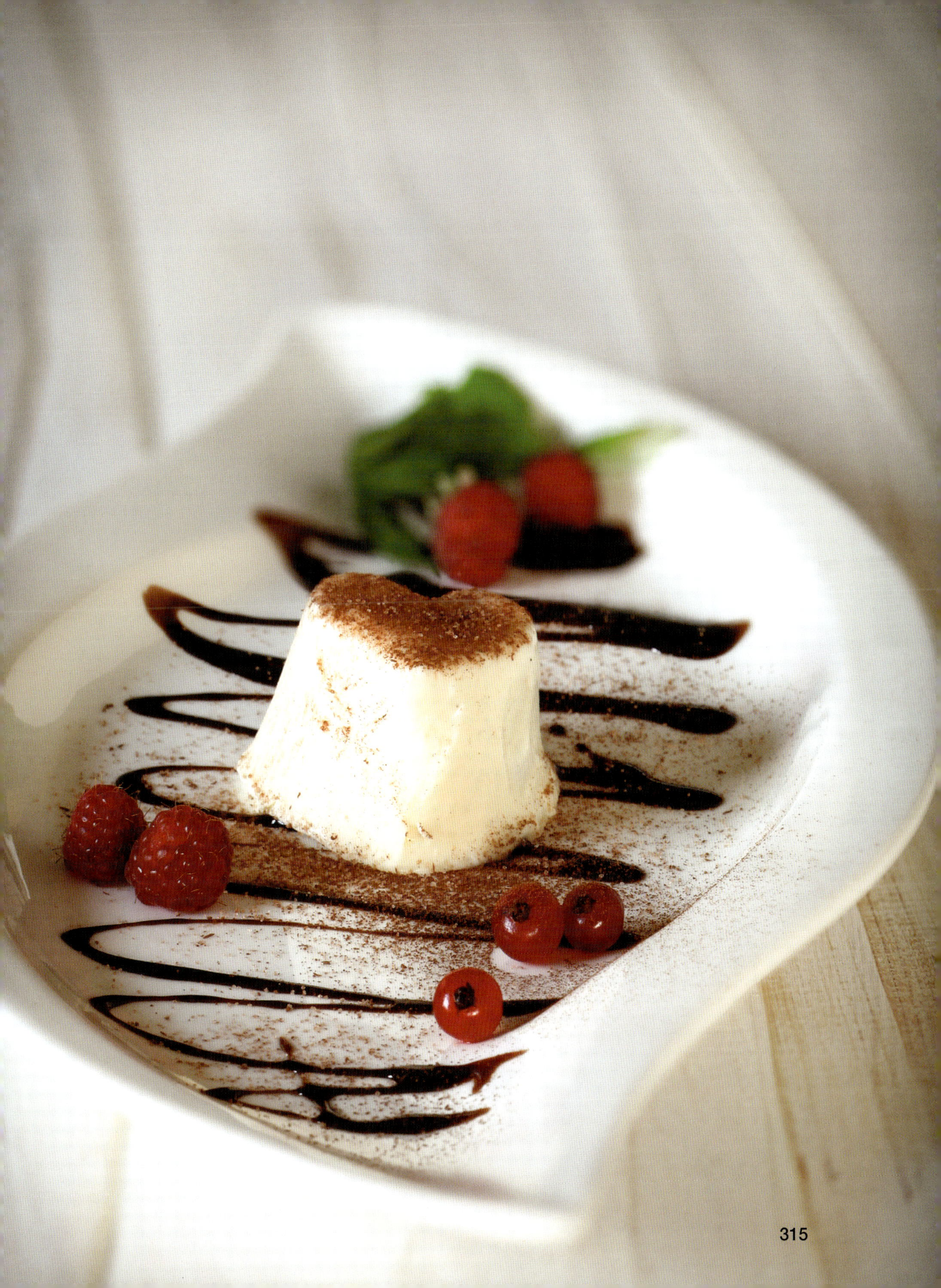

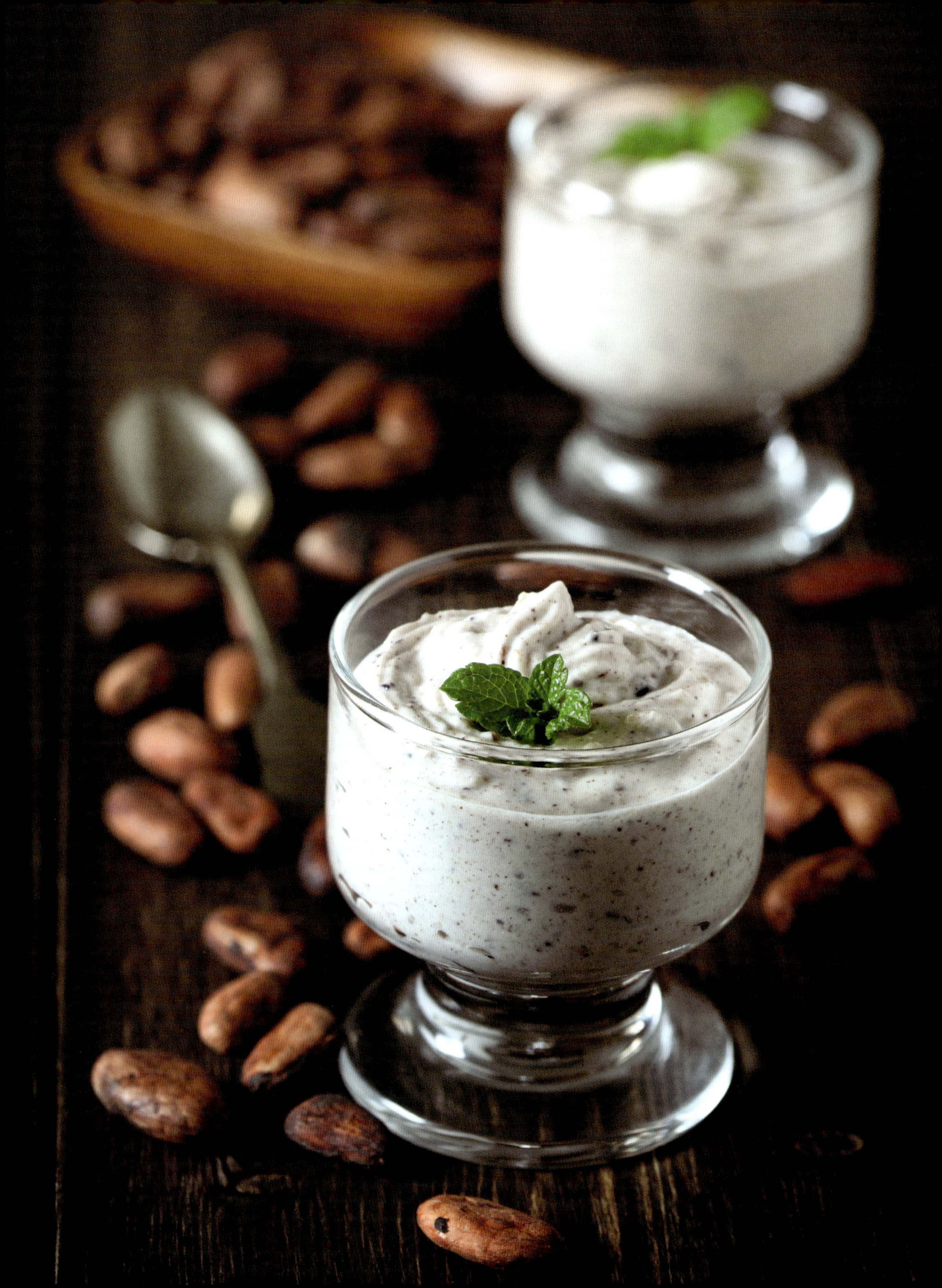

Yogurt Cocoa Mousse

20 g (¾ oz) whole cocoa beans
200 g (7 oz) low fat yogurt, strained
100 g (3½ oz) ricotta cheese
100 g (3½ oz) mascarpone
20 g (¾ oz) toasted hazelnuts, chopped
1 tablespoon brown sugar
50 ml (1½ fl oz) whisky, optional
some fresh mint leaves for decoration

In a blender combine the whole cocoa beans, toasted hazelnuts and blend until well crushed. Then pour in the strained yogurt add the ricotta cheese, mascarpone, brown sugar and whisky. Blend until smooth and divide into four bowls or glasses. Decorate with some fresh mint leaves. Leave the desserts to cool in the refrigerator for half hour or more and serve.

Serves 4

Per serving
263 kcal, 17.3 g fat (10.7 g saturated), 7.8 g protein, 13.3 g carbs (12.3 g sugar), 0.8 g fibre, 0.3 g salt

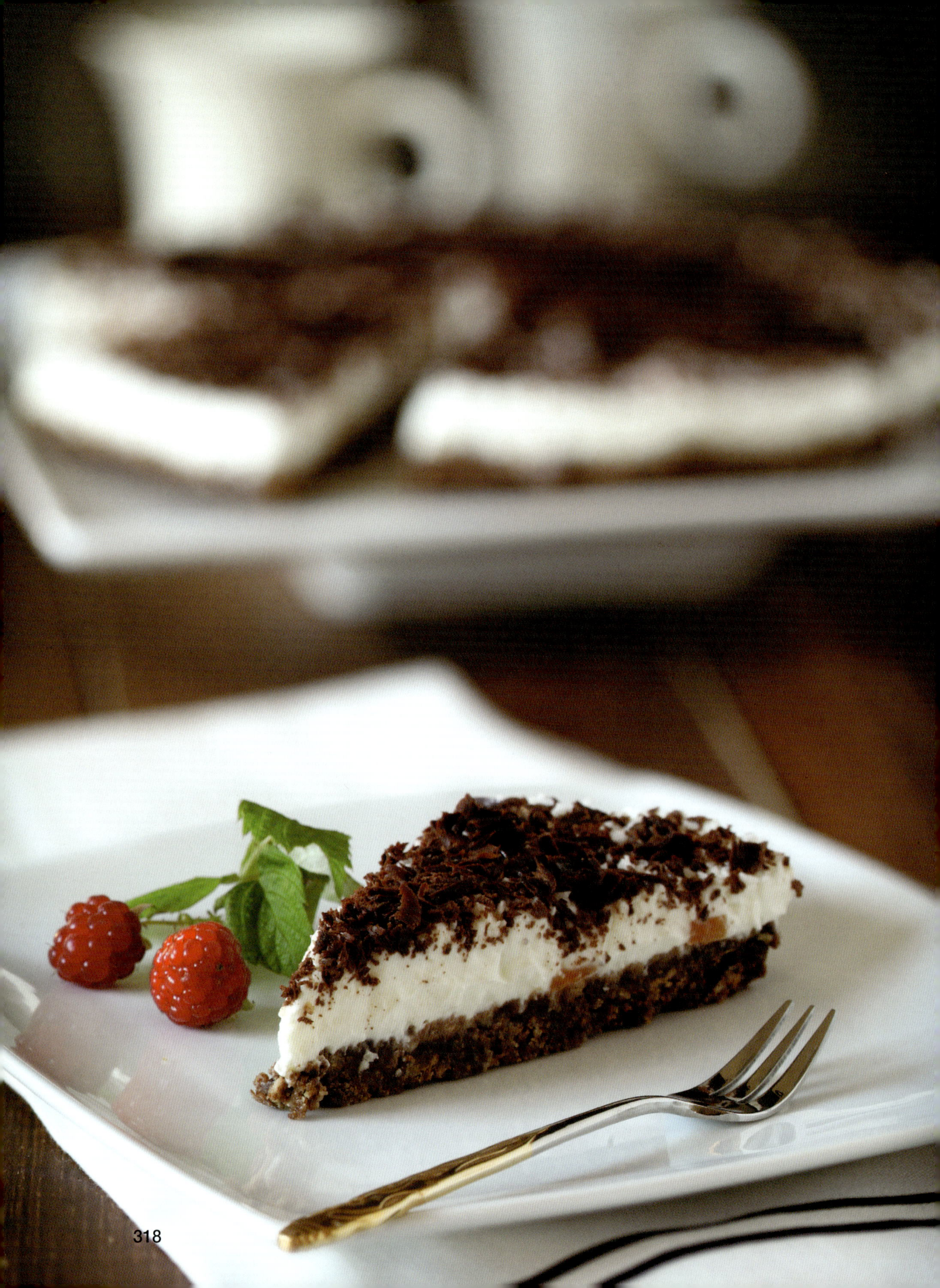

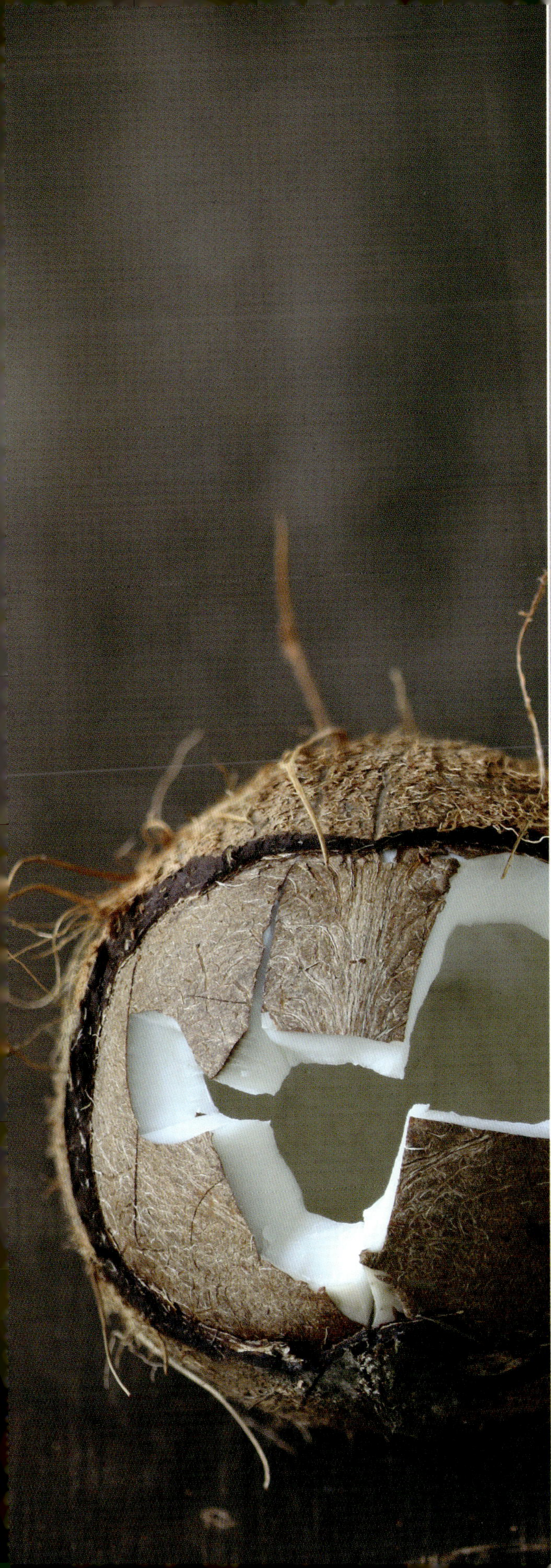

Coconut Cake

Base:
300 g (10½ oz) chocolate biscuits
125 g (4½ oz) butter, melted

Filling:
500 g (17½ oz) strained yogurt
30 g (1 oz) desiccated coconut
30 g (1 oz) citrus peel
12 g (½ oz) gelatin
30 g (1 oz) dark chocolate, shredded

Finely crush the chocolate biscuits and add the soft butter in a large bowl and stir until the mixture is compact. Then pour into a large parchment-lined cake pan and level well with a spoon. Let it cool in the refrigerator. Meanwhile, in a large bowl pour the strained yogurt, desiccated coconut and citrus peel and mix well. After that following the instructions on the packet, dissolve the gelatin and leave it to cool for a couple of minutes. Next add the gelatin to the yogurt mixture and stir with a whisk until well mixed. Pour the mixture over the biscuits base and leave it to chill in the refrigerator for 4 hours. Sprinkle over the shredded dark chocolate and serve.

Serves 6

Per serving
519 kcal, 35.6 g fat (22.2 g saturated), 10.2 g protein, 42.0 g carbs (30.9 g sugar), 1.4 g fibre, 0.8 g salt

Yogurt Panna Cotta with Raspberry Marmalade

50 g (2 oz) quinoa, boiled and drained
350 g (12 oz) low fat yogurt, strained
100 ml (3½ oz) semi skim milk
100 g (3½ oz) finely chopped pistachio nuts
12 g (½ oz) vegetarian gelatin, softened in water
2 tablespoons sugar
1 teaspoon vanilla flavoring
100 g (3½ oz) fresh raspberries to serve

Boil the quinoa seeds in 2 litres (4½ pints) water in a medium saucepan for about 15 minutes. Transfer into a cooking strainer and drain for about 5 minutes.
Next transfer it to a medium bowl and add the strained yogurt, milk, chopped pistachios, sugar, vanilla flavoring and mix well. Once mixed, add the softened in water vegetarian gelatin and stir with a whisk. Divide the mixture into four bowls or glasses by first pouring one tablespoon of raspberry marmalade and then add the yogurt mixture. Sprinkle over some chopped pistachios and arrange some fresh raspberries. Leave it to cool in the refrigerator for a minimum of 3 hours then serve.

Serves 4

Per serving
305 kcal, 15.8 g fat (2.8 g saturated), 14.1 g protein, 28.4 g carbs (21.6 g sugar), 2.9 g fibre, 0.5 g salt

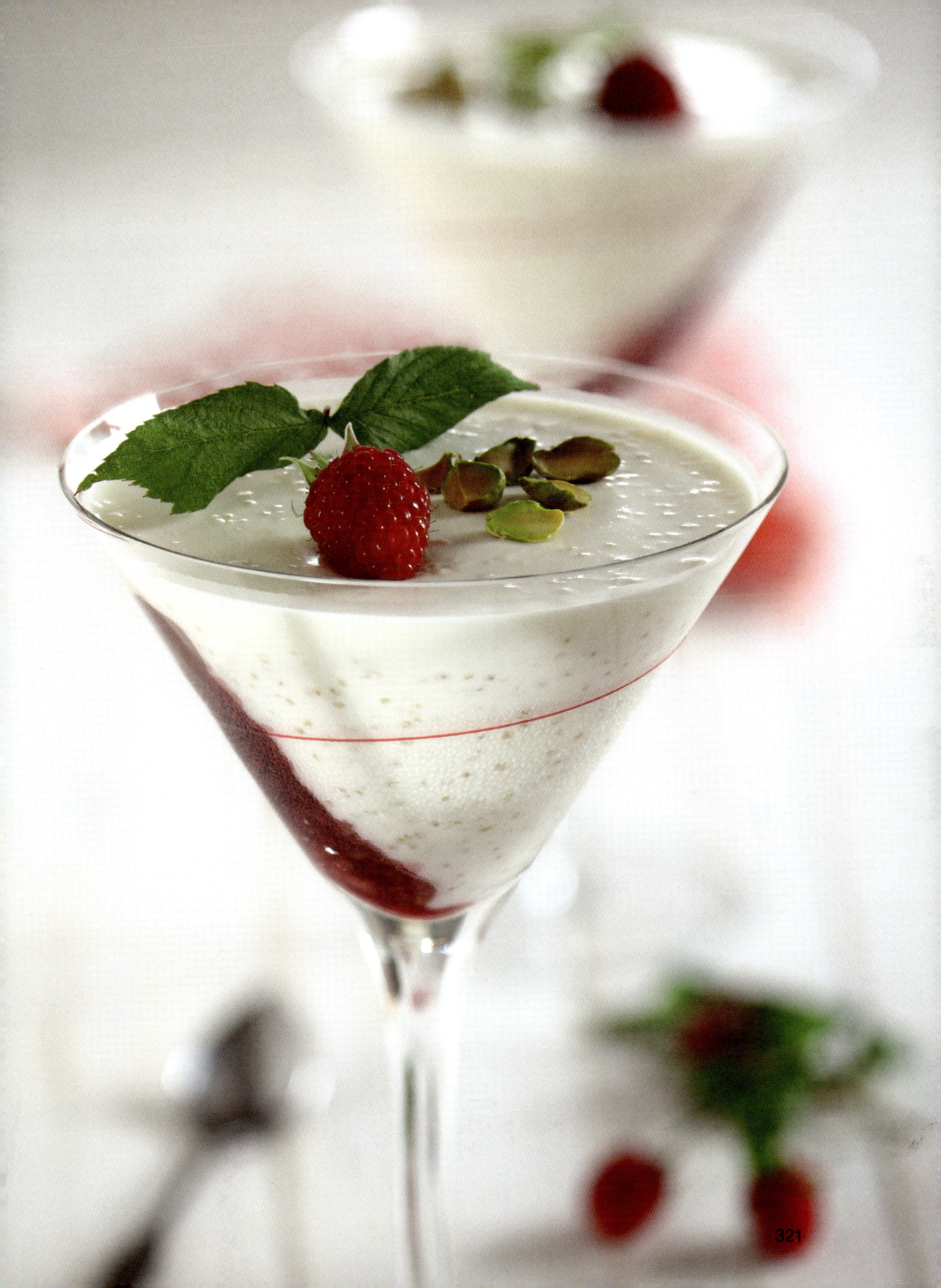

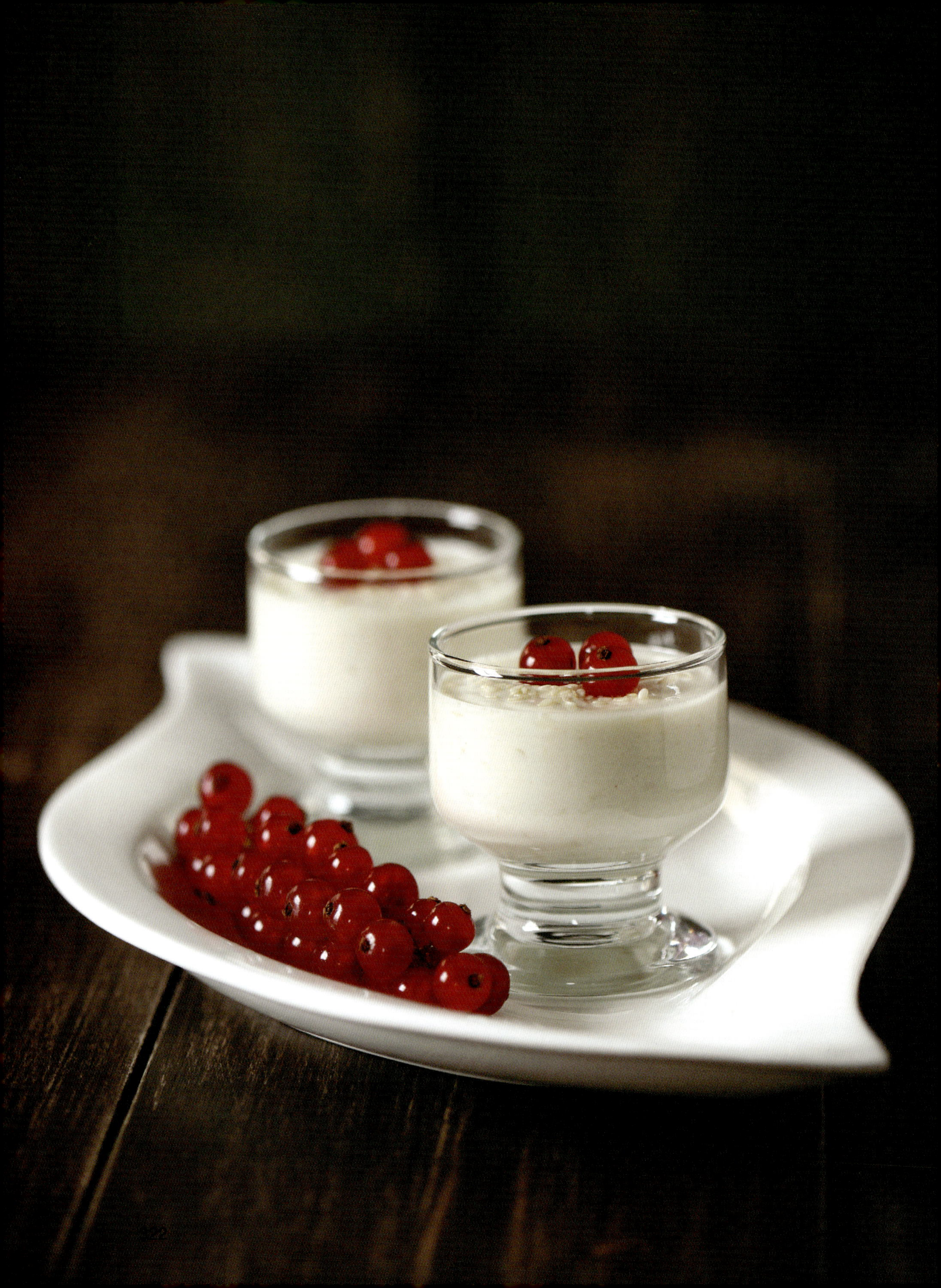

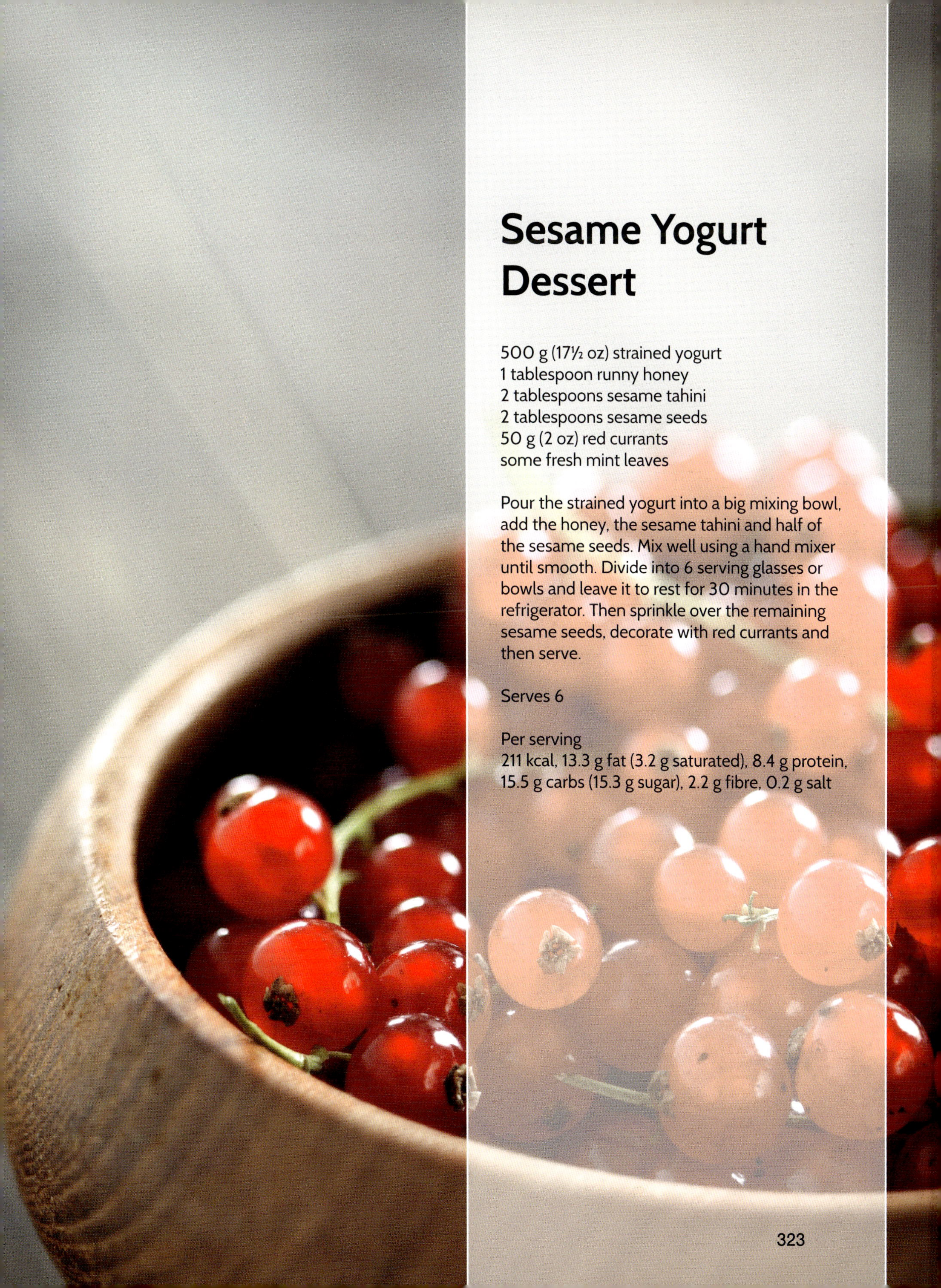

Sesame Yogurt Dessert

500 g (17½ oz) strained yogurt
1 tablespoon runny honey
2 tablespoons sesame tahini
2 tablespoons sesame seeds
50 g (2 oz) red currants
some fresh mint leaves

Pour the strained yogurt into a big mixing bowl, add the honey, the sesame tahini and half of the sesame seeds. Mix well using a hand mixer until smooth. Divide into 6 serving glasses or bowls and leave it to rest for 30 minutes in the refrigerator. Then sprinkle over the remaining sesame seeds, decorate with red currants and then serve.

Serves 6

Per serving
211 kcal, 13.3 g fat (3.2 g saturated), 8.4 g protein, 15.5 g carbs (15.3 g sugar), 2.2 g fibre, 0.2 g salt

Kumquats Yogurt Dessert

8 Kumquats, sliced and seeded
8 tablespoons granola
400 g (14 oz) low fat yogurt
4 tablespoons honey
2 tablespoons fresh mint leaves, chopped

Divide and put the granola into four glasses or small bowls then pour over four tablespoons of yogurt in each glass. Arrange the kumquat slices over the yogurt and pour some honey. Lastly decorate the top with some fresh mint leaves.

Serves 4

Per serving
272 kcal, 5.2 g fat (0.7 g saturated), 8.3 g protein, 49.6 g carbs (35.1 g sugar), 4.1 g fibre, 0.2 g salt

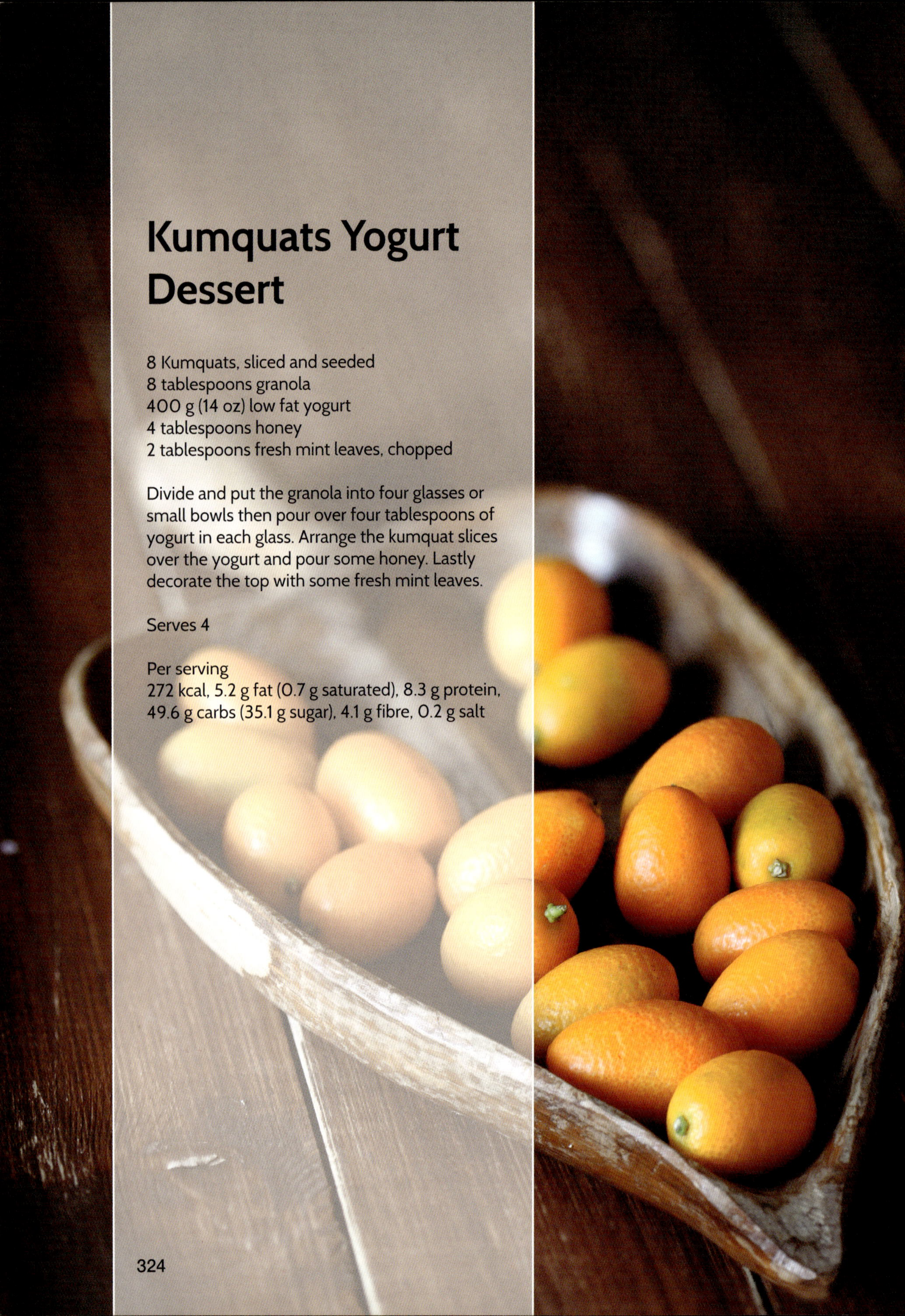

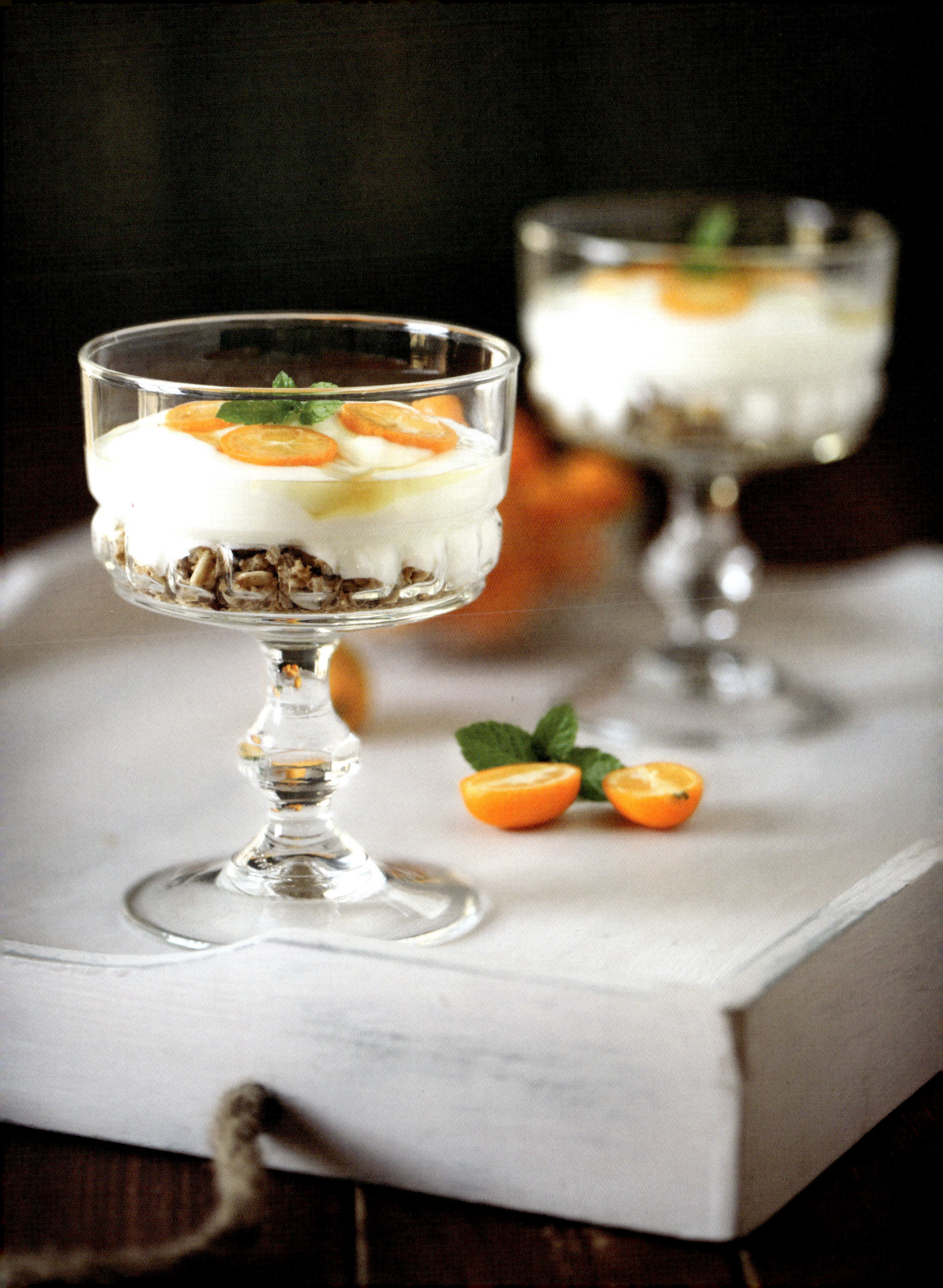

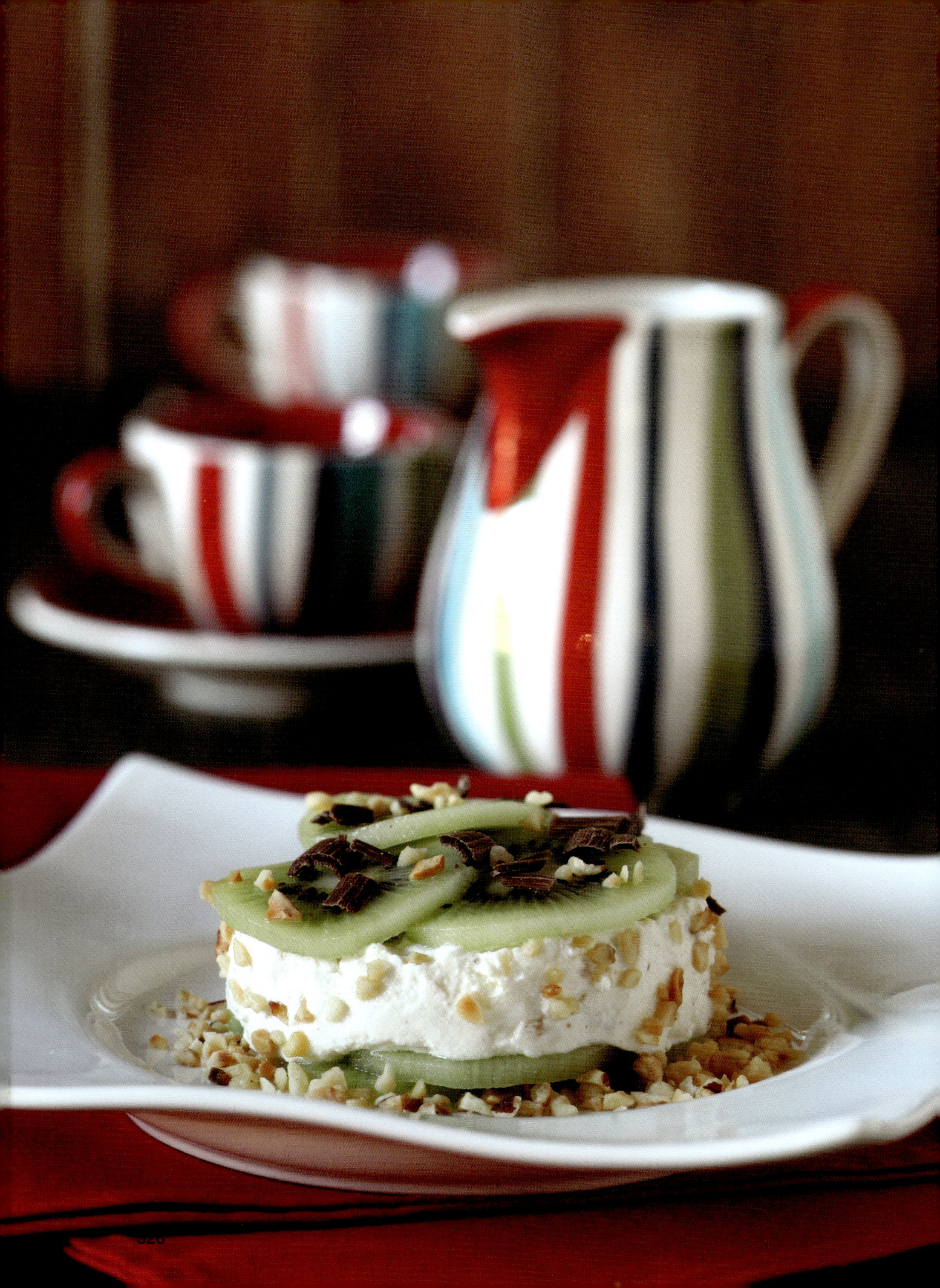

Kiwi Yogurt Dessert

6 ripe kiwis
200 g (7 oz) ricotta
200 g (7 oz) mascarpone
200 g (7 oz) low fat yogurt, strained
30 g (1 oz) dry dates, chopped
1 tablespoon of icing sugar
1 teaspoon ground cardamom
50 g (2 oz) hazelnuts, roasted and chopped
50 g (2 oz) dark chocolate, shredded

Combine together in a medium bowl the ricotta, mascarpone cheese, strained yogurt, sugar, ground cardamom, chopped dry dates and half of the finely chopped hazelnuts. Mix well and set aside. Peel the kiwis and cut them into thin slices. On a serving plate using a round cake ring make a kiwi layer on the bottom of the cake ring, fill it with the yogurt mixture and finish with another layer of kiwi slices. Take the round cake ring out and decorate with shredded chocolate and chopped roasted hazelnuts. Serve cold.

Serves 6

Per serving
349 kcal, 26.4 g fat (15.8 g saturated), 9.3 g protein, 19.4 g carbs (18.2 g sugar), 2.6 g fibre, 0.1 g salt

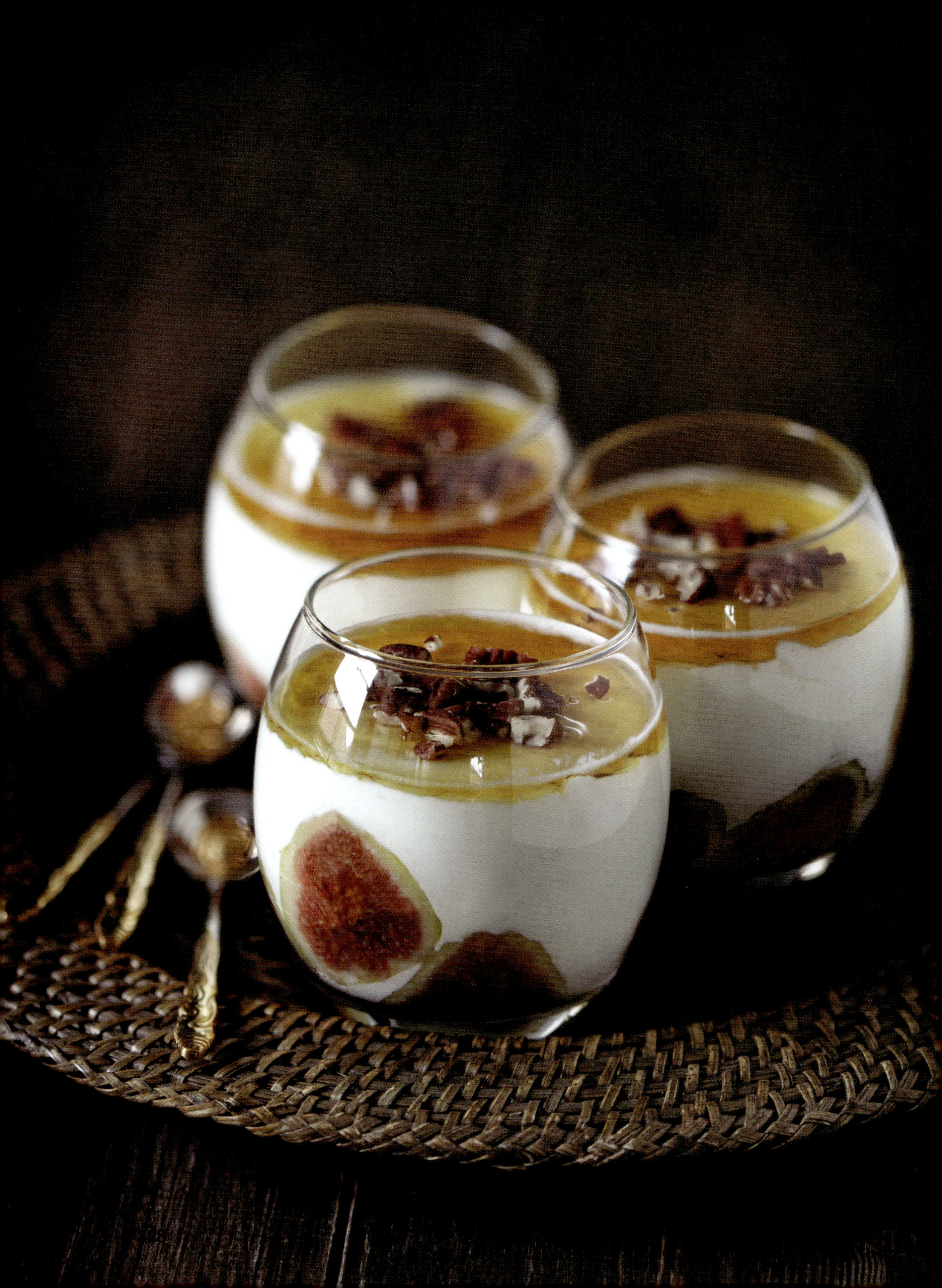

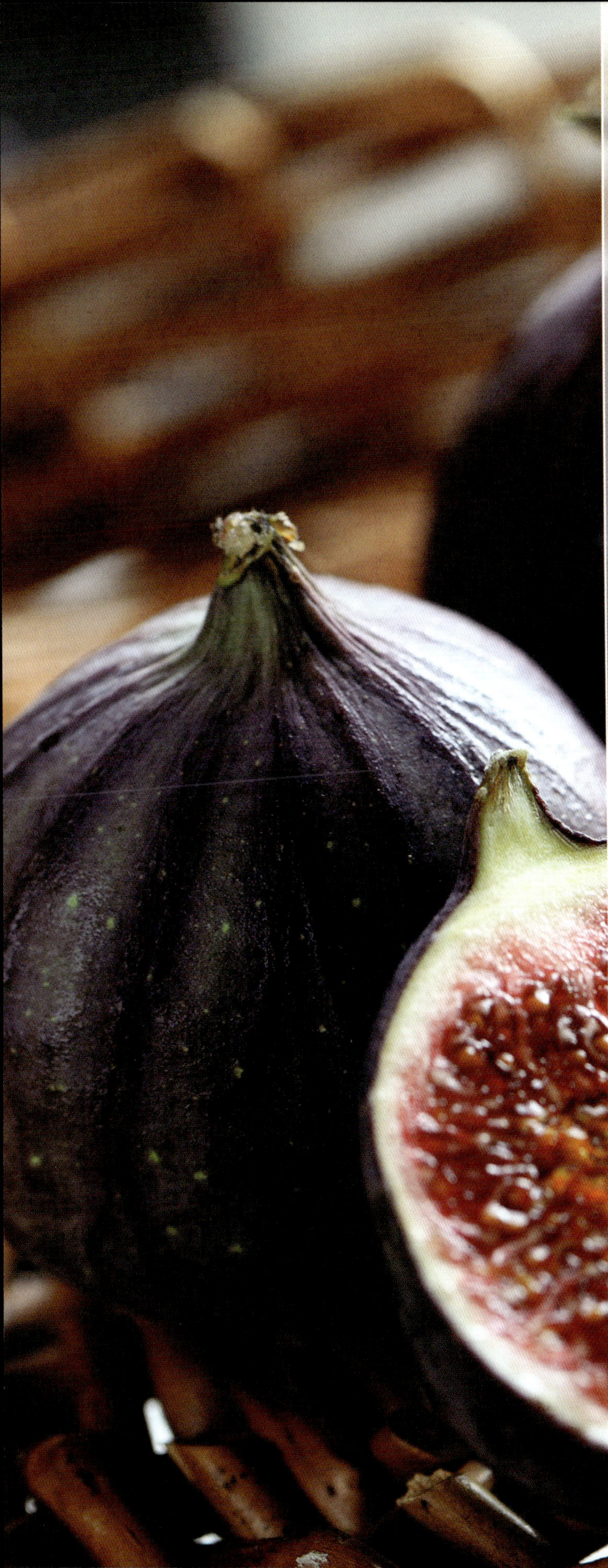

Figs and Yogurt Panna Cotta

500 g (17½ oz) low fat yogurt
300 ml (10 fl oz) cream
140 g (5 oz) fresh figs, peeled and sliced
12 g (½ oz) of vegetarian gelatin, softened
6 tablespoons honey
100 g (3½ oz) toasted walnuts, coarsely chopped

Arrange the washed and sliced figs at the bottom of glasses or bowls. Then pour the yogurt into a large bowl, add the cream and mix well. Next add the softened in water vegetarian gelatin and stir with a whisk. Pour the yogurt mixture gently over the figs to fill the glasses and cover up with kitchen cling film. Leave overnight int the refrigerator. Remove the film and pour over 2 tablespoons of honey in each glass and sprinkle over some chopped walnuts.

Serves 6

Per serving
344 kcal, 21.9 g fat (7.9 g saturated), 10.2 g protein, 28.5 g carbs (28.3 g sugar), 1.2 g fibre, 0.2 g salt

Stuffed Apple with Walnuts and Blackcurrants

4 apples
50 g (2 oz) walnuts, chopped
50 g (2 oz) dry black currants
2 tablespoons oatbran
2 tablespoons sugar
2 tablespoons cinnamon
2 tablespoons of grape seeds oil
2 tablespoons honey
250 g (9 oz) low fat yogurt, strained

Preheat the oven to 180°C (350°F). In a medium bowl make the stuffing mixture by combining the chopped walnuts, raisins, oat bran, grape seeds oil and mix well. Add the sugar and cinnamon, mix again and set aside. Wash the apples and cut the tops almost quarter or so. Then using a melon baller or teaspoon make apple bowls by scooping out the inside of the apple to make enough room for the stuffing. Fill the apples with the stuffing and place them in a casserole dish. Add 100 ml (3½ oz) water to the dish to make a water bath, cover with kitchen foil and bake the oven for about 45 minutes. Once cooked remove from the oven and leave it to cool a bit and serve together with a tablespoon of strained yogurt, pour over a teaspoon of runny honey and sprinkle some cinnamon.

Serves 4

Per serving
335 kcal, 15.6 g fat (2.1 g saturated), 6.6 g protein, 42.8 g carbs (40.5 g sugar), 4.7 g fibre, 0.1 g salt

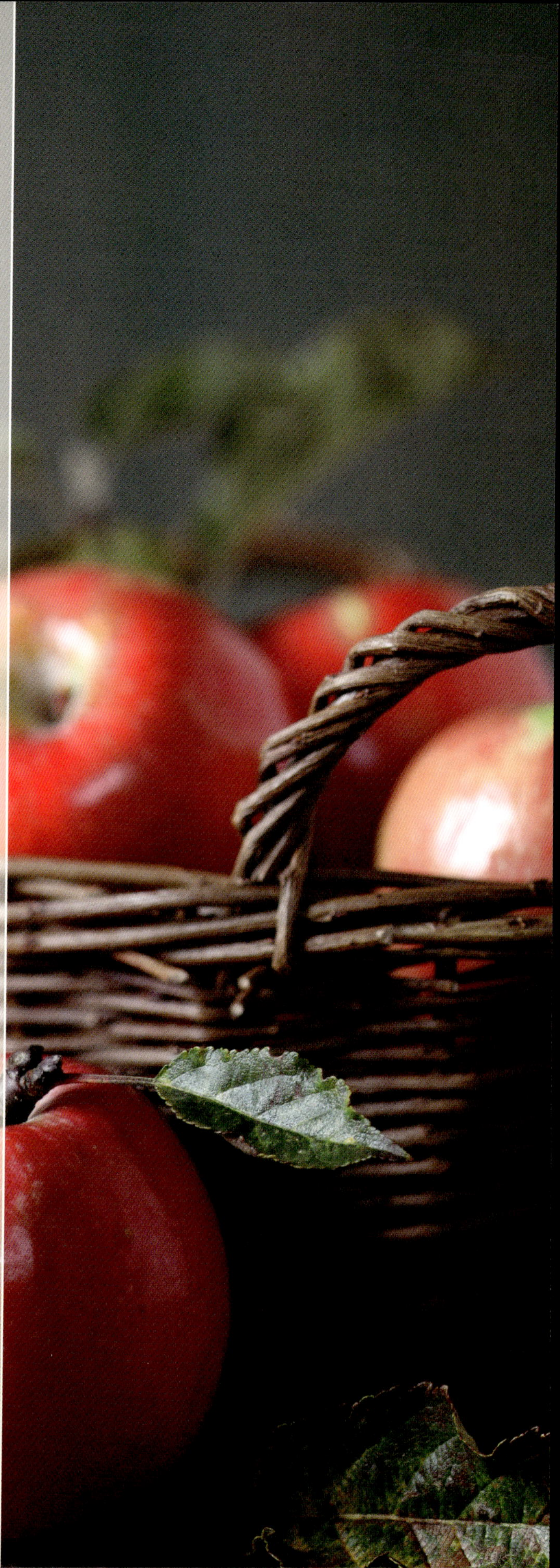

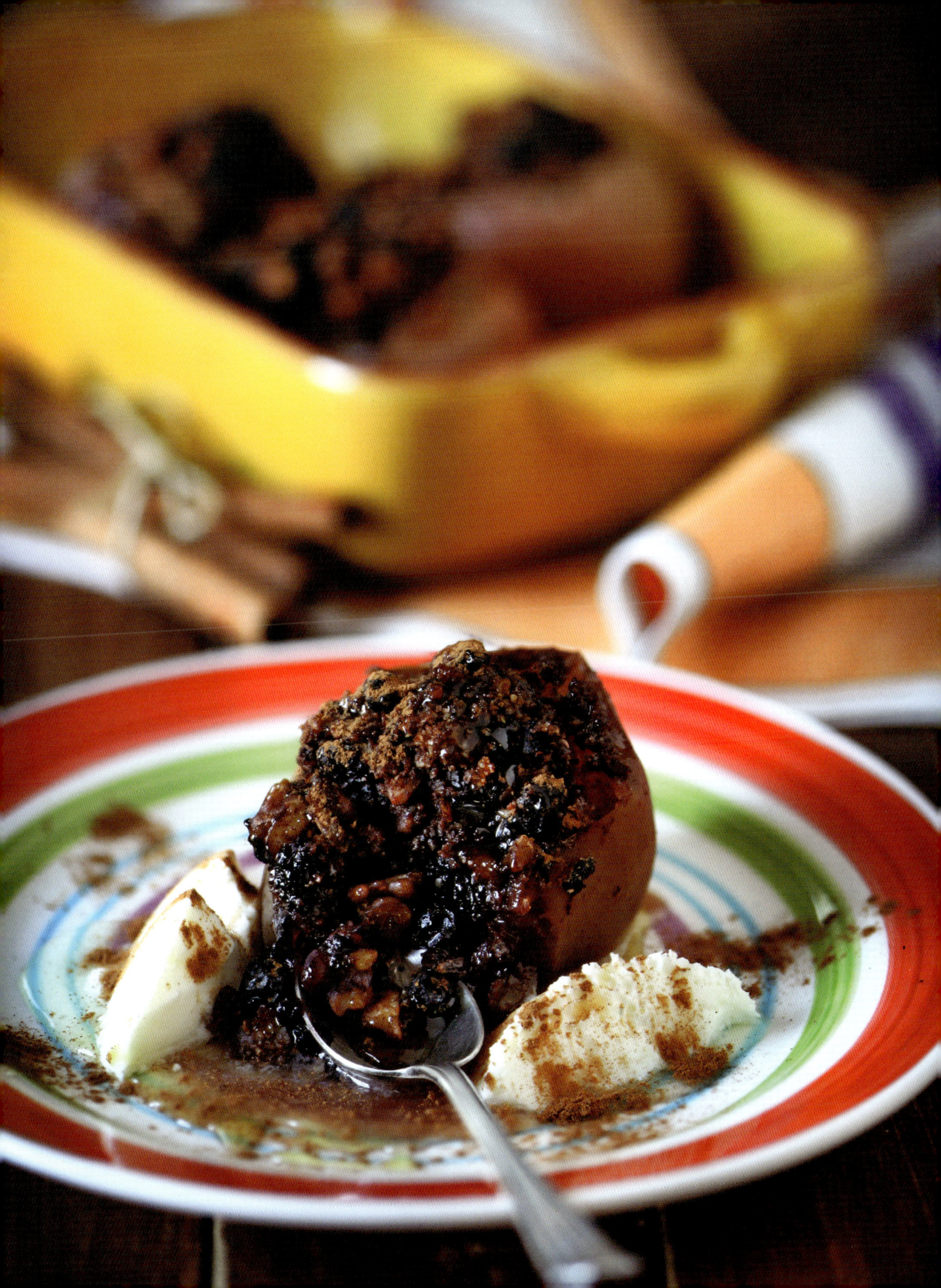

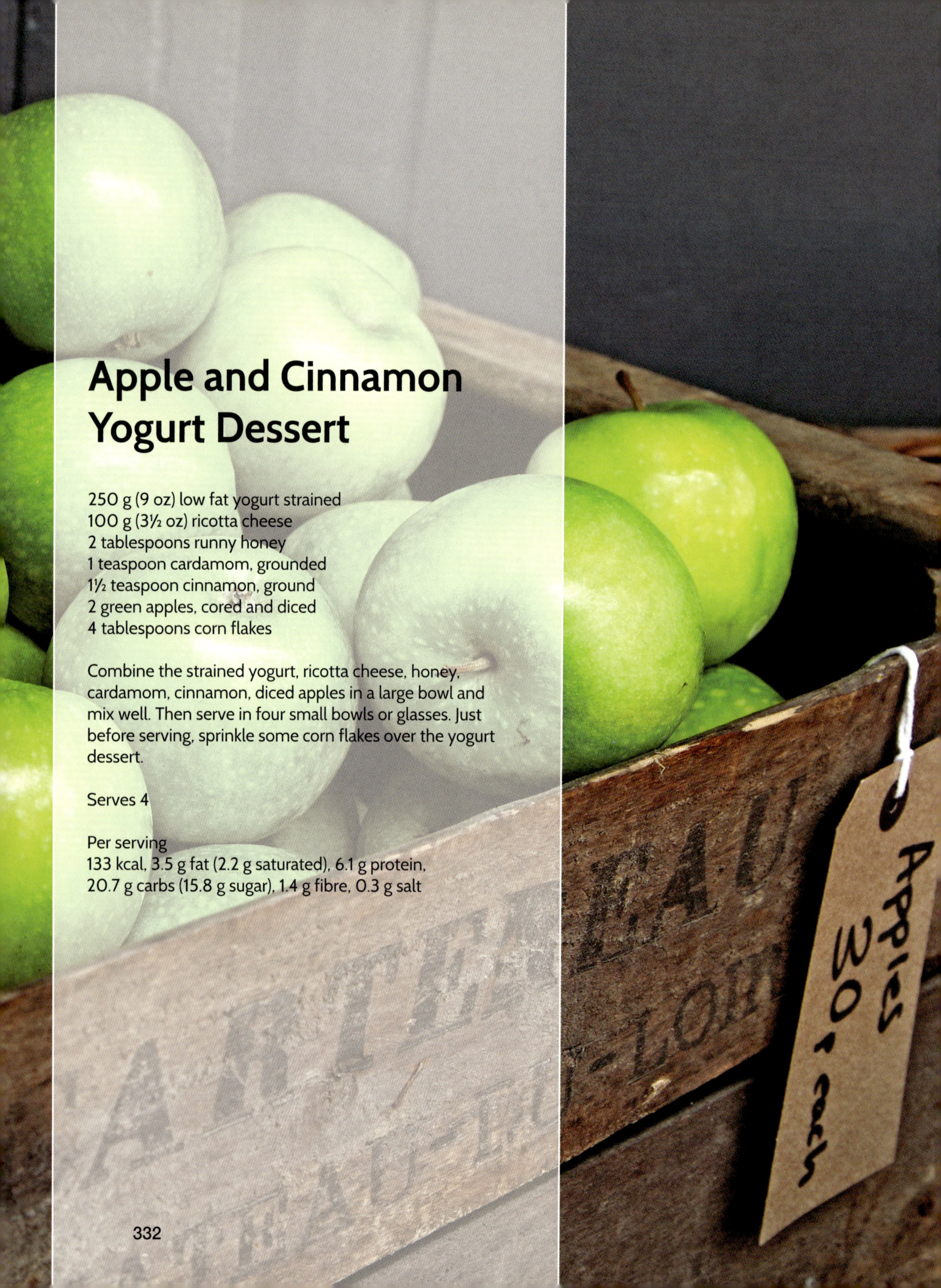

Apple and Cinnamon Yogurt Dessert

250 g (9 oz) low fat yogurt strained
100 g (3½ oz) ricotta cheese
2 tablespoons runny honey
1 teaspoon cardamom, grounded
1½ teaspoon cinnamon, ground
2 green apples, cored and diced
4 tablespoons corn flakes

Combine the strained yogurt, ricotta cheese, honey, cardamom, cinnamon, diced apples in a large bowl and mix well. Then serve in four small bowls or glasses. Just before serving, sprinkle some corn flakes over the yogurt dessert.

Serves 4

Per serving
133 kcal, 3.5 g fat (2.2 g saturated), 6.1 g protein, 20.7 g carbs (15.8 g sugar), 1.4 g fibre, 0.3 g salt

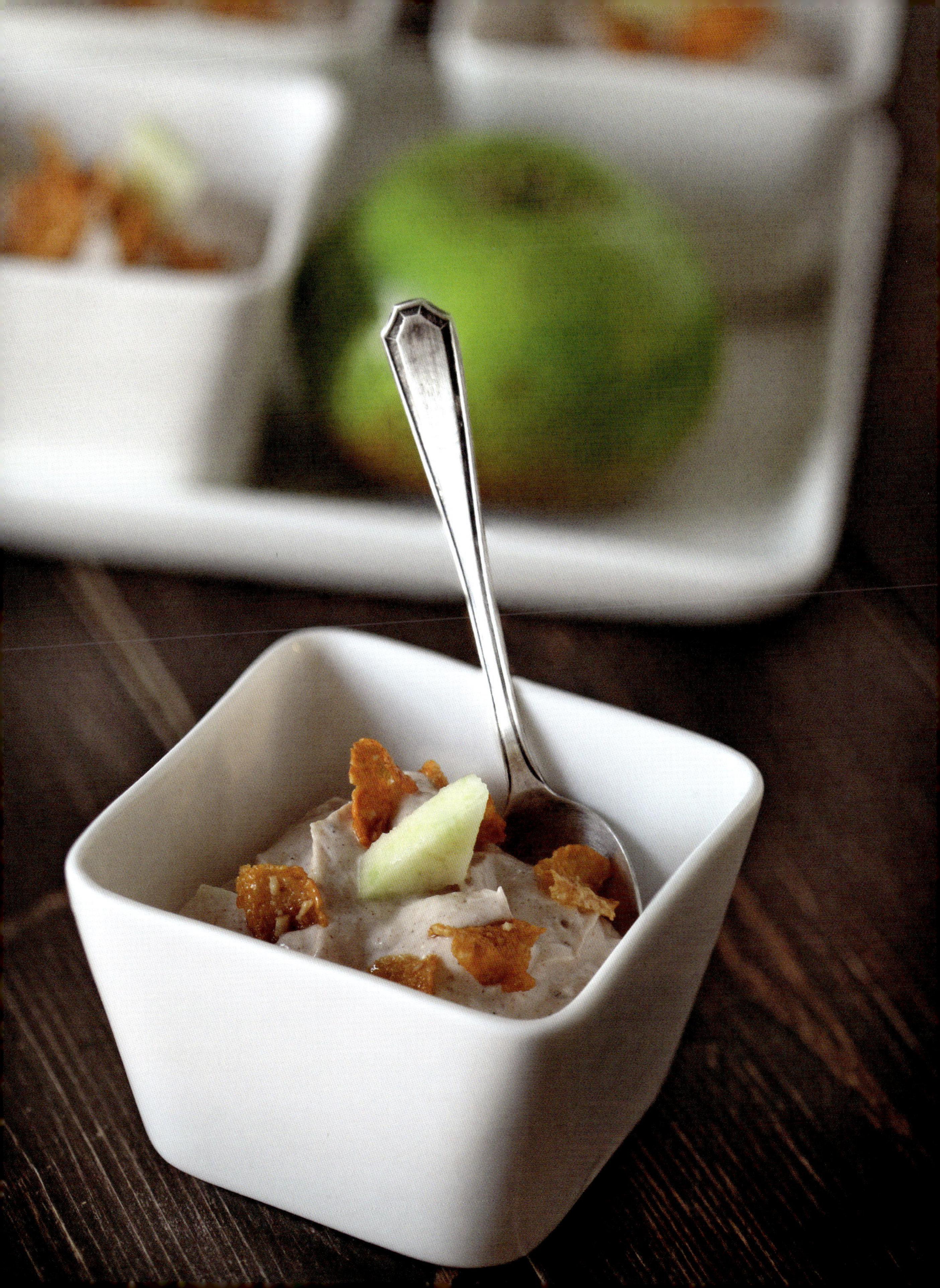

Baked Apple with Walnuts and Raisins

1 apple, finely diced
50 g (2 oz) walnuts, chopped
50 g (2 oz) raisins
2 tablespoons oatbran
2 tablespoons sugar
2 tablespoons cinnamon
2 tablespoons of grape seed oil
2 tablespoons honey
200 g (7 oz) low fat yogurt, strained

Preheat the oven to 180°C (350°F). Combine the diced apple, chopped walnuts, dry black currants and grape seed oil in a medium size bowl and mix well. Then add the oatbran, sugar, cinnamon, and mix it well again. Next transfer the mixture into six heatproof mini casserole dishes with lids. Close the lid and bake in the oven for about 40 minutes. Once ready, remove from the oven and leave it to cool a bit. Remove the lid and serve together with a tablespoon of strained yogurt. You can pour over a teaspoon of runny honey and sprinkle some cinnamon for more flavor.

Serves 6

Per serving
219 kcal, 10.3 g fat (1.3 g saturated), 4.0 g protein, 27.9 g carbs (26.4 g sugar), 3.1 g fibre, 0.1 g salt

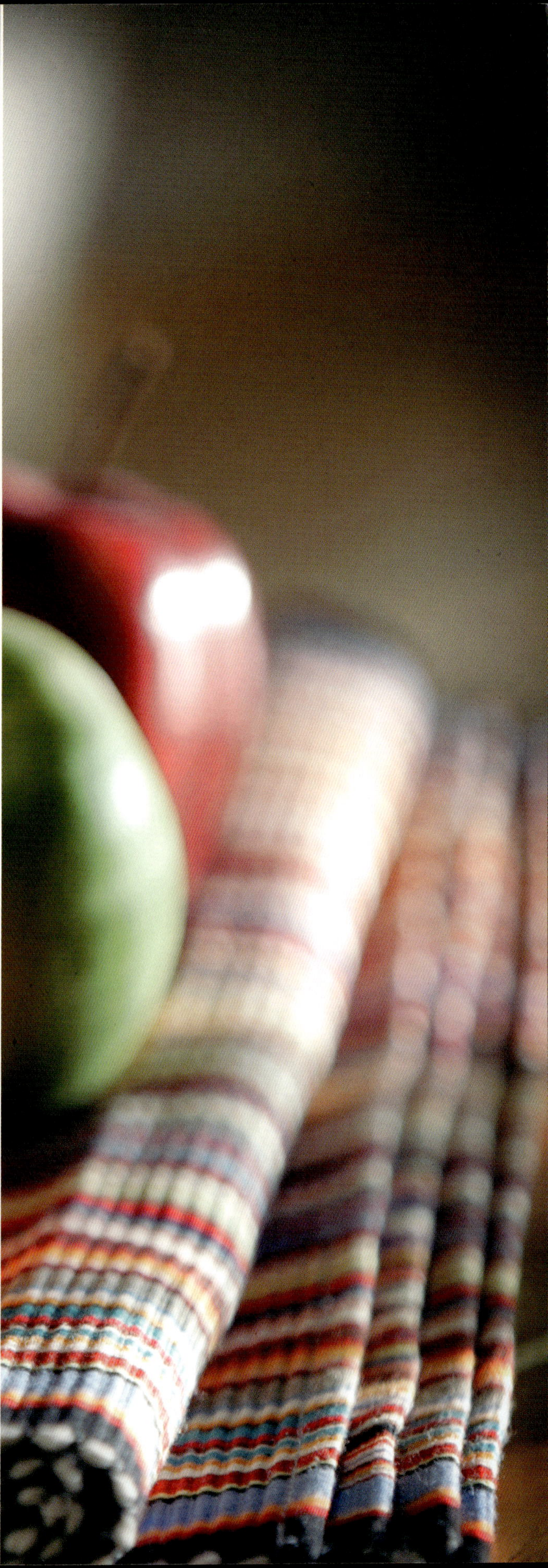

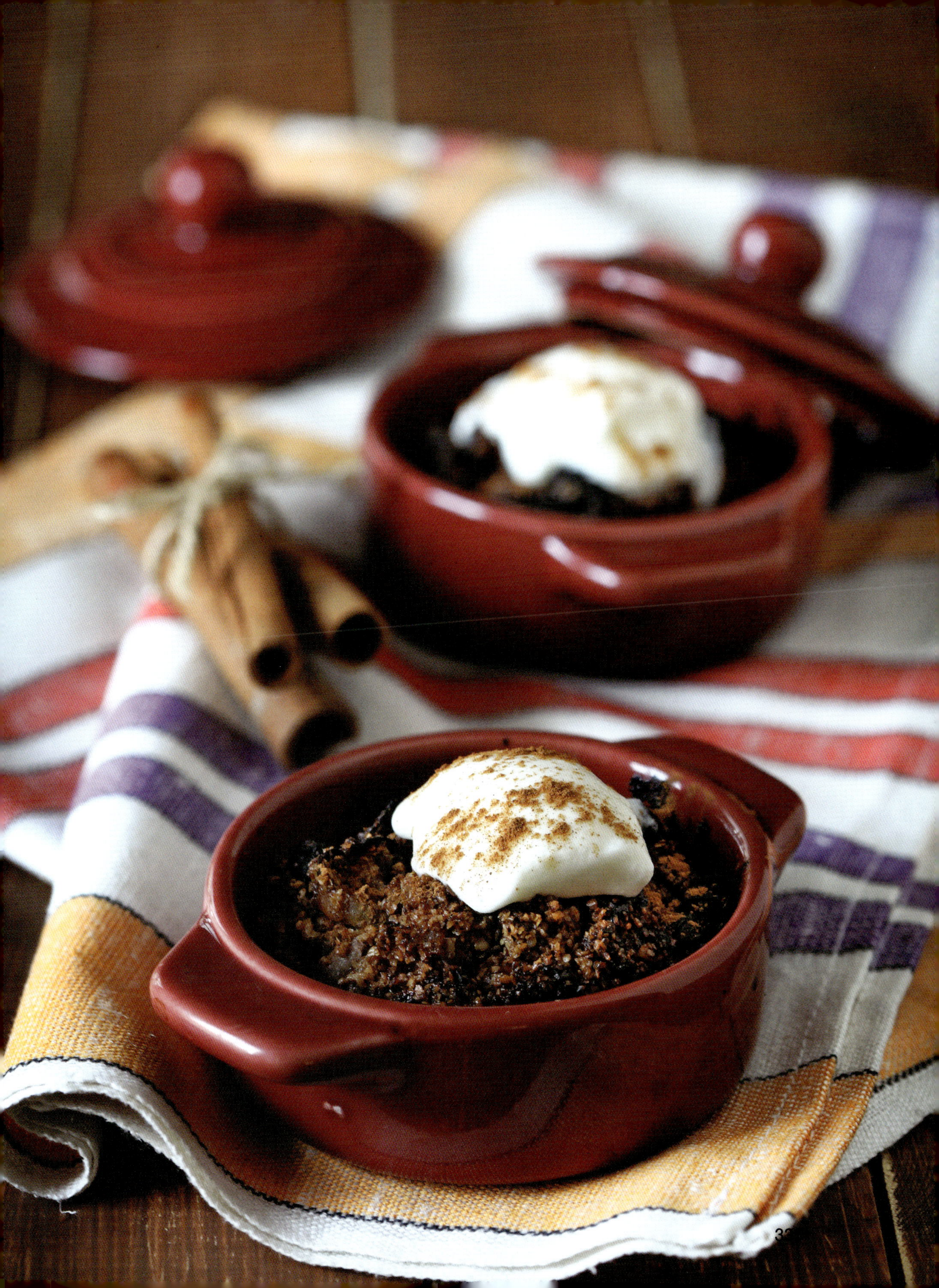

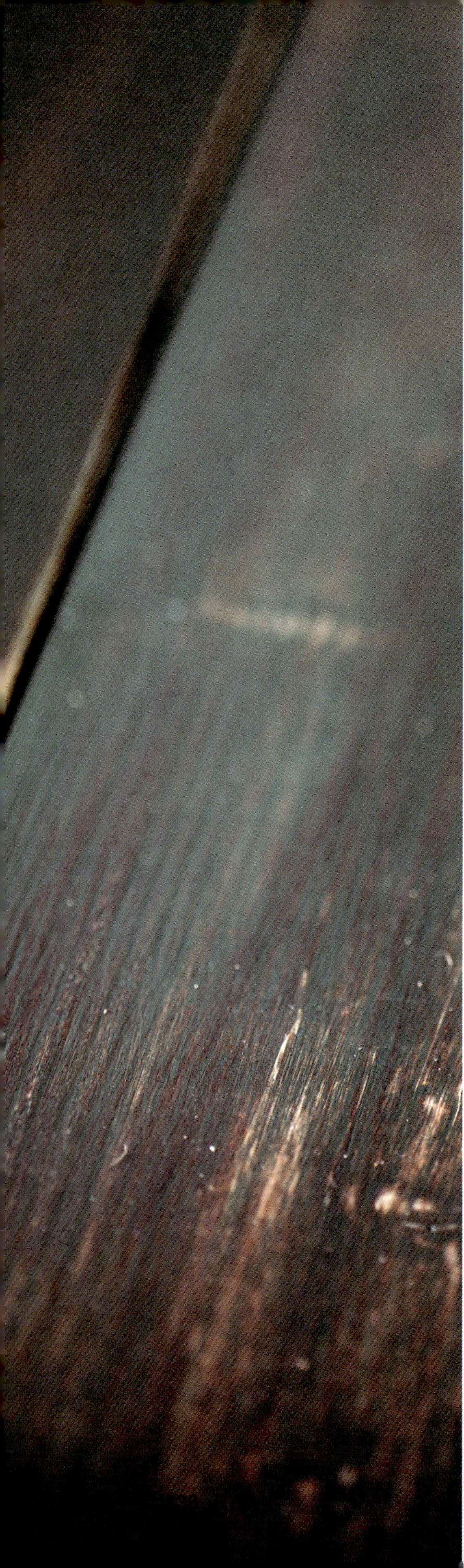

Almond and Date Tart with Kiwi Yogurt

300 g (10½ oz) low fat yogurt, strained
2 kiwis, peeled and sliced
100 g (3½ oz) almonds, chopped
50 g (2 oz) jumbo rolled oats
300 g (10½ oz) halawi dates, pitted
2 tablespoons runny honey
1 tablespoon cinnamon, ground
1 teaspoon cardamom ground
pinch of salt

Preheat the oven to 180°C (350°F). Combine the chopped almonds, jumbo rolled oats, pitted halawi dates, cinnamon and a pinch of salt in a blender bowl, blend until the mixture becomes like a dough. Place the dough onto four lightly oiled porcelain quiche pans and shape it down to the bottom and up the sides following the shape of the pan with your fingers. Bake in the oven for about 10 minutes or a bit more until browned. Remove from the oven and from the pans and leave to rest and cool completely for another 15 minutes or more over a rack. Meanwhile in a small bowl combine the strained low fat yogurt, grounded cardamom, runny honey and mix well. Pour the yogurt mixture over the cooled crusts, spread and level using a spoon and finally arrange over some of the sliced kiwis. Leave the tart to rest into the refrigerator for about 15 minutes or more and serve it cool. Delicious!

Serves 4

Per serving
310 kcal, 15.8 g fat (1.7 g saturated), 10.6 g protein, 33.0 g carbs (24.9 g sugar), 2.8 g fibre, 0.9 g salt

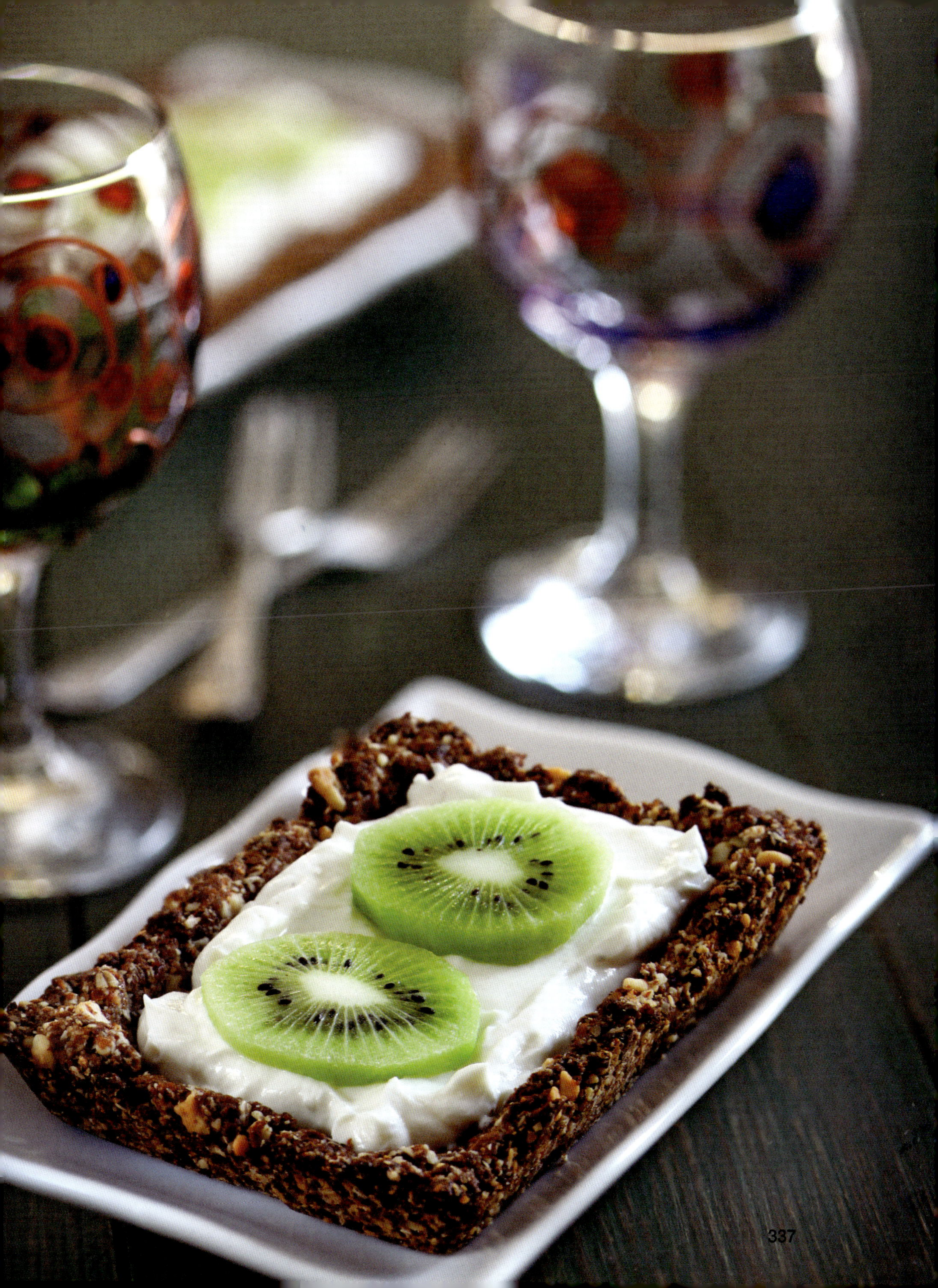

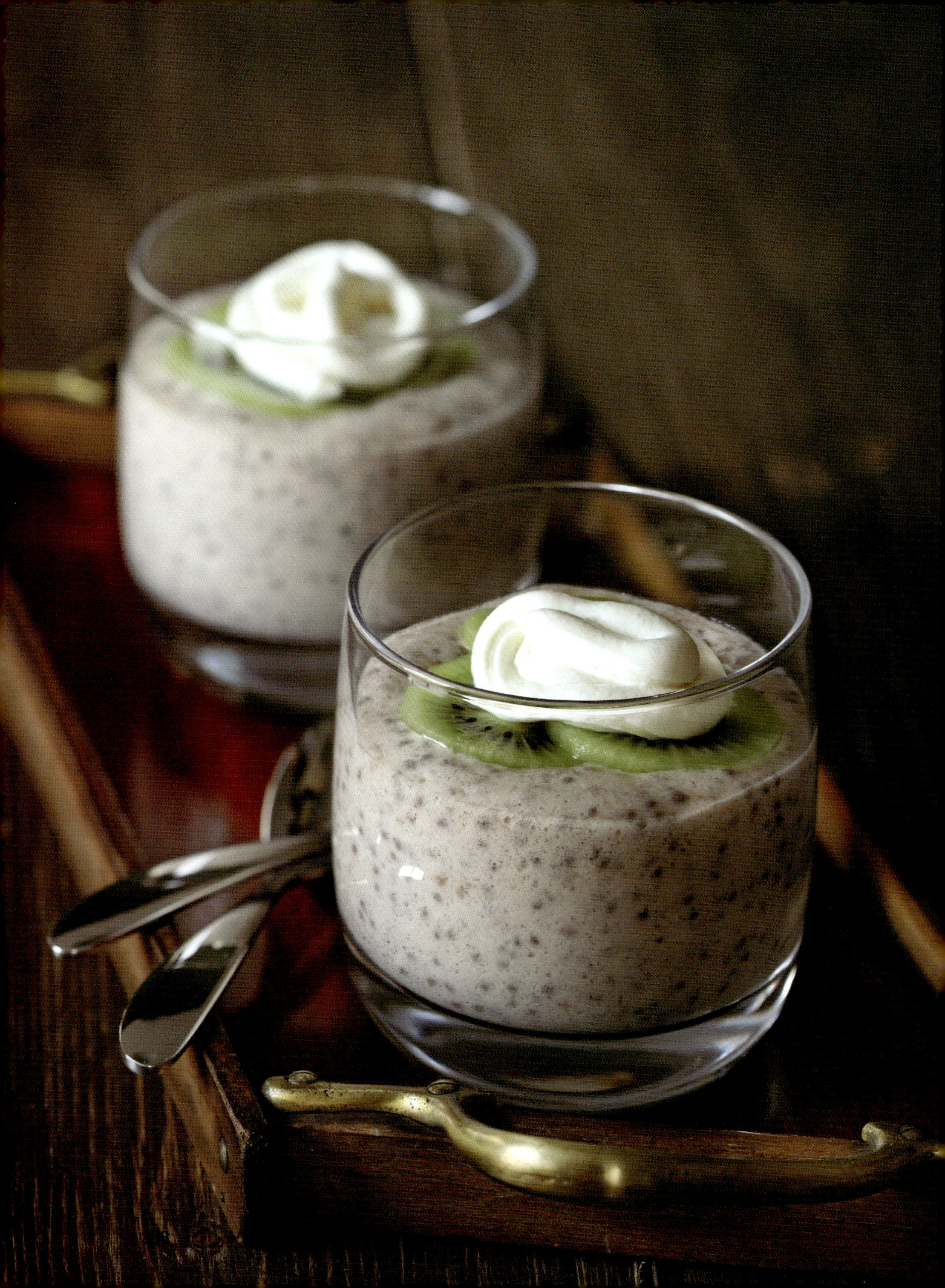

Banana and Chia Breakfast

200 ml (6¾ fl oz) semi-skimmed goats milk
1 small ripe banana, peeled
1 kiwi, peeled and sliced
3 tablespoons chia seeds
1 teaspoon cinnamon, ground
½ teaspoon cardamom ground
1 teaspoon runny honey
100 g (3½ oz) low fat yogurt, strained

Pour the semi-skimmed milk into the blender bowl, add peeled banana, the cinnamon and blend until smooth and no banana chunks remain. Then pour the mixture into a glass jar with a lid, add the chia seeds, cover with the lid and shake it well. Leave it to rest in the refrigerator for about one hour or more, keep shaking from time to time. Meanwhile combine the strained yogurt, runny honey and grounded cardamom in a small bowl and mix well, set aside for later to garnish. To serve divide chia mixture into two glasses or bowls. Arrange some kiwi slices over and add on the top some honey strained yogurt.

Serves 2

Per serving
207 kcal, 8 g fat (2 g saturated), 10 g protein, 34 g carbs (25 g sugar), 8.0 g fibre, 0.2 g salt

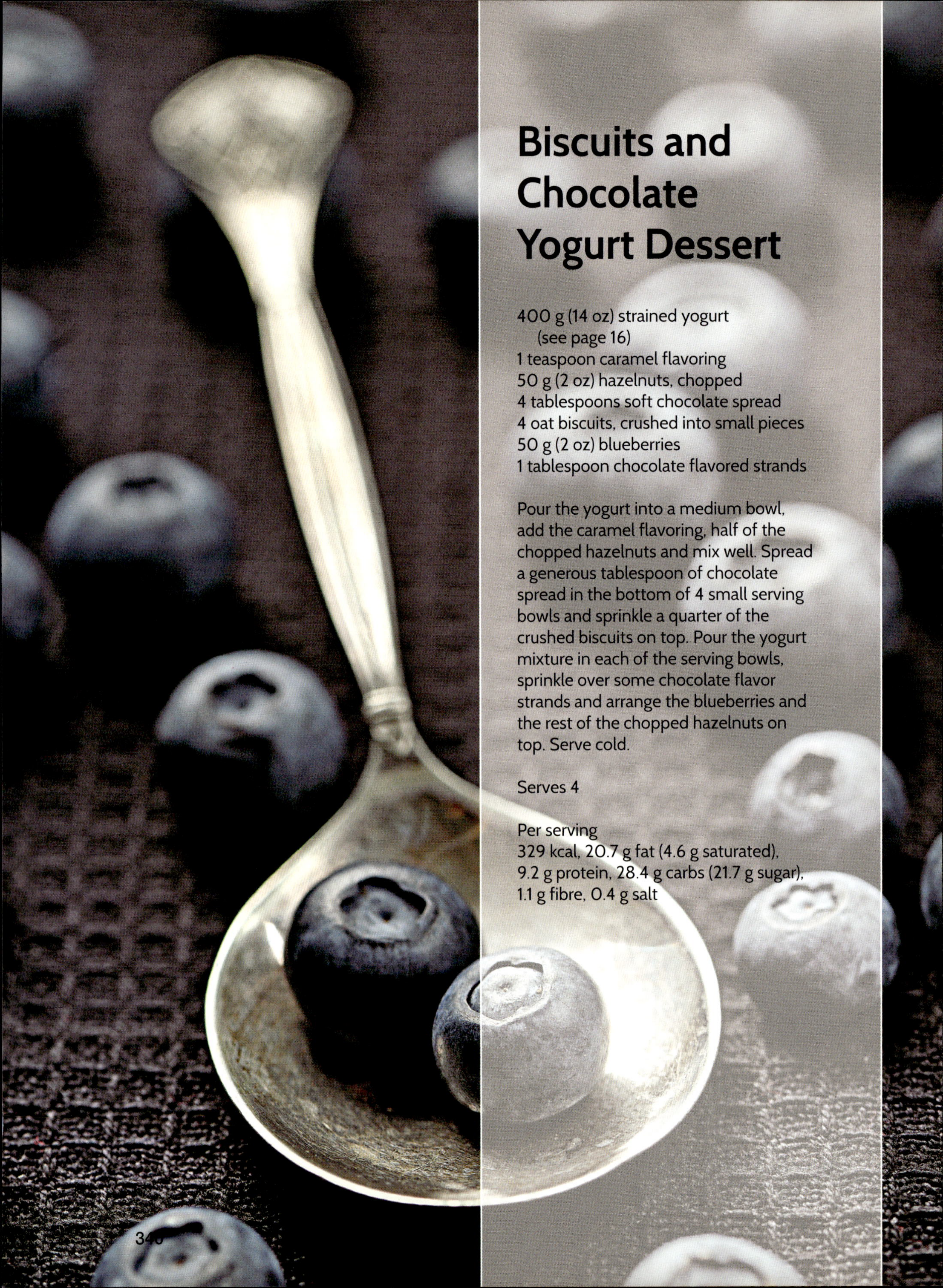

Biscuits and Chocolate Yogurt Dessert

400 g (14 oz) strained yogurt
(see page 16)
1 teaspoon caramel flavoring
50 g (2 oz) hazelnuts, chopped
4 tablespoons soft chocolate spread
4 oat biscuits, crushed into small pieces
50 g (2 oz) blueberries
1 tablespoon chocolate flavored strands

Pour the yogurt into a medium bowl, add the caramel flavoring, half of the chopped hazelnuts and mix well. Spread a generous tablespoon of chocolate spread in the bottom of 4 small serving bowls and sprinkle a quarter of the crushed biscuits on top. Pour the yogurt mixture in each of the serving bowls, sprinkle over some chocolate flavor strands and arrange the blueberries and the rest of the chopped hazelnuts on top. Serve cold.

Serves 4

Per serving
329 kcal, 20.7 g fat (4.6 g saturated), 9.2 g protein, 28.4 g carbs (21.7 g sugar), 1.1 g fibre, 0.4 g salt

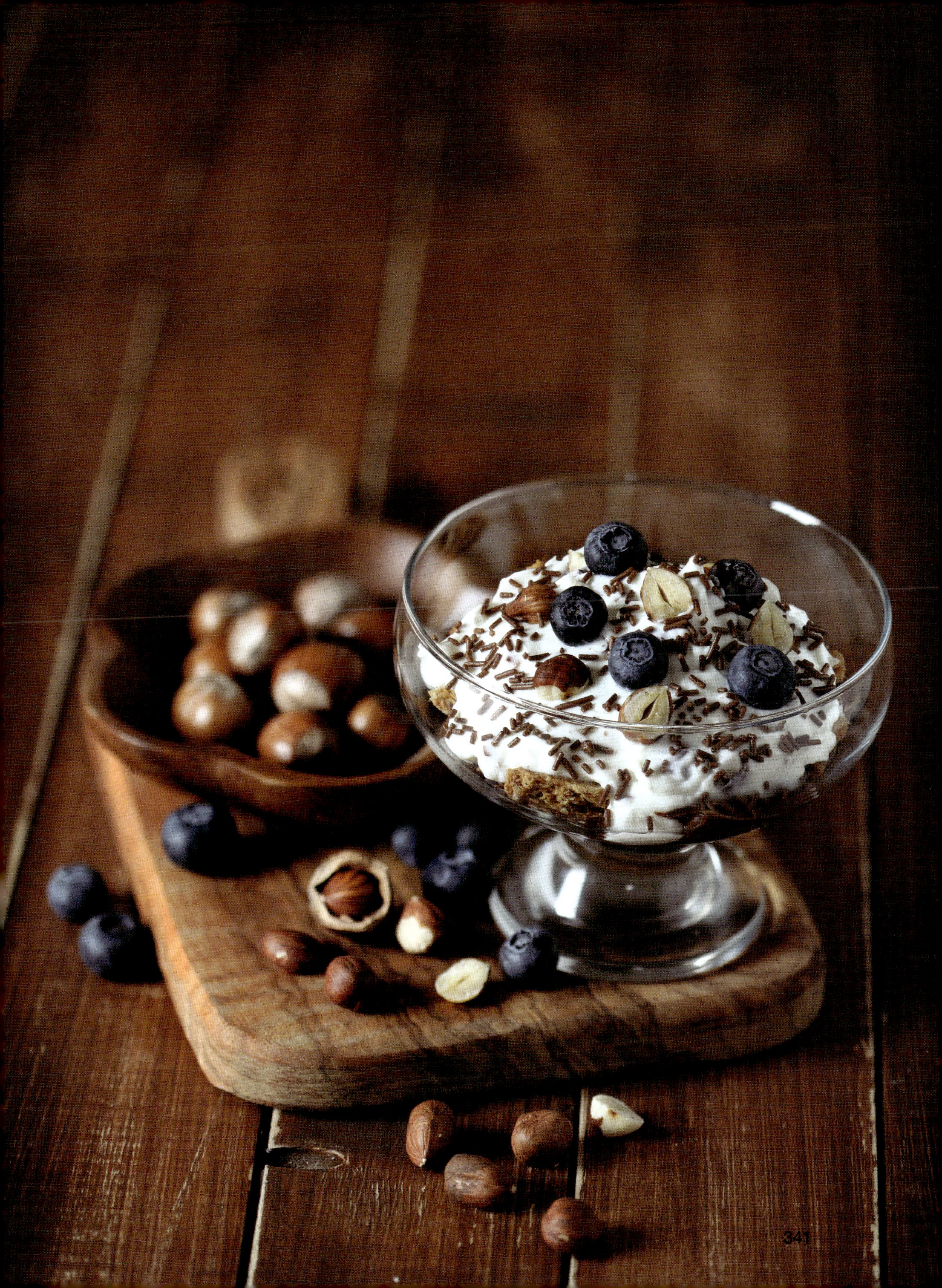

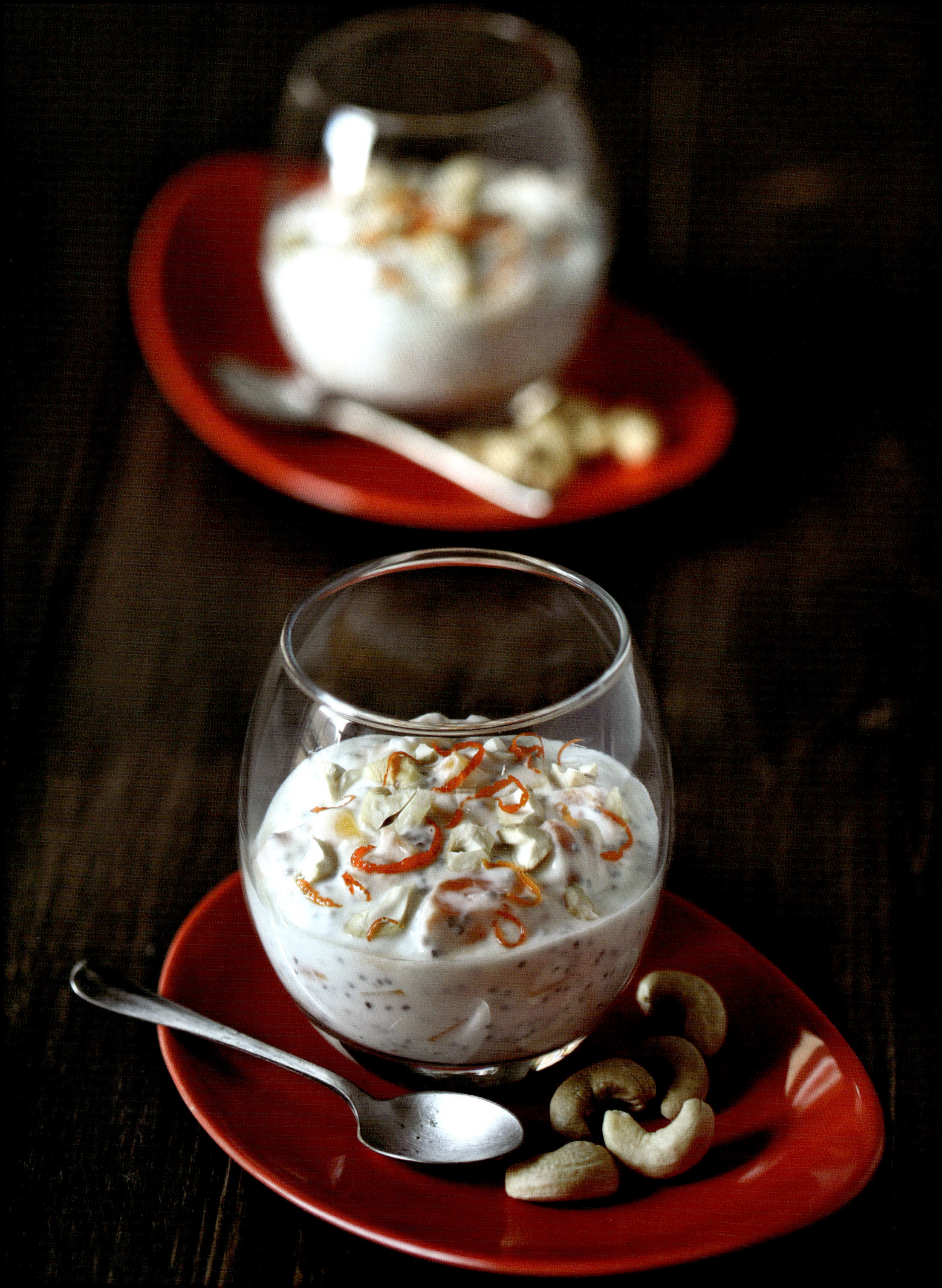

Chia Seed Pudding

500 g (17½ oz) low fat yogurt
2 tablespoons chia seeds
1 tablespoon of honey
1 mandarin peeled and diced on small pieces
1 small mango, peeled and diced on small pieces
3 tablespoons of chopped cashew nuts
1 teaspoon mandarin zest

Pour the yogurt into a large bowl and then add the chia seeds, honey, chopped mandarin and chopped mango. Mix well and separate the mixture into four small bowls or glasses and sprinkle over the cashew nuts and zest. Leave it to rest in the refrigerator for about 15 minutes and serve.

Serves 4

Per serving
195 kcal, 7.9 g fat (1.7 g saturated), 8.9 g protein, 25.2 g carbs (20.2 g sugars), 4.9 g fibre, 0.4 g salt

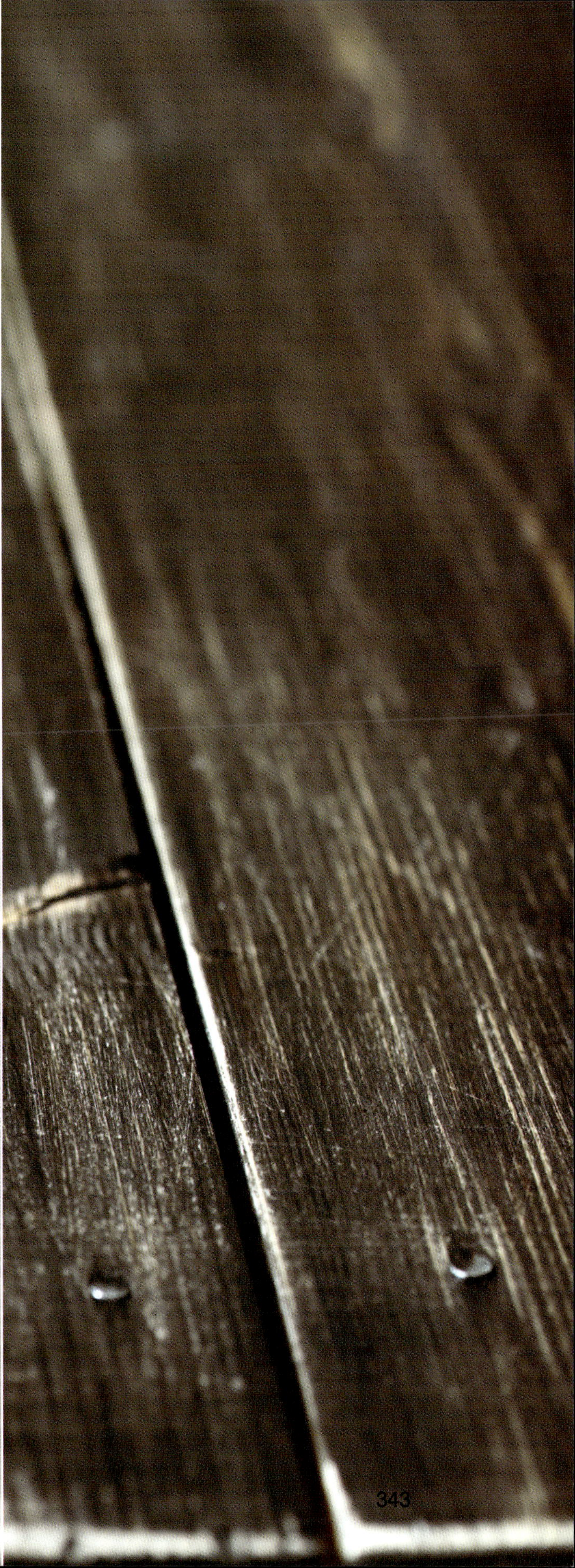

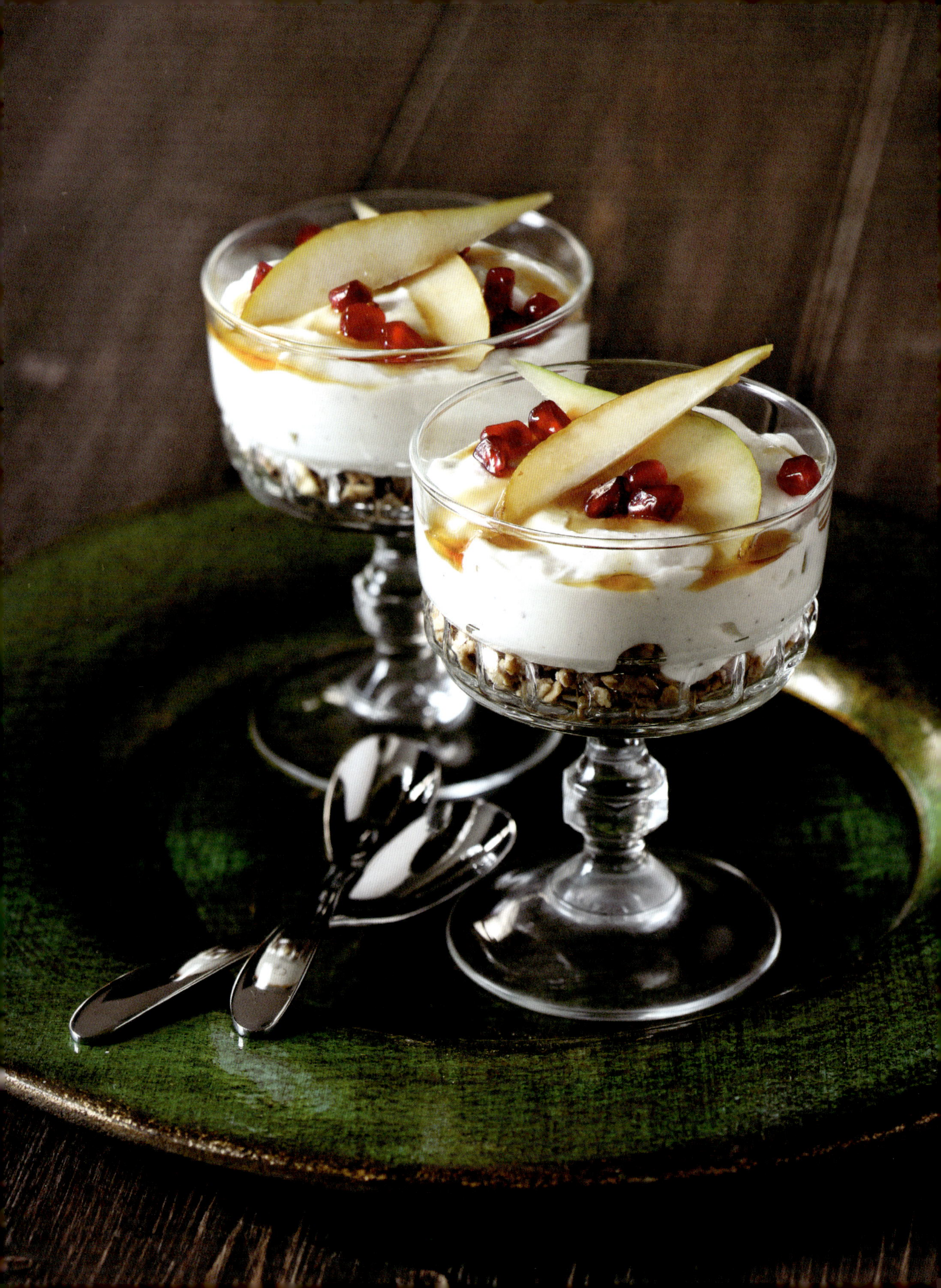

Pear and brandy yogurt dessert

200 g (7 oz) granola
1 teaspoon cardamom, ground
250 g (9 oz) low fat yogurt, strained
250 g (9 oz) ricotta cheese
4 tablespoons brown sugar
100 ml (3½ oz) brandy
1 large ripe pear, cored and diced
50 g (2 oz) pomegranate seeds

In a large bowl combine the strained yogurt, ricotta cheese, grounded cardamom, diced pear and mix well. Then divide and put the granola into six glasses or small bowls and pour over four tablespoons of yogurt mixture in each glass. Set aside. Then in a small saucepan bring the brandy to a simmer and add the sugar, stirring to dissolve the sugar for about 3 minutes, turn off the heat and leave it to rest for a couple of minutes. Meanwhile arrange some pear slices and pomegranate seeds on the top of the yogurt mixture and pour over the brandy.

Serves 6

Per serving
314 kcal, 9 g fat (3 g saturated), 12 g protein, 42 g carbs (26 g sugar), 3.5 g fibre, 0.1 g salt

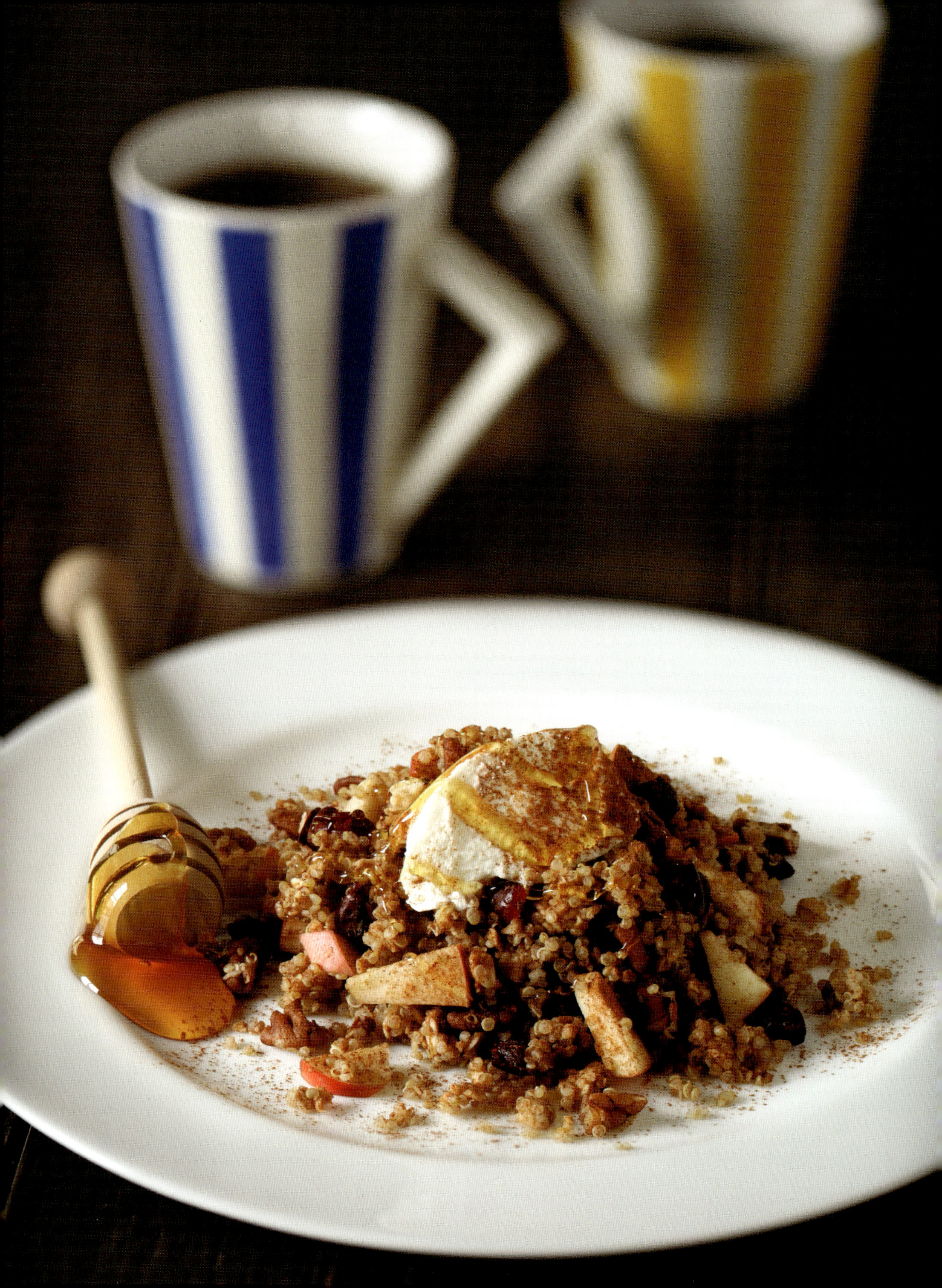

Quinoa, Apple and Cinnamon Morning

200 g (7 oz) quinoa
200 g (7 oz) low fat yogurt, strained
1 teaspoon cinnamon, ground
1 pink lady apple, diced
2 tablespoons honey
100 g (3½ oz) granola
30 g (1 oz) cranberries, dry and sliced
30 g (1 oz) pecans, chopped
100 g (3½ oz) blueberries

Boil the Quinoa seeds in 700 ml (23½ fl oz) water for about 10 minutes. Transfer into a cooking strainer and drain for 5 minutes. Next transfer it to a medium bowl and add the diced apple, granola, cinnamon, honey and mix well. Divide onto four small plates and spoon over some strained yogurt, top with the dry cranberries and some chopped pecans, sprinkle over some cinnamon and blueberries and then serve.

Serves 4

Per serving
370 kcal, 11.7 g fat (1.0 g saturated), 12.6 g protein, 56.2 g carbs (19.3 g sugar), 3.1 g fibre, 0.2 g salt

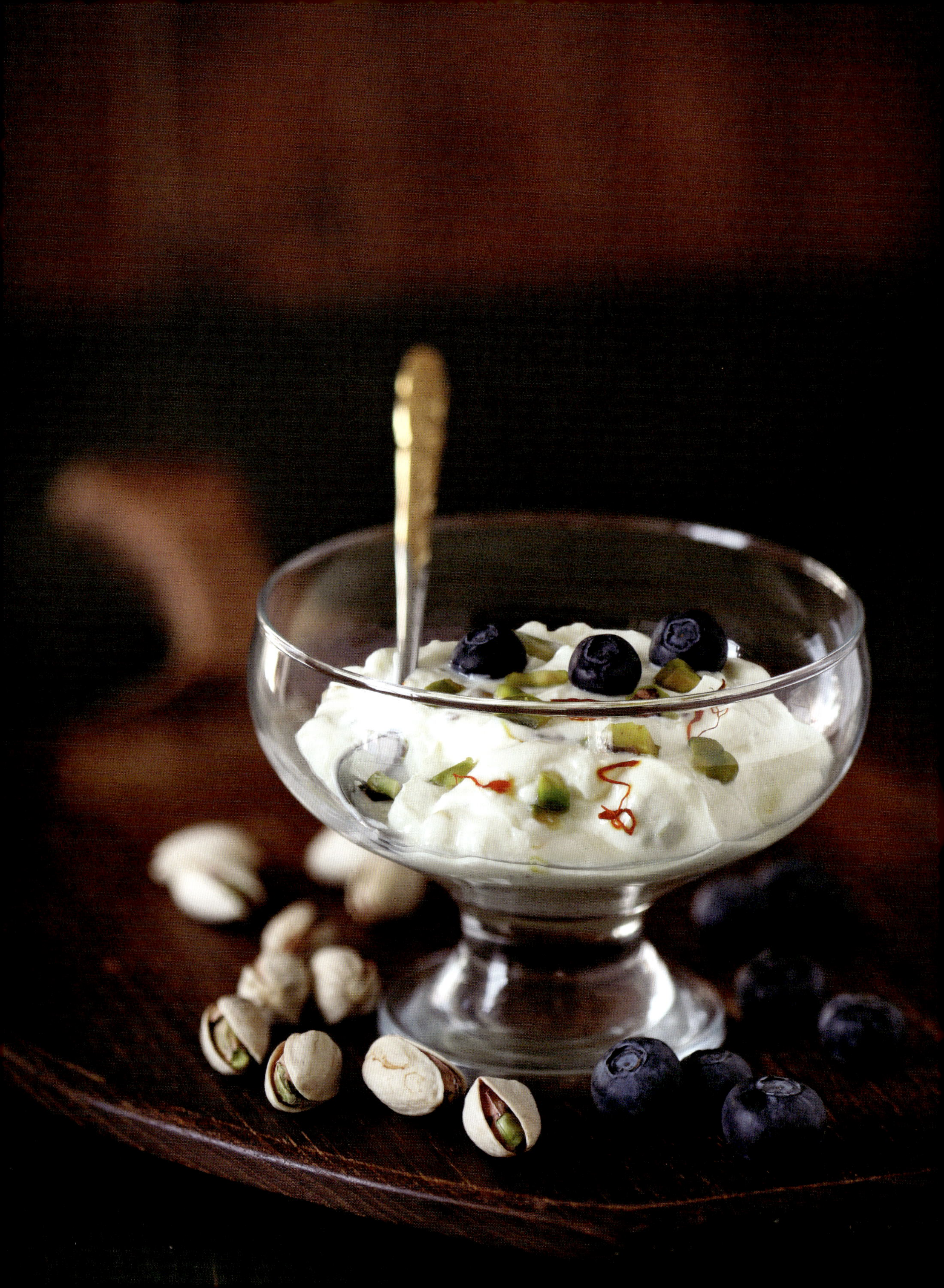

Saffron Sweet Yogurt

500 g (17½ oz) strained yogurt
1 teaspoon saffron threads, crushed
50 ml (1½ fl oz) worm milk
1 tablespoon icing sugar
½ teaspoon cardamom seeds, crushed
50 g (2 oz) pistachios, chopped
50 g (2 oz) fresh berries

In a small pan heat the milk but do not boil and add the saffron. Let it steep for about 20 minutes. Meanwhile pour the yogurt into a big mixing bowl, add the icing sugar and mix well. Next add the saffron mixture, stir and divide between 6 serving glasses or bowls. Decorate with some chopped pistachios and fresh berries.

Serves 6

Per serving
165 kcal, 7.4 g fat (2.9 g saturated), 8.5 g protein, 17.5 g carbs (17.2 g sugar), 0.8 g fibre, 0.3 g salt

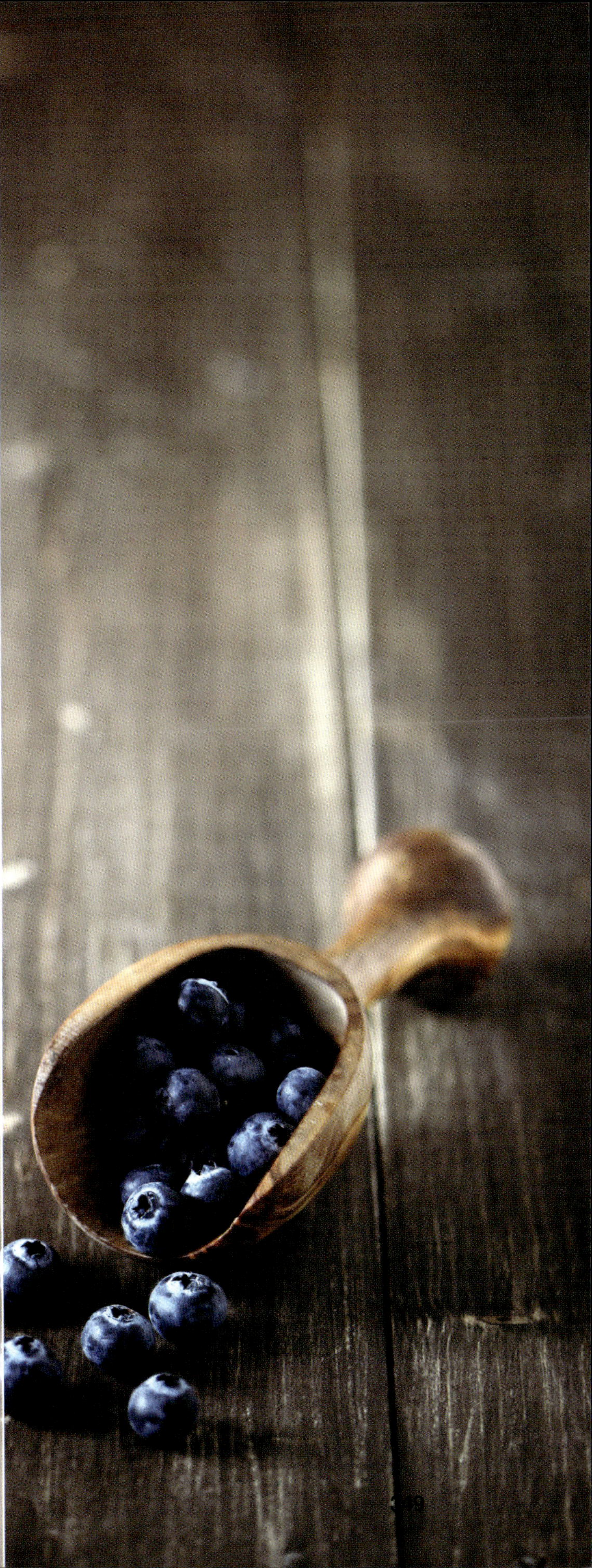

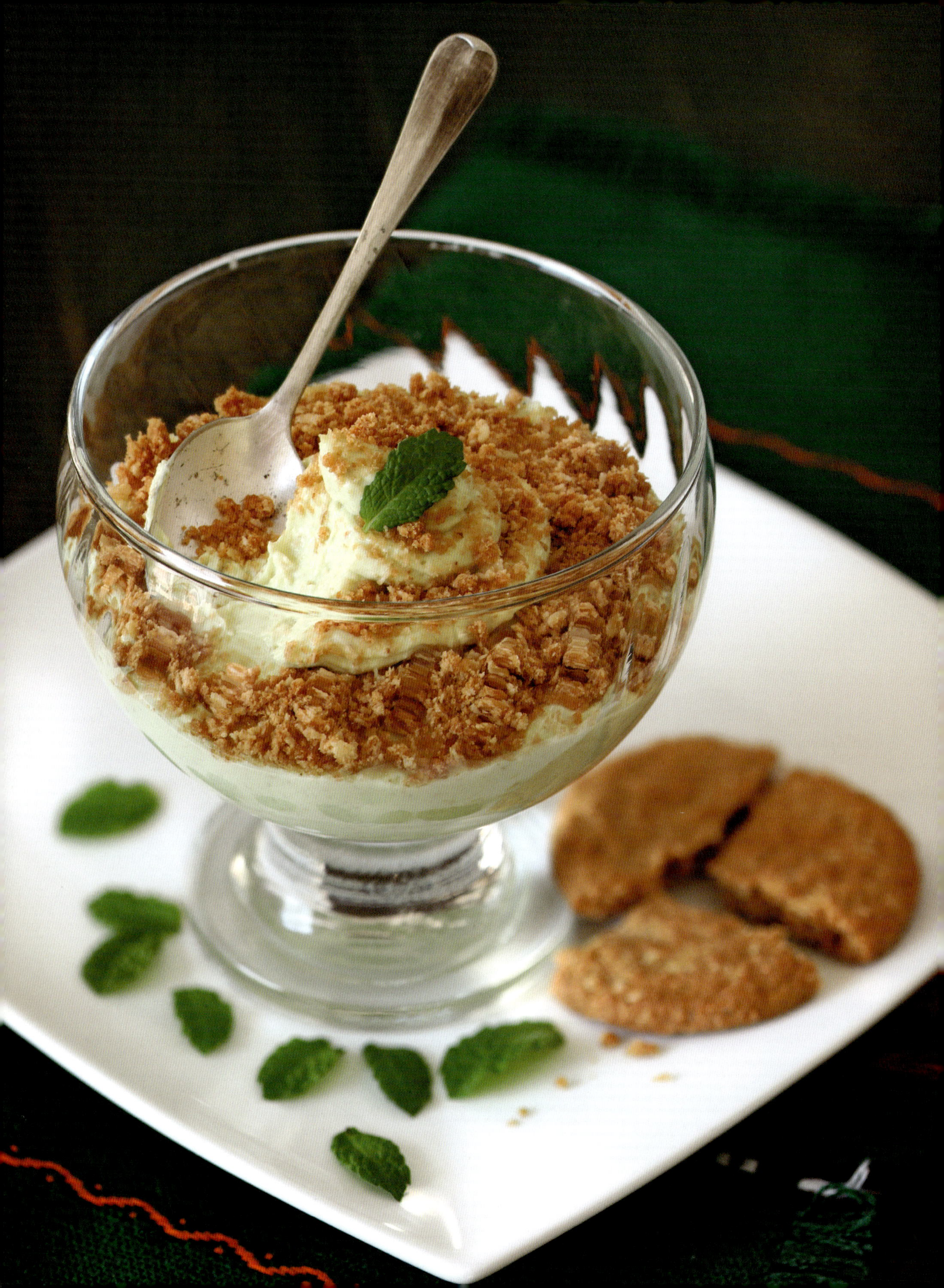

Minty Yogurt Mousse

350 g (12 oz) low fat yogurt, strained
150 g (5 oz) ricotta cheese
4 oat biscuits
1 teaspoon peppermint natural extract
½ teaspoon natural green food color

Break the oat biscuits into small crumbs in a mortar. Next in a medium bowl mix the strained yogurt, ricotta cheese, peppermint natural extract and natural green food color. Add the biscuit crumbs and mix again gently. Finally divide into four bowls or glasses and leave to rest for no more than 15 minutes in the refrigerator. Serve cool with some more crumbs over!

Serves 4

Per serving
197 kcal, 8 g fat (4g saturated),
14 g protein, 18 g carbs (10 g sugar),
0.8 g fibre, 0.4 g salt

Apple and Pecan Nut Strudel

4 pink lady apples, peeled, cored and chopped
freshly squeezed juice of ½ lime
150 g (5 oz) brown sugar
30 g (1 oz) caster sugar
3 tablespoons oatmeal
75 g (3 oz) butter, melted
200 g (7 oz) filo pastry, sheets
150 g (5 oz) pecan nuts, chopped
30 g (1 oz) blueberries, dry
250 g (9 oz) low fat yogurt, strained
1 tablespoon of ground cinnamon
tablespoon icing sugar
pinch of dried edible flower petals

Preheat the oven to 180°C (350°F). In a large bowl pour 1 litre (2 pints) cold water and the lime juice and set aside. Peel, core and finely chop the apples and add the pieces to the bowl with the water and lime for couple of minutes. Then transfer the apple pieces into a colander to drain and then put in a dry large bowl. Sprinkle over the caster sugar and oatmeal, mix well and set aside. Next in a small medium bowl mix together brown sugar, cinnamon and chopped pecan nuts. Finally using a brush, oil the bottom of a baking tray and lay the first filo pastry sheet. Then oil again with the melted butter using the brush and sprinkle over some of the pecan nuts mixture. Repeat with the next filo pastry sheet. Over the third and fourth filo pastry divide and sprinkle the apple pieces. Then continue with the rest of the filo pastry and pecan nuts. Oil the last sheet and transfer the baking tray to the oven and bake for about 20 minutes or until golden brown. Leave it to rest for a couple of minutes and cut into six pieces. Serve with a spoonful of strained yogurt and sprinkle over some icing sugar and dried edible flower petals.

Serves 6

Per serving
586 kcal, 30 g fat (8 g saturated), 11 g protein,
74 g carbs (45 g sugar), 4.9 g fibre, 0.2 g salt

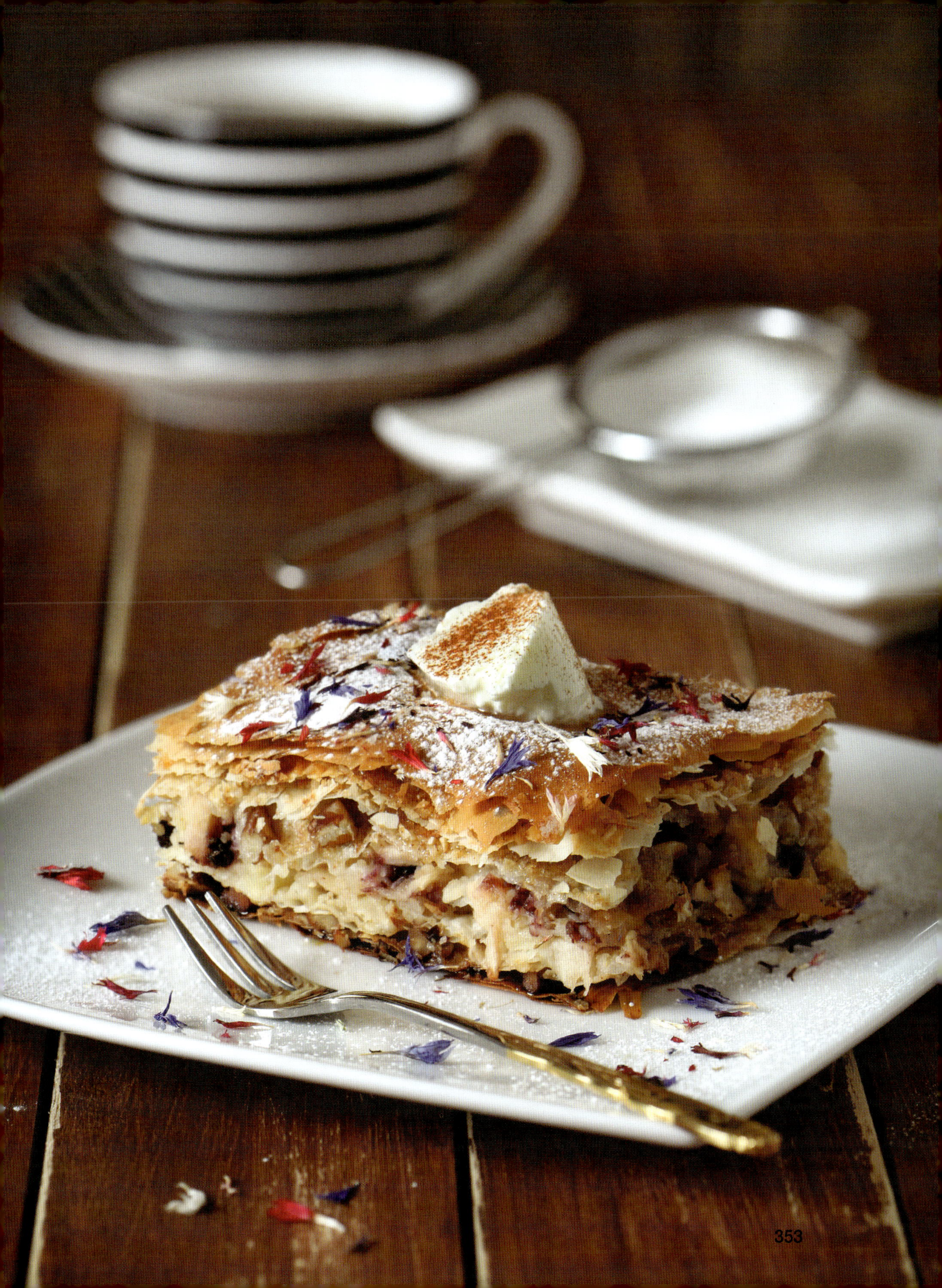

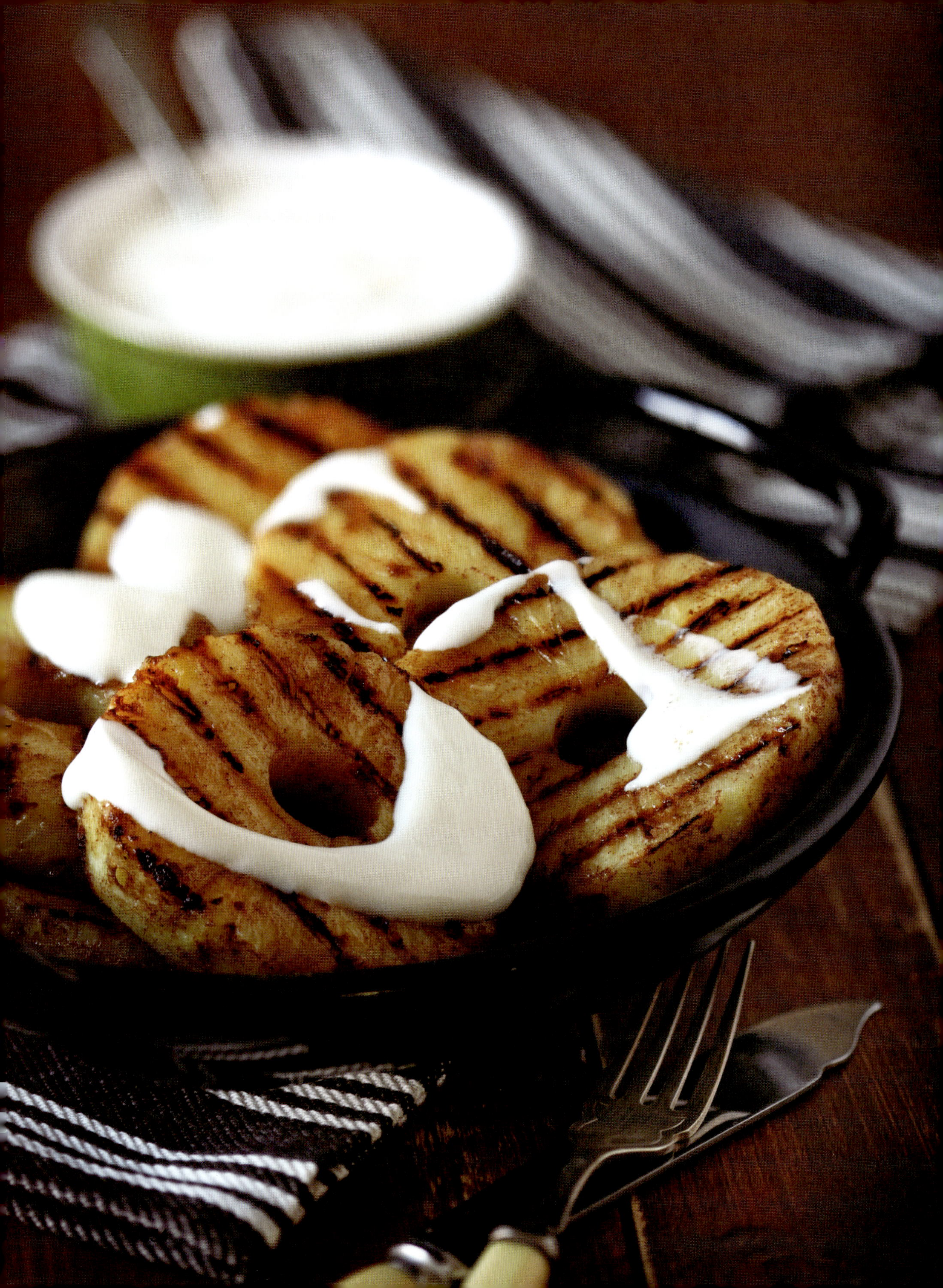

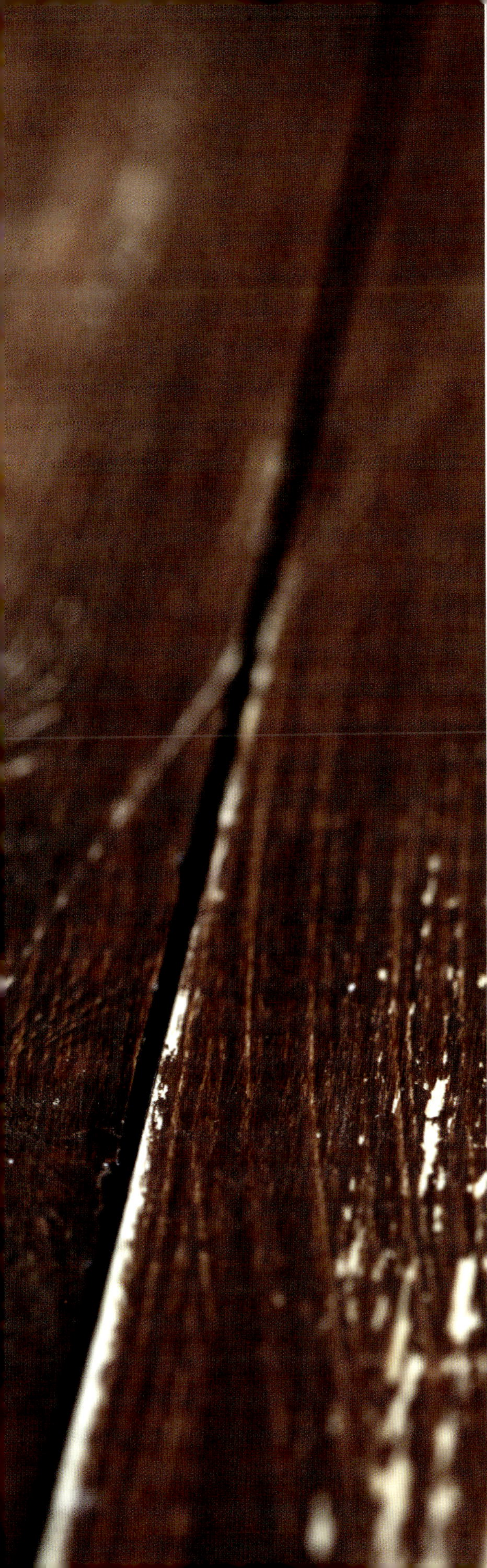

Grilled Pineapple

1 medium pineapple, trimmed, peeled, cored and sliced
3 tablespoons sunflower oil
freshly squeezed juice of ½ lime
1 teaspoon cinnamon, ground

To prepare marinade, combine the sunflower oil, lime juice and ground cinnamon in a large bowl and mix well. Then dip in the pineapple slices to marinate and mix all over. Leave them to rest and absorb the marinade for a couple minutes. After that, oil the grill or grill pan and bring to medium heat. Arrange the pineapple slices over the grill and cook for about 3 minutes on each side. Leave the pineapple rings to cool a bit and serve with the yogurt dip.

200 g (7 oz) low fat yogurt
1 tablespoons runny honey
3 drops vanilla flavoring

To make the yogurt dip, combine the low fat yogurt, runny honey and vanilla flavoring and mix well.

Serves 6

Per serving
94 kcal, 6 g fat (1 g saturated), 2 g protein, 9 g carbs (9 g sugar), 0.5 g fibre, 0.1 g salt

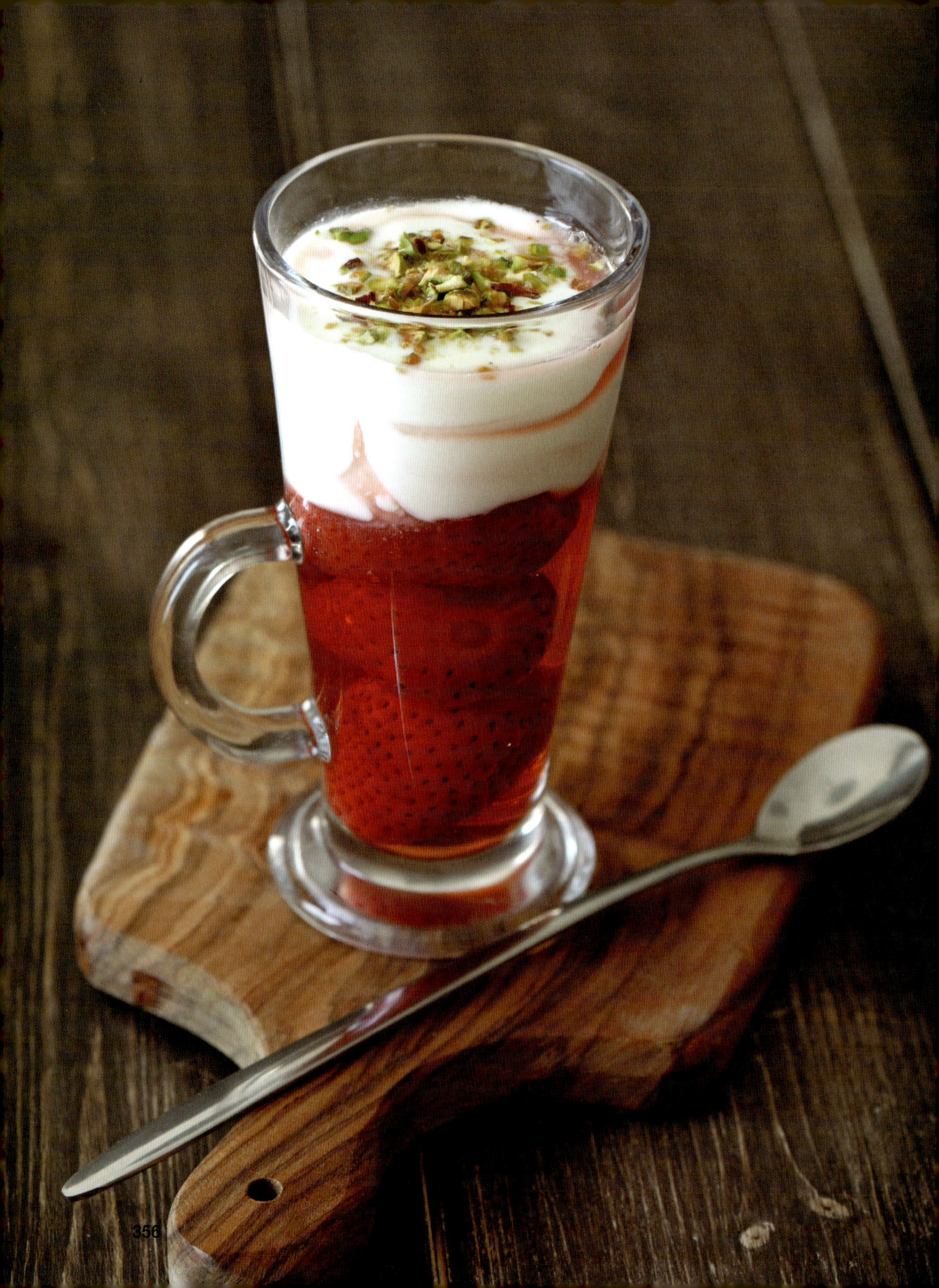

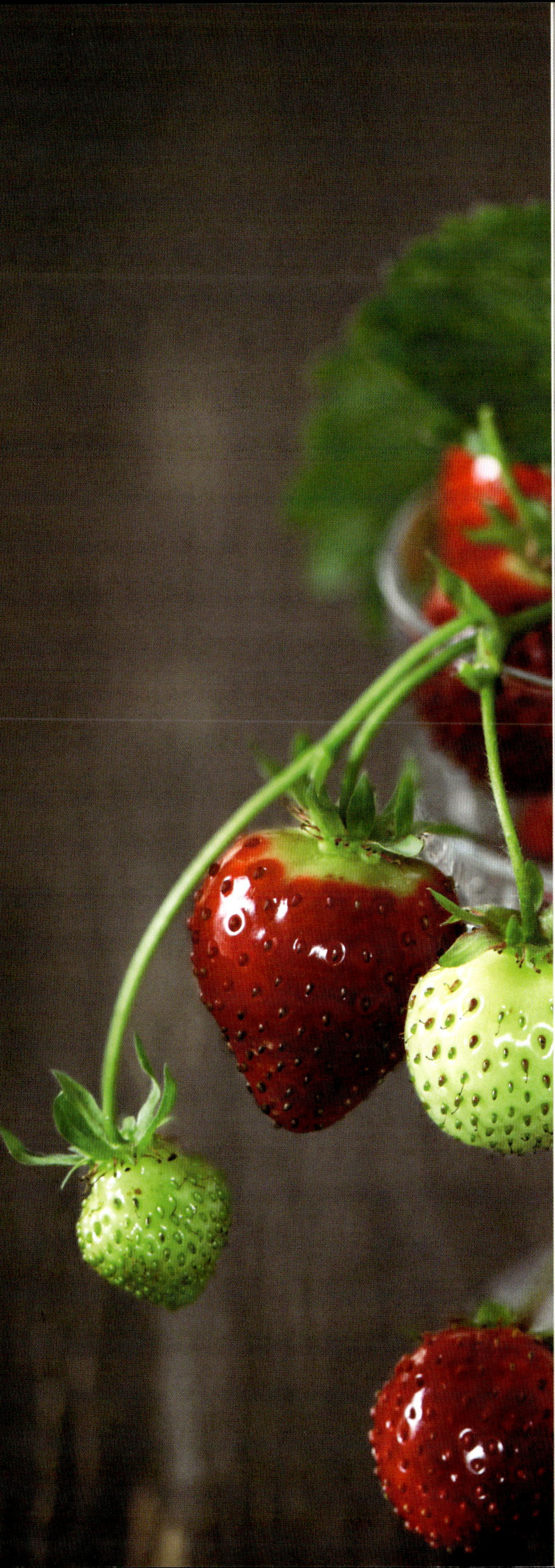

Poached Strawberries

450 g (16 oz) strawberries
300 ml (10 fl oz) boiling water
2 lemon scented geranium leaves
100 g (3½ oz) caster sugar

For the yogurt topping:
250 g (9 oz) low fat yogurt
½ teaspoon Madagascan vanilla extract
25 ml (¾ fl oz) brandy
30 g (1 oz) pistachios, toasted and chopped
10 fresh mint leaves

Wash and dry the strawberries then remove the husk. Cut in half if the strawberries are large and set aside. Combine the boiling water and caster sugar in a medium saucepan and simmer over a high heat for about 2 minutes until the sugar has dissolved. Add the geranium leaves and cook for 2 minutes. Finally add the strawberries and cook for another 2 minutes. Remove the pan from the heat and then remove the geranium leaves. Transfer the mixture to a bowl and leave in the refrigerator to cool. Meanwhile, combine the yogurt, vanilla extract and brandy together in a bowl. To serve, place a couple of strawberries into a tall glass and pour some of the liquid, just to cover the strawberries. Spoon over some of the yogurt topping and finish with a sprinkle of chopped pistachios and fresh mint leaves on top.

Serves 4

Per serving
225 kcal, 4 g fat (1 g saturated), 6 g protein, 41 g carbs (40 g sugar), 2.5 g fibre, 0.1 g salt

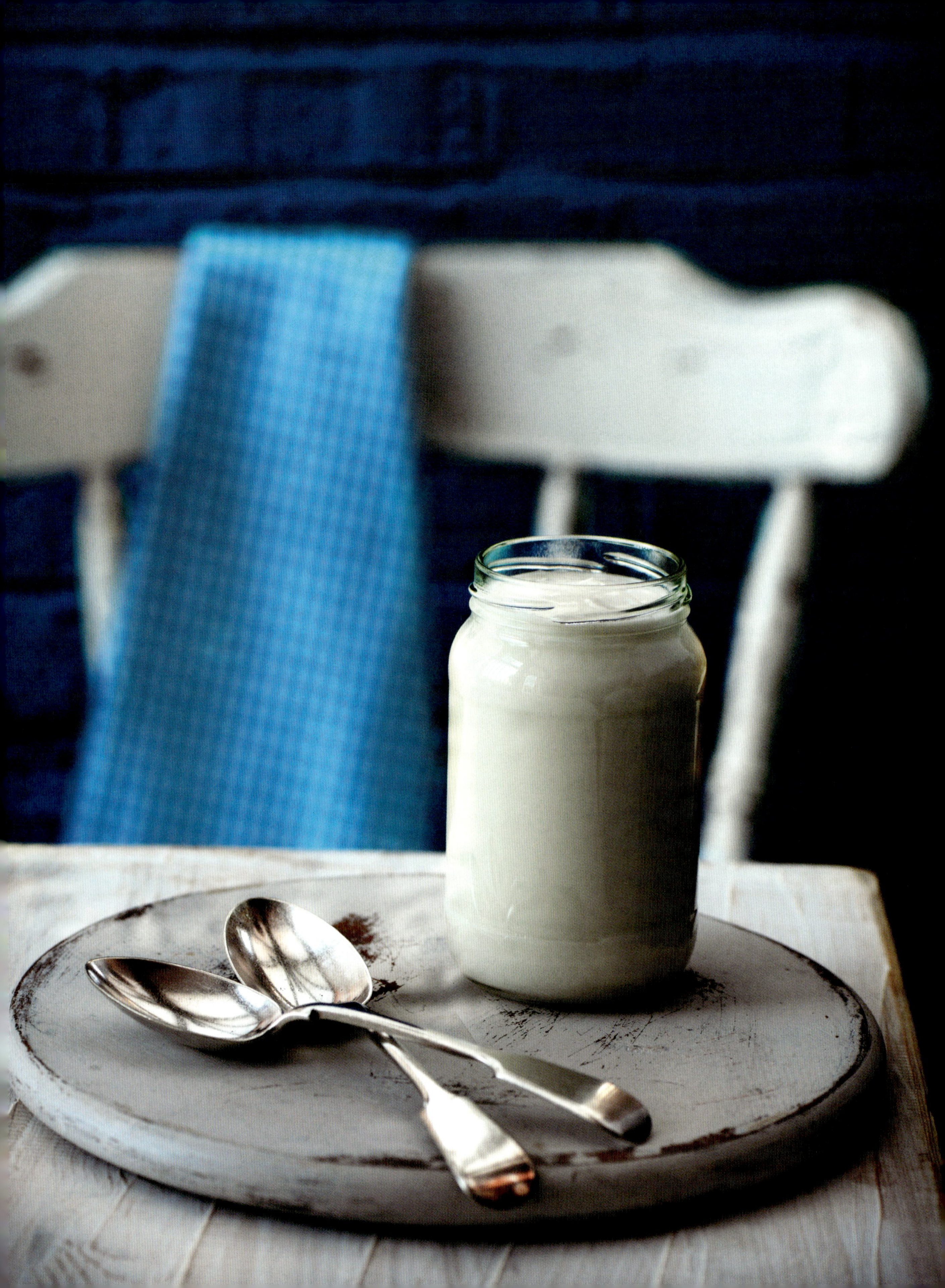

Frozen Yogurt

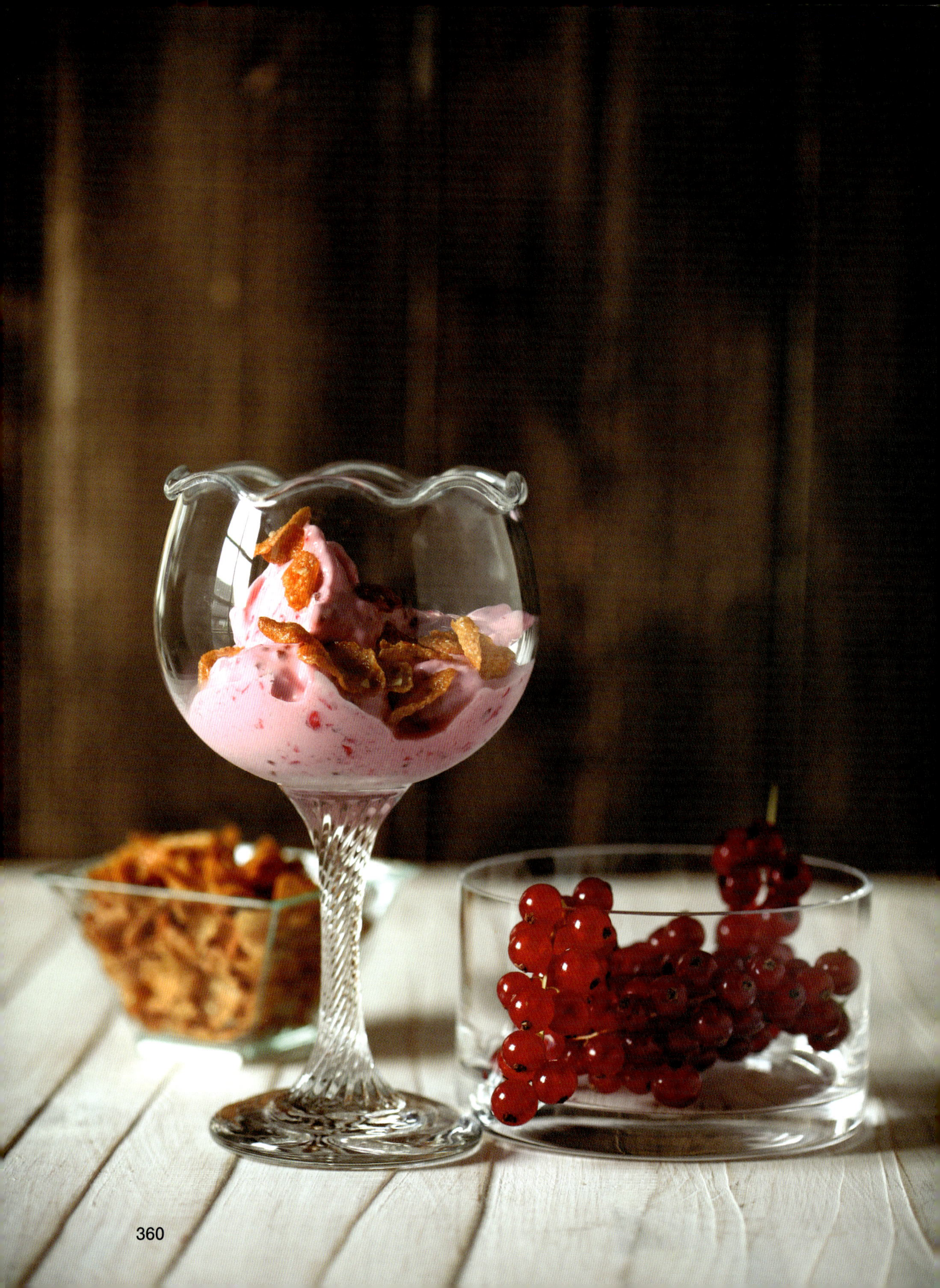

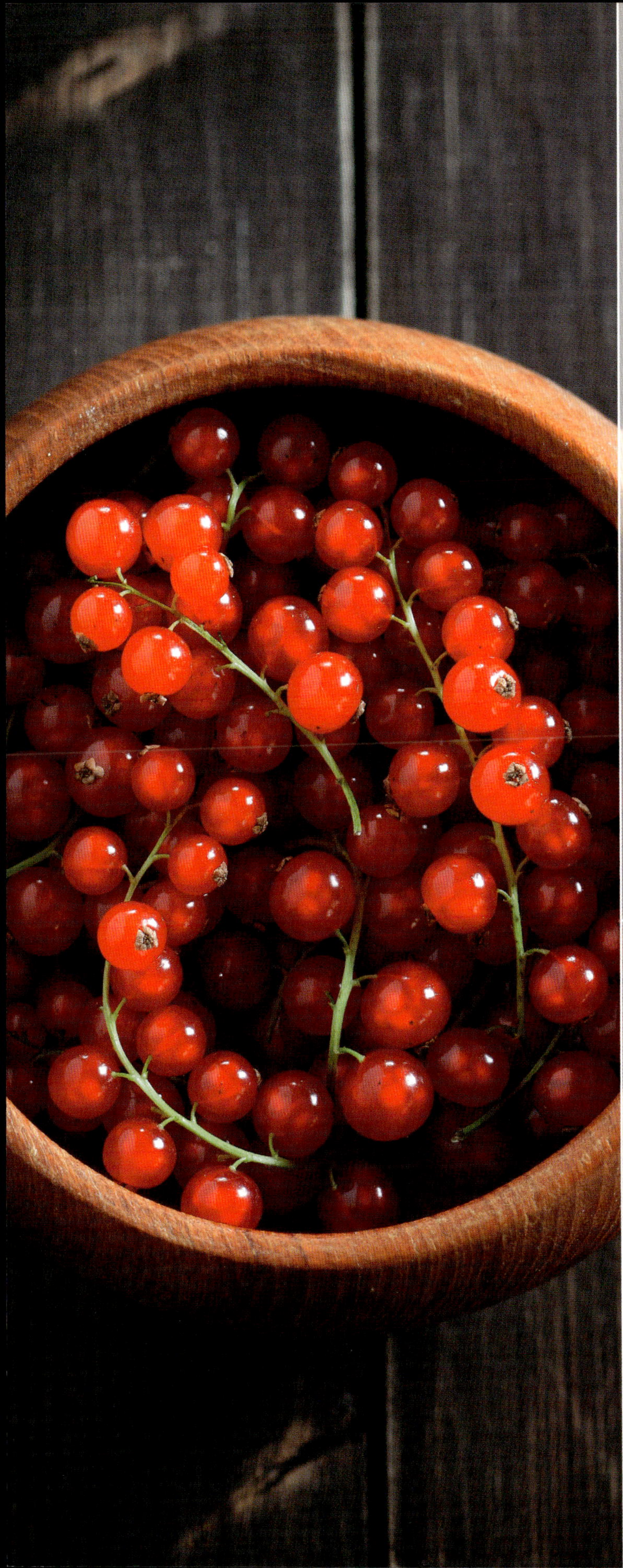

Redcurrant Frozen Yogurt

150 g (5 oz) redcurrants, frozen
250 g (9 oz) low fat yogurt, strained
30 g (1 oz) corn flakes
1 teaspoon vanilla flavoring

Throw the frozen redcurrants into to the blender, add the strained yogurt and vanilla flavoring and blend until smooth. Serve in bowls or glasses with some corn flakes on the top.

Serves 2

Per serving
142 kcal, 1.4 g fat (0.9 g saturated), 8.0 g protein, 26.1 g carbs (13.9 g sugar), 3.9 g fibre, 0.6 g salt

Mango and Kiwi Kulfi

1 mango, stoned, peeled and chopped
50 g (2 oz) pistachios, toasted and finely chopped, plus extra to decorate
2 kiwis, peeled and chopped
1 banana, peeled and chopped
50 g (2 oz) dried cranberries,
1 teaspoon ground cardamom
200 ml ($6\frac{3}{4}$ fl oz) evaporated milk
600 g (21 oz) strained yogurt
2 tablespoons icing sugar

Throw the mango pieces into a blender and whizz until smooth. Pour into a small bowl, add the finely chopped pistachios and set aside. Put the kiwi and banana pieces into the blender and whizz until smooth and pour into another small bowl and add the cranberries and cardamom and set aside. Pour the evaporated milk into a medium bowl, add the yogurt and the icing sugar and mix well. Add half the yogurt mixture to the mango bowl and half to the kiwi bowl and mix well.

Make 3 layers of the flavors in a medium sized (1 kg/ 2.2 lb) silicone loaf mould by pouring half of the kiwi mixture in first, then the mango mixture and then the rest of the kiwi mixture on top. Cover with cling film and leave for about 4 hours or overnight in the freezer. To serve, carefully invert the Kulfi out of the mould, and then slice it into 1 cm ($\frac{1}{2}$ inch) thick slices, rinsing the knife in a bowl of hot water and drying between each cut. Leave at room temperature for 20 minutes before serving. Serve sprinkled with some chopped toasted pistachios over the top.

Serves 10

Per serving
127 kcal, 4 g fat (2 g saturated), 9 g protein, 13 g carbs (12 g sugar), 1.8 g fibre, 0.1 g salt

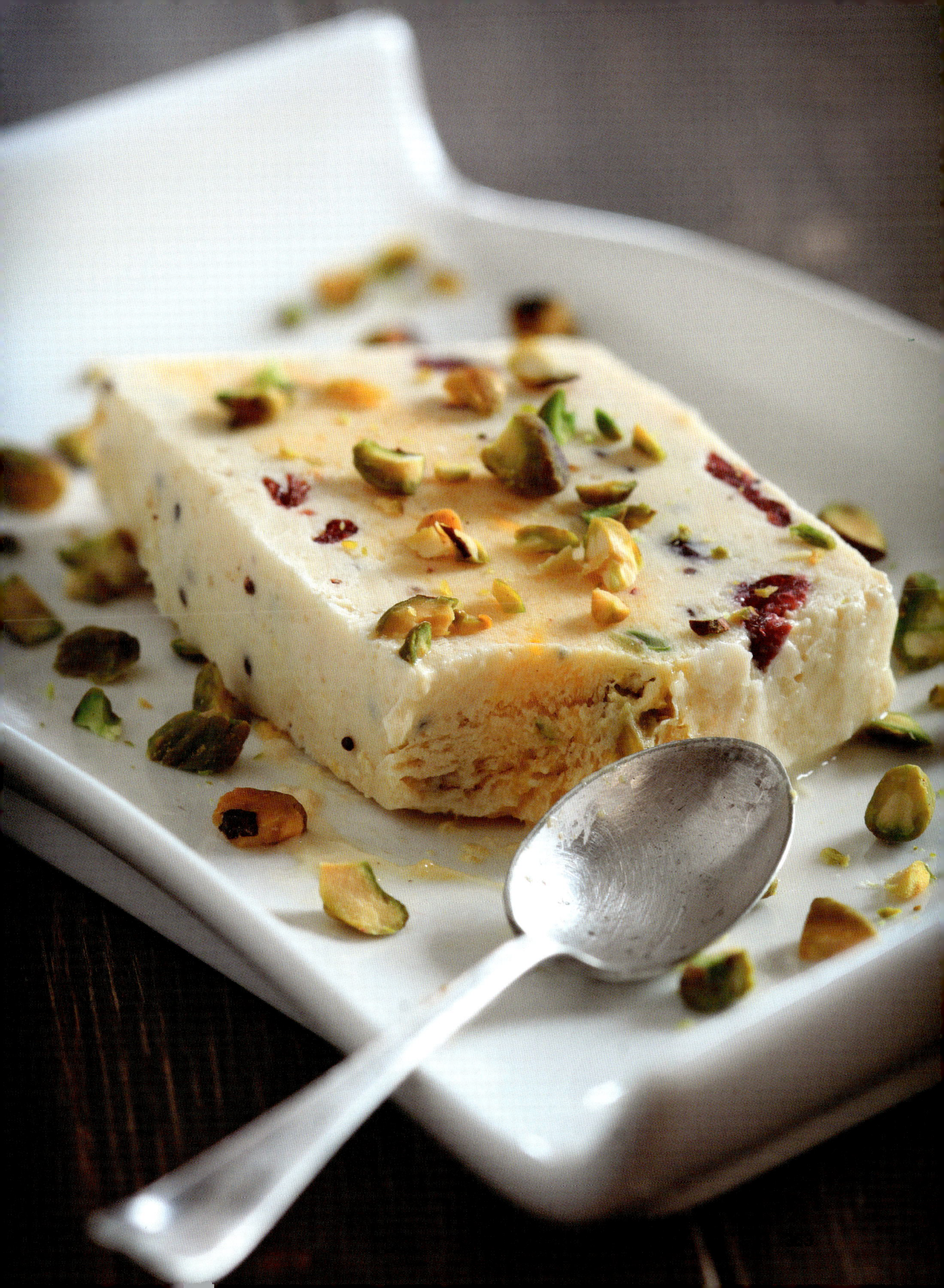

Blueberry Ice Pops

3 clementines
200 g (7 oz) blueberries
50 g (2 oz) caster sugar
400 g (14 oz) single cream
200 g (7 oz) low fat yogurt
2 tablespoons white chocolate drops

Squeeze the juice from the clementines. Put the blueberries in a saucepan and add the clementine juice. Bring to the boil, and then simmer over a high heat for about 5 minutes, stirring until the berries burst, soften and release their juice. Add the caster sugar and cook for another 5 minutes, stirring until the sugar has dissolved. Remove from the heat, transfer to a large bowl and leave at room temperature to cool. Add the cream, low fat yogurt and chocolate drops and mix it gently together so you still see the different colors. Gently spoon the mixture into ice pop moulds and freeze for about 4 hours or overnight.

Serves 8

Per serving
181 kcal, 11 g fat (7 g saturated), 4 g protein,
17 g carbs (16 g sugar), 0.6 g fibre, 0.1 g salt

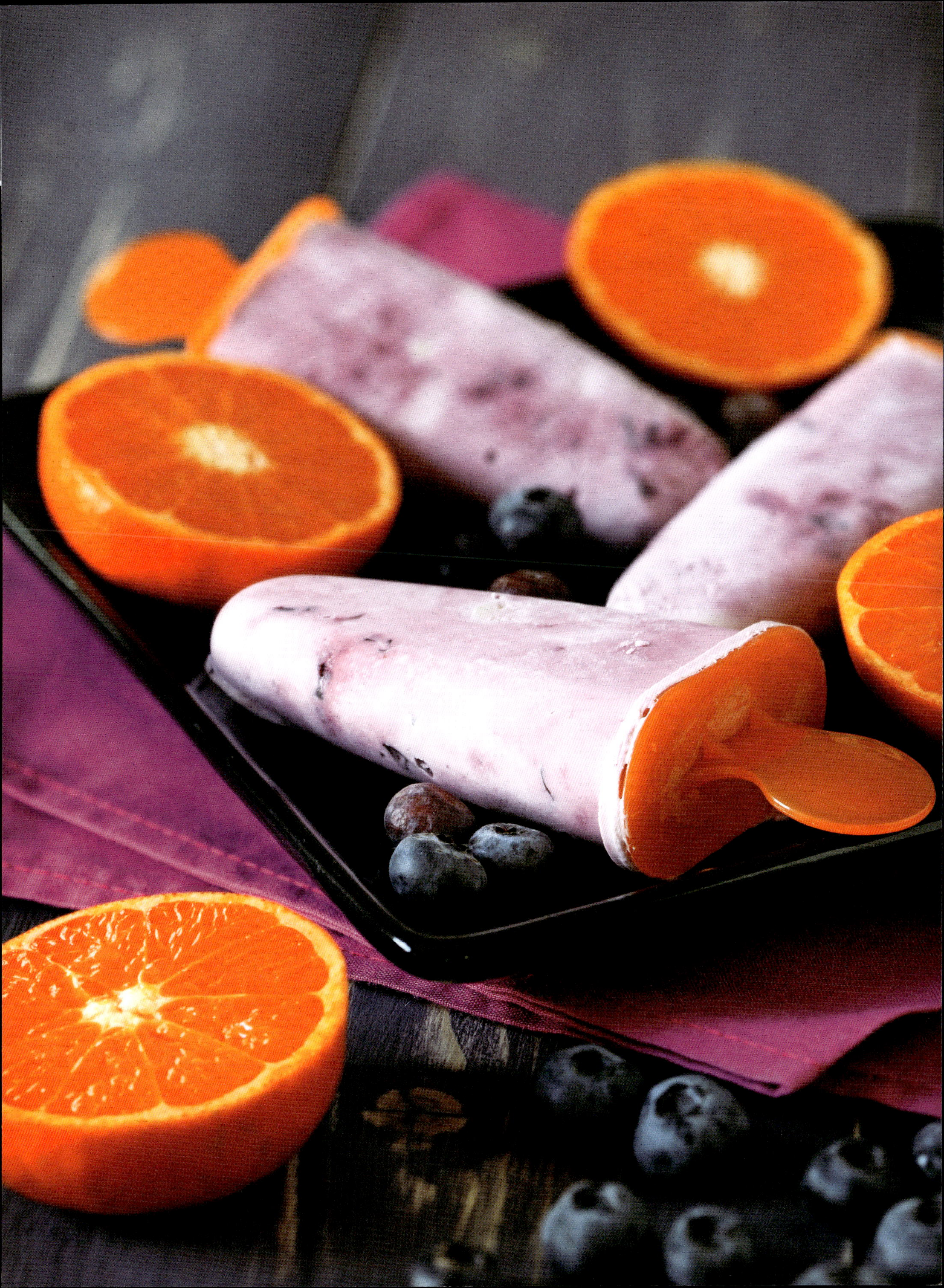

Kiwi and Red Cranberry Kulfi

300 g (10½ oz) low fat yogurt, strained
150 ml (5 fl oz) evaporated milk
2 kiwis, peeled and chopped
1 banana, peeled and chopped
1 tablespoons icing sugar
pinch of saffron threads
30 g (1 oz) red cranberries, dried
30 g (1 oz) almonds, toasted finely chopped

Throw the kiwi and banana pieces into the blender and whiz until smooth, pour into a small bowl. Next add the dried red cranberries and almonds and set aside. In a small saucepan pour the evaporated milk, add a pinch of saffron threads and stir gently while heating. Do not boil. Leave it to cool at room temperature. Once cool, add the yogurt, icing sugar and mix well. Next pour the kiwi mixture in and mix again. Finally pour the mixture into small kulfi silicone moulds. Cover with cling film and leave it to rest for about 4 hours or overnight in the freezer. Serve the kiwi and red cranberry kulfi cold topped with some chopped toasted almonds.

Serves 8

Per serving
98 kcal, 4 g fat (1 g saturated), 7 g protein,
10 g carbs (9 g sugar), 0.7 g fibre, 0.9 g salt

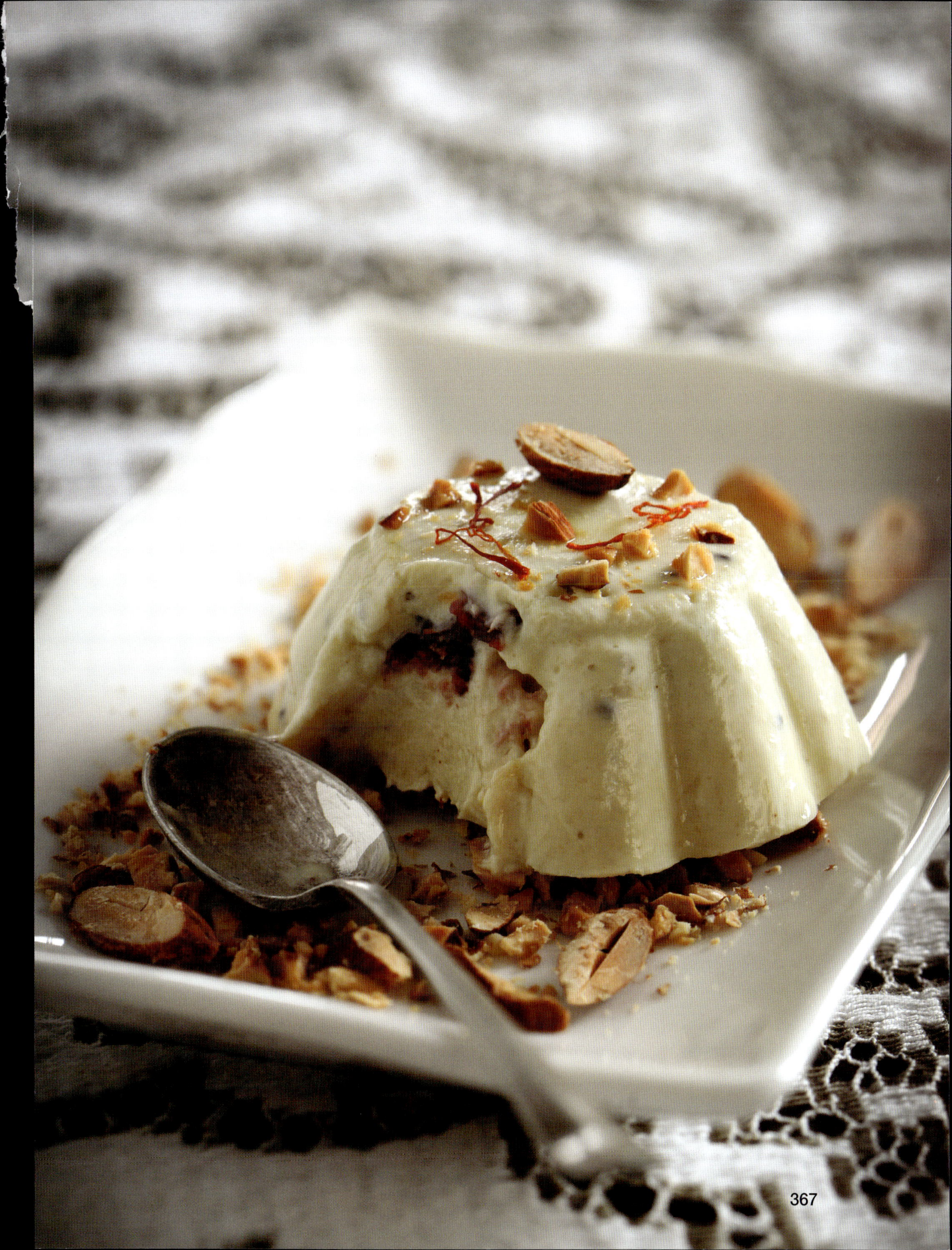

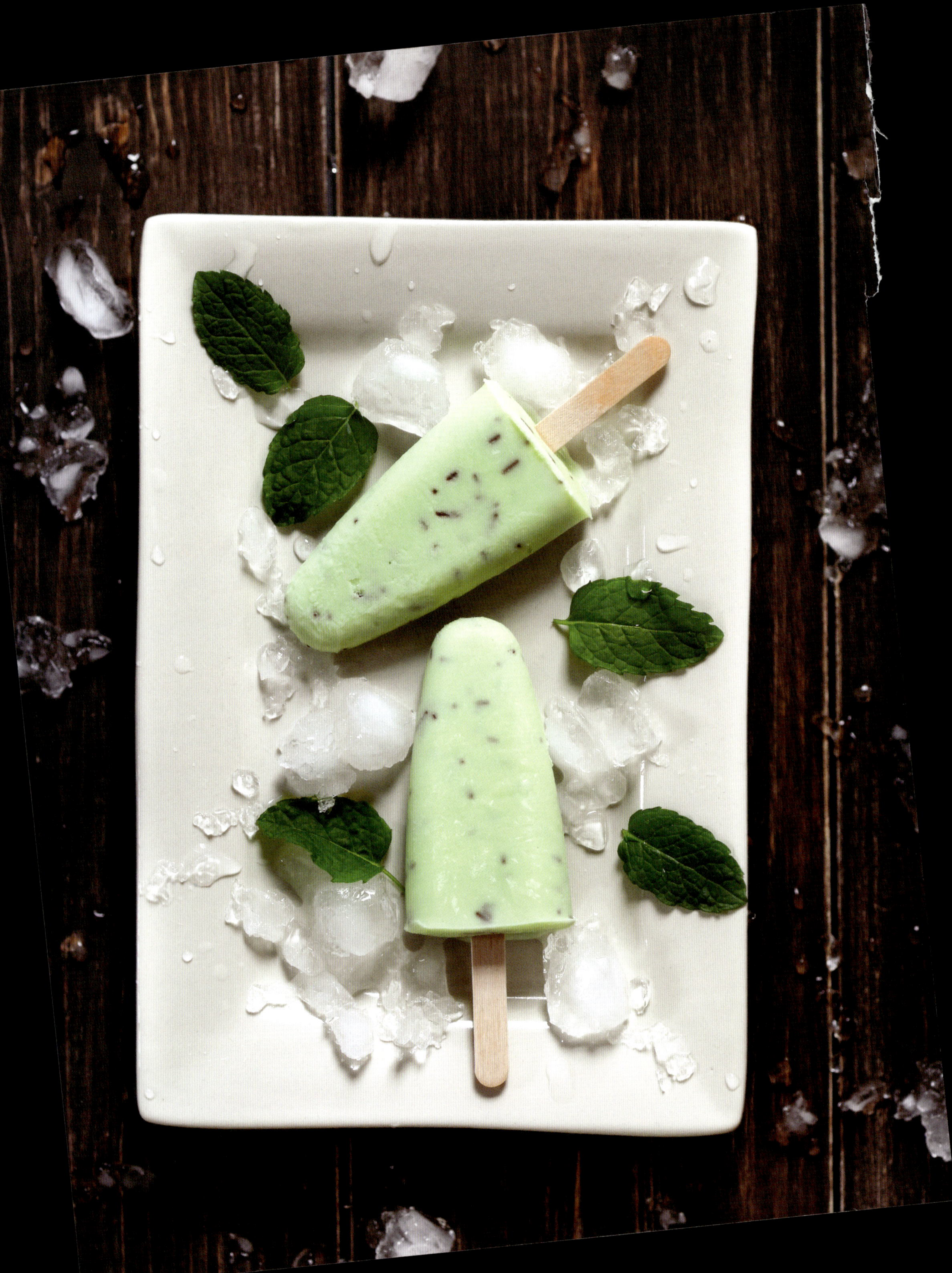

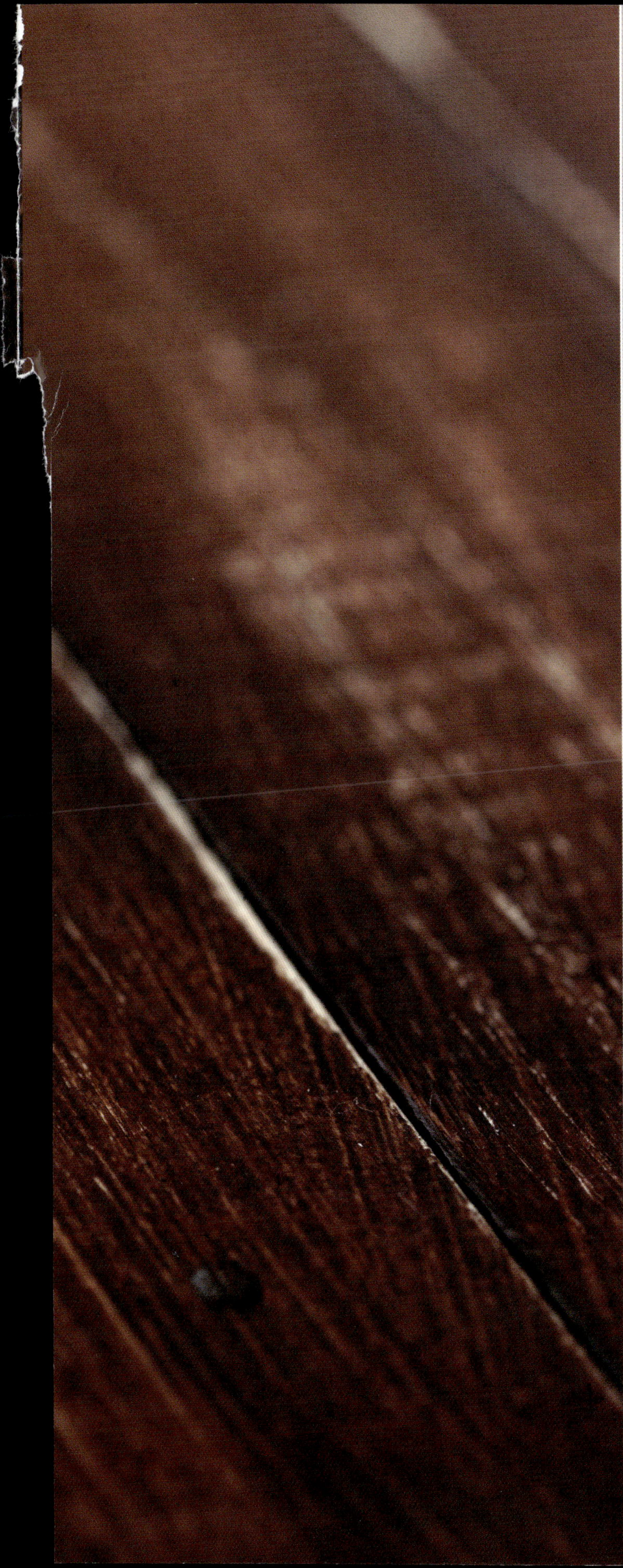

Yogurt Sorbet

250 g (9 oz) low fat yogurt, strained
100 g (3½ oz) mascarpone
100 g (3½ oz) caster sugar
3 tablespoon liquid glucose
1 teaspoon peppermint natural extract
½ teaspoon natural green food color
30 g (1 oz) chocolate flavor flakes

Pour 100 ml (3½ oz) boiling water into a medium bowl and add the liquid glucose, caster sugar and mix well to dissolve the sugar thoroughly then set aside to cool at room temperature. Meanwhile pour the strained yogurt into a large bowl and add the mascarpone, peppermint natural extract, natural green food color and mix well. Then add the sugar mixture and mix well. Make sure the sugar mixture is cooled at room temperature. Finally add the chocolate flavor flakes mix a bit very gently and pour the mixture in the popsicle molds, add wooden sticks and keep in the freezer for about 5 hours or overnight before it is ready to eat!

Serves 8

Per serving
162 kcal, 6 g fat (4 g saturated), 4 g protein, 24 g carbs (20 g sugar), 0.0 g fibre, 0.0 g salt

Banana and Mango Kulfi

2 medium mangos, stone off, peeled and chopped
2 ripe bananas, chopped
200 g (7 oz) low fat yogurt, strained
2 tablespoon icing sugar
2 teaspoon cardamom, grounded
50 g (2 oz) hazelnuts, roasted and finely chopped

Throw the mango pieces into the blender and whiz until smooth. Then add the bananas and blend until no lumps remain. Then add the strained yogurt, icing sugar, ground cardamom, chopped hazelnuts and blend again. Pour the kulfi mixture in the popsicle molds and keep in the freezer for about 4 hours or overnight before it is ready to eat!

Serves 8

Per serving
103 kcal, 4.8 g fat (0.6 g saturated), 2.2 g protein, 13.5 g carbs (11.1 g sugar), 2.0 g fibre, 0.1 g salt

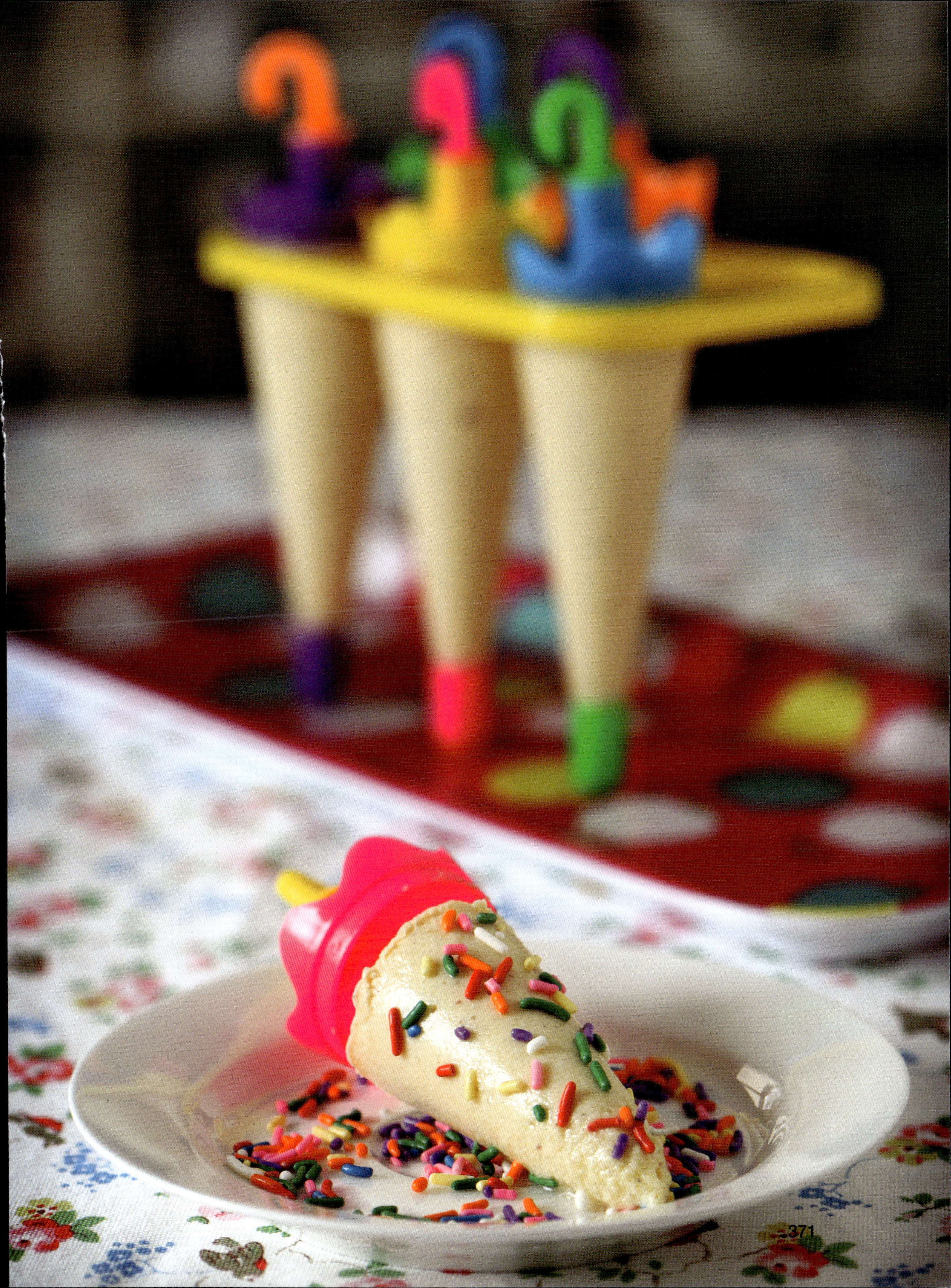

Recipe Index

Desserts

Frozen yogurt

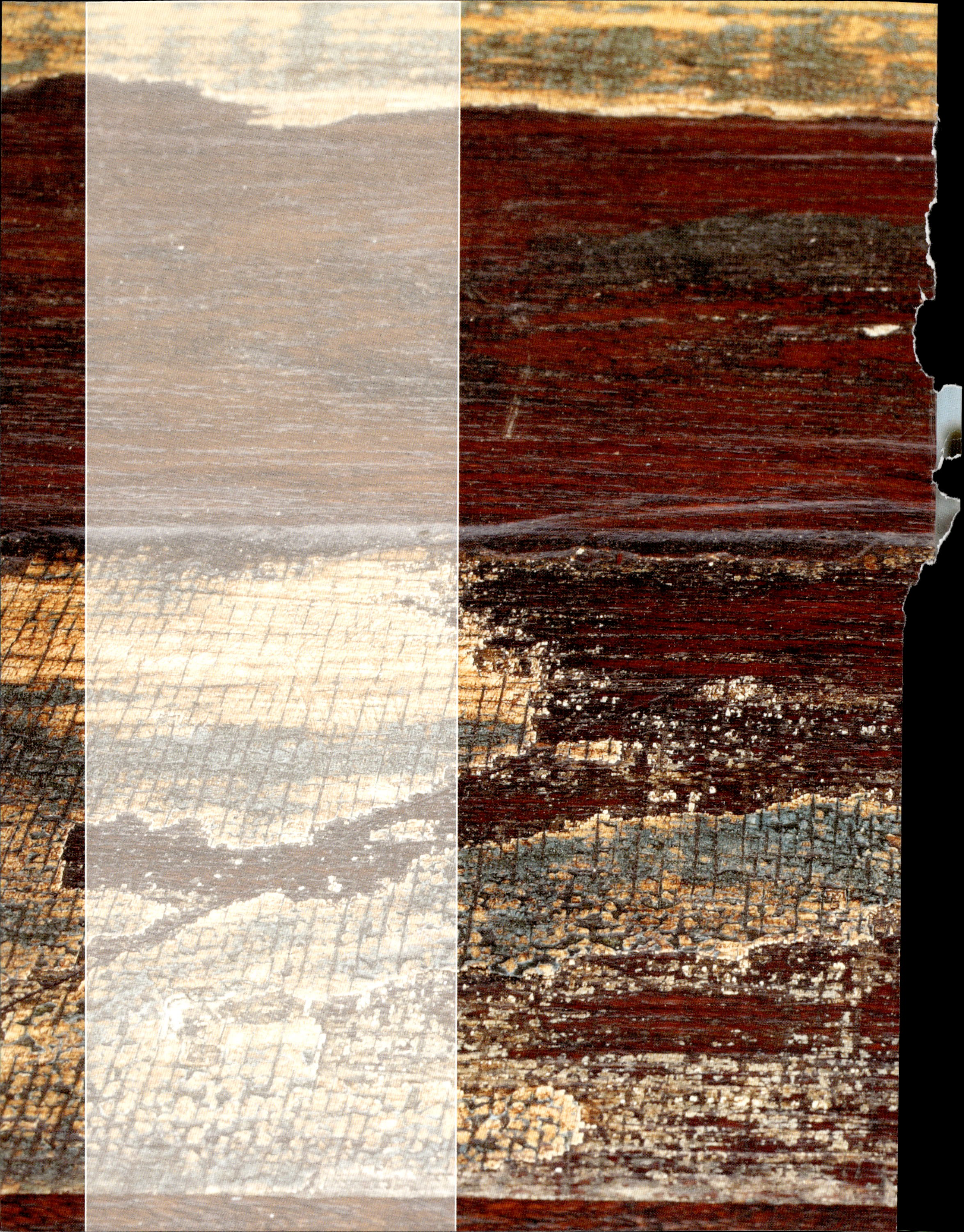

Disclaimer

The name of that white, creamy, sour dairy product - Yogurt came from the Turkish word "Jugurt". In my birth place (Bulgaria) people used to say "the yogurt is an elixir of longevity" but because I am not a scientific expert I can only guarantee that this book will give you really simple and healthy ways to cook for your family using the smartest food in the world - yogurt.

Reference

Yogurt - science and technology, 1985, by A.Y.Tamime and R.K.Robinson

It's always a pleasure to recommend a wonderful book especially when it includes great recipes, for you know that you are doing something special for others in highlighting an opportunity for them to enjoy healthy and nutritious food.
This book gives you the reader a myriad of healthy ways to incorporate yogurt into your lifestyle in a unique and entertaining visual journey from one recipe to another.
Ilian is a genius with the camera he is recognised worldwide as a perfectionist and the consummate professional, within the pages of this superb book you experience not only his passion for food but also how he brings food alive with his skill behind the lens.
As the editor of the magazine The Culinary Artist I appreciate when an author gives you recipes and guidelines that work out perfectly and the added delight at seeing the finished product so beautifully photographed.
Dr. Billy Gallagher HC. Certified Master Chef
Editor-in-chief The Culinary Artist Magazine

Ilian is a brilliant photographer who is now showing us his culinary talents and food styling techniques in his magnificent new book, Elixir. As he says, we do indeed eat with our eyes first, and he has shown his talent in that area with his creative styling and his artful, naturally relaxed food photography. He invites the viewer into the image, and we want to engage ourselves and step into the photo. Ilian is a masterful artist who has brought not only his styling and photogr aphy skills to the forefront, but also shared his love of a healthful lifestyle and welcomes us into his circle of family and friends. After reading his book, I would love to spend an evening with all of them, sharing in a wonderful meal and creating new friendships.
Cindy Epstein, Food Stylist and Culinary Consultant

I've known Ilian for several years now and have always enjoyed his work.
In his new project 'Elixir' his enthusiasm, craft and eye for detail really shine through.
The Bulgarians claim to have been the first people to use yogurt, so, as a son of Bulgaria Ilian has shown a great understanding and knowledge of his subject. Not only the beautiful photography but the styling, cooking and recipes have all been done by him and the result is everything a cookbook should be. Stylish, beautiful and full of recipes that make me want to get into the kitchen and start cooking!
Tim Clinch, Food Photographer

In the age of 'fast food' the need of homemade healthy food is vast. In this sense, Ilian's book is relevant and timely.
The recipes suggested by the author are based on yogurt, which is a must for the modern diet because of its favorable effect on the gastrointestinal microbes. All the recipes follow the rules of healthy living. They are clearly and precisely written, as well as easy and simple to follow. Being a master photographer, Ilian has provided brilliant illustrations to depict the culinary masterpieces. All this intrigues the reader to follow the recipes and share the final product with friends and family.
This book is of tremendous value. It brings about an enthusiasm to prepare our own delicious and healthy food, arranged in an eye-catching manner.
Let us all revel in this magic.
Prof. Borislav Vladimirov, MD, PhD,
Gastroenterology, Medical University-Sofia